CARIOLOGY FOR THE NINETIES

CARIOLOGY FOR THE NINETIES

EDITED BY

WILLIAM H. BOWEN AND LAWRENCE A. TABAK

UNIVERSITY OF ROCHESTER PRESS

First published 1993

University of Rochester Press
200 Administration Building, University of Rochester
Rochester, New York, 14627, USA
and at PO Box 9, Woodbridge, Suffolk IP12 3DF, UK

ISBN 1 878822 17 9

Library of Congress Cataloging in Publication Data

Cariology for the nineties / edited by William H. Bowen and Lawrence A. Tabak.
p. cm.
Includes bibliographical references and indexes.
ISBN 1-878822-17-9 (hardcover : alk. paper) :
1. Dental caries. I. Bowen, William H. II. Tabak, Lawrence A., 1951– .
[DNLM: 1. Dental Caries—epidemiology. 2. Dental Caries—prevention & control. WU 270 C2765 1993]
RK331.C35 1993
617.6'7—dc20
DNLM/DLC
for Library of Congress 92–48515

This publication is printed on acid-free paper
Printed in the United States of America

Table of Contents

List of Contributors

Dr. David W. Banting
University of Western Ontario, Faculty of Dentistry, London, Ontario, N6A 5C1 Canada

Dr. Ronald J. Billings
Associate Director for Clinical Affairs, Eastman Dental Center, 625 Elmwood Avenue, Rochester, NY 14620

Dr. Arnold S. Bleiweis
Graduate Research Professor and Chairman, University of Florida, Department of Oral Biology, College of Dentistry, Box J-424, Gainesville, FL 32610

Dr. George H.W. Bowden
Professor and Head, Oral Biology, Faculty of Dentistry, The University of Manitoba, Department of Oral Biology, Winnipeg, Manitoba, Canada R3E OW3

Dr. Robert A. Burne, Jr.
University of Rochester, Department of Dental Research, 601 Elmwood Avenue, Box 611, Rochester, NY 14642

Dr. Colin Dawes
Professor of Oral Biology, Faculty of Dentistry, The University of Manitoba, Department of Oral Biology, 780 Bannatyne Avenue, Winnipeg, Manitoba, Canada R3E OW3

Dr. Paul DePaola
Director, Cariology Center, Forsyth Dental Center, 140 Fenway, Boston, MA 02115

Professor Martin Downer
Eastman Dental Hospital, 256 Gray's Inn Road, London WC1X 8LD, England, U.K.

Dr. Jan Ekstrand
School of Dentistry, Karolinska Institutet, Department of Cariology, Box 4064, S-141 04 Huddinge, Sweden

Dr. Richard P. Ellen
Professor and Head, Department of Periodontics, Faculty of Dentistry, University of Toronto, 124 Edward Street, Toronto, Ontario, Canada M5G 1G6

DR. SUSAN J. FISHER
University of California at San Francisco, HSW 604, Department of Stomatology, Box 0512, San Francisco, CA 94143

PROFESSOR D A M GEDDES
Head of Oral Biology Group, University of Glasgow, Glasgow Dental Hospital and School, 378 Sauchiehall Street, Glasgow G2 3JZ, Scotland

DR. DONALD I. HAY
Head, Department of Biochemistry, Forsyth Dental Center, 140 Fenway, Boston, MA 02115

MS. DORTHEA A. JOHNSON
The University of Texas, Department of Community Dentistry, 7703 Floyd Curl Drive, San Antonio, TX 78284

DR. HOWARD K. KURAMITSU
Department of Pediatric Dentistry, The University of Texas, Health Science Center at San Antonio, Dental School, 7703 Floyd Curl Drive, San Antonio, TX 78284-7888

DR. MICHAEL J. LEVINE
Professor and Associate Chairman, Department of Oral Biology, University at Buffalo, State University of New York, School of Dental Medicine, Foster Hall, Buffalo, NY 14214-3092

DR. IRWIN D. MANDEL
Director, Center for Clinical Research in Dentistry, Columbia University in the City of New York, School of Dental and Oral Surgery, 630 West 168th Street, New York, NY 10032

DR. HENRY C. MARGOLIS
Forsyth Dental Center, Physical Chemistry Department, 140 Fenway, Boston, MA 02115

DR. ROBERT E. MARQUIS
University of Rochester, Department of Microbiology/Immunology, 601 Elmwood Avenue, Box 672, Rochester, NY 14642

DR. CYRIL MEYEROWITZ
Chair, Department of Clinical Dentistry, University of Rochester, 601 Elmwood Avenue, Box 705, Rochester, NY 14642

DR. GEORGE H. NANCOLLAS
SUNY at Buffalo, Department of Chemistry, Archeson Hall, Buffalo, NY 14214

PROFESSOR DENIS M. O'MULLANE
Oral Health Services Research Unit, University College Cork, Cork Farm Centre, Dennehys Cross, Cork, Ireland

DR. FRANK G. OPPENHEIM
Chairman and Professor, Boston University, School of Graduate Dentistry, Department of Periodontology & Oral Biology, 100 East Newton Street, Boston, MA 02118

DR. ROBERT G. QUIVEY, JR.
University of Rochester, Department of Dental Research, 601 Elmwood Avenue, Box 611, Rochester, NY 14642

DR. HAROLD C. SLAVKIN
School of Dentistry, University of Southern California, Center for Craniofacial Molecular Biology, 2250 Alcazar Street, CSA 103/HSC, Los Angeles, CA 90033

DR. MARTHA J. SOMERMAN
Department of Periodontics, University of Michigan, School of Dentistry, Ann Arbor, MI 48109

DR. JOHN W. STAMM
Dean, School of Dentistry, The University of North Carolina at Chapel Hill, CB# 7450, Room 104 Brauer Hall, Chapel Hill, NC 27599-7450

PROFESSOR K. W. STEPHEN
Chairman, Department of Oral Medicine and Pathology, University of Glasgow Dental School, 378, Sauchiehall Street, Glasgow; G2 3JZ, Scotland, U.K.

DR. LAWRENCE A. TABAK
University of Rochester, Department of Dental Research, 601 Elmwood Avenue, Box 611, Rochester, NY 14642

DR. JASON M. TANZER
University of Connecticut Health Science Center, School of Dental Medicine, Department of Oral Diagnosis, 263 Farmington Avenue, Farmington, CT 06032

DR. MARTIN A. TAUBMAN
Head, Department of Immunology, Forsyth Dental Center, 140 Fenway, Boston, MA 02115

DR. J. HANS VAN HOUTE
Forsyth Dental Center, 140 Fenway, Boston, MA 02115

DR. DOMENICK T. ZERO
Head, Division of Intraoral Studies and Senior Research Associate, Eastman Dental Center, Department of General Dentistry/Oral Biology, 625 Elmwood Avenue, Rochester, NY 14620

Preface

Epidemiological studies conducted in several countries in the Western world have revealed a marked decline in the prevalence of dental caries. In the United States, for example, approximately one-half of children aged 5 to 12 years have never experienced tooth decay. Of course, this means that 50% of children have had at least one cavity. These interesting observations have given rise to a misplaced tidal wave of euphoria. It is difficult to imagine any other circumstances where 50% of a population suffering a disease would evoke such an aura of success. Have we become so used to failure that a modicum of success engenders the impression that all of the problems pertaining to the etiology, pathogenesis and prevention of dental caries have been solved? Unfortunately, among a great number of researchers, such an impression appears all too prevalent.

To many, dental caries has become an intellectual bore—the disease is solved; there are no more exciting scientific challenges; it is time to move on to more challenging fields. Thus, this conference was conceived out of an erroneous notion. We set out to show that caries continues to be a public health problem worldwide; that enigma of dental caries is worthy of the attention of the finest scientific minds and the application of the most sophisticated techniques from epidemiology to molecular biology. In arranging the conference, we tried to avoid the obvious; several areas we chose to omit altogether because either they have been the subject of symposia elsewhere or we felt they were receiving sufficient attention. Their omission in no way belies their importance.

We are grateful to the participants for what we believe are outstanding contributions. We believe each one, in its own unique way, will stimulate or entice persons to enter this exciting field. We have yet to see the end of dental caries, despite some important advances. As Churchill observed, "It is not even the beginning of the end. But it is perhaps the end of the beginning."

Finally, we would like to express our gratitude to our sponsors and to the administrative staff of the Department of Dental Research (Ms. Carol Ann Stafford, Ms. Susan Andersen Lukas, Ms. Patricia J. Noonan, Ms. Hilary A. Fraser, and Ms. Tracy Stone) for their complete professionalism in organizing this conference.

William H. Bowen, B.D.S., Ph.D.
Lawrence A. Tabak, D.D.S., Ph.D.
Editors
Rochester, New York
June 1992

We are deeply grateful to the following for their support of this conference:

Block Drug Company, Inc.
Colgate-Palmolive Company
The Gillette Company
International Life Sciences Institute-Nutrition Foundation (ILSI-NF)
Johnson & Johnson CONSUMER PRODUCTS, INC.
Oral-B Laboratories
The Procter & Gamble Distributing Company
Unilever Research
Warner-Lambert Company
Wm. Wrigley Jr. Company

Dental Caries: Another Extinct Disease?

IRWIN D. MANDEL

Given the international character of the participants in the conference I think that an appropriate way to help put it in perspective is to quote from David Lodge's novel "Small World" (Lodge, 1984). Lodge, who retired a few years ago as Professor of Modern English Literature at the University of Birmingham, England, has combined his experience as an academic jet setter with his skills as a novelist in a very original fashion. Let us share his insights.

"The modern conference resembles the pilgrimage of medieval Christendom in that it allows the participants to indulge themselves in all the pleasures and diversions of travel while appearing to be austerely bent on self-improvement. To be sure, there are certain penitential exercises to be performed—the presentations of a paper, perhaps, and certainly listening to the papers of others. But with this excuse you journey to new and interesting places, meet new and interesting people, and form new and interesting relations with them; exchange gossip and confidences (for your well-worn stories are fresh to them, and vice versa); eat, drink and make merry in their company every evening; and yet, at the end of it all, return home with an enhanced reputation for seriousness of mind."

My penitential exercise is to predict the future of dental caries. Lately, predicting the future has become a growth industry; every group and every conference seems to be involved. Perhaps it is because the year 2000, that once mythical number, is within striking distance. Be that as it may, I am the designated predictor. When I was growing up the only people with the temerity to predict were gypsy fortune tellers. Every neighborhood seemed to have an empty store that was occupied from time to time by a gypsy lady of uncertain age who read cards, tea leaves or a crystal ball. It's not unlikely there may have been a rich gypsy enterpreneur behind the scenes who owned a chain of empty stores that he franchised to fortune tellers. I am an independent and I freely admit that predicting the future is a precarious business. I believe it was Confucius, or perhaps Walter Cronkite, his American counterpart, who said that: "He who looks into the crystal ball is destined to dine on ground glass." I fully agree. It

TABLE 1 *Dental caries prevalence and subsistence pattern**

Subsistence Pattern	n *Groups*	% *Carious Teeth*	Range % *Carious Teeth*
Hunting and Gathering	17	1.30	0.0-5.3
Mixed Economy	13	4.84	0.4-10.3
Agricultural	32	10.43	2.3-26.9

*From Moore and Corbett, 1971

is possible, however, by reviewing the past and examining the present, to make reasonable projections about the future and to respond to the challenging question about dental caries: To be or not to be?

A popular public misconception is that caries is one of the modern plagues, like smog and acid rain—that we have been paying for the sweet life through the teeth. In a quantitative sense this is true of course—epidemiologic data clearly demonstrated that the sugar-laden diets of many of the technologically advanced societies could be directly associated with caries incidence (Newbrun, 1982)—but caries is an ancient disease, perhaps a million years old, as is very evident from the skeletal record (Hardwick, 1960). Prior to the Iron Age probably no more than 2-4% of teeth examined exhibited decay (Hardwick, 1960) but its presence was widespread geographically. During the Iron Age and through the Roman period, caries increased modestly to about 10% of the teeth examined (Table 1). The English skeletal data, which are the most complete, indicate that the incidence of caries remained relatively constant during the Anglo-Saxon and Medieval periods and then dramatically increased toward the end of the seventeenth century (Brothwell 1959; Moore and Corbett 1971, 1973, 1975). In England and other Western countries caries has increased continually until a decade ago. The only break in this inflationary spiral was during World War II, when the occupied countries of Europe experienced a marked reduction in caries (Sognnaes 1948). With the resumption of sugar import the caries pattern reverted to the pre-war level. Epidemiologic studies have disclosed a worldwide pattern of caries that in a sense reflects the anthropological and historical findings (Russell 1966; Barmes 1977). The incidence of caries in the 1950s and 1960s was extremely low in underdeveloped countries, but increased rapidly with industrialization and exposure to the modern Western diet.

From ancient times until the end of the 16th century the most frequent site of caries in the permanent dentition was at the junction of cementum and enamel usually interproximally or at the facial line angle (Moore and Corbett, 1973)—very similar to the root caries seen today. It was a disease of the mature years and secondary to attachment loss. There were, however, some exceptions to the late onset root caries pattern. Jaws of the Anasazi Indians (the ancient ones) and the Zunis in the Southwestern United States exhibit occlusal and interproximal enamel caries similar to that seen in modern societies (Leigh, 1925). One very possible explanation is their use of partial mastication to mix certain foods with saliva, then allowing the mixture to ferment overnight to form sweetened foods—certainly a welcome relief from their usually monotonous diet.

Recipes transmitted orally over many generations and used in many tribes until relatively recent times indicate that fermentation was part of the preparation of a variety of sweet foods (Cushing, 1922). Datila, a long pulpy fruit, was converted by fermentation, than boiling and drying into a solid, gummy transparent candy-like material with a taste similar to black licorice. It was called tsu-pi-a-we and was highly prized in barter. Another delicacy was made from the mescal plant or mature agave. The most common fermented food, however, was stone cake or sweet cake (a-tea-mu-we). The recipe called for preparation of a batter of corn meal with scalding water, and then sweetening it by mastication and fermentation, followed by baking.

It is interesting that some present day Indian tribes in South America use a similar process of mastication and fermentation to prepare a thick sweet drink made from manioc, called chicha, which they slurp frquently. In one such tribe at least, the prevalence of caries is known to be very high (Larrick *et al.* 1979).

One of the important lessons from the historical record is that even though the overall caries level was very low during the pre-sugar periods there were instances in which the prevalance was very high, not only among those people that had discovered the properties of amylase and the attraction of premasticated foods, but even long before that. There is a report of a jaw specimen of an early hominid dating from 200-500,000 years ago that had carious lesions on 11 of 13 maxillary teeth (Brothwell, 1959). Jaws of children from the medieval period include cases with extensive caries apparently the result of using a piece of honeycomb wrapped in linen as a pacifier—an early predecessor of baby bottle caries. We are not newcomers to a dichotomous distribution of caries, or polarization as it has been called by others (Winter, 1990).

In the United States caries has been a serious concern since the early colonial period. There are numerous accounts in the diaries and letters of visitors of the abysmal state of the dentition of the American-born men and women (Asbell, 1985). "The inhabitants of this province (Massachusetts) are formed by symmetry, handsome and have delicate complexions . . . but, both sexes have universally and even proverbially bad teeth, which must probably be occasioned by their eating so much molasses." With the establishment of the American colonies, the infamous slave triangle of England, Africa, and the West Indies (the home of the very prosperous tobacco and sugar cane plantations) was modified to a rectangle that included the Northeast where molasses was converted to rum and then shipped to England (Mintz, 1985). By the time of the Revolutionary War most 18 year-olds had a smile like a picket fence and it was often difficult for recruits to pass the physical exam which required two matching front teeth, crucial for biting open a container of powder.

The high caries rate in the Northeastern part of the United States has prevailed until the present day. During the Civil War when formal data on dental status was first recorded it was not only evident that caries was high in this region but that it was substantially higher than in other parts of the country. In their review of ealy U.S. military data Graves and Stamm (1985) noted that in 1863-64 the overall rejection rate for dental reasons was 25/1,000; however, it was 5.4/1000 for men from Wisconsin, but 34.9/1000 for recruits from Massachusetts. In World War I the rejection rate because of dental conditions was 103/1000 for Vermont but only 3/1000 from Arkansas.

The military data dramatically highlight the continuing dental deterioration in the first half of this century. At the time of entry of the U.S. in World War II dental defects were the leading cause of rejection from service; 8.8% could not meet the minimum standard of 6 opposing teeth. Once again the Northeast had the highest rate of rejection (Britten and Perott, 1941). The requirements were very pragmatically changed to "enough teeth in the lower arch to hold a partial denture" and thus meet the oppositional requirements. By inducting enough dentists, by the end of 1942 recruits could be accepted if they could be fitted with full upper and lower dentures. The good news is that this sorry state of dismal dental health lead to the establishment of the National Institute of Dental Research.

The benchmark national survey of caries in the U.S. was the one conducted in 1961-2 and included a resonable cross-section of the urban and rural population, women and men, white and non white (Kelly, Van Kirk and Garst, 1967). This survey reaffirmed the geographic variation noted since the Civil War with caries rates highest in the Northeast and lowest in the Southwest. Less frequently noted was the finding that "one half of the total number of decayed teeth occurred in one-tenth of the population." Both geographic variation and polarization were characteristic of the caries pattern in the U.S., as well as in many other parts of the world. The reasons for the geographic variations are still unclear; most investigators considered differences in trace elements in the soil and water as the most likely possibility (Nizel and Pappas, 1989).

Surveys in the 1980's continued to support this pattern of caries. The national oral health surveys in children (De Paola, 1990) and the National Preventive Demonstration Program in the U.S. showed that 20% of the children had nearly 60% of the decay (Klein *et al.*, 1985). In the U.K. 60% of the DMFT was found in 25% of the children (Picton, 1986); in Syndey 12% of children had 50% of the DMFT (Burton *et al.* 1984). The dichotomous distribution of caries was very much evident.

In both of the children's surveys in the U.S., 1979-80 and 1986-87, the geographic variations followed the historical data (Carlos and Wolfe, 1988). The regional findings in the National Adult Survey found that coronal dental caries was highest in the northern and coastal areas and lowest in the southern and inland areas (Brunelle, Miller-Chisholm and Loe, 1987). Root surface caries by contrast, exhibited little regional difference for either the employed or the senior populations. However in the seniors prevalence was lowest in the Southwest, traditionally the area with least caries. In root caries factors such as previous coronal caries experience, periodontal status, oral hygiene and diet may overshadow geographic variables (Banting, 1986; DePaola *et al.* 1989; Hunt, 1990).

What the epidemiologic findings point up is the tyranny of the mean. One must not jump to conclusions based purely on mean values but be cognizant of the range and standard deviations as well. It is necessary to pay attention to fringe groups in health affairs as well as in politics. In addition to geographic variation it is clear that race, behavioral patterns and socio-economic status are important factors in determining who is at risk (Hunt, 1990; Winter, 1990), and who requires the most attention. There are obvious difficulties in reaching high caries groups in the underdeveloped countries but there are still problems in the developed world as well. In addition the recent increase in immigration to the developed countries poses a new set of challenges (DiAngelis, Feigal and Piztado, 1985; Bedi, 1989).

Given this thumb-nail sketch of caries status, and it will be considerably embellished this afternoon, what analogues can we find among other diseases that can help us project to the future? If we continue to follow the current concept of caries development as a result of the interplay of a susceptible host, a fermentable carbohydrate diet and a rather specific cariogenic plaque flora—the tilting of a precarious balance—the future strategies for extinction will continue to emphasize increasing host resistance, dietary modification and combatting the potentially destructive microflora.

Increasing Host Resistance

Since fluoride in various forms is obviously our major player in augmenting host resistance, its absence would constitute a breach in the defense system and we should look to deficiency diseases for direction. There are some similarities with goitre, a deficiency of iodide and the avitaminoses, especially Vitamin D and rickets and perhaps Vitamin C and scurvy. In all instances the strategy has been to provide supplements such as iodized salt and cod-liver oil or encourage appropriate dietary intake such as citrus fruits for Vitamin C. Fluoride does not neatly fit any of the classic deficiency diseases since a topical effect appears to be nearly as effective as a systemic one. In addition fluorides do not offer complete protection because of a somewhat limited effect on occlusal caries. Hence a combination of the use of multiple forms of fluoride and sealant application would be a necessary approach to caries eradication via heightened host resistance.

How successful can we be in world-wide use of fluorides and sealants? Clearly the effort would have to be enormous. The developed countries are moving in that direction, but not as rapidly as they might. Only 7.6% of the children in the U.S. are receiving sealants. A major educational campaign and changes in practice laws are necessary to make it economically feasible. Fluoride toothpaste use is widespread but socioeconomic and educational barriers still exist for other forms of self and professionally applied fluorides. Water fluoridation has reached a plateau and further implementation will require much greater efforts. In the developing countries oral health care will have to be given a much higher priority to generate national programs. It is very difficult to project a realistic time table as to when such a change could occur.

Dietary Modification

Another way at looking at caries is to think of it as an over-consumption, or an inappropriate consumption of sugars and other forms of fermentable carbohydrates. This view has gone out of fashion but it is worth re-examination in view of the tremendous attention being given to another dietarily modified plaque disease—artherosclerosis and its consequences. In the U.S. we have national campaigns to reduce fat and cholesterol levels and some indication that the message is affecting the media and maybe even the intima. When it was tried for sugars and caries in the mid-century period it had little impact. People accepted the information intellectually but not viscerally. When head and hedonism clash it is easy to predict the winner.

Today, in the post-modernist era, dietary modification for caries would be even more difficult to acccomplish on a broad basis. There seems to be a campaign to pardon sucrose, the arch criminal (Newbrun, 1967) and its accomplices. The increasing use of low fermentative or non fermentative sweeteners are a partial answer, but only reach a segment of the very populations that could benefit most. Xylitol-containing products, especially chewing gum appear to have cariostatic properties and field trials have been encouraging (Isokangas *et al.*, 1988). This is certainly an area to explore more fully especially since its effect seems to be augmentative to fluorides. Again a time-table is difficult to establish.

Combatting the Cariogenic Microflora

The most direct analogue for examing the question "Dental Caries: Another Extinct Disease?" is to consider it an infectious disease and to look for parallels with the victories in this area. The conventional wisdom holds that the marked increase in life expectancy during the 20th Century in the developed world was mainly due to the conquest of the infectious diseases. In technically advanced countries the pestilences of antiquity no longer plague us. However, as Paul

Hoeprich pointed out in the preface to his classic text on infections diseases, even in technologically advanced countries infectious diseases remain important contributors to illness and death (Hoeprich, 1972). He noted that in 1969 in the United States there were about 50 million cases of acute infective and parasitic diseases resulting in over 200 million days of restricted activity, 100 million days of bed disability and 21 million days lost from work. Today the impact of infectious diseases is undoubtedly much greater because of AIDS and numerous other new diseases. But even old diseases do not always die or even fade away. We see new geographic ranges for old diseases, new populations at risk and new forms, niches and modes of transmission (Lorber, 1988).

Well before the advent of antibiotics and widespread vaccination the infectious diseases that had been most devastating in previous centuries—typhoid, dysentery, typhus, plague—were brought under control by development of efficient sewage and water supply systems, plus greater concern with personal cleanliness. But they were never eradicated. They did not become extinct; witness outbreaks in South America and current concerns in the Middle East when sanitation breaks down. The protective barricade is easily breached. The situation is similar for dental caries. Personal oral hygiene would be comparable to sanitation. To consider oral hygiene as an effective means of controlling caries would necessitate a "Brave New World" in which plaque control would have to rank with Malthusian drill.

The classic success stories are of course smallpox and polio. The basis for smallpox eradication was established on May 15, 1796, when Edward Jenner successfully vaccinated James Phipps. Mass vaccination, however, did not begin for 75 years until the Franco-Prussian war, and the process of final eradication was not initiated until 1958 when the catastrophic consequences of the disease in 63 countries were reported to the World Health Assembly. There were 28 million victims, 30% of whom had died. These figures so stirred the international community that a globally coordinated program was developed and fully materialized in 1967, the 300 million dollar cost financed largely by the USSR and the U.S. (Bloch, 1984). In October 1977, "Ali Maow Maalin, a cook from Somalia, had the distinction of being the last victim of naturally acquired smallpox on the surface of this planet" (Lorber, 1988). Its disapperance was a triumph of biology, technology and international cooperation in preventive medicine.

The polio story, although also a happy one, does not have as dramatic a final scene as smallpox. In the United States, thanks to the inactivated and then the oral vaccine the disease has been virtually eliminated. But there have been pockets of outbreaks when there is under-immunization. Worldwide it has been estimated that approximately 200,000 cases per year still occur, primarily in developing countries with inadequate immunization programs. As Jonas Salk pointed out: "The limiting factor is in part developmental and economic and in part the need for political will" (Salk, 1983).

Eradication of a disease requires a combination of a potent weapon(s) against the disease, such as vaccination, a strong effective public health program worldwide, popular support and a sufficient surveillance system (Cockburn, 1967). Such a combination could be marshalled for smallpox, but so far not for poliomyelitis. Viewed from the perspective of these infectious diseases it is highly unlikely that dental caries will ever become extinct. Even with a highly effective vaccine or other strategy that suppresses *S. mutans* or inhibits its cariogenicity, we cannot be sure that other organisms such as *Lactobacillus casei* or *Actinomyces viscosus*, or other streptococci or combinations, could not initiate some caries. With a less than perfect vaccine *S. mutans* will stay around—it is a survivor. It is an ancient organism found in primitive populations with no exposure to outside contact (Coykendall, 1976). Even under the most adverse conditions such as in tube-fed patients where the organism is forced to subsist on a minimal liquid diet—saliva—it exists in plaque and retains its acidogenic potential (Ellison and Mandel, Unpublished Observations). In naturally caries resistant adults *S. mutans*, although in low numbers, are still present in plaques and can readily produce caries in animal models (Fitzgerald *et al.*, 1977).

If eradication is not feasible then to what degree can we control the disease? I think that it has already been demonstrated that when full advantage can be taken of the existing anticaries armentarium a marked decrease in caries can occur. To move beyond this point requires the will and the commitment of resources to reach the underserved and most vulnerable members of the population, both in the developed and undeveloped countries, since with caries it is the have nots who have most of the disease. It becomes a question of equity and public policy. It is also important to broaden the anticaries strategies to provide both greater effectiveness and a wider range of choices to accommodate the diversity of attitudes and receptivity as well as the variations in risk.

There is very definitely a need for continued research. Let the conference proceed.

REFERENCES

ASBELL, M.B. (1988): *Dentistry: A Historical Perspective*, Bryn Mawr: Derrance & Co., p. 82.

BANTING, D.W. (1986): Epidemiology of Root Caries, *Gerontology* 5:5-11.

BARMES, D.E. (1977): Epidemiology of Dental Disease, *J Clin Periodontol* 4:80-92.

BEDI, R. (1989): Ethnic Indicators of Dental Health for Young Asian School Children Resident in Areas of Multiple Deprivation, *Brit Dent J* 106:331-334.

BLOCH, H. (1983): A Disease That Disappeared, *Clin Pediat* 23:290-291.

BRITTEN, R.H. and PERROTT, G. (1941): Summary of Physical Findings of Men Drafted in the World War, *Pub Hlth Rep* 56:41-62.

BROTHWELL, D.R. (1959): Teeth in Earlier Human Populations, *Proc Nutr Soc* 18:59-72.

BURTON, J.B.; ROB, M.I.; CRAIG, C.G.; and LAWSON, J.S. (1984): Changes in Caries Experience of 12 Year Old Sydney School Children Between 1963 and 1982, *Med J Australia* 140:405-407.

CARLOS, J.P. and WOLFE, M.D. (1988): Dental Caries: Historic and Current Perspectives, *Compend Contin Educ*, Suppl No. 11:S360-364.

COCKBURN, A (1967): *Infectious Diseases: Their Evolution and Eradication*, Springfield: Charles C. Thomas.

COYKENDALL, A.L. (1976): On the Evolution of *S. mutans* and Dental Caries. In: *Microbial Aspects of Dental Caries*, H. Stiles, W. Loesche and T. O'Brien, Eds., Sp. Supp. *Microbiology Abstracts*, New York: Information Retrieval, Inc., pp. 703-712.

CUSHING, F.H. (1922): Zuni Bread Stuffs: Indian Notes and Monographs, Vol. 8, New York: Museum of the American Indian.

DE PAOLA, P.F. (1990): Measurement Issue in the Epidemiology of Dental Caries. In: *Risk Assessment in Dentistry*, J. Bader, Ed., Chapel Hill: Univ of North Carolina Dental Ecology, pp. 19-26.

DE PAOLA, P.F.; SOPARKAR, P.M.; TAVARES, M.; and KENT, R.L. Jr. (1989): The Clinical Profiles of Individuals With and Without Root Caries, *Gerontology* 8:9-15.

DI ANGELIS, A.J.; FEIGAL, R.J.; and PINTADO, M.R. (1985): Caries Prevalence In A Southeast Asian Population, *Quintessence Int* 10:727-730.

FITZGERALD, D.G.; STEVENS, R.; FITZGERALD, R.J.; and MANDEL, I.D. (1977): Comparative Cariogenicity of *S. mutans* Strains Isolated from Caries Active and Caries Resistant Adults, *J Dent Res* 56:894.

GRAVES, R.C. and STAMM, J.W. (1985): Oral Health Status in the United States: Prevalence of Dental Caries, *J Dent Educ* 49:341-351.

HARDWICK, J.L. (1969): The Incidence and Distribution of Caries Throughout the Ages in Relation to the Englishmen's Diet, *Brit Dent J* 108:9-17.

HOEPRICH, P.D. (1972): Preface. In: *Infection Diseases: A Guide to the Understanding and Management of Infectious Processes*, P. Hoeprich, Ed., Hagerstown: Harper & Row, p. xix.

HUNT, R.J. (1990): Behavioral and Sociodemographic Risk Factors for Caries. In: *Risk Assessment in Dentistry*, Chapel Hill: Univ of North Carolina Dental Ecology, pp. 29-34.

ISOKANGAS, P.; ALANEN, P., TIEKSO, J. and MAKINEN, K.K. (1988): Xylitol Chewing Gum in Caries Prevention: A Field Study in Children, *J Am Dent Assoc* 117:315-320.

KELLY, J.E.; VAN KIRK, L.E. Jr.; and GARST, C.C. (1967): Decayed, Missing and Filled Teeth in Adults—U.S. 1960-62, Washington, National Center for Health Statistics Series 11, No. 23.

KLEIN, S.P.; BOHANNEN, H.M.; BELL, R.M.; DISNEY, J.A.; FOCH, C.B.; and GRAVES, R.M. (1985): The Cost and Effectiveness of School Based Preventive Dental Care, *Am J Publ Health* 75:382-391.

LARRICK, J.W.; YOST, J.A.; KAPLAN, J.; KING, G.; and MAYHALL, J. (1979): Patterns of Health and Disease Among the Waorani Indians of Eastern Ecuador, *Med Anthropol* (Spring): 147-185.

LEIGH, R.W. (1925): Dental Pathology of Indian Tribes of Varied Environmental and Food Conditions, *Am J Phys Anthrop* 8:179-199.

LODGE, D. (1984): *Small World*, London: Secker & Warburg.

LORBER, P. (1988): Changing Disease Patterns of Infectious Diseases, *Amer J Med* 84:569-578.

MILLER, A.J.; BRUNELLE, J.A.; CARLOS, J.P.; BROWN, L.J.; and LOE, H. (1987): *Oral Health of United States Adults, National Findings*, N.I.H. Publ No. 87-2865.

MINTZ, S.W. (1985): *Sweetness and Power*, New York: Viking.

MOORE, W.E. and CORBETT, M.E. (1973): The Distribution of Caries in Ancient British Populations 2. Iron Age, Romano, British and Mediaeval Periods, *Caries Res* 7:139-153.

MOORE, W.J. and CORBETT, M.E. (1971): The Distribution of Caries in Ancient British Populations. 1. Anglo-Saxon Period, *Caries Res* 5:150-158.

MOORE, W.J. and CORBETT, M.E. (1975): The Distribution of Dental Caries in Ancient British Populations. 3. The 17th Century, *Caries Res* 9:163-172.

NEWBRUN, E. (1967): Sucrose, the Arch Criminal of Dental Caries, *Odontol Revy* 18:373-386.

NEWBRUN, E. (1982): *Sugar and Dental Caries: A Review of Human Studies, Science* 217:418-423.

NIZEL, A.E. and PAPPAS, A.S. (1989): *Nutrition in Clinical Dentistry*, Third Edition, Philadelphia: W.B. Saunders, pp 208-209.

PICTON, D.C.A. (1986): Basis for the Use of Topical and Systemic Fluorides in Caries Prevention, *J Royal Soc Med* 79 (Suppl 14):18-21.

RUSSEL, A.L. (1966): World Epidemiology and Oral Health. In: *Environmental Variables in Oral Disease*, S. J. Kreshover and F.J. Mclure, Eds., Washington: *Amer Assoc Adv Sci*, p. 21.

SALK, J. (1983): The Virus of Poliomyelitis: From Discovery to Extinction, *J Am Med Assoc* 250:808-810.

WINTER, G.B. (1990): Epidemiology of Dental Caries, *Archs Oral Biol* 35(Suppl): 1S-7S.

EPIDEMIOLOGY

Impact of Changing Patterns of Dental Caries

MARTIN C DOWNER

The decline in caries experience, particularly in the young, since the early 1970s in many industrialised countries has been extensively reported. The first comprehensive documentation of available data was collated by Glass (1982). This was followed by an examination of the implications of the changing pattern of disease by the Fédération Dentaire Internationale (1985). Recently, the distribution of caries in Europe, changes in caries experience that have determined current levels, and the reasons for those changes have been analysed (Downer, 1991a). Also the epidemiology of permanent tooth caries in the Americas has been brought up to date (Stamm, 1991).

Improvements in oral health, arising in particular from the decrease in caries and its sequelae, have important consequences for providers of dental care. At the same time, changes in the pattern of disease have created new challenges for research workers in the field of caries epidemiology and lead to a need to review the research agenda.

In considering the impact of changing patterns of dental caries, the present study looks at some indicators of dental health of relevance to current management information needs with particular reference to the recent survey of dental health of United Kingdom adults (Todd and Lader, 1991). The study also presents evidence of a cohort effect in the decline in caries, and examines the validity of the epidemiological data on caries experience. The challenge presented by particular groups within populations in whom relatively high caries levels persist is then considered, and finally the implications for research are discussed.

Professional Implications of Current Indicators of Dental Health

The data presented in this first section were derived from a recent overview of the United Kingdom national surveys of adult dental health (Downer, 1991b).

Since 1968 these surveys, based on weighted, multi-stage population samples and carried out by teams of trained and standardised examiners, have provided a detailed record at 10-year intervals of the dental status of the full adult age range. No country, apart from the United States, has such comprehensive time series data enabling trends in adult dental health to be observed.

For the detection of caries a predominantly visual examination technique was used with positive diagnosis confined to unequivocal cavitation and presumptive involvement of dentine. The methods and criteria have remained largely constant throughout the surveys. However, as well as using standard indices for recording the condition of the natural teeth, in the latest 1988 survey other key indicators of dental health were also reported which enabled the attainment of important goals to be assessed. These included the proportion of the population who had some natural teeth, the proportion who were substantially dentate, having 21 or more natural teeth, and mean numbers of sound untreated teeth.

The proportion of the UK adult population who retained some natural teeth rose from 70% in 1978 to 79% in 1988. By 1988, 96% of young middle aged adults in the 35-44 year age range were dentate. However, among the elderly, that is to say people of 65 years and over, only one third retained any natural teeth. The pattern of tooth loss in older people reflects the disease and irreversible treatment by extraction of earlier times and offers little scope for improvement. Nevertheless on the basis of present trends it is estimated that by the end of the first decade of the next century, 90% of the British population will be dentate including 65% of those aged 65 and over.

As regards the retention of 21 or more natural teeth, taken in the survey as an arbitrary indicator of a functional, predominantly natural dentition, 63% of all adults and 80% of dentate adults had achieved this goal in 1988. Moreover it was estimated that over 90% of the working age population would be substantially dentate, with 21 or more natural teeth, by 2008.

The mean number of sound untreated teeth among British adults also improved between 1978 and 1988. This was particularly noticeable in the youngest adult age group where 16-24-year-olds now have on average more than two thirds of their teeth sound and untreated.

The improvements in dental health documented in the surveys have taken place during a period in which the UK population has both expanded and aged. In order to illustrate the impact of changes in dental health between 1968 and 1988 in the growing adult population, selected key indicators are expressed in Table 1 as estimates of absolute numbers of teeth in different categories. These have been set against population estimates for England and Wales for the survey years.

Whereas population size increased by 11%, it can be seen that percentage changes in numbers of teeth in all categories were far greater. Thus there was a

TABLE 1. *Changes in the dental condition of adults in England and Wales.*

	1968 (millions)	*1978 (millions)*	*1988 (millions)*	*1968-88 (% change)*
Adult population	36.4	37.7	40.3	+11
Dentate adults	22.9	26.8	32.2	+41
No. of natural teeth	502	621	787	+57
No. of sound untreated teeth	294	353	484	+65
No. of filled (otherwise sound) teeth	158	217	268	+72
No. of decayed (or unsound) teeth	50	51	32	−36

rise of 65% in the number of sound untreated teeth, representing a considerable improvement in dental health. Nevertheless, a further 32 million teeth in 1988 were estimated to require either treatment for caries or the replacement of unsound restorations.

The pool of teeth at risk has substantially increased, yet it is difficult to assess the extent to which risk will be translated into overt disease. There is evidence that individuals who retain a large complement of natural teeth are disease resistant and, for example, the idea that decreasing rates of endentulism will necessarily result in more root caries has lately been called into question (Beck *et al.*, 1988).

It is recognised that dental health surveys are not capable of forecasting the detailed content of future professional activity with any degree of certainty (Nuttall and Davies, 1988). Nevertheless, it is possible by observing trends to make some general predictions. At the upper end of the age spectrum, many more people can now expect to remain substantially dentate. However, it is estimated that it will be 50 years at the earliest before the market for replacement dentures in the UK disappears. Meanwhile increasing preservation of natural teeth, many of them heavily restored, implies that the need for repair of existing restorations, work which evidence suggests may currently comprise two thirds of adult conservative treatment (Elderton and Davies, 1984), is likely to remain high. The 1988 survey indicated that root caries in the UK population was of relatively low prevalence averaging 0.7 teeth with root surface decay and 1.2 with root surface fillings at the peak age of 55-64 years. Providing replacement coronal restorations will probably be a considerably more onerous task than the treatment of root caries judging by present disease levels.

The profession will be carrying out restorative treatment on a steadily ageing population. Much of this may be more complex than the routine restorative work currently undertaken on younger age groups yet many of the patients will be less robust on account of age and disability. This has important implications for the profession and also highlights the need for increased research into the burdens that future patterns of disease will place upon the dental services.

Cohort Effect in Declining Caries Prevalence

In addition to the national surveys of adults, similar surveys of child dental health were undertaken in 1973 and 1983 (Todd and Dodd, 1985). Also, a national rolling programme of regionally co-ordinated surveys of dental caries in specific age groups of children was initiated in England and Wales in 1985 (Evans and Dowell, 1990) using diagnostic standards compatible with those of the national surveys (Palmer *et al.*, 1984). By combining data sets from these various surveys it is possible to obtain a comprehensive picture of secular trends in caries experience nationally.

In Table 2 and Fig. 1, data obtained from large population samples of 5-, 12-, and 14-year-olds examined in the regional program have been appropriately weighted (Downer, 1989a) and used to augment the ten-year national survey data in order to present mean percentage caries reduction rates for six different age groups of the population of England and Wales over two discrete periods of observation for each group. The survey years varied but the average reductions in caries have been normalised by expressing them as compounded annual reduction rates per annum rather than as absolute percentage reductions over the different time intervals. One difference in the method of computing the DMF indices for children and adults should, however, be noted. Whereas in children the 'missing' component comprised only teeth presumed lost because of caries, in adults all missing units in a dentition of 32 teeth were included.

Taking each age group in turn, it is apparent that in the period between 1973 and 1983, the decline in dmf primary teeth of 5-year-olds averaged 7.7% per annum. However, no further reduction occurred nationally between 1983 and 1985/86 and although the last observation period was short, the caries level in this youngest age group had apparently begun to bottom-out and stabilise. It is possible that this was due to growth in fluoride toothpaste sales having approached a plateau and little change in overall sugar consumption in the UK in recent years (Downer, 1991a). In 12- and 14-year-olds, on the other hand, reduction rates of 4.9% and 4.4% respectively between 1973 and 1983 accelerated to 11.3% and 8.8%, and at least doubled during two more recent periods since 1983. This represents a cohort effect of young children with reduced caries levels advancing into adolescence. However, the greatest relative percentage change occurred in 16-24- year-olds, although the reductions were much lower in absolute terms. Here an annual compound reduction rate of less than 1% between 1968 and 1978 accelerated more than threefold between 1978 and 1988.

TABLE 2. *Changes in caries experience of children and young adults in England and Wales between 1968 and 1988.*

Age group	*Caries index*	*Year*	*Base No. **	*Weighted mean*	*Compounded annual reduction rate (%)*
5-year-olds	dmft	1973	952	4.0	
		1983	719	1.8	7.7
		1985/86	72339	1.8	–
12-year-olds	DMFT	1973	956	4.8	
		1983	1036	2.9	4.9
		1988/89	101294	1.5	11.3
14-year-olds	DMFT	1973	923	7.4	
		1983	1109	4.7	4.4
		1986/87	38889	3.4	8.8
16-24-year-olds	DMFT	1968	375	15.8	
		1978	567	14.5	0.9
		1988	622	10.4	3.3
25-34-year-olds	DMFT	1968	478	19.4	
		1978	661	18.3	0.6
		1988	605	15.8	1.5
35-44-year-olds	DMFT	1968	508	22.3	
		1978	600	21.0	0.6
		1988	567	19.1	0.9

* Adjusted to include edentulous fractions of the population samples.

In the two older adult age groups, although it can be seen that annual caries reduction rates over the most recent ten years increased considerably compared with those of the preceding ten year period, the acceleration was less marked than in the late teens and early twenties age group where the most dramatic change has occurred in relative terms. Eventually as these young adults with greatly improved oral health mature and move into their thirties and forties, it is likely that marked decreases in caries levels will be seen in increasingly older age groups of the population. Restorative treatment needs in these age groups should be commensurately reduced.

Validity of the Data

Both the validity of the data collected in cross-sectional epidemiological investigations like the UK surveys and the inferences drawn from the findings have lately been questioned on the grounds that they underestimate the true

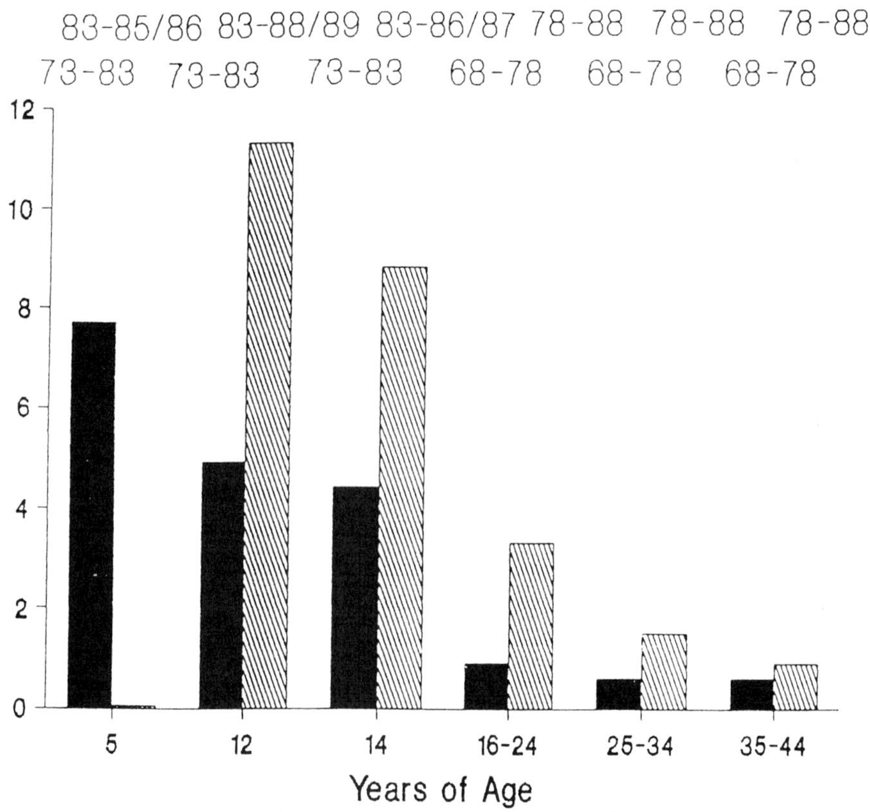

Figure 1. Compound annual reduction rates in caries experience over various observation periods in six different age groups of the population of England and Wales.

prevalence of caries in populations (Kidd, 1991; Manji *et al.*, 1991). Criticism has centered on the fact that the examinations are carried out under sub-optimal conditions, that enamel lesions are not recorded, and that primary and secondary caries of dentine are frequently underscored because radiography is not used.

However, such criticisms fail to take into account two factors. First, any diagnostic method will generate not only false-negative decisions where the presence of lesions is missed, but also false-positives where sound tooth surfaces or surfaces with enamel lesions only are misclassified as cavitated. Secondly, as the prevalence of caries declines, so the absolute number of false-positive decisions in relation to true positives becomes magnified (Downer, 1989b).

It is possible to illustrate these phenomena by taking data from experimental studies, in which caries diagnostic decisions have been validated histologically for example, and then interpolating them into assumed, albeit realistic, distributions of caries in populations. It is found that where true caries prevalence is low, recorded prevalence is likely to be artifically inflated by false-positive diagnoses. The frequency of these may exceed that of true positives and greatly exceed that of undetected lesions.

There is strong circumstantial evidence also, that the prevalence of caries has not been substantially underestimated in surveys. The reported decline in the disease has been taking place since at least 1970 so that the agents responsible must have been operating for some twenty years. By 1977, for example, over 95% of the toothpaste market in Britain consisted of fluoride containing products. If large numbers of lesions were missed in earlier surveys then many of these would surely have manifested themselves as frank cavitation some ten or more years later, even if initially these lesions were small and slowly progressing (Ekanayake and Sheiham, 1987). Yet mean DMFT scores at the cavitation level actually fell among young dentate adults in the UK by 28% in 16-24-year-olds and by 12% in 25-34-year-olds between 1978 and 1988. Moreover during the same period, edentulousness in the younger age group remained insignificant, and fell from 4% to 1% in 25-34-year-olds (Downer, 1991b). In the cohort which attained 25-34 years of age in 1988, DMFT had increased by a mean of less than 1.3 over the course of the preceeding ten-years. An upsurge in frank cavitation from the progression of previously undetected lesions therefore simply has not occurred.

Variations in Caries Levels in Populations

Data summarising age-specific caries levels differ between countries and often conceal, also, large regional and local geographic variations within them (Downer, 1991a). These reflect social, behavioural, cultural and economic characteristics of the populations concerned, although the influence of these factors on caries is indirect and not well defined (Beck *et al.*, 1988).

Caries experience as measured by DMF is related to age but not strongly associated with gender, race or socio-economic status. On the other hand, the separate components of DMF are clearly related to these factors. Thus females, whites, higher social classes and urban dwellers generally have the higher F scores and the lower D and M scores. These demographic variables cannot influence the disease process directly but operate indirectly through behavioural patterns and life-styles. Socio-economic status, for example, which is governed by education, occupation and income, determines the normative value placed on maintaining a natural dentition and influences the degree of knowledge, ability and personal commitment that individuals bring to bear in adopting health-promoting life-styles and protecting themselves against disease. Oral hygiene practices, dietary habits, including sugar intake in particular, and access to and use of dental care services are all known to have strong associations with socio-economic status (Downer, 1991a).

Table 3 presents DMFT and its components for five European populations in the 35-44 year age range for which dependable data were available (Marthaler,

TABLE 3. *Caries experience in selected 35-44-year-old populations of Europe.*

Population	*Decayed teeth*	*Missing teeth*	*Filled teeth*	*DMFT*	*Year*
East Germany	1.6	4.7	9.8	16.1	1989
West Germany	1.9	5.4	10.3	17.5	1989
Republic of Ireland	1.1	10.1	7.8	19.0	1989
Switzerland	0.7	6.2	15.4	22.3	1987/88
United Kingdom	1.0	6.9	11.0	19.0	1988

1990; Downer 1991b). It can be seen that Switzerland had the lowest D component, the highest F component and the highest mean DMFT. Ireland and the UK had the same DMFT levels but the UK had the higher F component and the lower M component. West Germany had a low M component but the highest D component and an F component in the intermediate range. The East German values were not dissimilar to the West German but all were lower. The data probably reflect cultural, social and economic differences between the populations concerned, and differences in prevailing health promotional policies and systems of dental care delivery.

Within the UK it is illuminating to examine the position in two regional subgroups of the same 35-44-year-old population with contrasting dental health profiles. Data abstracted from Todd and Lader (1991) are presented in Table 4 for males in Southern England, females in Scotland and for both genders in the whole UK. It can be seen that whereas the D and F components of mean DMFT were not markedly different between the two regional groups, the M component for Scottish females amounted to 10.9 compared with only 6.5 for Southern England males. The M component for females was inflated because 10% of that subgroup were edentulous compared with only 2% of the males. Such differences are repeated locally in different parts of the country and in different socioeconomic groups with particular subgroups having even more extreme age-specific index values.

Ironing out inequalities in dental health and raising standards in particular disadvantaged or high risk groups of the population is a formidable challenge to policy makers and to those commissioning or providing care. Two distinct oral health promotion strategies exist for approaching the task (Sheiham and Joffe, 1991). The so-called high risk strategy, which focuses on individual counselling, and small group health education and preventive programmes, is currently favoured in many countries. However, it is costly, relatively ineffective and often fails to reach those individuals most in need. The alternative approach, the whole population strategy, which relies on mass prevention methods such as fluoridation and the adoption of sugar substitution in food manufacturing and processing, has already proved highly effective. The gains from fluoridation in

TABLE 4. *Caries experience in 1988 of males in Southern England, females in Scotland, and males and females in the United Kingdom aged 35-44-years.*

Region and gender	*Decayed teeth*	*Missing teeth **	*Filled teeth*	*DMFT*
Southern England males	1.3	6.5	11.4	19.2
Scotland females	0.9	10.9	11.9	23.7
United Kingdom males and females	1.0	7.9	11.0	19.9

* Adjusted to include edentulous fractions of the population samples.

particular have been considerable but the implementation of whole population strategies requires a strong political will.

Research Opportunities

The present study has considered the impact of the changing pattern of dental caries and attempted to highlight some current areas of interest in the field of caries epidemiology arising as a consequence of the reported changes. The topics discussed have raised some pointers as to the directions which the next phase of research in the discipline should take. Evident reductions in the prevalence of the disease have given rise to new research challenges and a number of these can be enumerated. Thus there is a need to develop appropriate new outcome measures and to refine ways of forecasting the future tasks of dental health professionals and in particular the implications of ageing and oral health. There is a need to explore ways of improving the dental health outlook for those disadvantaged groups which continue to suffer high levels of disease. The cost-effectiveness, feasibility and suitability of high risk versus whole population strategies need more thorough investigation, and methods of predicting high caries risk need to be refined. There is also now a need to set new goals for oral health, capable of realistic achievement. Finally, it is essential to continue monitoring the dental health of populations on a regular, systematic basis in order to detect any changes in trends and to measure the attainment of goals.

These are only some of the important research challenges. Caries remains a ubiquitous disease and it is clear that there are many unanswered questions still to be addressed by the research community.

REFERENCES

BECK, J.D.; KOHOUT, F.; and HUNT, R.J. (1988): Identification of high caries risk adults: attitudes, social factors and diseases. *Int Dent J;* 38:231-238.

DOWNER, M.C. (1989a): Time trends in dental decay in young children. *Health Trends;* 21:7-9.

DOWNER, M.C. (1989b): Validation of methods used in dental caries diagnosis. *Int Dent J;* 39:241-246.

DOWNER, M.C. (1991a): Description and explanation of the distribution of caries in the populations of Europe: in Johnson, N.W. (ed): *Risk Markers for Oral Diseases Volume 1 Dental Caries.* Cambridge, Cambridge University Press, pp.100-131.

DOWNER, M.C. (1991b): The improving dental health of United Kingdom adults and prospects for the future. *Br Dent J;* 170:154-158.

EKANAYAKE, L.S. and SHEIHAM, A. (1987): Reducing rates of progression of dental caries in British schoolchildren. A study using bitewing radiographs. *Br Dent J;* 163:265-269.

ELDERTON, R.J. and DAVIES, J.A. (1984): Restorative treatment in the General Dental Service in Scotland. *Br Dent J;* 157:196-200.

EVANS, D.J. and DOWELL, T.B. (1990): The dental caries experience of 12-year-old children in Great Britain. *Community Dent Health;* 7:307-314.

FÉDÉRATION DENTAIRE INTERNATIONALE (1985): Changing patterns of oral health and implications for oral health manpower: Part 1. Technical Report No.24. *Int Dent J;* 35:235-251.

GLASS, R.L. (1982): The first international conference on the declining prevalence of dental caries. The evidence and the impact on dental education, dental research, and dental practice. *J Dent Res;* 61: suppl., 1301-1383.

KIDD, E.A.M. (1991): A critical evaluation of caries diagnostic methods and epidemiological methods. Can we trust the available data? in Johnson, N.W. (ed): *Risk Markers for Oral Diseases* Volume 1 Dental Caries. Cambridge, Cambridge University Press, pp.15-32.

MANJI, F.; FEJERSKOV, O.; BAELUM, V.; LUAN, W-M.; CHEN, X. (1991): The epidemiological features of dental caries in African and Chinese populations: implications for risk assessment. in Johnson, N.W. (ed): *Risk Markers for Oral Diseases* Volume 1 Dental Caries. Cambridge, Cambridge University Press, pp.62-99.

MARTHALER, T.M. (1990): Caries status in Europe and predictions of future trends. Symposium report. *Caries Res;* 24:381-396.

NUTTALL, N.M. and DAVIES, J.A. (1988): The capability of the 1983 children's dental health survey in Scotland to predict fillings and extractions subsequently undertaken. *Community Dent Health;* 5:355-362.

PALMER, J.D.; ANDERSON, R.J.; and DOWNER, M.C. (1984): Guidelines for prevalence studies of dental caries. *Community Dent Health;* 1:55-66.

SHEIHAM, A. and JOFFE, M. (1991): Public dental health strategies for identifying and controlling dental caries in high and low risk populations. in Johnson, N.W. (ed): *Risk Markers for Oral Diseases* Volume 1 Dental Caries. Cambridge, Cambridge University Press, pp.445-481.

STAMM, J.W. (1991): The epidemiology of permanent tooth caries in the Americas. in Johnson, N.W. (ed): *Risk Markers for Oral Diseases* Volume 1 Dental Caries. Cambridge, Cambridge University Press, pp.132-155

TODD, J.E. and DODD, T. (1985): Children's Dental Health in the United Kingdom 1983. London, Her Majesty's Stationery Office.

TODD, J.E. and LADER, D. (1991): Adult Dental Health 1988 United Kingdom. London, Her Majesty's Stationery Office.

Caries In Our Aging Population: What Are We Learning

PAUL F. DEPAOLA

For most of the lifetimes of just about everyone here, the major oral disease of children has been dental caries. Of course, it was widely known that dental caries did continue on into adulthood but it was generally believed that beyond the age of about 25, carious lesions developed much less frequently than in the earlier years. Incidentally, the reason often given for this was that by age 25 and beyond, most or all of the caries susceptible tooth surfaces were already carious, filled, or missing, and therefore no longer available for attack.

Now, we must discard this ancient and venerable wisdom, because we live in a changing world. What can we say today about the incidence and prevalence of dental caries in children as opposed to adults?

One of the best reports bearing directly upon this question is that entitled, "A 10 Year Longitudinal Study Of Caries Incidence Rates In A Sample of Male Adults in the USA", by Glass *et al.*, (1987). Table 1 shows some of the data from this particular study. A sample of 729 non-institutionalized dentulous adult males was followed for 10 years, with a series of 4 comprehensive oral and radiographic examinations carried out under standard conditions at intervals of about 3 years. Individual counts were made of new decayed and filled surfaces occurring during the intervals between examinations, as well as of sound surfaces at risk in order to calculate mean DFS rates per 100 surfaces at risk adjusted to a period of one year.

As the table shows, the whole mouth annual new DFS rates range from 1.03 to 1.92. The mean, which is not shown, is 1.36 per 100 surfaces at risk, per year.

The authors then compared these rates to those seen in children over the last several years. In order to make valid comparisons the caries experience of

The clinical trial reported in this paper was supported by NIH No. DE-07009 and the Colgate-Hoyt Company of Canton, MA.

The author wishes to express his deepest gratitude to Dr. Edgard Moreno whose expertise was the basis for the section on "basic questions".

TABLE 1 *Mean Age Group Annual DFS Rates Per 100 Surfaces at Risk (Modifed from Glass et al, (1987))*

	Ex 1 vs 2			*Ex 2 vs 3*			*Ex 3 vs 4*		
Age	*<45*	*45-54*	*>55*	*<45*	*45-54*	*>55*	*<45*	*45-54*	*>55*
DFS Rates Per 100 Surfaces Per Year	1.03	1.43	1.92	0.90	1.20	1.74	1.25	1.65	1.62

children was expressed, again, as rates per 100 surfaces per year. In the several studies shown in Table 2, annual caries incidence rates range from 1.08 to 2.47 new DFS per 100 surfaces at risk. This is well within the range shown in Table 2 for adults. This comparison is conservative, however, because with the larger number of filled surfaces in adults, the risk of secondary caries is greater. Therefore, the inherent underestimation of caries rates should be greater in adults than in children.

All in all, this report clearly suggests that in this group of adults the observed annual caries incidence rates are roughly similar to those experienced by children. As Glass *et al.* assert, therefore, the preventive procedures advocated today for children may also be applicable to adults.

This statement is obviously based upon the premise that fluoride inhibits caries (both coronal and root) in adults just as it does in children, and probably through a similar mechanism of action. However, as indicated in two reviews appearing in the proceedings of the recent workshop entitled, "Cost Effectiveness of Caries Prevention in Dental Public Health" (Burt, 1989) there is a scarcity of clinical trials in which either professionally or self-applied fluoride gels have been tested on subjects older than school age and, "only one study of the efficacy of fluoride mouthrinsing in adults has been published". In addition, few studies have assessed the anticaries effectiveness of fluoride containing dentifrices in adults.

TABLE 2 *DFS Rates, Per 100 Surfaces Per Year*

Age at start of study years	*Time period years*	*Mean annual*	*Reference rate*
6-11	3	1.94	Glass and Shiere, 1978
11-12	2	2.39	Naylor and Glass, 1979
7-11	2	2.17	Glass, 1981a
6-11	2-1/2	1.62	Glass, 1981b
7-11	2-1/2	1.08	Glass, Peterson and Bixler, 1983
7-11	2	2.47	Glass, 1983

Against this impoverished background of knowledge we recently undertook an investigation involving the use of fluoride in middle-aged and elderly adults. Drawing upon inspiration from work by Billings, *et al.* (1985) and Nyvad, and Fejerskov, (1986) we resorted to the strategy of using as the dependent variable not the usual increment in carious surfaces but rather, the number of early lesions which convert to an arrested state. In the study by Billings, *et al.*, 54 lesions of varying depth were exposed to fluoride therapy for 2 years. Seventy percent of the incipient lesions arrested. In the work by Nyvad and Fejerskov, a particular scheme of fluoride therapy produced arrestment in every lesion by the end of six months. While these were astonishing successes, the fact is that both studies were conducted without a placebo group. Notwithstanding, the results of these uncontrolled studies were so remarkable that it seemed appropriate to design and implement a double-blind trial with a proper control group to determine if total, or nearly total, arrestment of early root surface lesions could be demonstrated with appropriate scientific constraints in place.

The investigation was carried out by myself as principal investigator and Dr. Pramod Soparkar as both co-investigator and examiner. This was a very appropriate transition for Dr. Soparkar who had just completed a root surface caries effort in which he had examined over 300 subjects utilizing an extensive and refined diagnostic scheme of our own construction which had been thoroughly and successfully tested for reliability when it was created. What follows is a report of this study organized so as to achieve as succinct a format as possible.

I. Purpose

The purpose of the study was to determine the effect upon buccal root surface caries lesions of the daily self-application of 5000 ppm neutral NaF gel* in conjunction with the periodic professional application of 12000 ppm neutral NaF gel**.

II. Materials and Methods

1. Basic Study Design

The study was designed as a randomized double-blind clinical trial with a treatment and control group.

* Prevident Brush-On Gel, Colgate-Hoyt, Canton, MA

** Prevident Plus Gel, Colgate-Hoyt, Canton, MA

2. Study Sites

The effort was based at the Forsyth Dental Center in Boston and the Center for Community Dental Health (CCDH) in Portland, Maine. Respondents were screened at the Forsyth and the CCDH clinićs and at various field sites established with portable equipment.

3. Enrollment of Subjects

Subjects accepted into the program were those, (1) who had at least one unequivocally active early buccal surface root lesion, (2) who were, in the opinion of the examiner, free from oral or systemic conditions which contraindicated participation, and (3) who expected to maintain their place of residence for the duration of the study. Recruitment continued until eighty-three subjects were obtained of whom 41 were randomly assigned to the control group and 42 to the treated group.

4. The Clinical Procedures

The clinical examinations were conducted at the clinic of the Forsyth Dental Center, the dental clinic of the Maine Medical Center (across the street from the CCDH) and in portable clinics set up to screen subjects who resided outside the Greater Boston and Portland areas. The portable clinics were placed in senior centers, churches, and senior apartment complexes in a variety of widely scattered communities. Both the fixed and portable clinics contained state-of-the-art equipment including excellent lighting, suction, and air. At baseline, subjects were evaluated for coronal caries (DMF index), oral hygiene in the manner of Greene and Vermillion, (1960), gingival status in the manner of Loe-Sillness (1963), and root surface caries. The latter was divided into three phases designated as C_1, C_2, and AC, in the manner of DePaola *et al.* (1989). A C_1 lesion is a well defined softened area, yellowish or light brown in color, but without cavitation, i.e, the morphological integrity of the surface is undisturbed. Penetration by explorer is possible. A C_2 lesion is a softened area, yellowish or light brown in color with a disruption of the surface contour. Penetration by explorer is possible. An AC or, arrested caries lesion, is a darkly stained almost black area with a leathery consistency; there may or may not be cavitation. There is little if any penetration by explorer. For this study the potential subjects whose C_2 lesions were beyond the earliest stages were excluded.

After the clinical examination the early root lesions were isolated with cotton rolls and dried with compressed air. This was followed by application of either the active (12,000 ppm F) or placebo gel for two minutes. After the gel treatment, subjects received hands-on instruction in proper brushing, flossing, and the use of the self-applied gel formulation. The instructions were supplemented with take-home materials. The subjects were then provided with a four month

TABLE 3 *Age and Sex of Continuous Participants*

	Sample Size	*Mean Age(Yrs)*	*No. Males*	*No. Females*
Control	36	68.58	11	25
Treatment	35	72.54	10	25
Total	71	70.55	21	50

supply of Colgate dentifrice, brushes, and appropriate self-applied gel formulation. Upon leaving, subjects received a $10.00 remuneration. Follow-up examinations occurred at four months, eight months, and twelve months. At each follow-up, root lesion status was reassessed. The appropriate gel was re-applied to test lesions, the oral hygiene procedures were reviewed, home-care materials were re-supplied, and subjects were remunerated.

5. Use of Products and the Motivational Program

As indicated, each subject received home care instruction at the time of the baseline and follow-up visits. The home routine included brushing with Colgate MFP dentifrice at least twice daily, one of the brushings to be in the evening before bedtime. The evening brushing was followed by the self-application of the gel.

The need for meticulous oral hygiene with special attention to the diseased root surfaces, was stressed throughout the investigation. In Massachusetts, subjects were telephoned twice at equally spaced intervals between visits as a means of maintaining motivation and promoting the proper use of products. In Maine the motivational program included two letters sent to subjects between visits.

III. Results

Table 3 shows the numbers, the age and the sex of continuous participants, i.e., those subjects who presented at the baseline as well as at every follow-up. Thirty-six of 41 control subjects and 35 of 42 treated subjects were continuous participants. Subject losses were for reasons not associated with the study. The mean ages of the control and treated subjects were 68.58 and 72.54 years respectively. There were 11 males and 25 females in the control group while the treated group consisted of 10 males and 25 females.

The mean clinical indices at baseline for each group are given in Table 4. No significant differences between groups were found with respect to oral hygiene status, number of teeth present, DFS score, number of exposed root surfaces, numbers of C_I and C_2 lesions, arrested lesions (n=0), and number of root surface restorations. There was a significant difference, however, ($p = 0.02$) between mean gingivitis scores.

TABLE 4 *Mean Clinical Indices at Baseline for Treatment and Control Group*

Group	*OHI*	*Gingivitis Score*	*No. Teeth Present*	*DFS*	*No. Exposed Root Surfaces*	*Buccal C_1*	*Buccal C_2*	*Buccal AC Lesions*	*No. Root Surface Fillings*
Control	0.86	1.05	19.33	29.39	16.42	0.58	1.58		1.69
(n = 36)	(0.47)*	(0.45)	(6.16)	(21.54)	(11.94)	(0.73)	(1.36)	0.00	(2.04)
Treatment	0.72	0.76	18.43	32.37	19.31	0.86	1.51		2.26
(n = 35)	(0.58)	(0.48)	(7.18)	(23.60)	(9.81)	(1.00)	(1.31)	0.00	(2.50)
t value	0.99	2.48	0.20	0.56	1.12	1.32	0.22	—	1.04
p value	0.33	0.02	0.84	0.58	0.27	0.19	0.83	—	0.30

* Figures in parentheses are standard deviations

TABLE 5 *Percentage of Buccal C_1's Arrested at 4, 8, and 12 Month Follow-up Examinations*

	Group	*4 mos*	*8 mos*	*12 mos*
% C_1's	Control	18	28	40
Arrested	Treatment	39	95	91

chi-square at 4 mos = 4.67, p = 0.03*
chi-square at 8 mos = 22.61, p <0.01*
chi-square at 12 mos = 13.29, p <0.01*

* All chi-square analyses were conducted utilizing the Donner and Banting (1988) technique to compensate for possible intra-oral site correlation.

Table 5 contains the percentage of C_1 lesions arrested at each follow-up examination. In the control group 18% of the C_1 lesions had arrested after four months while the corresponding figure for the treatment group was 39%. At 8 months the values were 28% in the controls vs. 95% in the treated. By the end of the 12 month study interval 40% of C_1's had arrested in the controls and 91% in the treated subjects.

Table 6 shows the percentage of C_2 lesions arrested at 4, 8, and 12 months in the two groups. For the controls there were no lesions arrested at 4 months, 5% at eight months, and 8% at 12 months. The corresponding values in the treated group were 13% at 4 months, 53% at 8 months, and 57% at 12 months. Chi square analyses, conducted in the manner of Donner and Banting (1988) so as to take into account potential intraoral site correlations, suggest highly significant differences between groups both with respect to C_1 and C_2 lesions.

Table 7 shows the numbers of control and treated subjects who experienced arrestment vs. no arrestment after 12 months. Among the controls 10 experienced arrestment while 26 did not. In the treated subjects, the corresponding values were 31 with arrestment and 4 without. The chi-square of 24.45 is significant with $p < 0.025$.

TABLE 6 *Percentage of Buccal C_2's Arrested at 4, 8, and 12 Month Follow-up Examinations*

	Group	*4 mos*	*8 mos*	*12 mos*
%C_2's	Control	0	5	8
Arrested	Treatment	13	53	57

chi-square at 4 mos = 4.30, p = 0.04*
chi-square at 8 mos = 22.89, p <0.001*
chi-square at 12 mos = 29.32, p <0.001*

* All chi-square analyses were conducted utilizing the Donner and Banting (1988) technique to compensate for possible intra-oral site correlation.

TABLE 7 *The Proportion of Subjects Who Experienced Arrestment Over the Duration of the Study*

Group	*No. Who Experienced Arrestment*	*No. Who Did Not Experience Arrestment*	*Total*
Treatment	31	4	35
Control	10	26	36
Total	41	30	71

chi-square = 24.45, df = 1, $p < 0.025$

IV. Discussion

The baseline findings show that the random assignment of subjects to groups worked reasonably well. The groups were balanced with respect to age and sex, as well as to a variety of baseline indices including oral hygiene, number of teeth present, DF surfaces, number of C_l lesions, C_2 lesions, arrested lesions, and root fillings. There was one exception in that control subjects were found to have a higher gingivitis score at baseline but there is nothing to suggest that this one instance of group imbalance biased the outcome of the study in any manner.

It is apparent from the trend data that a substantially higher percentage of C_l lesions were found to be arrested in treated subjects than in the controls at each of the follow-up examinations. By eight months most (95%) treated lesions were arrested. At twelve months the percentage of arrested lesions in the treatment group dropped slightly (91%), which may reflect of diagnostic reversals on the part of the examiner.

A similar pattern was found with respect to the C_2 lesions. At each follow-up there were far more treated lesions arrested than control lesions. It is interesting to note, however, that in the case of the C_2, lesions which by definition are more advanced than the C_l's, the percentages arrested at each follow-up were distinctly lower than was the case with the C_l lesions at corresponding points in time. Thus, by the end of the study 91% of the C_l's had arrested vs 57% of the C_2 lesions. It is evident therefore that the earlier the fluoride therapy is initiated, the greater the likelihood of the desired outcome.

It is of interest that none of the subjects had arrested caries at baseline and yet we were able to produce a large percentage of arrested lesions over the course of the study. We attribute this to the intense oral hygiene motivational program which we think impelled subjects to brush more frequently, for a longer duration, and with special attention to test lesions.

Another point of interest is that there were a substantial number of lesions in the control group which underwent arrestment (forty percent of C_l's and 8% of C_2's). Although this is much less than was observed in the treated group, it is still noteworthy since lesion arrestment in controls was not a predicted outcome. After the fact, however, it is not difficult to explain. While control subjects were not exposed to the active fluoride gels they did participate in an intensive oral hygiene regime which included the twice daily use of a fluoride dentifrice. It is reasonable to assume, as stated above, that most, if not all subjects in this study brushed their teeth more meticulously, with greater regularity, and with greater attention to diseased areas, than was their usual custom. The very purpose of the periodic oral hygiene instruction was to produce this result. It appears, then, that the vigorous home care including the use of a fluoride dentifrice, by itself produced some caries arrestment, although this effect was confined almost entirely to early lesions, that is, the C_I's In a recent report (DePaola *et al.*, 1989), oral hygiene was identified as an exceptionally important determinant in the development of root surface lesions. The present findings are consistent with this observation.

The outcome of this study raises a series of interesting clinical research questions:

1. How much of the benefit observed in treated subjects was attributable to the self-applied fluoride agent vs. that which was professionally applied?
2. What would be the effect of the present treatment regime on interproximal lesions?
3. Are the benefits of the three fluoride agents, that is, the dentifrice, self-applied gel, and professionally applied gel additive or interactive?
4. What would be the outcome if patients followed the present treatment scheme twice a day instead of once a day? Under these conditions could the number of professional treatments be reduced or even eliminated? Would more C_2 lesions arrest?
5. Is there a point beyond which a C_2 lesion is irretrievable from the standpoint of arrestment? The clinical impression in this study was that the C_2 lesions which did arrest were for the most part in the very earliest stages of cavitation.
6. What would be the effect of the treatment regime described herein upon the *prevention* of lesions as opposed to arrestment? Unfortunately, the assessment of prevention requires much more time and many more subjects than is the case with arrestment.

It is clear from this list of clinical questions, which could no doubt be lengthened considerably, that a great deal more *in vivo* research is required and there is the potential for generating some answers of considerable practical usefulness. I am referring here primarily to the questions dealing with caries arrestment and secondarily to the closely related issue of prevention. However, if we widen our thinking to the entire domain of questions focusing upon root surface caries, the scope of the research effort required to provide the answers suggests a program of research which must be measured in terms of years. Consider merely the critical problem of risk assessment and its usual sequent, that of targeting. These are problems which are just beginning to receive some attention and the results generated to date suggest a long way yet to go (Disney, *et al.*, 1989, Kent *et al.*, 1991).

Furthermore, if we are to move expeditiously towards the eventual eradication of the disease, progress paralleling that required at the clinical level is also essential at the basic level. Indeed, it is most likely that without the development of certain crucial information at the basic level we may never totally achieve our ultimate objective. The following limited list of basic questions is intended to illustrate the point.

1. Why do caries-like lesions develop much faster in dentin than in enamel in a given demineralizing solution in the laboratory, whereas the opposite is true *in vivo*?
2. Are these rate differentials a function of intrinsic differences in the nature of the two minerals? Could this be a function of differences in porosity?
3. What is the composition of plaque and plaque fluid which develops on dentin as opposed to enamel?
4. Do topical fluorides repress cariogenic bacteria or decrease their acid production?
5. What are the driving forces for incipient dissolution of enamel and dentin? Can they be defined unambiguously. Is calcium fluoride involved in the process and if so, by what mechanism?
6. Is it possible to develop remineralizing procedures that would be equally effective for enamel and dentin?
7. Can laboratory tests be developed which provide some credible indication of the effectiveness of new prophylactic measures which are under consideration for costly, long-term evaluation in large samples of subjects?

Far more questions could be added to this but there is no need to belabor the point. There is a lot of work to do.

We hear over and over again that caries in children has declined significantly. No one seems to have made the point, though, that caries in adults has undergone an increase in relative importance. The meaning here is that while children's caries was endemic, research questions related primarily to adult caries had to be given a relatively lower priority. Now that the burden of children's caries has lightened, the adult caries questions demand attention, and so there is now an obligation for the research community to widen its efforts with respect to those aspects of caries which pertain in particular to adults.

REFERENCES

BILLINGS, R.J.; BROWN, L.R.; and KASTER, G.A. (1985): Contemporary Treatment Strategies for Root Surface Dental Caries, *Gerodontics* 1:20-27.

BRUNELLE, J.A. (1989): Oral Health of United States Children, *NIH Publication* No. 89-2247:5.

BURT, B.A. (1989): Proceedings for the Workshop: Cost Effectiveness of Caries Prevention in Dental Public Health, *J Pub Hlth Dentistry* 49:252-344.

DEPAOLA, P.F.; SOPARKAR, P.M.; and KENT, R.L. Jr. (1989a): Methodological Issues Relative to the Quantification of Root Surface Caries, *Gerodontology* 8:3-8.

DEPAOLA, P.F.; SOPARKAR, P.M.; TAVARES, M.; and KENT, R.L. Jr. (1989b): The Clinical Profiles of Individuals with and without Root Surface Caries, *Gerodontology* 8:9-15.

DISNEY, J.A.; STAMM, J.W.; GRAVES, R.C.; ABERNATHY, J.R.; BOHANNON, H.M.; and ZACK, D.D. (1989): Description and Preliminary Results of a Caries Risk Assessment Model, *Proceedings of a Conference,* June 2-3, 1989:204-214.

DONNER, A. and BANTING, D. (1988): Analysis of Site Specific Data in Dental Studies, *J Dent Res* 67:1392-1395.

FEJERSKOV, O.; THYLSTRUP, A.; and LARSEN, M.J. (1981): Rational Use of Fluorides in Caries Prevention, *ACTA Odontol Scand* 39:241-249.

GLASS, R.L.; ALMAN, J.E.; and CHAUNCEY, H.H. (1987): A 10-Year Longitudinal Study of Caries Incidence Rates in a Sample of Male Adults in the USA, *Caries Res* 21:360-367.

GREENE, J.C. and VERMILLION, J.R. (1960): A Method of Classifying Oral Hygiene Status, *J.A.D.A.* 61:172-179.

KENT, R.; SOPARKAR, P.; PAPAS, A.; and DEPAOLA, P.F. (1991): Factors Associated with Root Surface Caries, *J Dent Res* 70: Abstract No. 750.

LOE, H. and SILLNESS, J. (1963): Periodontal Disease in Pregnancy. I. Prevalence and Severity, *ACTA Odontol Scand* 21:532-551.

MILLER, A.J.; BRUNELLE, J.P.; CARLOS, L.; BROWN, L.J.; and LOE, H. (1987): Oral Health of United States Adults, *NIH Publication* No. 87-2868:35-68.

NYVAD, B. and FEJERSKOV, O. (1986): Active Root Surface Caries Converted into Inactive Caries as a Response to Oral Hygiene, *Scand J Dent Res* 94:281-284.

Caries In Young Populations—Worldwide

K.W. Stephen

In 1982, the World Health Organisation, in conjunction with the Fédération Dentaire Internationale, adopted the "Global goals for oral health by the year 2000" policy, which included the recommendation that 50% of 5/6-yr-olds should be caries-free (FDI-WHO, 1982). The WHO basic survey methods (WHO, 1987) also recommended caries diagnoses should involve the use of dental explorers, but did state that " . . . stained pits or fissures in the enamel that catch the explorer . . . should be coded as sound". However, the accuracy of any "caries-free" status accorded to deciduous teeth in 5/6-yr-olds, on the basis of a clinical-only examination, must be questioned, in view of the publications which highlight deciduous caries underscoring (approx. 60%) in the absence of bitewing radiographs (Murray & Majid, 1978; Stecksen-Blicks & Wahlin, 1983). Furthermore, the damage which such sharp probing can inflict upon slightly decalcified, but otherwise intact, occlusal surfaces (Bergman & Linden, 1969; Van der Laan - van Dorp *et al.*, 1986) led to the development of the "European" caries examination system, whereby blunted 0.7 mm probes (Todd & Whitworth, 1974), round-ended 0.6 mm Williams' periodontal probes (Stephen *et al.*, 1988) or, more recently, 0.5 mm ball-ended CPITN probes (SHBDEP, 1987/88) are utilized. In addition, caries assessments employing the "sticky fissure" method have been shown to be less reproducible than those in which cavitation below approximately 0.5/0.6 mm is ignored from the scoring sequence (McHugh *et al.*, 1964; Rugg-Gunn *et al.*, 1976). Other examination-related aspects which can affect clinical accuracy, have been highlighted by Kidd (1991) and include general examination conditions, lighting, whether or not teeth are dried, whether or not they are plaque-free, and whether or not restorations (with possible recurrent caries) are present.

Even in the presence of acceptable radiographs, using a simple elastomeric orthodontic tooth-separation technique, Rimmer & Pitts (1990) have demonstrated that 29.1% of deciduous approximal lesions which were not noted radiographically, were capable of detection by direct vision. Hence, if the 211 children and 756 deciduous tooth surfaces studied by these workers were to be deemed representative of that particular child population, perhaps it might be questioned (as did Silverstone, 1984) whether the truly caries-free tooth (i.e. never subjected to discernible attack) actually exists following a year or so of intra-oral approximal contact.

In view of the above, and the varying criteria applied to date, it is perhaps not surprising that such deciduous dentition epidemiological data as do exist, may be of questionable value from a comparative point-of-view. Unfortunately, much of the information available is not expressed as per the WHO/FDI 5/6-yr-old target i.e. the 50% caries-free statistic, even though it was collected after publication of these aims in 1982. In addition, although the results of substantial epidemiological effort are published annually, and much data exist with respect to world-wide trends for caries in 12-yr-olds (WHO, 1989), there is a relative paucity regarding deciduous details. This is due, possibly to a combination of the fact that children in many countries do not commence schooling until 6 (or even 7) years of age, and that most clinical trials relating to water fluoridation, topical fluoridation etc, concern themselves with caries development/inhibition in the permanent dentition. Nonetheless, in this text, an attempt has been made to summarize appropriate available information as it relates to mainly English-language Index Medicus-quoted literature sources.

Country/Regional Data

Shown in Table 1 are 1986 details relating to 27 European countries where, for 14 of these, 5/6-yr-old "caries-free" information existed (WHO, 1986). Here, nine were then below the stated target, with only Finland and Malta (50%), Denmark (54%) and The Netherlands and USSR (both 55%), meeting the demanded level. For the other 17 countries listed in Group B, no data of this sort were available. However, even by 1990, when facts relating to 31 European populations were reviewed by Møller, in spite of these guidelines, although mean deft scores were presented in 22 cases, no "caries-free" statistics were detailed. Furthermore, for nine of that group, no deciduous data of any sort were given.

At the more "individual" study level, other European data do exist for 3/6-yr-olds, where dmft/dft values ranged from England's 1989 mean of 0.96, with 75% of 5-yr-olds being assessed as caries-free (Dowell & Evans, 1989), to 1975 Hungarian data (Bruszt *et al.*, 1977) which indicated a mean dmft of 6.3 in Baja, and only 11% caries-free (Table 2). Here, two Irish data-sets were presented for fluoridated and non-fluoridated children, the respective dmft values being 1.8 and 3.0, with 52% and 38% respectively being judged "sound" (O'Mullane *et al.*, 1986).

With regards to North America, considering the long-standing interest in dental health which has been evident in the U.S.A. and Canada, relatively few

TABLE 1 *Details of "Caries-Free" 5-6 Yr Olds from 14 European Countries—Group (A). However, for 17 Countries in the Lower Group (B), No Such Data Were Available in 1986 (W.H.O. 1986).*

GROUP (A)

	C-F		*C-F*
Bulgaria	20%	Sweden	46%
Italy	20%	U.K.	49%
GDR	25%	Finland	50%
Hungary	25%	Malta	50%
Poland	25%	Denmark	54%
Luxembourg	36%	Netherlands	55%
Ireland	45%	USSR	55%

GROUP (B)

Albania	Monaco
Austria	Norway
Belgium	Portugal
Czechoslovakia	Romania
France	San Marino
GFR	Spain
Greece	Switzerland
Iceland	Turkey
	Yugoslavia

C-F = Caries-free

studies could be traced referring to the 5/6-yr-old group, and caries-free data were often absent (Table 3). In the NIDR-conducted U.S. National Children's Survey (U.S. DHHS, 1981), the mean dmft score was 2.16, while in 1989, an assessment of Mississippi "head-start" children showed 3-yr- olds to have a mean dft of 1.34, and 6-yr-olds to have 4.32 decayed or filled deciduous teeth (Trubman *et al.*, 1989). In 1986, a study by Irigoyen *et al.* in Mexico, reported a dft value of 6.08 in 6/7-yr-olds, while the similar 6-yr-old index in Guatemala was 5.38 three years later (McNulty & Foss, 1989). Labrador 5-yr-olds have been investigated by Messer (1990), in both 1969 and 1987, during which period the mean dmft value dropped overall from 7.4 to 4.9, with a corresponding "caries-free" rise from 7.4% to 17.4%. However, when these data were broken down by race, it was found the white ("settler") subjects' mean dmft had dropped from a 1969 value of 5.4 to 3.0 in 1987, with the caries-free rising from 14.3% to 30.8% over the same time. Unfortunately, with regards to Inuits, there was only a difference of 0.9 between the 1969 and 1987 mean dmft scores. During the same period, their caries-free prevalence had dropped from 5.3% in 1969, to 0% in 1987.

TABLE 2 *Deciduous Caries Prevalence Data Derived from Studies Undertaken in Various European Countries from 1975-1989.*

		Age	*dmft*	*C-F*	*Reference*
Iceland	1989	4 yr	2.4	46%	Holbrook *et al.* 1989
Ireland	1984	5 yr	1.8 (F)	52%	O'Mullane *et al.* 1986
			3.0 (non-F)	38%	" "
Hungary	1955	5 yr	4.5	24%	Bruszt *et al.* 1977
	1975		6.3	11%	" "
Scotland	1989	5.22	2.80	42%	Dowell & Evans 1989
England	1989	5.48/5.53	0.96/2.46	45-75%	" "
Wales	1989	5.50	2.27	46%	" "
France	1989	6 yr	3.5 (dft)	36%	Cahn *et al.* 1989

F = Fluoridated; Non-F = Non-fluoridated; C-F = Caries-free

From South America, little data exist for the deciduous dentition, although a dmft score of 3.2 has been accorded to Panamanian 1/4-yr-olds (P.A.H.O., 1991), while for Chileans aged 4/5 yr, their mean value was given as 5.5 (P.A.H.O., 1991).

TABLE 3 *Deciduous Caries Data (dmft) from Labrador 5 Yr Olds, Panamanian 1 - 4 Yr Olds, Chilean 4 - 5 Yr Olds and dft Data from Other North American 3 - 7 Yr Olds.*

		Age	*dft*	*C-F*	*Reference*
USA	1979/80	5 yr	2.16	?	U.S.D.H.H.S. 1981
Mississippi	1989	3 yr	1.34	?	Trubman *et al.* 1989
		6 yr	4.32	?	" "
Mexico	1986	6/7 yr	6.08	?	Irigoyen *et al.* 1986
Guatemala	1989	6 yr	5.38	?	McNulty & Fos 1989
			(dmft)		
Labrador					
(all)	1969	5 yr	7.4	7.4%	Messer 1990
	1987		4.9	17.4%	
(white)	1969	5 yr	5.4	14.3%	" "
	1987		3.0	30.8%	
(inuit)	1969	5 yr	8.1	5.3%	" "
	1987		7.2	0.0%	
Panama	1989	1/4 yr	3.2	?	P.A.H.O. 1991
Chile	1984/85	4/5 yr	5.5	?	P.A.H.O. 1991

C-F = Caries-free
P.A.H.O. = Pan-American Health Organisation
U.S. D.H.H.S. = U.S. Department of Health and Human Services

TABLE 4 *Deciduous Caries Data for Children of Various Countries in Asia*

		Age	*dmft*	*C-F*	*Reference*
INDIA					
North	1985	5 yr	U. 1.4/4.4	11-55%	Tewari *et al.*
			R. 1.3/2.8	25-45%	1991
East	1985	5 yr	U. 1.5/2.5	41-46%	" "
			R. 1.1/2.7	42-65%	" "
North East	1985/86	5 yr	5.3/6.4	10-19%	" "
West/					
Central/	1985	5 yr	U. 1.6/1.9	46-49%	" "
South			R. 0.6/1.6	59-75%	" "
BANGLADESH	1976	6 yr	6.4	9%	Tchernykh 1979
	1984	5/6 yr	2.4	38%	" 1985
NEPAL	1987	6 yr	2.0	42%	Ulenius 1987
BURMA	1977	6 yr	3.3	31%	Maung 1977
SRI LANKA	1984	6 yr	4.6	22%	Saparamadu 1984
THAILAND					
Chiang Mai	1987	6 yr	4.1	37%	Davis & Songpaisan
Mae Rim	1987	6 yr	8.4	9%	1987
INDONESIA	1984	6 yr	3.7	30%	Paulin 1984
MONGOLIA	1970	6 yr	1.7	35%	Vinogradova 1970
	1976	6 yr	3.2	23%	Bultcheva 1976
TIBET	1989	6 yr	5.8	6%	Robertson *et al.* 1989
		6 yr	3.7	25%	" "
VIETNAMESE (London)	1990	5 yr	8.3	0%	Todd & Gelbier 1990
CHINA (Beijing)	1989	6 yr	6.3 (d = 5.2)	?	Wright *et al.* 1989
JAPAN	1989	1.5 yr	0.4	89%	Nagatani 1989
		3.5 yr	4.4	33%	" "
			(dft)		
MALAYSIA	1985	3 yr	2.9	?	Meon & Nik Hussein 1985
		6 yr	5.9	?	" " "

U = Urban; R = Rural; C-F = Caries-free

With respect to South East Asia, deciduous data spanning the years 1970-1990 are presented in Table 4. Here, Tewari *et al.* (1991) detailed results of an Indian country-wide survey, undertaken in 1985/86, where data were often divided into urban and rural samples. Subjects from the North East of the sub-continent appear to have the highest prevalence, with dmft scores of 5.3/6.4, and only 10 - 19% caries-free. On the other hand, those from West/Central/South India were 59 - 75% caries-free, with dmft indices of 0.6/1.6, for rural populations, while the equivalent urban figures were 46 - 49% caries-free, and dmft scores of 1.6/1.9.

Information relating to Bangladesh revealed a dmft of 6.4 in 1976, and only 2.4 in 1984, the corresponding caries-free rates having risen from 9% to 48% (Tchernykh, 1979). In Nepal, Ulenius (1987) reported a 6-yr-old mean dmft index of 2.0, with 42% of this age-group being caries-free while, in Burma ten years earlier, Maung (1977) found 31% caries-free with a dmft value of 3.3. Sri Lankan 6-yr-olds (Saparamadu, 1984) were reported as having a 22% caries-free situation and a mean dmft of 4.6. In Thailand, Davis & Songpaisan (1987) found almost twice the caries prevalence in Mae Rim (8.4), as in Chiang Mai (4.1), with equivalent caries-free rates of 9% and 37% respectively. For Indonesia (Paulin, 1984); Mongolia (Bulchera, 1976) and Tibet (Robertson *et al.*, 1989), 6-yr-old dmft scores were not dissimilar, with 30%, 23% and 25% respectively being recorded as caries-free. However, in 1970, Vinogradova noted a Mongolian 6- yr-old dmft of 1.7, with 35% sound, and a separate Tibetan group had a dmft of 5.8 in 1989, with a prevalence of 94% (Robertson *et al.*).

For Vietnamese children (examined in London by Todd & Gelbier, 1990), a dmft of 8.3 (with zero caries-free) was found for 5-yr- olds, and a survey in Beijing (Wright *et al.*, 1989) indicated a Chinese 6-yr-old dmft of 6.3, the "d" component of which amounted to 5.2. A 1989 study in Japan, by Nagatani, had 89% of 1.5-yr- olds caries-free (dmft = 0.4), while only 33% of 3.5-yr-olds were not affected, the mean dmft being 4.4. Finally, a Malaysian survey by Meon & Nik Hussein (1985) reported a dmft of 2.9 in 3- yr-olds, and 5.9 in 6-yr-olds. No caries-free information was provided here, as was the case with the Beijing study.

The deciduous caries situation in several African countries is indicated by the data in Table 5. Of those listed, the Madagascar 6-yr-old dmft of 5.2 was by far the highest, with the values for Ugandan, Kenyan and non-fluoridated Tanzanian youngsters being almost identical. Furthermore, their caries-free proportions were not dissimilar. However, in relation to two Nigerian surveys (Olojugba & Lennon, 1977 & 1983), an apparent rise from a mean dmft value of 0.79 for 5-yr-olds in 1977, to 1.98 in 1983, was indicated. South African information is presented which shows a dmft reduction by one unit (from 2.97 to 1.97) for 5-yr-old whites (Booyens *et al.*, 1991) with a caries-free rise from 40.0% to 50.9%, over an eight year period. However, in Table 6, South African caries-free data for White, Indian, Coloured, Urban Black and Rural Black 3- and 4-yr-olds are shown, along with estimated caries-free information for 5-yr-olds (Cleaton-Jones *et al.*, 1989). Here it is evident that the Indian, Coloured and Urban Black children have the highest caries prevalence (from 97% - 83%), while

TABLE 5 *Deciduous Caries Data for Children Aged from 4-7 Yrs in Various African Countries*

		Age	*dmft*	*C-F*	*Reference*
UGANDA	1988	6 yr	1.52	49%	Tirwomwe *et al.* 1988
KENYA	1988	6 yr	1.55	56%	Manji *et al.* 1991
MADAGASCAR	1988	6 yr	5.2	?	Petersen & Steengaard 1988
TANZANIA	1989	5-7 yr	1.5 (non-F)	49%	Mosha & Robinson 1989
			0.7 (F)	75%	
NIGERIA	1977	5 yr	0.79	?	Olujugba & Lennon 1987
	1983		1.98	?	" "
SOUTH AFRICA	1979	5 yr	2.97	40.0%	Booyens *et al.* 1991
	1987		1.97	50.9%	" "

F = Fluoridated; Non-F = Non-fluoridated; C-F = Caries-free

the Rural Blacks had 68%, and these Whites, only 40% involvement. Unfortunately, no dmft information was given.

In the Middle East, a study by a Zadik (1978), found only 16% of Israeli 5-yr-olds were caries-free, with a dmft score of 4.7 (Table 7). A 6-yr-old survey in 1977 (Ran, 1989), reported 14% to be caries-free, with a dmft of 5.2 and, twelve years later, a similarly aged cohort had 22% caries-free ($p < 0.01$) and a dmft of 4.9. Saudi Arabian data indicated a mean dmft of 1.8 for 4-yr-olds in 1990 (Khan *et al.*) and a dmft of 5.1 for 7-yr-olds. One year later, Al Khateeb *et al.* (1991) found 21% of 6-yr-olds caries-free, with a dmft value of 4.6.

Australasian figures are listed in Table 8, which show that nationally in Australia, dmft scores dropped by approximately 30% for both 4- and 5-yr-olds between 1977 and 1985 (Carr, 1988). However, in 1987, Cooper *et al.* reported Aboriginal 5-yr-olds had a dmft of 4.6 with only 19% caries-free and, in New Zealand, the 1978 dmft of 3.5 was more than 50% less than that reported for 5-yr-olds in 1950, the caries-free percentage having doubled over that period (Brown, 1982).

TABLE 6 *Percentages of 3 and 4 Yr Old Caries-Free South African Children, (Cleaton-Jones et al., 1989) Broken Down by Ethnic Grouping. The 5 Yr Old Data Was Estimated by Extrapolation from the Data Relating to the Younger Cohorts.*

	White	*Indian*	*Coloured*	*Black-U*	*Black-R*
3 yr	70%	41%	27%	48%	63%
4 yr	62%	29%	38%	43%	46%
5 yr (est).	60%	3%	10%	17%	32%

U = Urban; R = Rural

TABLE 7 *Deciduous Caries and Caries-Free Data for Israeli and Saudi Arabian 4 - 7 Yr Olds*

		Age	*dmft*	*C-F*	*Reference*
ISRAEL					
	1978	5 yr	4.7	16%	Zadik 1978
	1977	6 yr	5.2	14%	Ran 1989
				**	
	1985	6 yr	4.9	22%	" "
SAUDI ARABIA					
	1990	4 yr	1.8	?	Khan *et al.* 1990
		7 yr	5.1	?	" "
	1991	6 yr	4.6	21%	Al-Khateeb *et al.* 1990

** P < 0.01 C-F = Caries-free

Lastly, in Table 9, five European data-sets of a more longitudinal nature are presented where, either the same examiners (Hargreaves & Cleaton-Jones, 1990; Frencken *et al.*, 1990) and/or the same population sampling and examination techniques (Stecksen-Blicks *et al.*, 1989; Todd & Dodd, 1985; Downer, 1989; SHBDEP 1987-88; SHBDEP 1989-90) have been employed in not less than three studies, over periods from 1967 - 1989. While, in each case, these reports indicate caries prevalence rates have fallen, only in Umeå, Sweden, has a dmft decrease been demonstrated in the last of these clinical and radiograpic examinations presented from 1967 - 1987. However, even here, the mean dmfs values plateaued at 2.0 in both 1980/81 and 1987 (Stecksen-Blicks *et al.*, 1989).

TABLE 8 *Australian and New Zealand Deciduous Caries Data*

		Age	*dmft*	*C-F*	*Reference*
AUSTRALIA					
National	1977	4 yr	2.86	?	Carr 1988
	1985		1.88	?	" "
	1977	5 yr	2.96	?	" "
	1985		1.85	?	" "
Aboriginal	1987	5 yr	4.6	19%	Cooper *et al.* 1987
NEW ZEALAND					
	1950	5 yr	7.5	14%	Brown 1982
	1978		3.5	28%	" "

C-F = Caries-free

TABLE 9 *Longitudinal Deciduous Caries Prevalence Data from Sweden, the Isle of Lewis Scotland), England & Wales, Scotland, and Friesland (The Netherlands), from 1971 - 1990*

	Age	*dmft*	*C-F*	*Reference*
SWEDEN				
1967	4 yr	5.3	17%	Stecksen-Blicks *et al.* 1989
1971		3.2	33%	" "
1976		2.4	36%	" "
1980/81		2.0	50%	" "
1987		1.6	58%	" "
ISLE OF LEWIS (Scotland)				
1971	5 yr	7.29	?	Hargreaves & Cleaton-Jones 1990
1981		4.57	?	" "
1984		4.95	?	" "
1987		4.43	25%	" "
ENGLAND & WALES				
1973	5 yr	4.0	28%	Todd & Dodd 1985
1983		1.8	51%	" "
1985-86		1.8	54%	Downer 1989
SCOTLAND				
1983	5 yr	3.9	25%	Todd & Dodd 1985
1987		2.7	42%	SHBDEP 1987-88
1989		2.8	41%	SHBDEP 1989-90
FRIESLAND (NL)				
1973	6 yr	14.4	?	Frencken *et al.* 1990
1982		3.8	?	" "
1988		4.0	?	" "

C-F = Caries-free
SHBDEP = Scottish Health Boards' Dental Epidemiological Programme

Discussion

While the vast majority of the data cited has referred to single point prevalence studies, in some instances, similar age groups have been sampled at different times and, although it cannot necessarily be assumed that criteria and/or standards were similar (*vide supra*), from Labrador (Table 3), Bangladeshi (Table 4), Israeli (Table 7), Australian and New Zealand data (Table 8) it could be construed that the deciduous caries rate in these youngsters was perhaps declining. However, inspection of the Hungarian information in Table 2, the Inuit (Table 3), Mongolian (Table 4) and Nigerian data (Table 5), might indicate that the problem could be increasing.

While it is fairly well-established that caries experience in the deciduous dentition is directly related to that of the permanent successors (Mansbridge, 1967/68; Adler, 1969; Poulsen, 1976; Holm, 1978; Grey *et al.*, 1991), it would seem unlikely the reverse relationship would not hold! Hence, given the increase in 12-yr-old caries experience which has been reported for countries such as Burma, the Central African Republic, Indonesia, Spain, Sudan, Western Samoa, Yemen Arab Republic and Zambia (WHO, 1989), the problem in their young children must surely be rising?

Certainly, non-reported observations of 5/6-yr-olds in Middle-East countries would emphasise the extent of the disease which now exists (Stephen, 1991). Furthermore, in such developing communities, an increasing percentage of the population survives the traditional epidemics to which they used to be subjected, e.g. in Oman 45% are less than 15 yrs of age (Brogan, 1989) and in Qatar 50% are reputed to be under 12 years old (Shorter, 1991). Thus, it is likely that ever-more caries-prone youngsters will present such Governments with dental difficulties of enormous proportions, unless suitable primary health care techniques are implemented. However, if the actual disease prevalence is not even being assessed in 5/6-yr-olds, their future well-being must be in doubt.

With respect to data from the more industrialized countries, unfortunately the caries differences reported as a result of such variables as population sampling procedures, examination techniques (*vide supra*), ethnicity (Bedi, 1989; Todd & Gelbier, 1990; Bedi & Elton, 1991), or even urban or rural origins (Cleaton-Jones *et al.*, 1989), must mean that the accuracy and comparability of many data-bases should be questioned. However, it is on the basis of such relatively imprecise information that governmental decisions are made to alter dental health-care systems, or close Dental Schools (Bohannan, 1982), albeit in countries where such actions have already been taken, the situation may be such that almost 50% of 5-yr-olds still do not attend for regular dental monitoring/care (Todd & Dodd, 1985).

Finally, as was demonstrated by the data in Table 9, such repeat deciduous studies as there are, might indicate that the caries-reductions which were occurring may well have ceased. Furthermore, other Scots' clinical and radiographic 5-yr-old figures illustrated their continuing need for a prevention-based philosophy, as a 27% dmft increase, and a 10% caries-free decrease was recorded only five years after water defluoridation in the town of Wick (Stephen *et al.*, 1987). However, only a series of repeat examinations of similarly-aged cohorts at each site detailed, will determine whether or not the pattern which was emerging in Table 9 shall be confirmed. Certainly, until the results of these are known, there are no grounds for complacent celebration that in "The West" even their caries onslaught of past years has now been conquered.

REFERENCES

ADLER, P. (1968): Correlation between dental caries prevalence at different ages. *Caries Res* 2:79-86.

AL-KHATEEB, T.L.; DARWISH, S.K.; BASTAWI, A.E.; and O'MULLANE, D.M. (1990): Dental Caries in Children Residing in Communities in Saudi Arabia With Differing Levels of Natural Fluoride in the Drinking Water. *Community Dental Health* 7:165-171.

BEDI, R. (1989): Ethnic Indicators of Dental Health for Young Asian Schoolchildren Resident in Areas of Multiple Deprivation. *Br Dent J* 166:331-334.

BEDI, R. and ELTON, R.A. (1991): Dental Caries Experience and Oral Cleanliness of Asian and White Caucasian Children Aged 5 and 6 Years Attending Primary Schools in Glasgow and Trafford, U.K. *Community Dental Health* 8:17-23.

BERGMAN, G. and LINDEN, L. (1969): The Action of the Explorer on Incipient Caries. *Svensk Tandlaek Tidskr* 62:629-634.

BOHANNAN, H.M. (1982): The Impact of Decreasing Caries Prevalence: Implications for Dental Education. *J Dent Res* 61 Spec Iss:1369-1377.

BOOYENS, S.J.; VAN ROOY, H.K.; and VAN DER MERWE, C.A. (1991): Caries Experience and Treatment Needs of Five-Year-Old Caucasian Nursery Schoolchildren in Pretoria. *J Dent Assoc South Africa* 46:213-216.

BROGAN, S. (1989): Personal Communication.

BROWN, R.H. (1982): Evidence of Decrease in the Prevalence of Dental Caries in New Zealand. *J Dent Res* 61 (Spec. Iss.):1327-1330.

BRUSZT, P.; BANOCZY, J.; ESZTARY, I.; HADAS, E.; MAROSI, I.; NEMES, J.; and ALBRECHT, M. (1977): Caries Prevalence of Pre Schoolchildren in Baja, Hungary in 1955 and 1975. *Community Dent Oral Epidemiol* 5:136-139.

BULTCHEVA (1976): Assignment Report on Mongolia. Geneva: WHO.

CAHEN, P.M.; TURLOT, J.C.; FRANK, R.M.; and OBRY-MUSSET, A.M. (1989): National Survey of Caries Prevalence in 6 - 15-Year-Old Children in France. *J Dent Res* 68:64-68.

CARR, L.M. (1988): Dental Health of Children in Australia, 1977 - 1985. *Aust Dent J* 33:205-211.

COOPER, M.H.; SCHAMSCHULA, R.G.; and CRAIG, G.G. (1987): Caries Experience of Aboriginal Children in the Orana Region of New South Wales. *Aust Dent J* 32:292-294.

CLEATON-JONES, P.E.; HARGREAVES, J.A.; ROBERTS, G.; WILLIAMS, S.D.L.; and LEIDAL, T.I. (1989): The dmfs and dmft of Young South African Children. *Community Dent Oral Epidemiol* 17:38-40.

DAVIS and SONGPAISAN (1987): International Centre for Oral Health, Chiang Mai, Thailand. (Data from Global Oral Data Bank). ORH/NCD - Geneva: WHO.

DOWELL, T.B. and EVANS, D.J. (1989): The Dental Caries Experience of 5-Year-Old Children in Great Britain. A Survey Coordinated by the British Association for the Study of Community Dentistry in 1987-88. *Community Dental Health* 6:271-279.

DOWNER, M.C. (1989): Time Trends in Dental Decay in Young Children, *Health Trends* 21:7-9.

FDI-WHO (1982): Global Goals for Oral Health in the Year 2000. *Int Dent J* 32:74-77.

FRENCKEN, J.E.; KALSBEEK, H.; and VERRIPS, G.H. (1990): Has the Decline in Dental Caries Been Halted? Changes in Caries Prevalence Amongst 6- and 12-Year-Old Children in Friesland, 1973 - 1988. *Int Dent J* 40:225-230.

GREY, M.M.; MARCHMENT, M.D.; and ANDERSON, R.J. (1991): The Relationship Between Caries Experience in the Deciduous Molars at 5 Years and in First Permanent Molars of the Same Child at 7 Years. *Community Dental Health* 8:3-7.

HARGREAVES, J.A. and CLEATON-JONES, P.E. (1990): Dental Caries Changes in The Scottish Isle of Lewis. *Caries Res* 24:137-141.

HOLBROOK, W.P.; KRISTINSSON, M.J.; GUNNARSDOTTIR, S.; and BRIEM, B. (1989): Caries Prevalence, Streptococcus mutans and Sugar Intake Among 4-Year-Old Urban Children in Iceland. *Community Dent Oral Epidemiol* 17:292-295.

HOLM, A-K. (1978): Dental Health in a Group of Swedish 8-Year-Olds Followed Since the Age of 3. *Community Dent Oral Epidemiol* 6:71-77.

IRIGOYEN, M.; VILLANEUVA, R.;and DE LA TEJA, E. (1986): Dental Caries Status of Young Children in a Suburban Community of Mexico. *Community Dent Oral Epidemiol* 14:306-309.

KHAN, M.U.; ABU-ZEID, H.A.; and FARAJ, H. (1990): Teething Pattern and Prevalence of Dental Caries. *Indian J Pediatr* 57:105-108.

KIDD, E.A.M. (1991): A Critical Evaluation of Caries Diagnostic Methods and Epidemiological Methods. Can We Trust the Available Data? In: Risk Markers for Oral Diseases, Vol 1, Dental Caries, N.W. Johnson, Ed., Cambridge: Cambridge University Press. pp 15-32.

KRUBMAN, A.; SILBERMAN, S.L.; and MEYDRECH, E.F. (1989): Dental Caries Assessment of Mississippi Head Start Children. *J Public Health Dent* 49:167-169.

McHUGH, W.D.; McEWEN, J.; and HITCHIN, A.D. (1964): Dental Disease and Related Factors in 13-Year-Old Children in Dundee. *Br Dent J* 117:246-253.

McNULTY, J.A. and FOS, P.J. (1989): The Study of Caries Prevalence in Children in a Developing Country. *J Dent Child* 56:129-136.

MANJI, F.; FEJERSKOV, O.; BAELUM, V.; LUAN, W-M.; and CHEN, X. (1991): The Epidemiological Features of Dental Caries in African and Chinese Populations: Implications for Risk Assessment. In: Risk Markers for Oral Diseases, Vol. 1, Dental Caries, N.W. Johnson, Ed., Cambridge: Cambridge University Press. pp 62-99.

MANSBRIDGE, J.N. (1967/68): The Relationship Between Caries of the Deciduous and Permanent Teeth in the Same Child. *Edin Hosp Gaz* 8:6-11.

MAUNG, T. (1977): National Pathfinder Survey (Data from Global Oral Data Bank). ORH/NCD - Geneva: WHO.

MEON, R. and NIK HUSSEIN, N.N. (1985): Dental Decay in Pre-School Chinese Children Aged 3 - 6 Years in Petaling Jaya. *Dent J Malays* 8:9-12.

MESSER, J.G. (1990): The Dental Service and Dental Health of Northern Newfoundland and Labrador - A Twenty Year Study. DDS Thesis, University of Glasgow.

MØLLER, I.J. (1990): Caries Status in Europe and Predictions of Future Trends. 2. Introduction. *Caries Res* 24:382-384.

MOSHA, H.J. and ROBISON, V.A. (1989): Caries Experience of the Primary Dentition Among Groups of Tanzanian Urban Pre School Children. *Community Dental Oral Epiemiol* 17:34-37.

MURRAY, J.J. and MAJID, Z.A. (1978): The Prevalence and Progression of Approximal Caries in the Deciduous Dentition in British Children. *Br Dent J* 145:161-164.

NAGATANI, N. (1989): (Dental Health Examination in Infancy and Early Childhood. Part 2. The Results of Dental Survey and Screening of Dental Caries). *Kanagawa Shigaku* 23:537-555.

O'MULLANE, D.; CLARKSON, J.; HOLLAND, T.; O'HICKEY, S.; and WHELTON, H. (1986): Childrens Dental Health in Ireland 1984. The Stationery Office, Dublin.

OLUJUGBA, O.O. and LENNON, M.A. (1987): Dental Caries Experience in 5- and 12-Year-Old Schoolchildren in Ondo State, Nigeria in 1977 and 1983. *Community Dental Health* 4:129-135.

Pan-American Health Organisation (1991): Unpublished data.

PAULIN (1984): Assignment Report on Indonesia (Data from Global Oral Data Bank). ORH/NCD - Geneva: WHO.

PETERSEN, P.E. and STEENGAARD, M. (1988): Dental Caries Among Urban Schoolchildren in Madagascar. *Community Dent Oral Epidemiol* 16:163-166.

POULSEN, S. and HOLM, A-K. (1980): The Relation Between Dental Caries in the Primary and Permanent Dentition of the Same Individual. *J Public Hlth Dent* 40:17-25.

RAN, F. (1989): Declining Dental Caries in Jerusalem Schoolchildren. *Community Dent Oral Epidemiol* 17:217.

RIMMER, P.A. and PITTS, N.B. (1990): Temporary Elective Tooth Separation as a Diagnostic Aid in General Dental Practice. *Br Dent J* 169:87-92.

ROBERTSON, J.A.McL.; READE, P.C.; STEIDLER, M.E.; and SPENCER, A.J. (1989): A Dental Survey of Tibetan Children in Dharamsala. *Community Dent Oral Epidemiol* 17:44-46.

RUGG-GUNN, A.J.; DOWNER, M.C.; and ASHLEY, F.P. (1976): Reliability of Caries Data in Three Clinical Trials. *Community Dent Oral Epidemiol* 4:15-18.

SAPARAMADU, K.D.G. (1984). Assignment Report on Sri Lanka, WHO/ORH/J2/539. Geneva: WHO.

SHBDEP - SCOTTISH HEALTH BOARDS' DENTAL EPIDEMIOLOGICAL PROGRAMME (1987-88) DENTAL HEALTH SERVICES RESEARCH UNIT, UNIVERSITY OF DUNDEE.

SHBDEP - SCOTTISH HEALTH BOARDS' DENTAL EPIDEMIOLOGICAL PROGRAMME (1989-90) DENTAL HEALTH SERVICES RESEARCH UNIT, UNIVERSITY OF DUNDEE.

SHORTER, J. (1991): Personal Communication.

SILVERSTONE, L.M. (1984): Experimental Caries Models and Their Clinical Implications. In: Cariology Today. B. Guggenheim, Ed. Basel: Karger, p 243.

STECKSEN-BLICKS, C. and WAHLIN, Y-B. (1983): Diagnosis of Approximal Caries in the Pre-School Children. *Swed Dent J* 7:179-184.

STECKSEN-BLICKS, C.; HOLM, A-K.; and MAYANAGI, H. (1989): Dental Caries in Swedish 4-Year-Old Children - Changes Between 1967 and 1987. *Swed Dent J* 13:39-44.

STEPHEN, K.W.; McCALL, D.R.; and TULLIS, J.I. (1987): Caries Prevalence in Northern Scotland Before, During and 5 Years After, Water Defluoridation. *Br Dent J* 163:324-326.

STEPHEN, K.W.; CREANOR, S.C.; RUSSELL, J.I.; BURCHELL, C.K.; HUNTINGTON, E.; and DOWNIE, C.F.A. (1988): A 3-Year Oral Health Dose-Response Study of Sodium Monofluorophosphate Dentifrices With and Without Zinc Citrate: Anti-caries Results. *Community Dent Oral Epidemiol* 16:321-325.

STEPHEN, K.W. (1991): Unpublished Data.

TCHERNYKH (1979): Assignment Report on Bangladesh, ORH/J2/531 (Data from Global Oral Data Bank). ORH/NCD - Geneva: WHO.

TCHERNYKH (1985): Assignment Report sea/dh/72/Avril on Bangladesh (Data from Global Oral Data Bank). ORH/NCD - Geveva: WHO.

TEWARI, A.; GOYAL, A.; MEHTA, K.; and GAUBA, K. (1991): Distribution of Dental Caries in India and South-East Asia. In: *Risk Markers for Oral Diseases,* Vol 1, Dental Caries, N.W. Johnson, Ed., Cambridge: Cambridge University Press, pp. 35-42.

TIRWOMWE, F.; EKOKU, Y.; MANJI, F.; BAELUM, V.; and FEJERSKOV, O. (1988): Oral Health in Uganda: Results of a National Survey (1987). Nairobi: Ministry of Health; Uganda/Kenya Medical Research Institute.

TODD, J.E. and WHITWORTH, A. (1974): Adult Dental Health in Scotland 1972. London: HMSO.

TODD, J.E. and DODD, T. (1985): Children's Dental Health in the United Kingdom 1983. London: HMSO.

TODD, R. and GELBIER, S. (1990): Dental Caries Prevalence in Vietnamese Children and Teenagers in Three London Boroughs. *Br Dent J* 168:24-26.

ULENIUS (1987): Assignment Report on Nepal. ORH/J2/569 (Data from Global Oral Data Bank). ORH/NCD - Geneva: WHO.

U.S. Department of Health and Human Services (1981): The Prevalence of Dental Caries in United States Children, 1979 - 1980. N.I.H. Publication No. 82-2245.

VAN DER LAAN-VAN DORP, C.S.E.; EXTERKATE, R.A.M.; and TEN CATE, J.M. (1986): Effect of Probing on Progression of Fissure Caries. *Caries Res* 20:151.

VINOGRADOVA (1970): Assignment Report on Mongolia (Data from Global Oral Data Bank). ORH/NCD - Geneva: WHO.

WORLD HEALTH ORGANISATION (1986): Country Profiles on Oral Health in Europe. ICP/ORH 120 Regional Office for Europe, Copenhagen.

WORLD HEALTH ORGANISATION (1987): Oral Health Surveys. Basic Methods. 3rd Ed. World Health Organisation - Geneva.

WORLD HEALTH ORGANISATION (1989): Dental Caries Levels at 12 Years (Mimeograph of Data from Global Oral Data Bank) - Geneva: WHO.

WRIGHT, F.A.C.; DENGH, H. and SHI, S-T. (1989): The Dental Health Status of 6 and 12 Year Old Beijing Schoolchildren in 1987. *Community Dental Health* 6:121-130.

ZADIK, D. (1978): Epidemiology of Dental Caries in 5-Year-Old Children in Israel. *Community Dent Oral Epidemiol* 6:91-96.

Are We Using Epidemiology Effectively?

D.M. O'MULLANE

Epidemiology is concerned with the patterns with which disease or physiological conditions occur in human populations and with the factors that influence these patterns. The information obtained from epidemiological studies can be used in 3 basic ways (Lilienfield and Lilienfield 1980).

- To elucidate the etiology of a specific disease by combining epidemiologic data with information on for example, demography, genetics, microbiology and biochemistry.
- To evaluate the consistency of epidemiologic data with etiological hypotheses developed either experimentally or clinically.
- To provide the basis for developing and evaluating preventive procedures and public health practices.

Epidemiology has been an important tool in medical science for more than a century. It evolved to be a legitimate science as a result of a public health response to the great epidemics of the 19th century. The cholera epidemic in London in 1848 and the subsequent pinpointing of drinking water as the source of infection by John Snow is often quoted as one of the classical examples of the epidemiologist in the role of the "health detective". Although dental epidemiology has been used for a relatively shorter period, nevertheless its value has been proven on many occasions, none more dramatically than in the development of water fluoridation as an effective public health measure in the control of dental caries (Dean *et al.* 1950). The story of water fluoridation, beginning with the first clinical observations of McKay and Black (1916), is regarded as a classic example of the epidemiological method at work in the advancement of knowledge for the benefit of the community. Epidemiology is an eclectic discipline involving application of the principles of sociology, demography and statistics, hence the development of epidemiology as a science has paralleled developments in these disciplines. For example, statisticians such as Galton, Pearson, Yule and Fisher have had a major influence on the development of epidemiologic science over the last century.

TABLE 1 *Ireland, 1989. Mean number of surfaces present (ns) and mean number of decayed and filled surfaces (coronal caries) (DFS) and mean number of decayed surfaces (DS) by age.*

Age Group	*ns*	*DFS*	*DS*
16 - 24	124.2	7.9	2.2
25 - 34	114.3	15.2	1.9
35 - 44	95.5	17.2	2.4
45 - 54	65.3	13.8	2.8
55 - 64	41.4	8.7	2.1
65 +	31.8	7.3	3.2

There are various classifications of epidemiologic studies but for the purposes of this paper, concerned with the epidemiology of dental caries, the division into descriptive and analytical studies is most useful (Burt el al, 1989). Descriptive studies are mainly used to monitor disease trends in populations allowing comparisons to be made over time and between communities. Using such studies, the recent decline in dental caries prevalence in many developed communities has been established by national and local surveys. Geographic and other variations in caries levels within and between communities have lead to hypotheses being developed regarding the causes of caries which are subsequently tested in analytical studies. There are three basic types of analytical study: cross-sectional (prevalence), cohort (prospective or longitudinal) and case control (retrospective). As pointed out by Burt *et al.* (1989), the pioneering studies in the U.S. investigating the relationship between artificial fluoridation of water supplies and caries prevalence (Arnold *et al.* 1962, Ast and Fitzgerald, 1962, Blayney and Hill, 1967 and Hutton *et al.*, 1956) were a series of sequential cross-sectional studies rather than cohort designs. The Tiel-Culemburg study, conducted by the Utrecht team is the best known example of a longitudinal cohort fluoridation study (Backer Dirks *et al.* 1961). This study has had a major influence on the subsequent development of clinical trials for testing the effectiveness of fluoride and other agents in the control of caries (Rugg-Gunn *et al.*, 1973, De Paola *et al.* 1977, Stephen *et al.* 1988). Retrospective or case control studies have been used less frequently in dental caries research. This is probably due to the questionable precision of independent variables; for example in the study of the relationshop between diet and dental caries, the lengthy time-span between exposure to the independent variable and the appearance of dental caries causes problems in interpreting the association. Recently, retrospective studies have been used in investigations in an area associated with dental caries, namely the relationship between the age at which children began to have fluoride toothpastes applied to their teeth and the level of enamel opacities, including fluoride associated diffuse opacities in permanent teeth (Osujii *et al.*, 1988, Milsom and Mitropoulos 1989).

In attempting to answer the question "Are we using epidemiology effectively". I will firstly interpret it to mean "Are we using the science of epidemiology effectively" and three issues relevant to both descriptive and analytical studies will be considered; sample selection, measurement of caries and analysis of data. I will also address the question "Are we using epidemiological information effectively" in which I will briefly discuss the role of dental epidemiologists in the field of Oral Health Services Research and our contribution to the formulation of public health policy.

It is important to point out that the questions being posed in a study, or the aims and objectives of the study, dictate sample selection, measurement, analysis and the subsequent interpretation adopted. Whilst "data dredging" is a legitimate exercise on completion of a study for the development of further ideas and hypotheses, these should not be confused with the questions which the study was specifically designed to answer in the first place.

Selection of Sample

Since the late 1930's numerous descriptive studies of the level and pattern of dental caries in various communities have been published. The majority of samples selected for study are children and adolescents mainly due to the ease with which representative samples of these groups are contactable in schools. Obtaining a representative sample of adults however is considerably more difficult and expensive. In many instances the response rate amongst adults varies with age, sex and social class depending on the work patterns in the community being studied. In these instances it is important that the population being studied be clearly defined and that any bias in caries estimates due to unequal uptake by strata within the sample are taken into account by appropriate weighting procedures. It is important for epidemiologists to be aware that being chosen as the "lucky one" to have ones teeth examined in a survey is often not fully appreciated by the examinee despite being told that by doing so he/she will be contributing to science in general and particularly to public dental health. Other incentives may be necessary, as in the case of the recent National Survey of Adults Dental Health in Ireland (O'Mullane and Whelton, 1990) when those selected and who subsequently presented for examination, were included in a raffle, the first prize for which was a trip for two to Disneyland in Florida, U.S.A.

Sample selection for analytical caries studies has also been largely confined to children. Cross-sectional prevalence designs of the type reported in the early studies of water fluoridation, in which similar age groups of children but not the same cohorts were examined at 5-year intervals are less acceptable. This is mainly due to the occurence of secular changes in caries levels, which cannot be directly attributable to the agent being tested, and which makes interpretation of the results difficult. Currently the most widely used example of cohort (longitudinal, prospective) caries studies are the 2 or 3-year clinical trials of toothpastes, mouthrinses and other caries preventive agents and strategies (F.D.I. 1982). Panelists recruited to these studies are almost entirely confined to children and teenagers up to the age of 15 or 16 years. These studies have generally two aims, firstly to test an hypothesis regarding the effectiveness of an agent in the prevention of caries and secondly to estimate the extent of any effect. These studies are designed to give the agent every chance to demonstrate an effect. Children and teenagers are selected to participate for three main reasons. Firstly the caries increment over the 2- or 3-year-period of the study is likely to be sufficient to allow the agent to demonstrate an effect if the agent is capable of doing so. (It would be pointless attempting to demonstrate the effectiveness of an agent to alleviate headaches in a group who do not get headaches). Secondly children are easily contactable in school where annual clinical examinations for caries can be organised efficiently. Thirdly, in the case of home use studies, home addresses are easily obtainable, allowing the participants and their parents and siblings to be fully supportive of the study and encourage compliance. In theoretical terms these are explanatory clinical trials (Schwartz *et al.* 1980, O'Mullane, 1976). In the published reports of these studies the significance levels and confidence intervals are generally clearly described, and as is theoretically required (Fisher 1973) the inferences to be drawn relate to an infinite population of similar trials using the same age groups, compliance incentives and all other circumstances of the trial. Whilst this restricted interpretation may be adopted by the scientific world, in practice the results of such studies are used much more generally to promote use of the agent or strategy in the population as a whole. It is likely that such interpretations are largely correct in that if children and teenagers benefit, under artificial conditions, there is a strong possibility that adults also will benefit, though perhaps with some attenuation since the agent or strategy is used under real life conditions. Nevertheless it is this reviewer's opinion that in future, some pragmatic or field studies of dentifrices and mouthrinses and other agents should be conducted amongst both children and adults. Experience gained in studies aimed at preventing root caries may be helpful in designing adult studies. Recent work in the Oral Health Services Research Unit in University College Cork indicate that adults may be more willing to cooperate in such studies than was heretofore believed. It is worth considering that the caries increment in adults aged 16 to 34 may be of sufficient magnitude over a 4 - 5 year period to demonstrate a worthwhile effect with reasonable numbers. In the recent survey of Irish Adults (Table 1) (O'Mullane and Whelton, 1990) the mean DFS at age 16 - 24 was 7.9 and at a 25 - 34 was 15.2 with few teeth lost. Figures obtained in the U.S. and U.K. are similar (U.S. Public Health Service 1987; Downer 1991). Admittedly, caution is required when using the data to estimate incidence due to secular changes in caries levels which are likely to occur in future years. Nevertheless more and more teenagers are entering there 20s with an increasing number of smooth and interproximal tooth surfaces at risk to new caries attack. In many communities the increasing use of sealants will render pit and fissure surfaces of little value in caries studies, hence other surfaces will assume more importance.

Guidelines prepared by various regulatory and other bodies rightly play a major role in the design of caries clinical trials. The decline in the prevalence of caries and the need to use positive controls have resulted in an enormous increase in the size of samples required to meet these guidelines (Council on Dental Therepeutics 1988). The resultant increase in the cost and complexity of these trials could lead to a reduction in the number of such trials being conducted and the application of new knowledge for the benefit of the public. It is this reviewer's opinion that this issue should be addressed immediately with a view to finding ways of satisfying the requirements of regulatory agencies and at the same time maintaining sample sizes at a sensible level.

Measurement of Caries

The most widely used index of caries is the DMF which has undergone considerable refinements since it was first described by Klein and Palmer (1937). Differences in opinion amongst epidemiologists still exist notably between researchers in the U.S. who use a sharp probe to record sticky fissures in contrast to the European system where a blunt probe is only advocated to confirm diagnosis of a carious lesion if required and to clean tooth surfaces. Whether using teeth (dmft/DMFT) or surfaces (dmfs/DMFS) as the unit of measurement within the mouth, caries is usually graded from "caries incipiens", (Backer Dirks, 1951) or the early carious lesion including white spots, to a small cavity, to gross cavitation, a filling or extraction. When reporting on the study however, all scores from a particular grade upwards (e.g. cavitation) are aggregated giving a tooth or surface count for each subject as a measure of caries experience. Whilst this method of aggregating scores may have been reasonable when caries levels were higher, it would seem to be an inefficient method of using information on the progress of caries so diligently collected. In longitudinal cohort studies (e.g. clinical trials) discriminatory power is likely to be enhanced if progress of lesions from one grade to the other (including reversals) were included in the analysis (Backer Dirks, 1966). The pattern of change in lesions from one grade to the next is also likely to be helpful in explaining the method of action of an agent. It is worth noting that caries epidemiologists have made an important contribution to our understanding of the development of the carious lesion. In longitudinal studies prior to 1970 when the early caries lesion was included in the method of diagnosing caries, it was found that white spot lesions changed in one of three ways between annual examinations; the surface enamel either broke down and a cavity was formed, it remained unchanged or it disappeared (reversed). These observations helped cariologists to understand how the carious process is in fact a balance between demineralisation and remineralization. More recent studies have tended not to include the early carious lesion as an outcome variable. This is likely to be due in part to the resulting increase in the length of the clinical examination and the questionable reproducibity of examiners in the diagnosis of early carious lesions. Perhaps this decision should be reconsidered. Admittedly the measurement used is determined by the aims of the study. Nevertheless the value of including the early carious lesion was illustrated recently in the paper by Groeneveld (1990) who, on re-analysing the Tiel-Culemborg data was in a position to show that fluoridation was mainly effective through preventing progress of the early enamel lesion to dentine.

For safety and ethical reasons, caries epidemiologists do not use radiographs to quantify approximal caries to the same extent as in the 1960s and 1970s. The use of Fibre Optic Transillumination has to some extent overcome this difficulty (Mitropoulos, 1985). However a more complete estimate of caries incidence is obtained if radiographs are used. Hence, where local circumstances permit, it is desirable in longitudinal cohort studies, to take radiographs at the baseline and final examinations.

Analysis and Reporting Caries Data

Advances in computer technology has had a major influence in dental epidemiology in recent years. Direct data entry using lap-top computers in the field is now being employed on a regular basis reducing the time-span between data collection and the availability of accurate results. More importantly computerization allows the researcher to make use of standard complex statistical analyses which are necessary to make full use of the many independent variables associated with caries incidence. Various saliva and plaque parameters can now be included in regression and discriminant analyses with ease for example. Despite these advances this reviewer is not convinced that the standard of reporting basic epidemiological data in the dental literature has improved. For example in both descriptive and analytical studies when reporting mean DMFT / DMFS levels together with standard deviations for different sub-groups, the corresponding sample size for these sub-groups is often omitted even though the overall numbers included in the study may be reported. Also whilst the standard deviations give some indication of the variations in caries scores, they are not sufficient to inform the reader of the skewed nature of many caries data sets. Editors should insist that frequency distributions are presented either graphically or in tabular form which will of course also include the proportion free of caries. Lack of such information could hide important distribution patterns such as the bimodal distribution for DMFT found in 12-year-old children in Ireland in 1984 (Fig. 1) (O'Mullane *et al.*, 1986). Another common omission in published reports of studies of preventive agents is a description of the power of the test used; often no information is provided on α and β levels.

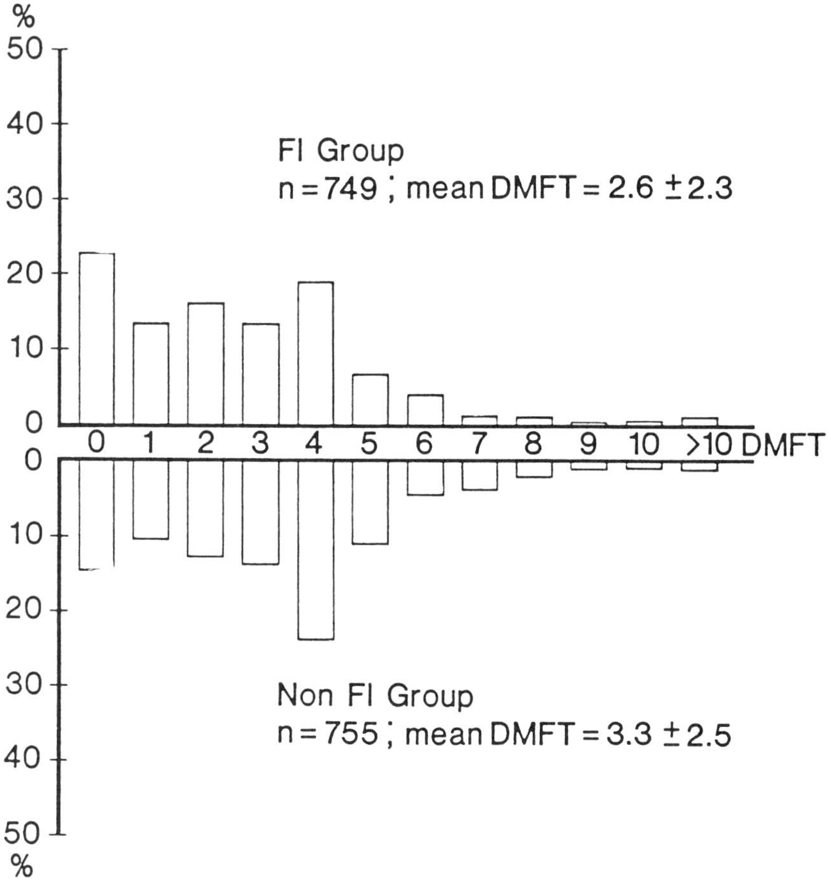

FIGURE 1 Ireland, 1984. 12-year-old children, percentage frequency distribution of DMFT scores.

Oral Health Services Research

In the past decade more and more caries epidemiologists have become involved in oral health services research which is concerned with study of the application of new knowledge for the benefit of the community. The information which we collect as epidemiologists is of value to those who make public health policy. More and more health agencies are seeking answers to questions on the effectiveness and cost of competing treatment and preventive strategies (Lennon *et al.* 1984). Whilst this is a welcome development there are some pitfalls which we as dental researchers should be aware of. As an example of these, one can mention the studies reported over the last ten years or so which have documented a decline in the prevalence of dental caries in many developed communities. These studies have been reported with a justifiable pride and perhaps some overstatement by dental epidemiologists. Unfortunately however we did not always comment or get fully involved in the policy implications of these findings, but others did. As a result decisions were taken regarding funding for caries research and for dental services which could not be justified if the changes in the prevalence and pattern of caries were more objectively viewed with public health policy implications in mind. For example, a careful assessment of the data for Ireland in 1984 shows that despite the fact that caries had declined by over 50% in the previous 20 years (O'Mullane *et al.*, 1986), 34% of 12-year-old lifetime residents of fluoridated communities continue to have 4 or more carious teeth (Fig.1), a sizeable public health problem. It is essential that epidemiologists in the field of health services research give equal emphasis to the policy implications of their results as to the results themselves. Over the years the results of many major epidemiologic caries studies, including national surveys, have been published with little or no comments or recommendations to guide policy makers on how to interpret the results and help decide on appropriate public health action.

In conclusion, whilst advances in dental epidemiology have to a large extent kept pace with general medical epidemiology, sample selection, measurement of caries and analyis and reporting of results in caries studies are aspects in which epidemiologic science is not being used effectively. The entry of caries epidemiologists into the field of oral health services research is a relatively new one which will demand a new approach to study design, analysis of data and interpretation of results. Study reports will require clear statements of the implications of results for public dental health.

REFERENCES

ARNOLD, F.A. Jr.; LIKINS, R.C.; RUSSELL, A.L.; and SCOTT, D.B. (1962): Fifteenth year of the Grand Rapids Fluoridation Study, *J.A.D.A.* 65:780-785.

AST D.B.; and FITZGERALD, B. (1962): Effectiveness of Water Fluoridation, *J.A.D.A.* 65:581-588.

BACKER DIRKS, O.; VAN AMERONGEN, J.; and WINKLER, K.C. (1951): A Reproducible Method for Caries Evaluation, *J Dent Res* 30:346-359.

BACKER DIRKS, O. (1966): Posteruptive changes in Dental Enamel, *J Dent Res* 45: Supplement to No.3, 503-511.

BACKER DIRKS, O.; HOUWINK, B.; and KWANT, G.W. (1961): The Results of 6½ years of Artificial Fluoridation of Drinking Water in the Netherlands; the Tiel-Culerborg Experiment, *Arch Oral Biol* 5:284-300.

BLAYNEY, J.R.; and HILL, I.M. (1967): Fluorine and Dental Caries, *J.A.D.A.* 74 (Sp. Iss.):233-302.

BURT B.A.; ALBINO, J.E.; CARLOS, J.P.; COHEN, L.K.; DUBNER, R.; GERSHEN, J.A.; and GREENE, J.C. (1989): Advances in the Epidemiological Study of Oral-Facial Diseases, *Advances in Dental Research* 3:30-41.

Council on Dental Therepeatics, American Dental Association (1988): Report on Workshop Aimed at Defining Guidelines For Caries Clinical Trials: Superiority and Equivalency Claims for Anti-caries Dentifrices, *J.A.D.A.* 117:663-665.

DEAN, H.I.; ARNOLD, F.A. Jr. and KNUTSON, J.W. (1950): Studies on Mass Control of Dental Caries Through Fluoridation of Public Water Supply, *Public Health Rep.* 65, 1403-1408.

DE PAOLA, P.F.; SOPARKAR, P.; FOLEY, S.; BOOKSTEIN, F.; and BAKHUS, Y. (1977): Effects of High Concentrations Arsonium and Sodium Fluoride Rinses in Dental Caries in Schoolchildren, *Comm Dent Oral Epidemiol* 5:7-14.

DOWNER, M.C. (1991): The Improving Dental Health of United Kingdom Adults and Prospects for the Future, *Br Dent J* 170:154-158.

Fédération Dentaire Internationale (F.D.I.) (1982): Principal Requirements for Controlled Clinical Trials of Caries Preventive Agents and Procedures, *Int Dent J* 32:292-310.

FISHER, R.A. (1973): *Statistical Methods and Scientific Inference:* Hafner Press: New York.

GROENEVELD, A.; VAN ECK, A.A.M.J.; and BACKER DIRKS, O. (1990): Fluoride in Caries Prevention; is the Effect pre- or posteruptive? *J Dent Res* 69 (Sp. Iss.): 751-755.

HUTTON, W.L.; LINESOTT, B.W.; and WILLIAMS, D.B. (1956): Final Report of Local Studies on Water Fluoridation in Brantford, *Canadian Journal Public Health* 47:89-92.

KLEIN, H.; and PALMER, C.E. (1937): Dental Caries in American Indian Children Public Health Bulletin No.239 U.S. Government Printing Office.

LENNON, M.A.; O'MULLANE, D.M.; and TAYLOR, G.O. (1984): A Pragmatic Clinical Trial of Fissure Sealants in a Community Dental Service Programme for 6 - 10 year-old children, *Comm Dent Health* 1:101-109.

LILIENFIELD, A.M.; and LILIENFIELD, D.E. (1980): *Foundations of Epidemiology,* Oxford University Press: New York.

MCKAY, F.S.; and BLACK, G.V. (1916): An Investigation of Mottled Enamel, *Dental Cosmos* 58:477-484.

MILSOM, K.; and MITROPOULOS, C.M. (1990): Enamel Defects in 8-year-old children in Fluoridated and Non-Fluoridated Parts of Cheshire, *Caries Res.* 24:286-289.

MITROPOULOS, C.M. (1985): A comparison of Fibre-optic Transillumination with Bitewing Radiographs, *Br Dent J* 159:21-23.

O'MULLANE, D.M. (1976): Efficiency in Clinical Trials of Caries Preventive Agents and Methods, *Comm Dent Oral Epidemiol* 4:190-194.

O'MULLANE, D.M.; CLARKSON, J.; HOLLAND, T.; O'HICKEY, S.; and WHELTON, H. (1986): Childrens Dental Health in Ireland 1984, Stationery Office, Dublin.

O'MULLANE, D.M.; and WHELTON, H. (1990): National Survey of Adults Dental Health in Ireland 1989/90: Preliminary Report, University College, Cork, Ireland.

OSUJII, O.O.; LEAKE, J.L.; CHIPMAN, M.L.; NIKIFOROUK, G.; LOCKER, D.; and LEVINE, N. (1988): Risk factors for Fluorosis in a Fluoridated Community, *J Dent Res* 67:1488-1492.

RUGG-GUNN, A.J.; HOLLOWAY, P.J.; and DAVIES, T.G.H. (1973): Caries Prevention by Daily Fluoride Mouthrinsing, *Br Dent J* 135:353-360.

SCHWARTZ, D.; FLAMONT, R.; and LELLOUCH, J. (1980): *Clinical Trials:* Translated by M.J.M. Healy, Academic Press, London.

STEPHEN, K.W.; CREANOR, S.L.; RUSSELL, J.I.; BURCHELL, C.K.; HUNTINGTON, E.; DOWNIE, C.F.A. (1988): A 3-year Oral Health Dose - Response Study of Sodium Monofluorophosphate Dentifrices with and without Zine Citrate: Anti-Caries Results, *Comm Dent Oral Epidemiol* 16:321-325.

U.S. Public Health Service (1987): Oral Health of United States Adults, N.I.H. Publication No. 87-2868.

SALIVA

Molecular Biological Approaches to Caries: Role of Saliva

LAWRENCE A. TABAK

It has long been appreciated that catastrophic loss of salivary function leads to an increased risk of dental caries (Fox *et al.*, 1985). Indeed, it is largely through the examination of patients lacking adequate salivary function that we have gained insight into the many roles that saliva must play in protecting against potential insults to the oral environment (Table 1). Evidence which supports the various functional roles proposed for saliva will be summarized in the papers which follow.

It is much less clear, however, if: (1) caries experience can be correlated with the expression of specific-salivary components, and (2) caries experience can be correlated with "sub-catastrophic" forms of salivary hypofunction.

In this paper we will briefly review the evidence which supports the idea that subtle forms of salivary hypofunction may lead to an increased risk of dental caries. Moreover, we will propose experiments which can be used to test this hypothesis directly using methods recently described. Finally, we will suggest several approaches where molecular biological approaches might be used to aid individuals who are suffering from salivary hypofunction.

Salivary Proteins Are Highly Polymorphic

Most of the acinar products of salivary glands have been shown to be members of protein families, and many of these display genetic polymorphisms (Azen, 1989; Karn, 1991; Tabak, 1991). The best studied of these families is the proline-rich proteins (PRPs).

PRPs are encoded by six genes located on chromosome 12 (p 13.2) over a stretch of approximately 700 kbp of DNA (Kim *et al.*, 1990). The six loci encode families of acidic, basic, and glycosylated PRPs which are subjected to an almost bewildering array of co- and post-translational modifications (Table 2). Attempts have been made to correlate caries experience with the PRP

TABLE 1 *Proposed Functions of Salivary Secretions*

1. Physico-mechanical flushing of the oral cavity
2. Tissue Coating: lubrication, hydration and formation of a permeability barrier
3. Modulation of the oral flora
4. Regulation of calcium/phosphate equilibrium
5. Antacid and neutralization of deleterious materials
6. Digestion: formation of a food bolus and deglutition

phenotype, but unfortunately, conflicting results have been reported (Table 3). Additionally, several preliminary studies have reported tantalizing findings. Johnson *et al.* (1991) indicated that there is a lower concentration of basic PRPs in caries-active subjects. Earlier work suggested a correlation of histatin levels in caries resistance (Iacono *et al.*, 1983). Collectively, these findings fit well with the view that dental caries can be considered a disease in which inadequate base production occurs (i.e. failure of the host to produce a needed [salivary] substrate which is subsequently metabolized to yield base) as opposed to the more prevailing view of the disease being related to acid production (for further discussion see paper by Marquis).

Detailed analysis of other salivary genes is rapidly emerging. Given these tools, molecular scanning methods (Rossiter and Caskey, 1990) can be applied to genotype large numbers of relevant patient populations. This should spring forth a new generation of epidemiological studies which will allow analysis of a wider range of independent variables.

TABLE 2 *Proline-rich Proteins**

Locus	*Allele*	*Proteins*
PRH1	$PRH1^1$	Db fast, Db slow
	$PRH1^2$	Pa1
	$PRH1^4$	PLF fast, PLF slow
PRH2	$PRH2^1$	PRP1, PRP3
	$PRH2^2$	PRP2, PRP4
	$PRH2^3$	$PRP1^1$, $PRP3^1$
PRB1	$PRB1^M$	Pe, (IIB-2)
	PRB^S	Pe, PmF (IB-9), PmS (IB-6)
PRB2	$PRB2^L$	Ps, PmS (IB-6)
PRB3	$PRB3^L$	GI^1 (PRG)
	$PRB3^S$	GI^3
	$PRB3S^{cys}$	GI^8
PRB4	$PRB4^L$	CON1, CON2

*adapted from Azen *et al.* (1990) and Lyons *et al.* (1988).

TABLE 3 *Association of PRP and Dental Caries*

Phenotype	*Population*	*Observation*
1. Db	Adult (N=92), black	Db^+ subjects had significantly higher DMFS than Db^- subjects
2. Pr, Pa, Db, Ps, Pm, Pb	Adults (46CF; 47CA)	Distributions of Pr, Pa, Db, Ps, Pm, and Pb were similar in CF and CA subjects
3. Pr, Pa, Pb	Adults (28CR; 26CA)	Familial nature of CR observed, but no differences in phenotype distribution
4. Pa	Adults	Pa^- phenotype more prevalent (68%) in caries for individuals than the Pa^+ phenotype (52%)
5. Db, Ps, PIF, PmF, Pa, Pr	Children (N = 306, 100 black)	Significant increase in DMFS of permanent teeth with age in children with Pa^+ and Pr22

1. Friedman *et al.*, (1980).
2. Anderson *et al.*, (1982).
3. Anderson and Mandel, (1982).
4. Azen, unpublished, as cited in Yu *et al.*, (1986).
5. Yu *et al.*, (1986).

Historically, medical science has capitalized on "complex surveillance systems" that exist for humans (White and Caskey, 1988). Indeed, many more traits have been mapped in humans than in any other species. Additionally, powerful genetic analysis can be used to look at family units or twins (Potter, 1990). However, one of the points expressed by both Drs. Mandel and O'Mullane at this conference is not to fall slave to the "tyranny of the mean." Just as there is considerable polymorphism in salivary protein expression, so too is there enormous variation in the level of expression (for example, see Rudney, 1989; and Denny *et al.*, 1991). A recent study by Shipp *et al.* (1991) points out how dramatically different salivary output is among healthy individuals. Each individual must serve as their own control, a fact that is rarely considered in design of caries studies.

Superimposed over this normal variation and function is the wide range of conditions that may compromise salivary output. Each of these conditions is different; that is, all salivary hypofunction is not the same (Fox *et al.*, 1985). For example, it is well documented that a leading cause of salivary hypofunction is the use of pharmaceuticals which have a secondary untoward effect called "dry mouth." These agents not only alter salivary output, but can also change salivary composition.

Independently, Johnson and Cortez (1988) and Watson *et al.* (1990) have observed that in rodents, chronic exposure to β-blockers such as propranolol leads to a dramatic decrease in two proline-rich proteins termed peak A and SP-3. Further, chronic propranolol treatment leads to an increased level of dental caries (Watson *et al.*, 1990). It remains to be determined whether the loss of these basic PRPs has anything to do with the increased prevalence of disease.

Transgenic Animal Models Could Provide Direct Evidence of Salivary Function

Direct proof for the role of specific salivary components in protection of dental caries could be obtained using recent technological advances which permit design of transgenic animals (Jaenisch, 1988; Hanahan, 1989). I propose that this technology be exploited to prove directly cause and effect relationships. For example, specific cell types could be genetically ablated by targeting (via cell-specific promoters) the expression of a toxin which would kill off selected populations of cells. This approach has been successfully used to delete terminally differentiated fiber cells of the eye (Breitman, 1987; Breitman, 1990). Similar studies are feasible now for the salivary glands. For example, work from our lab has identified a promoter which drives expression of a family of PRP-related proteins termed glutamine/glutamic acid-rich proteins in the acinar cell of the submandibular gland (Cooper and Tabak, 1991). By using this promoter to direct expression of a toxin, one could selectively destroy the acinar cells of the submandibular gland without perturbing other cell lineages. The next generation of studies could involve the classical "knockout" approach which has been used so successfully in bacteria and lower eukaryotes such as *Saccharomyces cerevisiae* (Lumsden and Wilkinson, 1990). Null alleles can be created to specifically eliminate expression of a gene product (Capecchi, 1989). In this manner, the question can be asked whether absence of a specific constituent has any influence on subsequent disease. Ultimately, subtle mutations in specific macromolecules of interest could be introduced to ascertain *in vivo* which domains of proteins are required for activity. Recently, two groups have independently reported the successful creation of transgenic rats (Mullins *et al.*, 1990; Hammer *et al.*, 1990). Given the wide use of rats as a model system to study dental caries, creation of salivary defective rats offers great promise for the future.

Approaches to the Treatment of Salivary Hypofunction

In general, the strategy used to treat salivary hypofunction is dependent upon whether or not residual, functional parenchymal tissue remains. In the former case, the presence of such functional remaining tissue can be exploited through the use of several intrinsic therapies. For example, dietary bulk can be used to enhance the masticatory stimulation and thereby influence salivary flow (see Johnson, this volume). Similarly, selective use of secretagogues has been shown to be effective (Fox *et al.*, 1986). This approach has its origins in the many animal studies conducted by physiologists in the fifties and sixties and studies in humans in the mid-sixties by Dawes (1966) and Mandel (1968). It was clearly shown by each of these investigators that pilocarpine delivered by different methods increases salivary flow from both the human parotid and submandibular/sublingual glands. In persons with the subjective complaint of xerostomia, pilocarpine treatment yields a transient increase in flow over that observed with the placebo alone. More recently, Wolff *et al.* (1990) have used pilocarpine in an attempt to preserve parotid function during irradiation for treatment of head and neck carcinoma. In a pilot study they have shown that injection of pilocarpine one hour prior to irradiation is helpful in maintaining parotid function (1990). Interestingly, the submandibular/sublingual gland is not affected. In a preliminary study, O'Connell and Bowen have shown that pilocarpine can be used as a means to protect against caries in partially desalivated rats (see this volume). Exposure to β-adrenergic agonists such as isoproterenol leads to hypertrophy and hyperplasia of rodent parotid and submandibular glands (Schneyer, 1969). To date, the underlying mechanism of these cellular changes have remained elusive, although several proto-oncogenes have been shown to be induced (Kousvelari *et al.*, 1990). The details of the biochemical regulation of the cell cycle are rapidly emerging (Freeman and Donoghue, 1991), and it is conceivable that this information could be used to facilitate the "regeneration" of salivary gland parenchyma in the future.

In cases where there is no remaining functional parenchymal tissue, extrinsic approaches must be used to treat the salivary hypofunction. In its simplest form this involves replacement of saliva with functional substitutes (a subject reviewed earlier, Levine *et al.*, 1987). More recently, workers have found some success in the creation of artificial organs in which cells are entrapped into "organoid"-like structures (Thompson *et al.*, 1989), which can then secrete needed macromolecules (e.g., Sullivan *et al.*, 1991). While the culture of salivary epithelium has proven difficult, perhaps immortalized cells (He *et al.*, 1990) or heterologous cells engineered to produce recombinant salivary molecules could be used to provide needed salivary function.

REFERENCES

ANDERSON, L.C.; LAMBERTS, B.L.; and BRUTON, W.F. (1982): Salivary Protein Polymorphisms in Caries-free and Caries-active Adults, *J Dent Res* 61:393-396.

ANDERSON, L.C. and MANDEL, I.D. (1982): Salivary Protein Polymorphisms in Caries-resistant Adults, *J Dent Res* 61:1167-1168.

AZEN, E.A. (1989): Genetic Protein Polymorphisms of Human Saliva. In: *Human Saliva: Clinical Chemistry and Microbiology,* Vol. 1, J. Tenovuo, Ed., Boca Raton: CRC Press, Inc., pp. 161-195.

AZEN, E.A.; MINAGUCHI, K.; and KIM, H.-S. (1990): Alleles at the *PRB*3 Locus Coding for a Disulfide-bonded Human Salivary Proline-rich Glycoprotein (Gl 8) and a Null in an Ashkenazi Jew, *Am J Hum Genet* 47:686-697.

BREITMAN, M.L.; CLAPOFF, S.; ROSSANT, J.; TSUI, L.-C.; GLODE, L.M.; MAXWELL, I.H.; and BERNSTEIN, A. (1987): Genetic Ablation: Targeted Expression of a Toxin Gene Causes Microphthalmia in Transgenic Mice, *Science* 238:1563-1565.

BREITMAN, M.L.; ROMBOLA, H.; MAXWELL, I.H.; KLINTWORTH, G.K.; and BERNSTEIN, A. (1990): Genetic Ablation in Transgenic Mice with an Attenuated Diphtheria Toxin A Gene, *Mol and Cell Biol* 10:474-479.

CAPECCHI, M.R. (1989): The New Mouse Genetics: Altering the Genome by Gene Targeting, *Trends Genet* 5:70-76.

COOPER, L.F. and TABAK, L.A. (1991): Characterization of the Gene Encoding the Salivary Gln/Glu-rich C-terminal Variant A Protein, *GENE,* 106:261-266

DAWES, C. (1966): The Composition of Human Saliva Secreted in Response to a Gustatory Stimulus and to Pilocarpine, *J Physiol* 183:360-368.

DENNY, P.C.; DENNY, P.A.; KLAUSER, D.K.; HONG, S.H.; NAVAZESH, M.; and TABAK, L.A. (1991): Age-Related Changes in Mucins from Human Whole Mouth Saliva, *J Dent Res,* 70:1320-1327.

FOX, P.C.; VAN DER VEN, P.F.; BAUM, B.J.; and MANDEL, I.D. (1986): Pilocarpine for the Treatment of Xerostomia Associated with Salivary Gland Dysfunction, *Oral Surg Oral Med Oral Pathol* 61:243-245.

FOX, P.C.; VAN DER VEN, P.F.; SONIES, B.C.; WEIFFENBACH, J.M.; and BAUM, B.J. (1985): Xerostomia: Evaluation of a Symptom with Increasing Significance, *J Am Dent Assoc* 110:519-525.

FREEMAN, R.S. AND DONOGHUE, D.J. (1991): Protein Kinases and Protooncogenes: Biochemical Regulators of the Eukaryotic Cell Cycle, *Biochemistry* 30:2293-2302.

FRIEDMAN R.D.; AZEN, E.A.; YU, P.L.; GREEN, P.A.; KARN, R.C.; and MERRITT, A.D. (1980): Heritable Salivary Proteins and Dental Disease, *Hum Hered* 30:372-375.

HAMMER, R.E.; MAIKA, S.D.; RICHARDSON, J.A.; TANG, J.-P.; and TAUROG, J.D. (1990): Spontaneous Inflammatory Disease in Transgenic Rats Expressing HLA-B27 and Human β_2m: An Animal Model of HLA-B27-Associated Human Disorders, *Cell* 63:1099-1112.

HANAHAN, D. (1989): Transgenic Mice as Probes into Complex Systems, *Science* 246:1265-1275.

HE, X.; FRANK, D.P.; and TABAK, L.A. (1990): Establishment and Characterization of 12S E1A Immortalized Rat Submandibular Gland Epithelial Cells, *Biochem Biophys Res Commun* 170:336-343.

IACONO, V.J.; MACKAY, B.J.; DENEPITIYA, L.; POLLOCK, J.J.; PETROPOULOU, K.; and MANDEL, I.D. (1983): Salivary Histidine-rich Polypeptide Profiles of Caries-resistant and -susceptible Adults, AADR *Abst* 62: No. 516.

JAENISCH, R. (1988): Transgenic Animals, *Science* 240:1468-1474.

JOHNSON, D.A. AND CORTEZ, J.E. (1988): Chronic Treatment with Beta Adrenergic Agonists and Antagonists Alters the Composition of Proteins in Rat Parotid Saliva, *J Dent Res* 67:1103-1108.

JOHNSON, D.A.; DODDS, M.W.J.; and ROMEU, J. (1991): Parotid Saliva Protein Profiles in Caries-active Versus Caries-free Subjects, IADR *Abst* 70: No. 314.

KARN, R.C. (1991): Genetic Control of Mammalian Salivary Proteins. In: *Aspects of Oral Molecular Biology,* Vol. 8, D.B. Ferguson, Ed., Basel: Karger, pp.117-140.

KIM, H.-S.; SMITHIES, O.; and MAEDA, N. (1990): A Physical Map of the Human Salivary Proline-Rich Protein Gene Cluster Covers over 700 kbp of DNA, *Genomics* 6:260-267.

KOUSVELARI, E.; YEH, C.-K.; MERTZ, P.M.; and CHINCHETRU, M. (1990): Regulation of Proto-oncogenes and Salivary Gland Cell Proliferation, *Adv Dent Res* 4:61-68.

LUMSDEN, A. and WILKINSON, D. (1990): The Promise of Gene Ablation, *Nature* 347:335-336.

LYONS, K.M.; AZEN, E.A.; GOODMAN, P.A.; and SMITHIES, O. (1988): Many Protein Products from a Few Loci: Assignment of Human Salivary Proline-Rich Proteins to Specific Loci, *Genetics* 120:255-265.

MANDEL, I.D.; KATZ, R.; ZENGO, A.; KUTSCHER, A.H.; GREENBERG, R.A.; KATZ, S.; SCHARF, R.; and PINTOFF, A. (1968): The Effect of Pharmacologic Agents on Salivary Secretion and Composition in Man I. Pilocarpine, Atropine and Anticholinesterases, *J Oral Therapeut and Pharm* 4:192-199.

MULLINS, J.J.; PETERS, J.; and GANTEN, D. (1990): Fulminant Hypertension in Transgenic Rats Harbouring the Mouse *Ren-2* Gene, *Nature* 344:541-544.

POTTER, R.H. (1990): Twin Half-sibs: A Research Design for Genetic Epidemiology of Common Dental Disorders, *J Dent Res* 69:1527-1530.

ROSSITER, B.J.F. and CASKEY, C.T. (1990): Molecular Scanning Methods of Mutation Detection, *J Biol Chem* 265:12753-12756.

RUDNEY, J.D. (1989): Relationships Between Human Parotid Saliva Lysozyme Lactoferrin, Salivary Peroxidase and Secretory Immunoglobulin A in a Large Sample Population, *Arch oral Biol* 34:499-506.

SCHNEYER, C.A. (1969): β-Adrenergic Effects by Autonomic Agents on Miosis and Hypertrophy in Rat Parotid, *Proc Soc Exp Biol Med* 131:71-75.

SHIP, J.A.; FOX, P.C.; and BAUM, B.J. (1991): How Much Saliva is Enough? 'Normal' Function Defined, *J Am Dent Assoc* 122:63-69.

SULLIVAN, S.J.; MAKI, T.; BORLAND, K.M.; MAHONEY, M.D.; SOLOMON, B.A.; MULLER, T.E.; MONACO, A.P.; and CHICK, W.L. (1991): Biohybrid Artificial Pancreas: Long-Term Implantation Studies in Diabetic, Pancreatectomized Dogs, *Science* 252:718-721.

TABAK, L.A. (1990): Structure and Function of Human Salivary Mucins, *Crit Rev Oral Biol Med* 1:229-234.

THOMPSON, J.A.; HAUDENSCHILD, C.C.; ANDERSON, K.D.; DIPIETRO, J.M.; ANDERSON, W.F.; and MACIAG, T. (1989): Heparin-binding Growth Factor 1 Induces the Formation of Organoid Neovascular Structures *In Vivo, Proc Natl Acad Sci* 86:7928-7932.

WATSON, G.E.; PEARSON, S.K.; FALANY, J.L.; TABAK, L.A.; and BOWEN, W.H. (1990): The Effect of Chronic Propranolol Treatment on Salivary Composition and Caries in the Rat, *Arch oral Biol* 35:435-441.

WHITE, R. AND CASKEY, C.T. (1988): The Human as an Experimental System in Molecular Genetics, *Science* 240:1483-1488.

WOLFF, A.; ATKINSON, J.C.; MACYNSKI, A.A.; and FOX, P.C. (1990): Pretherapy Interventions to Modify Salivary Dysfunction, *NCI MONOGR* 9:87-89.

YU, P.-I.; BIXLER, D.; GOODMAN, P.A.; AZEN, E.A.; and KARN, R.C. (1986): Human Parotid Proline-rich Proteins: Correlation of Genetic Polymorphisms to Dental Caries, *Genet Epidemiol* 3:147-152.

Hydroxyapatite-Interactive Proteins

DONALD I. HAY, EDGARD C. MORENO

Certain macromolecules present in the oral fluid interact with dental hard tissue surfaces to form a thin, closely adherent organic film termed the acquired enamel pellicle (Dawes *et al.*, 1963). The pellicle has several properties and activities which are important in dental health and disease (Mandel, 1976, 1979). Thus, it contains the specific receptors which mediate the highly selective initial colonization (Gibbons and vanHoute, 1975; Gibbons, 1980, 1984) of tooth surfaces by both commensal and pathogenic organisms, so making an important contribution to determining the organisms which form dental plaque. The pellicle remains interposed between the tooth and plaque, where it acts as a barrier to acid attack (Meckel, 1965). Although it influences ion movement between dental mineral and the tooth's external environment in a permselective fashion (Burke and Moreno, 1975; Zahradnik *et al.*, 1976), it permits the recalcification of many early carious lesions (Backer-Dirks, 1966; von der Fehr *et al.*, 1970) but limits this remineralization to subsurface sites (Hay, *et al.*, 1979). Thus, the pellicle helps regulate interactions between dental enamel and calcium and phosphate in saliva, which is supersaturated with respect to dental minerals (Hay *et al.*, 1982), to provide a protective and reparative environment which is important for the integrity of teeth. Also, the pellicle and the salivary mucous film provide lubrication between opposing teeth, soft tissue surfaces and abrasive foods (Tabak *et al.*, 1982), a property which for opposing tooth surfaces appears to be associated mainly with statherin (Douglas *et al.*, 1991).

The foregoing points emphasize the significance of the pellicle and its constituent HA-interactive proteins in several biologically important processes which occur at tooth surfaces. Although significant advances have been made in understanding pellicle formation, the precursor molecules which form pellicle, their quantitative contribution to this structure, and the functions of the pellicle are not completely understood. Consequently, we lack knowledge in several areas which is important for understanding important processes and activities which contribute to dental health, and others which cause dental caries and periodontal disease. This paper will describe some aspects of HA-interactive

TABLE 1 *Selected mineral-interactive macromolecules.*

HA-interactive proteins in bone
Amelogenins and phosphophoryns
HA-interactive salivary proteins, e.g., statherin, acidic proline-rich proteins (PRPs) & others
Polyaspartate and poly-glutamate
Pancreatic calcium carbonate-precipitation inhibitor
Urinary calcium oxalate-precipitation inhibitor
Caseins and phosvitins
Molluskan calcium carbonate-matrix proteins
Diatom and higher plant biomineral matrix proteins
Protein inhibitors of ice formation in polar fish

(Hukins, 1989; Sikes and Wheeler, 1991)

salivary proteins which appear to be involved in pellicle formation and function, and will attempt to outline deficiencies in knowledge in this area.

Mineral-Interactive Macromolecules

HA-interactive proteins can be considered as a subset of a larger group of macromolecules which act to modify events at solid-solution interfaces in many biological systems (Lowenstam, 1989). Since studies of these systems can provide information directly relevant to understanding tooth-salivary protein interactions, selected members of this broader group will be considered briefly.

Table 1 is intended to show their variety and to emphasize that information on structures, activities and structure-activity relationships of these macromolecules is likely to be valuable for understanding proteins with related activities in the oral cavity. They include several proteins involved in bone and tooth mineralization, different types of salivary proteins involved in regulating the chemistry of calcium phosphate in saliva and also considered to be involved in enamel pellicle formation, and two seemingly similar synthetic macromolecules, polyaspartate and poly-glutamate, the former interacting strongly with HA while the other does not, which are included here to emphasize the incompletely understood role of protein conformation in HA-reactivity.

Like saliva, other body fluids such as pancreatic fluid and urine contain macromolecules which are important as specific inhibitors of mineral precipitation, such as calcium phosphates, carbonate and oxalate (Nakagawa *et al.*, 1981; Multigner *et al.*, 1983), and have activities analogous to statherin and other salivary macromolecules which inhibit calcium phosphate precipitation (Moreno *et al.*, 1979). Caseins in milk and phosvitins in egg yolks (Holt and Kemenade, 1991) appear to act to transport or store calcium and phosphorus in stable, but biologically available forms and may provide insights into the action of statherin and related molecules.

Also, important information is available from studies of invertebrate systems, particularly mollusks (Addadi and Wiener, 1985; Addadi *et al.*, 1987), from other biominerals which do not contain calcium, such as those present in diatom (Swift and Wheeler, 1991) and higher plant biomineral matrices (Perry *et al.*, 1991). It is interesting to note that anti-freeze proteins in arctic fish appear to act by inhibiting growth on specific ice crystal faces (Raymond and deVries, 1991), in a fashion which may be related to that proposed for control of mineral formation by biomineral-interactive macromolecules (Moreno *et al.*, 1984).

A common thread linking this diverse group of proteins is that their activities are generally associated with acidic amino-acid residues such as aspartate and glutamate, phospho-serine, phospho-threonine, gamma-carboxy-glutamate and probably sulfate (Bernardi and Kawasaki, 1968; Bernardi *et al.*, 1972). This single common feature, however, is insufficient to explain the diversity of biological effects exhibited by these proteins. These include initiation and selective control of biomineral formation, such as generating different crystalline forms of the same salt or selectively controlling growth on specific crystal faces, stabilization, transport and storage of constituent ions of minerals, and inhibition of mineral formation in several body fluids. This is a remarkable array of biological phenomena ranging from initiation to inhibition of mineralization. It seems highly improbable that these specific and highly controlled activities depend only on the simple compositional properties of the proteins involved. Rather, this specificity is now beginning to be understood in terms of the state of such molecules or their conformations.

It has been shown (Campbell *et al.*, 1989; Linde *et al.*, 1989; Addadi *et al.*, 1991) that the type of activity exhibited by some mineral-interactive molecules, in solutions supersaturated with respect to the mineral of interest, depends on whether the molecule is free in solution, where it may inhibit mineral formation, or whether it is immobilized on a substrate, where it may promote mineral formation. The mechanisms underlying these differences in behavior are not well understood. Addadi *et al.* (1991) have emphasized the likely importance of specific molecular conformations in interactions of proteins with crystal surfaces. Thus, the closely related polymers, poly-aspartate and poly-glutamate, exhibit markedly different behaviors in modulating calcium phosphate chemistry. The only difference between these polymers is an additional methylene group between the side-chain carboxyl and the polypeptide chain in poly-glutamate, otherwise they are compositionally and electrostatically similar. Poly-aspartate, however, adsorbs strongly onto apatitic minerals and is a highly effective inhibitor of both primary and secondary precipitation of basic calcium phosphate salts from their supersaturated solutions (Hay *et al.*, 1979). In contrast, polyglutamate adsorbs poorly to apatitic minerals (Juriaanse *et al.*, 1980) and is a much weaker inhibitor of calcium phosphate precipitation (Hay *et al.*, 1979).

Addadi *et al.* (1991) showed from circular dichroism measurements that poly-aspartate possesses a beta-sheet conformation, under relevant conditions, while poly-glutamate of the same molecular weight adopts a "random coil" conformation under the same conditions. It is apparent that there is greater potential for a beta-sheet conformation to interact with crystal surface, compared with other possible conformations. It is not yet clear how the beta-sheet structure acts in solution systems, but its potential to order arrays of calcium ions, or to exert an influence over a significant volume of electrolyte and modify solution conditions to enhance mineral formation, are useful starting points for understanding this activity.

The potential significance of molecular conformation in protein-mineral interactions is also indicated by Aoba *et al.* (1989), who showed that the intact amelogenin molecule strongly modulates HA crystal growth. However, a simple cleavage of the amelogenin molecule, into its amino-terminal hydrophobic and carboxy-terminal acidic segments, led to loss of this activity. This strongly suggests that it is the conformation of the intact amelogenin molecule which is important in crystal growth regulation, rather than the simple chemistry of particular molecular segments.

The results from these two selected studies indicate the likely significance of this area of research and emphasize both the importance, and present lack of knowledge, regarding structural features of salivary proteins involved in interactions with tooth surfaces to form the enamel pellicle. An additional related important aspect is that certain bacteria attach to specific salivary proteins adsorbed onto HA, but do not interact with the same proteins in solution (Gibbons and Hay, 1988), suggesting that significant conformational changes occur as these proteins adsorb to tooth surfaces to form pellicle. Thus, although the pellicle is an important oral interface, knowledge of its precursors and the understanding of its mechanism of formation and properties are still incomplete. This lack of knowledge seriously hampers the understanding of key events which are, presumably, important factors in the initiation and severity of caries and periodontal disease, such as initial microbial colonization of teeth and its influence on subsequent plaque development, the influence of the pellicle on ingress of acid and egress of calcium and phosphate ions during acid attack, and the reverse movement of calcium and phosphate ions during the remineralization of early carious lesions.

Pellicle Precursors

Numerous candidate macromolecules have been proposed as possible pellicle precursors. These include salivary proteins such as acidic PRPs (Hay, 1973a;

Kousvelari *et al.*, 1980; Bennick *et al.*, 1983; Lamkin *et al.*, 1991), statherin (Hay, 1973b; Schlesinger and Hay, 1977; Lamkin *et al.*, 1991), histatins (Hay, 1973a; Lamkin *et al.*, 1991), a *Streptococcus mutans*-interactive protein (Ericson and Magnusson, 1976; Ericson and Rundegren, 1983), cystatins (Shomers, *et al.*, 1982a,b; Al-Hashimi and Levine, 1989; Lamkin *et al.*, in press), amylase (Rolla *et al.*, 1983; Al-Hashimi and Levine, 1989), lysozyme (Pruitt *et al.*, 1969; Rolla *et al.*, 1983), IgA and IgG (Rolla *et al.*, 1983), salivary mucin (Leach, 1963, 1964; Ericson 1967; McGaughey and Stowell, 1967) blood group-reactive glycoprotein (Rolla and Jonsen, 1968; Rolla *et al.*, 1969), salivary glycoprotein MG1 (Tabak *et al.*, 1985; Al-Hashimi and Levine, 1989; Lamkin *et al.*, 1991), salivary glycoprotein MG2 (Prakobphol *et al.*, 1982; Fisher *et al.*, 1987), salivary lipids and lipoproteins (Slomiany *et al.*, 1986), serum proteins (Kramer and Ramanathan, 1966) such as serum albumin (Orstavik and Kraus, 1973; Rolla *et al.*, 1983) and fibronectin (Takeuchi *et al.*, 1984) amongst others, and bacterial products (Armstrong 1966, 1967; Mayhall, 1970, 1977) including glucans and glycosyltransferases (Rolla and Mathiesen, 1970; Orstavik and Kraus, 1973; Rolla *et al.*, 1983), and lipoteichoic acid (Hogg and Lightfoot, 1989).

This extensive but incomplete list represents a remarkable array of possible precursors. It emphasizes the probable dominance of salivary proteins in pellicle as well as contributions from crevicular fluid constituents and bacterial products. It seems highly improbable, however, that all of these molecules make significant quantitative contributions to pellicle, and illustrates the inadequate state of knowledge regarding both the qualitative and quantitative contributions of different possible precursors to pellicle. There appear to be few quantitative data. Two exceptions to this are that Bennick *et al.* (1983) quantified PRPs in pellicle formed *in vivo* on removable enamel pieces, and Lamkin *et al.* (1991) studied pellicle formed on teeth *in vivo* using high performance liquid chromatography to purify pellicle constituents and micro-sequencing techniques to characterize the purified materials, an approach which has quantitative potential.

Mechanisms of Pellicle Formation

The understanding of the mechanisms by which pellicle forms is also incomplete. Thus, the view that pellicle forms by selective adsorption of salivary proteins onto tooth surfaces (Ericson, 1967; Hay, 1967, 1973a) with a contribution from serum proteins (Orstavik and Kraus, 1973) and microbial macromolecules (Rolla *et al.*, 1983) appears to be a sound starting point but several secondary factors are involved about which little is known. Thus, the different salivary concentrations and adsorption properties (affinity constant for HA and the number of adsorption sites (Moreno *et al.*, 1982, 1984)) of different pellicle precursors will be the primary determinants of their relative quantitative contribution to pellicle. However, although concentrations of salivary proteins are known to vary with glandular source and flow rate, actual quantitative knowledge is sparse. Thus, salivary concentrations of different HA-interactive proteins vary from gland to gland (Kousvelari *et al.*, 1980; Baum *et al.*, 1982; Mandel and Bennick, 1983; Hay *et al.*, 1984), vary with flow rate, exhibit circadian variations in animal models (Denny and Denny, 1984) and may vary with other physiological states. Although this is recognized, there is little quantitative information in spite of its importance for understanding and predicting selective protein adsorption. Given this information, however, novel models for studying adsorption from multi-component systems using a thermodynamic approach are available (Moreno *et al.*, 1987, in press).

There are also highly intriguing special effects, such as the partial post-translational cleavage of the PRPs, but this has not been investigated quantitatively. Wong *et al.* (1983) identified kallikrein as an enzyme with an appropriate specificity to effect this cleavage, but whether kallikrein is the enzyme involved, the cellular site at which cleavage takes place, and how the extent of cleavage of the PRP gene products is controlled, are not known. These are important issues because the PRPs have several important activities in the oral environment. Also, the recently discovered occurrence of genetically determined protein polymorphisms of statherin (Jensen *et al.*, 1991), the known polymorphisms of amylase (Keller *et al.*, 1971) and of the bacterial adhesion-promoting proteins described by Kishimoto *et al.*(1989, 1990) and the PRPs (Azen and Denniston, 1981; Azen *et al.*, 1985, 1987; Maeda *et al.*, 1985; Maeda, 1985), the heterogeneity and properties of mucins (Tabak *et al.*, 1982), which are discussed elsewhere in these proceedings (Levine, M.J. and Fisher, S.J.), and probably others are important topics in pellicle formation, because even small differences in composition and structure affect the way proteins interact with HA (Moreno *et al.*, 1982, 1984).

It is also necessary to understand the processes which yield a pellicle structure which has a large insoluble component, to be able to explain how pellicle controls ionic transport, particularly of hydrogen, calcium and phosphate ions, between tooth mineral and its fluid environment, how crystallization of calcium phosphates onto tooth surfaces is controlled *in vivo,* and to identify and explain how native pellicle constituents mediate bacterial attachment to teeth and to understand the molecular basis of this activity. A further significant area which is relatively unexplored is that the fluoride content of the adsorbate mineral has a marked effect on adsorption of macromolecules (Moreno *et al.*, 1978), implying effects on pellicle formation. Also, while well-defined model systems to study protein adsorption relative to pellicle formation have been devised, it is necessary to consider that this process involves adsorption of proteins from complex and probably non-homogeneous mixtures of salivary proteins (incompletely mixed serous and mucous phases and different glandular secretions), that kinetic factors may complicate thermodynamic predictions in that faster-adsorbing proteins may preempt adsorption of slower-adsorbing molecules with higher affinity, that conditions at tooth surfaces may not represent a system at equilibrium because adsorption is rapid and desorption is slow, and that pellicle precursors may be modified in saliva (Cowman *et al.*, 1975, 1976; Choih *et al.*, 1979) as well as after adsorption onto tooth surfaces (Bennick *et al.*, 1983).

This is a formidable array of complexities and it is legitimate to ask if pellicle formation is a consistent and controlled process, and whether it is amenable to investigation. Amino-acid analyses of pellicle proteins in several laboratories, however, have shown that pellicle composition is reasonably constant (Armstrong 1966, 1967; Armstrong and Hayward, 1968; Mayhall, 1970, 1977; Sonju and Rolla, 1973) and differs from the amino-acid composition of the total salivary proteins from which it is considered to form. This is important encouragement that pellicle formation involves specific and consistent processes. This notion is supported by the fact that the mineral in tooth surfaces has never been shown to nucleate calcium phosphate crystal growth from the supersaturated saliva, indicating the consistent presence of specific inhibitors of calcium phosphate crystal growth at the mineral surface, and that the initial bacterial colonization of newly formed pellicle is remarkably reproducible, indicating the consistent presence of specific attachment sites for the early tooth microflora.

Regarding modulation of bacterial adhesion to teeth, there are several ways in which salivary macromolecules may influence such adhesion, one of which is to act as bridging molecules between the tooth mineral surface and the bacterial cells. Studies of the adhesion-promoting activities of specific salivary proteins adsorbed onto HA have revealed a remarkable degree of specificity (Gibbons and Hay, 1988, 1989b) in that the adhesion of different bacteria is promoted by few salivary proteins which typically differed for the different strains or species tested. *Streptococcus mutans* JBP, for example, adheres strongly to HA-adsorbed proteins in the mucin fraction and, to a lesser extent, to adsorbed PRPs. The adhesion of *Actinomyces viscosus* LY7 is promoted by PRPs and statherin. *Porphyromonas gingivalis* adheres to adsorbed PRPs and to a second as yet unidentified molecule. Thus, different species appear to have evolved highly specific adhesion mechanisms, a phenomenon which explains the well-established highly selective bacterial colonization of teeth.

A further observation was that samples of saliva from the same subject, collected on different days, differed considerably in their abilities to promote adhesion of organisms to pellicles formed on HA in vitro (Gibbons and Hay, 1989a,b). This can be interpreted in terms of compositional differences in the pellicles with respect to the specific adhesion-promoting proteins for the organism studied, reflecting differences in the different saliva samples used to form the pellicles. These results emphasize the importance of characterizing salivas with respect to bacterial adhesion-promoting proteins, and the resulting compositional differences in pellicles, for understanding initial bacterial colonization of teeth.

In some bacterial species, highly novel adaptive mechanisms appear to have developed to effect adhesion to pellicles. Gibbons and Hay (1988) found that although *Actinomyces viscosus* cells bind strongly to PRPs adsorbed onto HA, adhesion is not inhibited by PRPs in solution. This is an important issue because saliva contains large amounts of PRPs which would be expected to inhibit LY7 cell adhesion and prevent colonization. It was suggested that *A. viscosus* has adapted to recognize sites in the PRP molecules which are exposed or which present a particular conformation only when PRPs are adsorbed onto HA. This mechanism represents a powerful adaptive step which allows LY7 cells to recognize unique adhesion sites in adsorbed PRPs yet avoid inhibition of adhesion by the same molecules in saliva. The term ''cryptitope'' (Gibbons *et al.*, 1990) has been proposed to describe such adhesion sites, which occur in several other systems.

Evidence regarding conformational changes of this kind has come from physical chemical studies of PRP adsorption onto HA (Moreno *et al.*, 1982, 1984). It was shown that this adsorption is endothermic and, therefore, driven by changes in entropy. Such entropic changes would include conformational changes of the protein molecule. Further evidence for post-adsorption conformational changes has been obtained from Fourier transform infra-red studies (Moreno *et al.*, 1991), which compared the spectra of PRP in the adsorbed state with their spectra when in solution. The results showed that the structures of PRP molecules are changed by adsorption, in that the proportions of beta-sheet, helix, etc. present in a PRP molecule when in solution, differ considerably from the proportions observed when the molecule is in the adsorbed state.

In conclusion, although substantial advances have been made with respect to identifying possible pellicle precursors, in understanding some aspects of their adsorption behavior onto hydroxyapatite, and towards identifying important biological activities of the pellicle and its constituent macromolecules, large gaps still exist in this knowledge. These include identifying and quantifying the contributions of the salivary, serum and bacterial macromolecules which are considered to form pellicle, advancing the understanding the mechanisms involved in pellicle formation, including the role of macromolecular conformation in adsorption behavior onto HA, and clarifying the biological functions of pellicle constituents and the molecular mechanisms involved in their activities. With this knowledge, an improved understanding of important steps which help maintain dental health, or which lead to dental disease, will be obtained.

REFERENCES

ADDADI, L. and WEINER, S. (1985): Interactions between acidic proteins and crystals: stereochemical requirements in biomineralization. *Proc Nat Acad Sci* (USA). 82:4110-4114.

ADDADI, L.; MORADIAN, J.; SHAY, E.; MAROUDAS, N.; and WEINER, S. (1987): A chemical model for the cooperation of sulfates and carboxylates in calcite crystallization. Relevance to biomineralization. *Proc Nat Acad Sci* (USA). 84:2732-2736.

ADDADI, L.; MORADIAN-OLDAK, J; and WEINER, S. (1991): Macromole-crystal recognition in biomineralization studies. In: *Surface Reactive Peptides and Polymers* Sikes, C.S. and Wheeler, A.P. Eds. American Chemical Society, Washington, DC. pp. 13-27.

AL-HASHIMI, I. and LEVINE, M.J. (1989): Characterization of *in vivo* salivary-derived enamel pellicle. *Arch Oral Biol* 34:289-95.

AOBA, T.; MORENO, E.C.; KRESAK, M. and TANABE, T. (1989): Possible roles of partial sequences at N- and C- termini of amelogenin in protein-enamel mineral interaction. *J Dent Res* 68:1331-1336.

ARMSTRONG, W.G. (1966): Amino acid composition of the acquired pellicle of human tooth enamel. *Nature* 210:197-198.

ARMSTRONG, W.G. (1967): The composition of organic films formed on human teeth. *Caries Res* 1:89-103.

ARMSTRONG, W.G. and HAYWARD, A.F. (1968): Acquired organic integuments of human enamel; a comparison of analytical studies with optical, phase contrast and electron microscope examination. *Caries Res* 2:294-305.

AZEN, E.A. and DENNISTON, C. (1981): Genetic polymorphism of PIF (parotid isoelectric focusing variant) proteins with linkage to the PPP (parotid proline-rich protein) gene complex. *Biochem Genetics* 19:475-485.

AZEN, E.A.; GOODMAN, P.A.; and LALLEY, P.A. (1985): Human salivary proline-rich protein genes on chromosome 12. *Am J Hum Genet* 37:418-424.

AZEN, E.A.; KIM, H.S.; GOODMAN, P.; FLYNN, S.; and MAEDA, N. (1987): Alleles at the PRH1 locus coding for the human salivary acidic proline-rich proteins Pa, Db and PIF. *Am J Hum Genet* 41:1035-1047.

BACKER DIRKS, O. (1966): Post-eruptive changes in enamel. *J Dent Res* 45:503-511.

BAUM, B.J.; KOUSVELARI, E.E.; and OPPENHEIM, F.G. (1982): Exocrine protein secretion from human parotid glands during aging: stable release of the acidic proline-rich proteins. *J Gerontol* 17:392-395.

BENNICK, A.; CHAU, G.; GOODLIN, R.; ABRAMS, S.; TUSTIAN, D.; and MADAPALLIMATTAM, G. (1983): The role of human salivary acidic proline-rich proteins in the formation of acquired dental pellicle *in vivo* and their fate after adsorption to the human enamel surface. *Arch Oral Biol* 28:19-27.

BERNARDI, G. and KAWASAKI, T. (1968): Chromatography of polypeptides and proteins on hydroxyapatite columns. *Biochim Biophys Acta* 160:301-310.

BERNARDI, G.; GIRO, M.G.; and GAILLARD, C. (1972): Chromatography of polypeptides and proteins on hydroxyapatite columns: some new developments. *Biochim Biophys Acta* 278:409-420.

BURKE, E.J. and MORENO, E.C. (1975): Diffusion fluxes of tritiated water across human enamel membranes. *Arch Oral Biol* 20:327-332.

CAMPBELL, A.A.; EBRAHIMPOUR, A.; PEREZ, L.; SMESKO, S.A.; and NANCOLLAS, G.H. (1989): The dual role of polyelectrolytes and proteins as mineralization promoters and inhibitors of calcium oxalate monohydrate. *Calcif Tissue Int* 45:122-128.

CHOIH, S.; SMITH, Q.T.; and SCHACHTELE, C.F. (1979): Modification of human parotid saliva proteins by oral *Streptococcus sanguis*. *J Dent Res* 58:516-523.

COWMAN, R.A.; PERELLA, M.M.; ADAMS, B.O.; and FITZGERALD, R.J. (1975): Amino-acid requirements and proteolytic activity of *Streptococcus sanguis*. *Applied Microbiology* 30:374-380.

COWMAN, R.A.; PERELLA, M.M.; and FITZGERALD, R.J. (1976): Caseinolytic and glyco-protein hydrolase activity of *Streptococcus mutans*. *J Dent Res* 55:391-399.

DAWES, C.; JENKINS, G.N.; and TONGE, C.H. (1963): The nomenclature of the integuments of the enamel surface of the teeth. *Br Dent J* 115:65-68.

DENNY, P.C. and DENNY, P.A. (1984): Diurnal variation of sialomucin concentration in female mouse submandibular glands measured by radioimmunoassay. *Arch Oral Biol* 29:1033-40.

DOUGLAS, W.H.; REEH, E.S.; RUDNEY, J.; RAMASUBBU, N.; BHANDARY, K.; and LEVINE, M.J. (1991): Heterogeneous equilibrium, self-association and boundary lubrication of salivary statherin. *J Dent Res* 70:499. Abstract 1866.

ERICSON, T. (1967): Adsorption to hydroxyapatite of proteins and conjugated proteins from human saliva. *Caries Res* 1:52-58.

ERICSON, T. and MAGNUSSON, I. (1976): Affinity for hydroxyapatite of salivary substances inducing aggregation of oral streptococci. *Caries Res* 10:8-18.

ERICSON, T. and RUNDEGREN, J. (1983): Characterization of a salivary agglutinin reacting with a serotype c strain of *Streptococcus mutans*. *Eur J Biochem* 133:255-261.

FEHR, F.R. von der; LOE, H.; and THEILADE, E. (1970): Experimental caries in man. *Caries Res* 4:131-148.

FISHER, S.J.; PRAKOBPHOL, A.; KAJISA, L.; and MURRAY, P.A. (1987): External radiolabelling of components of pellicle on human enamel and cementum. *Arch Oral Biol* 32:509-517.

GIBBONS, R.J. and VAN HOUTE, J. (1975): Bacterial adherence in oral microbial ecology. *Ann Rev Microbiol* 29:19-44.

GIBBONS, R.J. (1980): "Adhesion of Bacteria to Surfaces of the Mouth." In: *Microbial Adhesion to Surfaces*, Soc. Chem. Industry, p. 351-388.

GIBBONS, R.J. (1984): Adherent interactions which may affect microbial ecology in the mouth. *J Dent Res* 63:378-385.

GIBBONS, R.J. and HAY, D.I. (1988): Human salivary acidic proline-rich proteins and statherin promote the attachment of *Actinomyces viscosus* LY7 to apatitic surfaces. *Infection and Immunity* 56:439-445.

GIBBONS, R.J. and HAY, D.I. (1989a): Adsorbed salivary proline-rich proteins contribute to the adhesion of *Streptococcus mutans* JBP to apatitic surfaces. *J Dent Res* 68:1303-1307.

GIBBONS, R.J. and HAY, D.I. (1989b): Adsorbed salivary proline-rich proteins as bacterial receptors on apatitic surfaces. In *Molecular Mechanisms of Microbial Adhesion*. Switalski, L., Hook, M. and Beachey, E. (Eds.) Springer-Verlag. pp. 143-163.

GIBBONS, R.J.; HAY, D.I.; CHILDS, W.C.; and DAVIS, G. (1990): Role of cryptic receptors (cryptitopes) in bacterial adhesion to oral surfaces. *Arch Oral Biol* 35:107S-114S.

HAY, D.I. (1967): The adsorption of salivary proteins by hydroxyapatite and enamel. *Arch Oral Biol* 12:937-946.

HAY, D.I. (1973a): The interaction of human parotid salivary proteins with hydroxyapatite. *Arch Oral Biol* 20:1517-1529.

HAY, D.I. (1973b): The isolation from human parotid saliva of a tyrosine-rich acid peptide which exhibits high affinity for hydroxyapatite surfaces. *Arch Oral Biol* 18:1531-1541.

HAY, D.I.; MORENO, E.C.; and SCHLESINGER, D.H. (1979): Phospho-protein inhibitors of calcium phosphate precipitation from salivary secretions. *Inorg Persp in Biol and Med* 2:271-285.

HAY, D.I.; SCHLUCKEBIER, S.K.; and MORENO, E.C. (1982): Equilibrium dialysis and ultrafiltration studies of calcium and phosphate binding by human salivary proteins. Implications for salivary supersaturation with respect to calcium phosphate salts. *Calcif Tiss Int* 34:531-538.

HAY, D.I.; SMITH, D.J.; SCHLUCKEBIER, S.K.; and MORENO, E.C. (1984): Relationship between concentration of human salivary statherin and inhibition of calcium phosphate precipitation in stimulated human parotid saliva. *J Dent Res* 63:857-863.

HOGG, S.D. and LIGHTFOOT, I. (1989): Interaction of streptococcal lipoteichoic acid with artificial tooth pellicle. *Arch Oral Biol* 34:615-20.

HOLT, C. and VAN KEMENADE, M.J.J.M. (1991): The interactions of phosphoproteins with calcium phosphate. In: *Calcified Tissue*. Hukins, D.W.L., Ed. CRC Press, Boca Raton, FL. pp. 175-214.

HUKINS, D.W.L. (1989): *Calcified Tissue*. CRC Press, Boca Raton, FL.

JENSEN, J.L.; LAMKIN, M.S.; TROXLER, R.F.; and OPPENHEIM, F.G. (1991): Multiple forms of statherin in human salivary secretions. *Arch Oral Biol* 36(7):529-534.

JURIAANSE, A.C.; ARENDS, J.; and TEN BOSCH, J.J. (1980): The adsorption of acidic and basic homopolypeptides to whole bovine dental enamel. *J Coll Int Sci* 76:212-219.

KELLER, P.J.; KAUFFMAN, D.L.; ALLAN, B.J.; and WILLIAMS, B.L. (1971): Further studies on the differences between the iso-enzymes of human parotid amylase. *Biochemistry* 10:4867-4874.

KISHIMOTO, E.; HAY, D.I.; and GIBBONS, R.J. (1989): A human salivary protein which promotes adhesion of *Streptococcus mutans* serotype c strains to hydroxyapatite. *Infection and Immunity* 57:3702-3707.

KISHIMOTO, E.; HAY, D.I.; and KENT, R. (1990): Polymorphism of a human submandibular-sublingual salivary protein which promotes adhesion of *Streptococcus mutans* serotype c strains to hydroxyapatite. *J Dent Res* 69:1741-1745.

KOUSVELARI, E.E.; BARATZ, R.S.; BURKE, B.; and OPPENHEIM, F.G. (1980): Immunochemical identification and determination of proline-rich proteins in salivary secretions, enamel pellicle and glandular tissue specimens. *J Dent Res* 59:1430-1438.

KRAMER, I.R.H. and RAMANATHAN, K. (1966): The investigation of deposits on the surface of human enamel by means of a fluorescent antibody technique. *Arch Oral Biol* 11:1047-1048.

LAMKIN, M.S.; SETAYESH, M.R.; TROXLER, R.F.; and OPPENHEIM, F.G. (1991): Amino-acid sequence of peptides isolated from acquired enamel pellicle. *J Dent Res* 70:499. Abstract 1861.

LAMKIN, M.S.; JENSEN, J.L.; SETAYESH, M.R.; TROXLER, R.F.; and OPPENHEIM, F.G. (In press): Salivary cystatin SA-III, a potential precursor of the acquired enamel pellicle, is phosphorylated at both its amino- and carboxy-terminal regions. *Arch Biochem Biophys*

LEACH, S.A. (1963): Release and breakdown of sialic acid from human salivary mucin and its role in the formation of dental plaque. *Nature* 199:486-487.

LEACH, S.A. (1964): Some observations of the state of sialic acid in human saliva. *Arch Oral Biol* 9:461-467.

LINDE, A.; LUSSI, A.; and CRENSHAW, M.A. (1989): Mineral induction by immobilized polyanionic proteins. *Calcif Tissue Int* 44:286-295.

LOWENSTAM, H.A. and WIENER, S. (1989): *On Biomineralization* Oxford University Press, New York, NY.

MAEDA, N. (1985): Inheritance of the human salivary proline-rich proteins: a reinterpretation in terms of six loci forming two subfamilies. *Biochem Genet* 23:455-464.

MAEDA, N.; KIM, H.S.; AZEN, E.A.; and SMITHIES. O. (1985): Differential RNA splicing and post-translational cleavages in the human salivary proline-rich protein gene system. *J Biol Chem* 260:11123-11130.

MANDEL, I.D. (1976): Non-immunologic aspects of caries resistance. *J Dent Res* 55:22-31.

MANDEL, I.D. (1979): In defense of the oral cavity. In: *Saliva and Dental Caries*. Kleinberg, I., Ellison, S.A. and Mandel, I.D. (eds.), p. 473-491.

MANDEL, I.D. and BENNICK, A. (1983): Quantitation of human salivary acidic proline-rich proteins in oral diseases. *J Dent Res* 62:943-945.

MAYHALL, C.W. (1970): Concerning the composition and source of the acquired pellicle of human teeth. *Arch Oral Biol* 15:1327-1341.

MAYHALL, C.W. (1977): Amino acid composition of experimental salivary pellicles. *J Periodont* 48:78-91.

MCGAUGHEY, C. and STOWELL, E.C. (1967): The adsorption of human salivary proteins and porcine submaxillary mucin by hydroxyapatite. *Arch Oral Bio.* 12:815-828.

MECKEL, A.H. (1965): The formation and properties of organic films on teeth. *Arch Oral Biol* 10:585-597.

MORENO, E.C.; KRESAK, M.; and HAY, D.I. (1978): Adsorption of two human parotid salivary macromolecules on hydroxy-, fluorhydroxy- and fluorapatites. *Arch Oral Biol* 23:525-533.

MORENO, E.C.; VARUGHESE, K.; and HAY, D.I. (1979): Effect of human salivary proteins on the precipitation kinetics of calcium phosphate. *Calcif Tiss Int* 28:7-16.

MORENO, E.C.; KRESAK, M.; and HAY, D.I. (1982): Adsorption thermodynamics of acidic proline-rich human salivary proteins onto calcium apatites. *J Biol Chem* 257:2981-2989.

MORENO, E.C.; KRESAK, M.; and HAY, D.I. (1984): Adsorption of molecules of biological interest onto hydroxyapatite. *Calcif Tiss Int* 36:48-59.

MORENO, E.C.; KRESAK, M.; KANE, J.J.; and HAY, D.I. (1987): Adsorption of proteins, peptides and organic acids onto hydroxyapatite. *Langmuir* 3:511-519.

MORENO, E.C.; KRESAK, M.; and HAY, D.I. (1991): Adsorption of salivary proteins onto calcium apatites. *Biofouling* 4:3-24.

MULTIGNER, L.; DE CARO, A.; LOMBARDO, D.; CAMPESE, D.; and SARLES, H. (1983): Pancreatic stone protein, a phosphoprotein which inhibits calcium carbonate precipitation from human pancreatic juice. *Biochem Biophys Res Comm* 110:69-74.

NAKAGAWA, Y.; MARGOLIS, H.C.; YOKOYAMA, S.; KEZDY, F.J.; KAISER, E.T.; and COE, F.L. (1981): Purification and characterization of a calcium oxalate monohydrate crystal growth inhibitor from human kidney tissue culture medium. *J Biol Chem* 256:3936-3944.

ORSTAVIK, D. and KRAUS, F.W. (1973): The acquired pellicle: Immunofluorescent demonstration of specific proteins. *J Oral Path* 2:68-76.

PERRY, C.C.; FRASER, M.A.; and HUGHES, N.P. (1991): Macromolecular assemblages in controlled biomineralization. In: *Surface Reactive Peptides and Polymers* Sikes, C.S. and Wheeler, A.P. (Eds.) American Chemical Society, Washington, DC. pp. 316-339.

PRAKOBPHOL, A.; LEVINE, M.J.; TABAK, L.A.; and REDDY, M.S. (1982): Purification of a low-molecular-weight, mucin-type glycoprotein from human submandibular-sublingual saliva. *Carbohydrate Res* 108:111-122.

PRUITT, K.M.; CALDWELL, R.C.; JAMIESON, A.D.; and TAYLOR, R.E. (1969): The interaction of salivary proteins with tooth surface. *J Dent Res* 48:818-823.

RAYMOND, J.A. and DEVRIES, A.L. (1991): Inhibition of ice crystal growth by fish antifreezes. In: *Surface Reactive Peptides and Polymers* Sikes, C.S. and Wheeler, A.P. (Eds.) American Chemical Society, Washington, DC. pp. 249-255.

ROLLA, G. and JONSEN, J. (1968): A glycoprotein component from human sublingual submaxillary saliva. *Caries Res* 2:306-316.

ROLLA, G.; KORNSTAD, L.; MATHIESEN, P.; and POVATONG, L. (1969): Selective adsorption of an acidic glycoprotein from human saliva to tooth surfaces. *J Periodont Res* 4:8-9.

ROLLA, G. and MATHIESEN, P. (1970): The adsorption of salivary proteins and dextrans to hydroxylapatite. In: *The Dental Plaque* McHugh, Ed. Livingstone. Edinburgh. Pages 129-140.

ROLLA, G.; CIARDI, J.E.; and BOWEN, W.H. (1983): Identification of IgA, IgG, lysozyme, albumin, amylase and glucosyltransferase in the protein layer adsorbed to hydroxyapatite from whole saliva. *Scand J Dent Res* 91:186-190.

SCHLESINGER, D.H. and HAY, D.I. (1977): Complete covalent structure of statherin, a tyrosine-rich acidic peptide which inhibits calcium phosphate precipitation from human parotid saliva. *J Biol Chem* 252:1689-1695.

SHOMERS, J.P.; TABAK, L.A.; LEVINE, M.J.; MANDEL, I.D.; and HAY, D.I. (1982a): Properties of cysteine-containing phosphoproteins from human submandibular-sublingual saliva. *J Dent Res* 61:397-399.

SHOMERS, J.P.; TABAK, L.A.; LEVINE, M.J.; MANDEL, I.D.; and ELLISON, S.A. (1982b): The isolation of a family of cysteine-containing phosphoproteins from human submandibular-sublingual saliva. *J Dent Res* 61:973-977.

SIKES, C.S. and WHEELER, A.P. (1991): *Surface Reactive Peptides and Polymers* American Chemical Society, Washington, DC.

SLOMIANY, B.L.; MURTY, V.L.; ZDEBSKA, E.; SLOMIANY, A.; GWOZDZINSKI, K.; and MANDEL, I.D. (1986): Tooth surface-pellicle lipids and their role in the protection of dental enamel against lactic-acid diffusion in man. *Arch Oral Biol* 31:187-91.

SONJU, T. and ROLLA, G. (1973): Chemical analyses of the acquired pellicle formed in two hours on cleaned human teeth *in vivo*. *Caries Res* 7:30-38.

SWIFT, D.M. and WHEELER, A.P. (1991): Some structural and functional properties of a possible organic matrix from the frustules of the fresh water diatom *Cyclotella meneghiniana*. In: *Surface Reactive Peptides and Polymers* Sikes, C.S. and Wheeler, A.P. (Eds.) American Chemical Society, Washington, DC. pp. 340-353.

TABAK, L.A.; LEVINE, M.J.; MANDEL, I.D.; and ELLISON, S.A. (1982): Role of salivary mucins in the protection of the oral cavity. *J Oral Path* 11:1-17.

TABAK, L.A.; LEVINE, M.J.; JAIN, N.K.; BRYAN, A.R.; COHEN, R.E.; MONTE, L.D.; ZAWACKI, S.; NANCOLLAS, G.H.; SLOMIANY, A.; and SLOMIANY, B.L. (1985): Adsorption of human salivary mucins to hydroxyapatite. *Arch Oral Biol* 30:423-427.

TAKEUCHI, H.; HORI, Y.; YU, S.F.; FUJII, T.; SATO, M.; NAMIKAWA, I.; TATSUMI, M.; and TAKAGI, N. (1984): Mechanisms of dental plaque and calculus formation due to fibronectin. 2. Demonstration of fibronectin in the enamel pellicle. *Nippon Shishubyo Gakkai Kaishi* (Journal of the Japanese Association of Periodontology) 26:257-61.

WONG, R.S.; MADAPALLIMATTAM, G.; and BENNICK, A. (1983): The role of glandular kallikrein in the formation of a salivary proline-rich protein A by cleavage of a single bond in salivary protein C. *Biochem J* 211:35-44.

ZAHRADNIK, R.T.; MORENO, E.C.; and BURKE, E.J. (1976): Effect of salivary pellicle on enamel subsurface demineralization in vitro. *J Dent Res* 55:664-670.

Salivary Mucins and Dental Plaque Formation

F.A. SCANNAPIECO AND M.J. LEVINE

Mucins are by definition glycoproteins that are unique to mucosal secretions and contain > 40% carbohydrate. These molecules are multifunctional and protective in their native form. The charge from the conference organizers was to review the role of salivary mucins in the etiology of dental caries. This presented a difficult challenge since few investigations have rigorously addressed this issue due to problems inherent to the study of mucins. For example, the amount of mucin in saliva has not been accurately determined owing to the difficulty in obtaining mucin preparations substantially free of other components such as secretory IgA and lysozyme. As a result, pure mucins have not been readily available for preparation of immunological reagents for quantitative studies. In addition, many studies have found that the flow rate of saliva and the concentration of selected components varies considerably between individuals (Mandel, 1980; Ship *et al.*, 1991). Consequently, it is difficult to make any correlation between these factors and disease activity. Saliva is a complex mixture of macromolecules, many of which have overlapping functions. Therefore, it is possible that an individual may be quantitatively deficient in mucin with no obvious clinical effect because another component provides a compensatory role. Despite these difficulties, a few studies have attempted to evaluate the relationship between mucins and caries. Early surveys, using crude methods for mucin quantitation found no correlation between the mucin content of whole saliva and caries status (Dewar and Parfit, 1954; Kapsimilis *et al.*, 1966). There appears to be no difference in the oligosaccharide composition of mucins isolated from caries resistant and caries susceptible individuals (Reddy *et al.*, 1984). It was suggested that caries susceptibility may be related to an individual's blood-group secretor status, possibly through the influence of blood-group reactive mucins in modulating the oral flora (Arneberg *et al.*, 1976). However, other researchers

Supported, in part, by USPHS grants DE08240 and DE07585.

have found that binding of mucin to cariogenic bacteria was not dependent on the blood group-specific carbohydrate determinants (Gibbons and Quereshi 1976; Kondo *et al.*, 1978). Quantitive differences in mucins and mucin-associated lipids between caries active and caries resistant populations have been reported (Slomiany *et al.*, 1982; 1986; 1989b; 1990). However, the significance of these data relative to an individual's caries susceptibility remains unclear. In summary, the few studies that have attempted to correlate the quantity or quality of mucins in saliva with caries activity have provided conflicting or inconclusive results.

Due to the paucity of information regarding the relationship of salivary mucins to caries, the scope of this review was broadened to describe the role of mucins in dental plaque formation. It is well established that dental plaque is essential to the development of dental caries (Gibbons and van Houte, 1975; van Houte, 1980). Furthermore, it has long been recognized that saliva and mucins, in particular, interact with bacteria to modulate dental plaque formation (Mandel, 1974). Plaque formation can be broadly divided into three stages: 1) acquired enamel pellicle (AEP) formation; 2) initial microbial adherence; and 3) plaque maturation. This review will briefly describe general aspects of human salivary mucin structure and function and their role in plaque formation. Recent concepts concerning the possible mechanisms of mucin-bacterial interactions will also be presented. Finally, the goals of mucin research will be discussed as they pertain to dental plaque formation and the development of artificial salivas.

Mucin Structure and Function

Due to their rheological properties and tendency to associate with other components, salivary mucins have proved difficult to purify and characterize (Loomis *et al.*, 1987; Prakobphol *et al.*, 1982; Ramasubbu *et al.*, 1991). Earlier studies found that salivary mucin occurred as a single high molecular weight ($>$ 500 kDa) species containing blood group reactivity (Rölla and Jonsen, 1968; Hay *et al.*, 1971). More recent investigations, which used dissociating conditions to disrupt intra- and intermolecular hydrogen bonds and hydrophobic interactions between mucins and other salivary molecules, demonstrated the presence of two distinct mucins in human saliva. The larger species ($\sim 10^3$ kDa) has been designated mucin glycoprotein 1 (MG1) while the smaller mucin (130-150 kDa) is designated MG2 (Loomis *et al.*, 1987). Recently, MG2 has been found to exist as two glycoforms (MG2a and MG2b) which differ in their content of sialic acid and fucose (Ramasubbu *et al.*, 1991; Reddy *et al.*, 1992). Immunohistochemical studies have shown that MG1 is produced by submandibular, labial and palatine glands while MG2 is only produced in submandibular and labial glands (Cohen *et al.*, 1990; 1991; Rathman *et al.*, 1990). Additional evidence suggests that these two mucins may be secreted by distinct mucous cell populations (Cohen *et al.*, 1991). By Northern blot analysis, an oligonucleotide probe generated from the amino acid sequence of MG2 glycopeptides specifically hybridized to two mRNA species from human submandibular and sublingual glands (Reddy *et al.*, 1992). In the same study, a cDNA clone for MG2 from a human submandibular gland expression library also hybridized to these two mRNA species. In both cases, the larger mRNA was polydisperse, and the hybridization signal was more intense in the sublingual gland. Further details of the chemical structure of the human salivary mucins can be found in several recent reviews (Levine *et al.*, 1987; Cohen and Levine, 1989).

It has been suggested that MG1 and MG2 may play different roles in the oral cavity (Tabak *et al.*, 1982; Levine *et al.*, 1985; Cohen and Levine, 1989). However, as experimental data accumulate, it is apparent that these molecules have overlapping functions. The general function of mucins can be summarized as follows. Their high degree of glycosylation and potential for hydration allows mucins to combat the dessication or drying of oral surfaces. Mucins can bind to various toxins and chemical constituents to protect oral surfaces against environmental insult (Mandel, 1987). Their viscoelastic properties permit the lubrication of hard and soft tissues to minimize abrasion and facilitate speech and swallowing (Hatton *et al.*, 1985; Aguirre *et al.*, 1989). Mucins may also interact with host cells such as gingival fibroblasts to modulate wound healing (Heaney *et al.*, 1986). These glycoproteins play a role in mineralization (Nieuw Amerongen *et al.*, 1987). A significant function of salivary mucins is their propensity to complex or associate with other salivary molecules, particularly antimicrobials such as lysozyme, sIgA, cystatins and carbonic anhydrases (Prakobphol *et al.*, 1982; Biesbrock *et al.*, 1991). In this regard, mucins may act as carriers to concentrate these various antimicrobial components at different intraoral surfaces. Perhaps the most important role of salivary mucins is their ability to modulate the oral colonization of a wide variety of microorganisms.

Role of Mucins in Dental Plaque Formation

Mucins held a crucial place in early theories of dental plaque formation. One theory suggested that plaque formed as a result of mucin precipitation caused by a decrease in salivary pH following bacterial acid production (Kirk, 1910). Currently, it is thought that mucins (and other salivary proteins) function to promote plaque formation in two ways: 1) as receptors for bacterial adhesion to acquired enamel pellicle (AEP) and plaque, and 2) as a nutritional substrate for plaque bacterial growth and division. To simplify the study of mucin-bacterial interactions, these events are isolated as they would occur in the oral cavity; that is, in saliva, on AEP, or during plaque maturation. In saliva, mucins can bind to specific adhesins on bacteria to cause their clumping or agglutination that most frequently results in microbial clearance from the oral cavity. Alternatively, mucins in the AEP may facilitate bacterial adhesion onto the tooth surface or to other bacteria in dental plaque. It is likely that these events are not mutually exclusive and mucins probably function simultaneously as agglutinins as well as host tissue receptors for bacterial adhesion. These events can involve a complex series of interactions involving mucins, other salivary components, different bacteria, as well as various types of adhesins on the bacterial surface. Our present knowledge of mucin-bacterial interactions is the culmination of work carried out by many investigators over the last two decades. Earlier studies that examined salivary-bacterial interactions used intact secretions, most commonly whole saliva. More recently, a number of salivary components, including mucins, have been purified and biochemically characterized. The availability of these reagents and a wide array of assays has permitted investigators to gain an insight into the mechanisms involved in salivary-bacterial interactions.

Mucins in dental pellicles - Bacteria can attach to a layer of proteins which almost instantaneously forms on a freshly cleaned enamel surface (Busscher *et al.*, 1989). This protein layer is termed the acquired enamel pellicle (AEP). Analogous biofilms are also formed on other oral surfaces such as cementum (Fisher *et al.*, 1987), dental materials (Edgerton *et al.*, 1987) and soft tissues (Bradway *et al.*, 1989). The composition of pellicles may be different from surface to surface. However, further studies are needed to verify this point. Morphologically, the AEP was shown to be 0.5 - 0.8 μ in thickness (McDougall, 1963). The presence of carbohydrate in the AEP, first demonstrated by histochemical methods, was assumed to be derived from salivary glycoproteins (mucins) or bacterial products (McDougall, 1963). McGaughey and Stowell (1967) found that high molecular weight salivary materials (> 160 kDa) rapidly bound to hydroxyapatite (HAP). These components were presumed to be mucins since they stained with periodic acid-Schiff and Alcian blue. Blood-group reactive substance was also reported in AEP, supporting the presence of mucins (Sönju *et al.*, 1974). Other studies noted that salivary components that adsorbed onto the tooth surface contained galactose, mannose, fucose, glucosamine and galactosamine but lacked sialic acid. This suggested that adsorbed components were altered or degraded, possibly by enzymes of host or bacterial origin (Hay, 1967). Further studies by Hay (1969) suggested that AEP formation may occur in two stages. Initially, only proteins that bind to HAP with high affinity, such as the proline-rich proteins, are adsorbed. Next, other components such as mucins may adsorb with lower affinity to the preceding layer. Other studies found that the amino acid composition of AEP differed from saliva, suggesting that pellicle forms through selective adsorption of salivary components (Mayhall, 1970). *In vivo* AEP differed from the *in vitro* counterpart, indicating that some processing or alteration of the AEP components occurred *in vivo*. Both *in vivo* and *in vitro* pellicle contained galactose, mannose, fucose, glucose and rhamnose (Mayhall and Butler, 1976). However, sialic acid was not found in *in vivo*

AEP further supporting the observation of Hay (1967). The presence of glucose and rhamnose may reflect the contribution of bacterial components or glycolipids in AEP formation (Mayhall, 1970; Mayhall and Butler, 1976).

Recently, with the availability of more sensitive radiolabelling techniques, *in vivo* studies have demonstrated that MG1, but not MG2, was present in 2-hour AEP (Al-Hashimi and Levine, 1989). Fisher *et al.* (1987) verified the lack of MG2 in AEP, but found this mucin on cementum *in vivo*. This tissue specific tropism of mucins may be explained by degradation of MG2 on enamel surfaces *in vivo* or by a difference in the adsorptive behavior of these two mucins. *In vitro* studies have evaluated the adsorption of MG1 and MG2 to HAP. Langmuir adsorption isotherms indicated that MG1 had a greater affinity for HAP than MG2 and may preferentially function at tissue surfaces (Levine *et al.*, 1985; Tabak *et al.*, 1985). These *in vitro* studies suggest that small amounts of MG2 may adsorb to AEP *in vivo* but the techniques for detecting this mucin may have been inadequate.

Interaction of mucins with bacteria - In saliva, high molecular weight blood-group reactive glycoproteins have been shown to interact with a wide variety of oral microorganisms usually resulting in agglutination (Gibbons and Spinell, 1970; Hay *et al.*, 1971; Ericson *et al.*, 1976; Magnusson and Ericson, 1976; Kondo *et al.*, 1978; Levine *et al.*, 1978; Hogg and Embery, 1979; Eggert, 1980; Ellen *et al.*, 1983; Malamud *et al.*, 1984; Rundegren, 1986; Brack and Reynolds, 1987; Ebisu *et al.*, 1988). Gibbons and coworkers were among the first to describe a salivary bacterial agglutinin that was considered to be a high molecular weight blood-group reactive glycoprotein (Gibbons and Spinell, 1970; Hay *et al.*, 1971). A similar substance was extracted from dental plaque suggesting a role for this material in plaque formation. Bacteria such as *Streptococcus mutans* bound blood-group reactive components from whole saliva and mucin-like components isolated from submandibular-sublingual saliva (Gibbons and Quereshi, 1976). The ability of submandibular-sublingual saliva, but not parotid saliva, to agglutinate selected bacterial strains further supports the role of mucins in this activity (Ligtenberg *et al.*, 1991). Solid phase overlay assays using isolated bacterial components and/or individual salivary molecules also indicated that mucins may serve as receptors for specific bacterial adhesins on oral streptococci (Lamont *et al.*, 1988; Russell and Rahemtulla, 1989; Haraszthy *et al.*, 1991). Further investigations expanded the number of bacterial species capable of binding blood-group reactive substance preparations to include other streptococci and *Actinomyces* (Gibbons and Quereshi, 1978). Highly purified monkey salivary mucin and enriched preparations of human salivary mucins were both found to agglutinate strains of *S. mutans* and *S. sanguis* (Levine *et al.*, 1978). Interestingly, removal of mucin sialic acid residues abolished the agglutination activity for *S. sanguis* but not *S. mutans*. Mucin glycopeptides failed to induce agglutination of any of the strains tested, indicating that a certain density of oligosaccharides units may be required for agglutinating activity.

Due to the large number and distribution of O-linked oligosaccharides, MG2 was considered to be responsible for agglutination of *S. sanguis* and other species of bacteria (Tabak *et al.*, 1982; Levine *et al.*, 1985; Scannapieco *et al.*, 1987; Haraszthy *et al.*, 1991). Indeed, glycoproteins resembling MG2 have been shown to agglutinate *Eikenella corrodens* (Ebisu *et al.*, 1988) and *S. sanguis, S. oralis* and *S. rattus* (Koop *et al.*, 1990). Incubation of a variety of bacterial species with submandibular-sublingual saliva revealed MG2 to be a principal component of the "salivary pellicle" which coats or binds to bacteria in solution (Scannapieco *et al.*, 1987). Furthermore, depletion of MG2, but not MG1, from submandibular-sublingual saliva with immobilized antimucin antibody resulted in the loss of agglutination activity for *S. sanguis* and *S. mitis* (Jones *et al.*, 1987).

Although MG2 may be the major agglutinin in submandibular-sublingual saliva, MG1 has also been shown to mediate calcium-dependent agglutination of *S. sanguis* but not *S. mutans* (Hogg and Embery, 1979). The presence of a similar sulphated glycoprotein in human calculus would suggest a role for this material in plaque formation (Embery, 1977). In addition to mucins, saliva contains other components capable of agglutinating bacteria. These include a fucose-rich glycoprotein from parotid saliva (Ericson and Rundegren, 1983; Rundegren, 1986; Demuth *et al.*, 1990;), lysozyme (Pollock *et al.*, 1976; Iacono *et al.*, 1985) and sIgA (Williams and Gibbons, 1972; Liljemark *et al.*, 1979; Wold *et al.*, 1990).

Bacterial adherence to mucin in dental pellicles - The *in vitro* saliva-coated hydroxyapatite (sHAP) system is now widely used to study the interaction of bacteria with teeth (Gibbons *et al.*, 1976). This system has shown that viridans streptococci such as *S. sanguis* bind to at least two components in AEP; a sialic acid-containing receptor through a high-affinity interaction (Williams and Gibbons, 1972; Gibbons *et al.*, 1985a,b; Cowen *et al.*, 1987b; Liljemark *et al.*, 1989) and a hydrophobic and/or pH-sensitive receptor by a low-affinity, nonspecific interaction (Morris and McBride, 1984). These data are supported by kinetic studies of *S. sanguis* binding to sHAP where the initial reversible stage of adhesion to pellicle was unaffected by neuraminidase treatment, while the second stage of more firm adhesion was sialic acid dependent (Cowen *et al.*, 1987a). The desorption of *S. sanguis* from control pellicles exhibited two sequential rates, but desorption from neuraminidase-treated pellicles took place at a single rate equivalent to the initial rate constant for the control desorption. These findings suggest that sialic acid of AEP glycoproteins plays little role in the initial stage of bacterial adhesion, but does participate in the transition to higher-affinity interactions. Since mucins contain considerable amounts of terminal sialic acid (Prakobphol *et al.*, 1982; Loomis *et al.*, 1987) and have been identified in AEP (Al-Hashimi and Levine, 1989), it is reasonable to suggest that they serve as a high-affinity pellicle receptor for bacterial attachment. Indeed, other studies have demonstrated that the MG2 promotes *S. sanguis* adherence to glass, and that this interaction was abolished by the removal of this mucins sialic acid residues (Stinson *et al.*, 1982).

In contrast to sialic acid dependent adhesion, the adhesion of *S. mutans* and certain strains of *S. sanguis* to AEP appears to involve a galactose-containing receptor (Gibbons *et al.*, 1985b; Liljemark *et al.*, 1989). Galactose is often the terminal or penultimate sugar found on salivary mucin oligosaccharides (Reddy *et al.*, 1984) and is exposed following the removal of sialic acid by neuraminidase-producing organisms (Costello *et al.*, 1979; Ellen *et al.*, 1980; Murray *et al.*, 1984). Mucins may therefore serve as pellicle receptors for the adhesion of cariogenic streptococci to hydroxyapatite (Gibbons *et al.*, 1986; Gibbons and Hay, 1989). If sialic acid containing residues are modified by bacterial neuraminidases, more galactose residues would become available to bind increasing numbers of *S. mutans*.

Role of mucins in plaque maturation - Following the initial adhesion of bacteria to AEP, dental plaque may develop by at least two mechanisms: 1) the adhesion of additional bacteria to AEP-bound pioneer bacteria, and 2) growth and division of adherent bacteria. There is little experimental evidence to support the potential role of mucins in both processes. The first mechanism, known as interbacterial aggregation or coaggregation, is rather well studied when considering bacterial interactions by themselves (Kolenbrander, 1988). However, the role of saliva in this process has received little attention. Initial studies suggested that saliva may have little effect on these interactions (Kolenbrander and Phucas, 1984). In contrast, other studies suggest that salivary components may indeed modulate selective interactions (Komiyama and Gibbons, 1984; Ellen *et al.*, 1988; Nagata *et al.*, 1990; Stinson *et al.*, 1991). To date, the specific role of mucins in modulating coaggregation is essentially unexplored.

With respect to growth and division of adherent bacteria in plaque, salivary components could provide a significant nutritional source for oral bacteria and several studies support this contention. In fact, it has been proposed that bacteria specifically bind salivary molecules in order to capture nutritional substrates (De Jong and van der Hoeven, 1987; Ligtenberg *et al.*, 1991). When dental plaque was cultivated on defined media having saliva as the sole nutrient source, certain species such as *S. sanguis*, *Peptostreptococcus micros* and *Fusobacterium nucleatum* grew and were enriched, while other species such as *Actinomyces viscosus* were lost despite being present in the original inoculum (De Jong and van der Hoeven, 1987). The glycosidases and proteases produced by these enriched species resulted in their complete consumption from the culture medium. Further studies demonstrated that pig gastric mucin can act as the sole nutrient source for strains of *S. mitis*, *S. sanguis* and *S. mitior*, but not for strains of mutans streptococci (van der Hoeven *et al.*, 1990). These strains produced exoglycosidases capable of degrading mucin oligosaccharides. Such findings are interesting since *S. mitis*, *S. sanguis* and *S. mitior* are pioneer species in plaque and become established independently of dietary substrate availability.

Mutans streptococci, on the other hand, seem to require dietary carbohydrate to survive in appreciable numbers in the oral environment (Hamada and Slade, 1980). In fact, organisms possessing glycosidases may enable other organisms lacking such enzymes to use mucins as a nutrient source (van der Hoeven and Camp, 1991).

Mechanisms of Mucin-Streptococcal Interactions

Following initial random contact, bacteria adhere to enamel pellicles by at least two complementary mechanisms. The first involves nonspecific ionic and hydrophobic forces which align the bacterial surface components with pellicle constituents. The second involves stereochemical interactions which lock and stabilize bacterial surface adhesins to host receptors. A number of oral bacteria have lectin-like adhesins which bind to mucin oligosaccharides. For example, removal of sialic acid diminished the ability of mucins to agglutinate *S. sanguis* but not *S. mutans*, suggesting a specific interaction between sialic acid and *S. sanguis* (McBride and Gisslow, 1977; Levine *et al.*, 1978). The acidic trisaccharide of MG2 (Neuα2,3Galβ1,3GalNAc) is a potent inhibitor of *S. sanguis*-mediated hemagglutination (Murray *et al.*, 1982). These findings indicate that certain oral streptococci (including *S. sanguis*, *S. mitis*, *S. gordonnii* and *S. oralis*) have a surface lectin specific for sialic acid-containing structures (Murray *et al.*, 1986).

The aformentioned studies demonstrate that mucins in saliva can agglutinate bacteria while mucins in AEP can promote bacterial adherence. These events appear to be dependent upon whether mucin's interaction with bacteria, particularly viridans streptococci, takes place in solution (agglutination) or on solid surfaces (adherence). For example, solid phase assays using glass (Stinson *et al.*, 1982) or Immobilon^{TM} membranes (Haraszthy *et al.*, 1991) demonstrated that *S. gordonii* G9B binds to highly purified immobilized MG2. In solution phase assays, however, highly purified MG2 does not bind appreciably to these bacteria. In contrast, MG2 in native submandibular-sublingual saliva (e.g. in the presence of other salivary components) can interact with *S. gordonii* G9B in either type of assay. Comparable findings are obtained in the case of MG2 binding to mucosal pathogens such as *Pseudomonas aeruginosa* and *Staphylococcus aureus* (Biesbrock *et al.*, 1991). A similar observation was also made with a rat sialic acid-containing mucin complex which mediates calcium-dependent *S. mutans* agglutination (Brack and Reynolds, 1987). Removal of the mucin's sialic acid residues had no effect on *S. mutans* agglutination. However, when this mucin complex was dissociated into several components, each of these components alone no longer possessed agglutinating activity. It was postulated that mucin subunits are assembled into a macromolecular, agglutinating complex by the formation of calcium bridges between negatively charged bacterial surface

TABLE 1 *Future Directions of Salivary Mucin Research*

1. Continue structural studies
   a. oligosaccharides
   b. proteins
   c. lipids
   d. macromolecular structure
   e. conformation
2. Function of these domains
   a. AEP formation
   b. initial colonization
   c. plaque maturation
   d. rheological and viscoelastic properties
3. Nature and function of mucin complexing with other salivary molecules
4. Develop and design biocompatible antiplaque agents (artificial salivas)
   a. enhance function
   b. molecular mimicry: carbohydrate → peptide
   c. immortalize conformation
   5. Genetic manipulation of mucin function

components and mucin sialic acid or sulphate residues. Perhaps, the local microenvironment affects either the conformation of mucin or complexation of mucin with other salivary components; events which can subsequently play a role in selected mucin-microbial interactions.

Future Directions in Mucin Research

Some future directions for salivary mucin research are outlined in Table 1. There must be a continuation of efforts toward elucidation of structure-function relationships. Areas requiring additional studies include structural characterization of oligosaccharides, protein moieties (apomucin), associated lipids, macromolecular structure, and conformation.

Oligosaccharides and peptides - Previous studies dealing with human salivary mucins have focused on the role of their carbohydrate units since these comprise a major portion of the molecule (for review, see Cohen and Levine, 1989). More information is available on the oligosaccharide units of MG2 than MG1. Very little is known about the peptide portions of these molecules. Classical biochemical approaches have proved difficult due to the mucin's high molecular weight, high density of carbohydrate, unique amino acid composition and physico-chemical properties. However, molecular biological approaches have deduced the partial or complete amino acid sequences of mucins from human trachea (Gerard *et al.*, 1990), human intestine (Gum *et al.*, 1989), porcine submaxillary gland (Timpte *et al.*, 1988; Eckhardt *et al.*, 1991) mucin-like proteins from bovine submaxillary gland (Bhargava *et al.*, 1990), human breast or episialin (Gendler *et al.*, 1987; 1990; Ligtenberg *et al.*, 1990) and pancreatic tumor cells (Lan *et al.*, 1990). An interesting feature of the amino acid sequences of most of these mucins is the presence of tandem repeats. In general, these repeated sequences can be highly glycosylated and appear to have little or no secondary structure. While the function of tandem repeats remains unclear, it has been proposed that long stretches of highly glycosylated polypeptides may contribute to the viscoelastic properties of mucins in solution (Eckhardt *et al.*, 1991). In addition to tandem repeats, other portions of mucin's peptide may have functional significance. In a recent study, Eckardt *et al.* (1991) found that porcine submaxillary mucin contains a cystine-rich carboxyl terminal domain with a predicted secondary structure consistent with globular peptides. They postulate that this domain may be involved in intermolecular disulfide bonds that help the formation of mucin's multimeric or macromolecular structure. Future studies with human salivary mucins will be directed toward deducing their complete amino acid sequence and ascertaining the presence and function of tandem repeats.

Lipids - Several studies by Slominany and co-workers have focused on the nature of covalent and noncovalently bound lipids of salivary mucins (Slomiany *et al.*, 1989b). It appears that lipids are associated primarily with MG1 rather than MG2. These associations, particularly those of covalently bound fatty acids, occur in nonglycosylated domains (Loomis *et al.*, 1987; Slomiany *et al.*, 1989b). Studies are required to understand mechanisms and sites of acylation. Kasinathan *et al.* (1990) has shown that fatty acyltransferase activity is a cotranslational event. Investigations such as these will be facilitated by molecular biological studies on apomucins. Both covalent and non-covalently bounds lipids contribute to the viscoelastic properties of mucins in solution (Slomiany, 1989b). In particular, the content of covalently bound fatty acids may determine the extent of mucin interaction with non-covalently bound lipids (Slomiany *et al.*, 1989b). These investigators have attempted to correlate functional consequences of these lipid-mucin associations with caries resistance and caries susceptibility (for review, see Slomiany *et al.*, 1989a). However, additional studies are needed with sufficient numbers of subjects to correlate these parameters with caries and periodontal disease activity.

Macromolecular structure - Another area of needed research involves the characterization of mucin's macromolecular structure or association of mucin subunits through covalent and/or noncovalent forces into polymeric forms. Mucins can self-associate into homomers or associate with other molecules such as "link" (glyco)proteins to form heteromers. These polymeric forms are usually assembled intracellularly and may dictate mucin's viscoelastic and rheological properties. The presence of N-linked oligosaccharides may be essential for the formation of mucin's macromolecular structure while O-glycosylation may not be critical for these events (Dekker and Strous, 1990). In the case of heteromers, molecules associated with mucins may have their own distinct functions. For example, piliated strains of *Escherichia coli* can bind to the N-linked oligosaccharides located on the link glycopeptide of rat intestinal mucin (Sajjan and Forstner, 1990).

Conformation - Over the last decade, the majority of studies relating to mucin conformation have focused on the oligosaccharide units and have been facilitated by high resolution NMR (Vliegenthart *et al.*, 1983; van Halbeek, 1990) and mass spectroscopy techniques (also see chapter by Susan Fisher). Recently, protein crystallography has been used to study the stereospecific interaction between oligosaccharides bound to lectins or monoclonal antibodies. For example, Wright (1990) has examined the structure of a N-acetylneuraminyl-lactose-wheat germ agglutinin complex at 2.2 Å resolution while Cygler *et al.* (1991) determined the crystal structure of *Salmonella* dodecasaccharide-Fab complex at 2.05 Å resolution. Both studies were designed to explore the conformation of oligosaccharides in the bound state since these compounds exhibit a high degree of flexibility in solution. The role of Van der Waals forces, hydrogen bonding, and hydrophobic interactions between saccharide and saccharide and protein and saccharide were assessed. In an elegant study by Weis *et al.* (1988), the three-dimensional structure of influenza virus hemagglutinin complexed with sialyllactose found that sialic acids bound to a pocket of conserved amino acids surrounded by antibody binding sites. The proximity of the antibody binding sites indicated that the antibodies can neutralize virus infectivity by preventing virus binding to sialic acid receptors on cells. Similar studies are required with human salivary mucins, particularly to evaluate the mechanism of interaction between mucin oligosaccharides and bacterial lectins. In order to achieve this goal, the conformation of mucin oligosaccharides as well as the purification and biochemical characterization of relevant bacterial adhesins are required. The information obtained could suggest approaches for the design of antiplaque agents that could block attachment of bacteria to mucin coated surfaces.

Only a few studies have examined the conformation of an entire mucin molecule. Gerken *et al.* (1989), using carbon-13 NMR and light scattering techniques, found that the peptide linked GalNAc residue of ovine submaxillary mucin is a major determinant of peptide core conformation and mucin solution structure in general. Similar studies with human salivary mucins will provide valuable information on the conformation of these molecules. Collectively, these data can be used to more precisely define the role of mucins in the different stages of dental plaque formation.

Function - While mucins can now be assumed to participate in the formation of AEP *in vivo,* there are few direct data that describe the amount and fate of mucin in *in vivo* AEP over time. The "gold standard" regarding the time-frame for *in vivo* AEP collection has been 2 hours. Several questions remain unanswered. Are mucins degraded over time? What is the nature of this degradation?

We have recently prepared a monospecific polyclonal antibody to MG2 (Cohen *et al.*, 1991) that was used in SDS-PAGE/Western transfer analysis to evaluate MG2 in 20-minute, 2-hour, and 12-hour *in vivo* AEP. While intact MG2 was present in 20 AEP, it was partially degraded in 2-hour AEP, and completely in 12-hour AEP. Other issues to be addressed include the quality and quantity of pellicles on various oral surfaces (*e.g.* buccal versus lingual and interproximal enamel surfaces, different soft tissues and dental materials). These findings should be correlated with the occurrence of cariogenic or periodontopathic bacteria on these surfaces. Also, the variation of mucin deposition in AEP between individuals should be assessed and correlated with caries and periodontal disease activity.

An important property of AEP is to provide a lubricating surface between hard and soft tissues under dental incisal function, light and heavy mastication, and dental bruxing. Salivary glycoproteins, including mucins, have been shown to be effective lubricants under light masticatory conditions (Hatton *et al.*, 1985; 1987; Aguirre *et al.*, 1989). These glycoproteins and their complexes provide thin film lubrication under dental conditions of low occlusal load and high sliding speed. Physicochemical factors that contribute to this lubrication may be water retention due to solvation of carbohydrate residues with consequent effects on colligative properties and viscosity modification of saliva (Reeh *et al.*, 1990). Further studies are needed to define the structural requirements for these activities.

The majority of information on the role of mucins in microbial interactions has been discussed earlier in light of mucin's oligosaccharide interactions with carbohydrate binding adhesins on various oral bacteria. However, several questions remain unanswered regarding the function of these oligosaccharides in initial bacterial colonization and plaque maturation. What is the specificity and number of carbohydrate binding adhesins on different bacteria? Can these adhesins react with different mucins or other salivary glycoproteins and to what extent? Are these interactions the same when the mucins are adsorbed to oral surfaces as compared to their presence in solution? Similar questions can be asked regarding mucin's peptide, lipid, macromolecular structure and conformation. Indeed, it is likely that certain functions (*e.g.* viscoelastic properties) are dependent upon more than one aspect of mucin structure.

Heterotypic complexing - An active area of mucin research involves the significance of heterotypic complexing between mucins and molecules of salivary origin or otherwise. These types of interactions take place within the salivary ducts or the oral cavity and are therefore distinguished from intracellular associations involved in mucin's macromolecular structure. Complexing usually involves ionic forces, hydrogen bonding, and/or hydrophobic interactions. These may function on different intraoral surfaces or in solution. For example, mucins may function as a carrier to localize antimicrobials (*e.g.* lysozyme, cystatins, and sIgA) to oral hard and soft tissue interfaces. The noncovalent complexing of phospholipids with mucin in AEP may protect enamel from demineralization by acids from cariogenic bacteria (Slomiany *et al.*, 1989). In solution, the binding of a MG2-sIgA complex to mucosal pathogens may represent a nonspecific host defense mechanism (Biesbrock *et al.* 1991). A complex of mucins with lipids or albumin may have enhanced viscoelastic or rheological properties. In addition, the complex itself may have unique functional properties. All of these points require further investigation.

Development and design of artifical salivas - Ultimately, the long range goal of our salivary studies is to enhance the protective properties of saliva. This can be achieved by the design and development of antiplaque agents or artificial salivas. We propose to use the structural information on salivary molecules as a template for design since the compounds to be developed should be biocompatible as well as biodegradable. Two general patient populations should be considered; those with normal salivary flow and those with decreased salivary output. With regard to mucins, an important concern is their intraoral site of action. For example to minimize abrasion in individuals with decreased salivary flow, a mucin-like lubricant might be desirable for application to the enamel surface. Several points must then be considered. What part(s) of the molecule is involved in lubricity? Is the whole molecule needed for effective lubrication? Do these domains undergo a conformational change when adsorbed to enamel? If so, should this conformation be immortalized to insure its lubricity? Can these domains be engineered to insure that they lubricate on the enamel surface for an adequate period of time? Approriate decisions will be based upon the available information of mucin structure and function. Another potentially important function of mucins in artificial salivas is their ability to mask carbohydrate binding adhesins on the bacterial surface and thereby prevent microbial attachment. It may be possible to inhibit the microbial attachment of selected bacteria or their involvement in plaque maturation by artificial salivas consisting of oligosaccharides. Again, several practical considerations must be addressed. Which bacteria should be targeted and does their principal mode of attachment involve carbohydrates on salivary glycoproteins? Does the specificity of these interactions involve complex oligosaccharides and is their conformation important? The large-scale use of complex oligosaccharides as inhibitors of plaque formation may not prove practical since they are not easily manufactured and are therefore costly to produce. One possible alternative is the design and engineering of small peptides which mimic the oligosaccharide's conformation. This approach will require comparing the three-dimensional structure of the oligosaccharide in solution and in a bound state by co-crystallization with the relevant microbial adhesin. The information obtained can be used in conjunction with computer modeling to design and synthesize appropriate peptides. If successful, these peptides could be subsequently manufactured by conventional synthetic means or by recombinant technologies.

A final direction of mucin research involves the genetic manipulation of mucin synthesis to modify or enhance function. This type of approach has been discussed in greater detail by Dr. Tabak.

In summary, salivary mucin research is at an important threshold. The laboratory tools are now available to pursue and perhaps complete the structure-function studies on these molecules within the next decade. During this time, available information will be applied to clinical modalities aimed at modulating dental plaque formation and subsequent caries and periodontal disease activity.

REFERENCES

AGUIRRE, A.; MENDOZA, B.; REDDY, M.S.; SCANNAPIECO, F.A.; LEVINE, M.J.; and HATTON, M.N. (1989): Lubrication of Selected Salivary Molecules and Artificial Salivas, *Dysphagia* 4:95-100.

AL-HASHIMI, I. and LEVINE, M.J. (1989): Characterization of *In Vivo* Salivary-derived Enamel Pellicle, *Arch Oral Biol* 34:289-295.

ARNEBERG, P.; KORNSTAD, L.; NORDBØ, H.; and GJERMO, P. (1976): Less Dental Caries Among Secretors than Among Non-secretors of Blood Group Substance, *Scand J Dent Res* 84:362-366.

BHARGAVA, A.K.; WOITACH, J.T.; DAVIDSON, E.A.; and BHAVANANDAN, V.P. (1990): Cloning and cDNA Sequence of a Bovine Submaxillary Gland Mucin-like Protein Containing Two Distinct Domains, *Proc Natl Acad Sci USA* 87:6798-6802.

BIESBROCK, A.; REDDY, M.S.; and LEVINE, M.J. (1991): Interaction of a Salivary Mucin-secretory IgA Complex with Mucosal Pathogens, *Infect Immun*, 59:3492-3497.

BRACK, C.M. and REYNOLDS, E.C. (1987): Characterization of a Rat Salivary Sialoglycoprotein Complex which Agglutinates *Streptococcus mutans, Infect Immun* 55:1264-1273.

BRADWAY, S.D.; BERGEY, E.J.; JONES, P.C.; and LEVINE, M.J. (1989): Oral Mucosal Pellicle. Adsorption and Transpeptidation of Salivary Components to Buccal Epithelial Cells, *Biochem J* 261:887-896.

BUSSCHER, H.J.; UYEN, H.M.W.; STOKROOS, I.; and JONGEBLOED, W.L. (1989): A Transmission Electron Microscopy Study of the Adsorption Patterns of Early Developing Artificial Pellicles on Human Enamel, *Arch Oral Biol* 34:803-810.

COHEN, R.E.; AGUIRRE, A.; NEIDERS, M.E.; LEVINE, M.J.; JONES, P.C.; REDDY, M.S., and HAAR, J. G. (1990): Immunochemistry of High Molecular-weight Salivary Mucin, *Arch Oral Biol* 35:127-136.

COHEN, R.E.; AGUIRRE, A.; NEIDERS, M.E.; LEVINE, M.J.; JONES, P.C.; REDDY, M.S.; and HAAR, J. G. (1991): Immunochemistry and Immunogenicity of Low Molecular-weight Human Salivary Mucin, *Arch Oral Biol* 36:347-356.

COHEN, R.E. and LEVINE, M.J. (1989): Salivary Glycoproteins. In: *Human Saliva: Clinical Chemistry and Microbiology*, J.O. Tenouvo, Ed., Boca Raton: CRC Press, pp.101-130.

COSTELLO, A.H.; CISAR, J.O.; KOLLENBRANDER, P.R.; and GABRIEL,O. (1979): Neuraminidase-dependent Hemagglutination of Human Erythrocytes by Strains of *Actinomyces viscosus* and *Actinomyces naeslundii, Infect Immun* 26:563-572.

COWEN, M.M.; TAYLOR, K.G.; and DOYLE, R.J. (1987a): Energetics of the Initial Phase of Adhesion of *Streptococcus sanguis* to Hydroxylapatite, *J Bacteriol* 169:2995-3000.

COWEN, M.M.; TAYLOR, K.G.; and DOYLE, R.J. (1987b): Role of Sialic Acid in the Kinetics of *Streptococcus sanguis* Adhesion to Artificial Pellicle, *Infect Immun* 55:1552-1557.

CYGLER, M.; ROSE, D.R.; and BUNDLE, D.R. (1991): Recognition of a Cell-Surface Oligosaccharide of Pathogenic *Salmonella* by an Antibody Fab Fragment, *Science* 253:442-445.

DE JONG, M.H. and VAN DER HOEVEN, J.S. (1987): The Growth of Bacteria on Saliva, *J Dent Res* 66:498-505.

DEKKER, J. and STROUS, G.J. (1990): Covalent Oligomerization of Rat Gastric Mucin occurs in the Rough Endoplasmic Reticulum, is N-Glycosylation-Dependent, and Precedes Initial O-Glycosylation, *J Biol Chem* 265:18116-18122.

DEMUTH, D.R.; LAMMEY, M.S.; HUCK, M.; and MALAMUD, D. (1990): Comparison of *Streptococcus mutans* and *Streptococcus sanguis* Receptors for Human Salivary Agglutinin, *Microb Path* 9:199-211.

DEWAR, M.R. and PARFIT, G.J. (1954): Physical Properties of Saliva and Caries Activity, *J Dent Res* 33:756.

EBISU, S.; FUKUHARA, H.; and OKADA, H. (1988): Purification and Characterization of *Eikenella corrodens* Aggregating Factor from Submandubular-Sublingual Saliva, *J Periodont Res* 23:328-333.

ECKHARDT, A.E., TIMPTE, C.S., ABERNETHY, J.L., ZHAO, Y.; and HILL R.L. (1991): Porcine Submaxillary Mucin Contains a Cystine-rich, Carboxyl-terminal Domain in Addition to a Highly Repetitive, Glycosylated Domain, *J Biol Chem* 266:9678-9686.

EDGERTON, M.; TABAK, L.A.; and LEVINE, M.J. (1987): Saliva: a Significant Factor in Removable Prosthodontic Treatment., *J Prosthet Dent* 57:57-66.

EGGERT, F.M. (1980): The Nature of Secretory Agglutinins and Aggregating Factors. I. Secretory Conglutinin-like Factor, Secretory Bacterial Aggregating Factors and Secretory IgA Antibody in Human Saliva and Amniotic Fluid, *Int Arch Aller Appl Immunol* 61:192-202.

ELLEN, R.P.; FILLERY, E.D.; CHAN, K.H.; and GROVE, D.A. (1980): Sialidase-enhanced Lectin-like Mechanism for *Actinomyces viscosus* and *Actinomyces naeslundii* Hemagglutination, *Infect Immun* 27:335-343.

ELLEN, R.P.; BRATTHALL D.; BORGSTRÖM, M.; and HOWLEY, T.P. (1983): *Actinomyces viscosus* and *Actinomyces naeslundii* Agglutinins in Human Saliva, *Scand J Dent Res* 91:263-273.

ELLEN, R.P.; SCWARZ-FAULKNER, S.; and GROVE, D.A. (1988): Coaggregation Among Periodontal Pathogens, Emphasizing *Bacteroides gingivalis-Actinomyces viscosus* Cohesion on a Saliva-coated Mineral Surface, *Can J Microbiol* 34: 299-306.

EMBERY, G. (1977): A Sulphated Glycopeptide in Human Supragingival Calculus Extracts, *Calc Tiss Res* 23:13-17.

ERICSON, T.; CARLÉN, A.; and DAGERSKOG, E. (1976). Salivary Aggregating Factors. In: *Microbial Aspects of Dental Caries*, Vol 1, H.M. Stiles, W.J. Loesche and T.C. O'Brian, Eds. Washington: Information Retrival, pp. 151-162.

ERICSON, T. and RUNDEGREN, J. (1983): Characterization of a Salivary Agglutinin Reacting with a Serotype c Strain of *Streptococcus mutans*, *Eur J Biochem* 133:255-261.

FISHER, S.J.; PRAKOBPHOL, A.; KAJISA, L.; and MURRAY, P.A. (1987): External Radiolabelling of Components of Pellicle on Human Enamel and Cementum, *Arch Oral Biol* 32:509-517.

GENDLER, S.J.; BURCHELL, J.M.; DUHIG, T.; LAMPORT, D.; WHITE, R.; PARKER, M.; and TAYLOR-PAPADIMITRIOU, J. (1987): Cloning of Partial cDNA encoding Differentiation and Tumor-associated Mucin Glycoproteins Expressed by Human Mammary Epithelium, *Proc Natl Acad Sci USA* 84:6060-6064.

GENDLER, S.J.; LANCASTER, C.A.; TAYLOR-PAPADIMITRIOU, J.; DUHIG, T.; PEAT, N.; BURCHELL, J.; PEMBERTON, L.; LALANI, E-N.; and WILSON, D. (1990): Molecular Cloning and Expression of Human Tumor-associated Polymorphic Epithelial Mucin, *J Biol Chem* 265:15286-15293.

GERARD, C.; EDDY, R.L.; and SHOWS, T.B. (1990): The Core Polypeptide of Cystic Fibrosis Tracheal Mucin Contains a Tandem Repeat Structure, *J Clin Invest* 86:1921-1927.

GERKEN, T.A.; BUTENHOF, K.J.; and SHOGREN, R. (1989): Effects of Glycosylation on the Conformation and Dynamics of O-Linked Glycoproteins: Carbon-13 NMR Studies of Ovine Submaxillary Mucin, *Biochemistry* 28:5536-5543.

GIBBONS, R.J.; COHEN, L.; and HAY, D.I. (1986): Strains of *Streptococcus mutans* and *Streptococcus sobrinus* Attach to Different Pellicle Receptors, *Infect Immun* 52:555-561.

GIBBONS, R.J.; ETHERDEN, I.; and MORENO, E.C. (1985a): Contribution of Stereochemical Interactions in the Adhesion of *Streptococcus sanguis* C5 to Experimental Pellicles, *J Dent Res* 64:96-101.

GIBBONS, R.J.; ETHERDEN, I.; and PEROS, W. (1985b). Aspects of the Attachment of Oral Streptococci to Experimental Pellicles. In: *Molecular Basis of Oral Microbial Adhesion*, S.E. Mergenhagen and B. Rosan, Eds. Washington: American Society for Microbiology, pp.77-84.

GIBBONS, R.J. and HAY, D.I. (1989): Adsorbed Salivary Acidic Proline-rich Proteins Contribute to the Adhesion of *Streptococcus mutans* JPB to Apatitic Surfaces, *J Dent Res* 68:1303-1307.

GIBBONS, R.J.; MORENO, E.C.; and SPINELL, D.M. (1976): Model Delineating the Effects of a Salivary Pellicle on the Adsorption of *Streptococcus miteor* onto Hydroxyapatite, *Infect Immun* 14:1109-1112.

GIBBONS, R.J. and QUERESHI, V. (1976). Interactions of *Streptococcus mutans* and Other Oral Bacteria with Blood Group Reactive Substances. In: *Microbial Aspects of Dental Caries*, Vol 1, H.M. Stiles, W.J. Loesche and T.C. O'Brian, Eds. Washington: Information Retrival, pp.163-181.

GIBBONS, R.J. and QUERESHI, J.V. (1978): Selective Binding of Blood Group-reactive Salivary Mucins by *Streptococcus mutans* and Other Oral Organisms, *Infect Immun* 22:665-671.

GIBBONS, R.J. and SPINELL, D.M. (1970). Salivary-induced Aggregation of Plaque Bacteria. In: *Dental Plaque*, W.D. McIlugh, Ed. Edinburgh, E. and S. Edinborough, Livingstone, Ltd., pp. 207-216.

GIBBONS, R.J. and VAN HOUTE, J. (1975): Dental Caries, *Ann Rev Med* 26:121-136.

GUM, J.R.; BYRD, J.C.; HICKS, J.W.; TORIBARA, N.W.; LAMPORT, D.T.A.; and KIM, Y.S. (1989): Molecular Cloning of Human Intestinal Mucin cDNAs. Sequence Analysis and Evidence for Genetic Polymorphism, *J Biol Chem* 264: 6480-6487.

HAMADA, S. and SLADE, H.D. (1980): Biology, Immunology and Cariogenicity of *Streptococcus mutans*, *Microbiol Rev* 44:331-384.

HARASZTHY, G.G.; SCANNAPIECO, F.A.; BERGEY, E.J.; REDDY, M.S.; BOBEK, L.A.; and LEVINE, M. J. (1991): Characterization and Molecular Cloning of a Salivary Mucin Binding Component from *Streptococcus gordonii* G9B, Abstracts of the Annual Meeting, Washington: American Society for Microbiology.

HATTON, M.N.; LEVINE, M.J.; MARGARONE, J.E.; and AGUIRRE, A. (1987): Lubrication and Viscosity Features of Human Saliva and Commercially Available Saliva Substitutes, *J Oral Maxillofac Surg* 45:496-499.

HATTON, M.N.; LOOMIS, R.E.; LEVINE, M.J.; and TABAK, L.A. (1985): The Role of Carbohydrate in the Lubricating Property of a Salivary Glycoprotein-Albumin Complex, *Biochem J* 230:817-820.

HAY, D.I. (1967): The Adsorption of Salivary Proteins by Hydroxyapatite and Enamel, *Arch Oral Biol* 12:937-946.

HAY, D.I. (1969): Some Observations on Human Saliva Proteins and Their Role in the Formation of the Acquired Enamel Pellicle, *J Dent Res* 48(Suppl. 5):806-810.

HAY, D.I.; GIBBONS, R.J.; and SPINELL, D.M. (1971): Characteristics of Some High Molecular Weight Constituents with Bacterial aggregating Activity from Whole Saliva and Dental Plaque, *Caries Res* 5:111-123.

HEANEY, T.G.; EMBERY, G.; and GREEN, D. (1986): Saliva and Salivary Sulphated Glycoprotein Inhibit Adhesion and Locomotion of Human Gingival Fibroblast-like Cells *In Vitro*, *J Periodont Res* 21:266-278.

HOGG, S.D. and EMBERY, G. (1979): The Isolation and Partial Characterization of a Sulphated Glycoprotein from Human Whole Saliva Which Aggregates Strains of *Streptococcus sanguis* but not *Streptococcus mutans*, *Arch Oral Biol* 24:791-797.

IACONO, V.J.; ZOVE, S.M.; GROSSBARD, B.L.; POLLOCK, J.J.; FINE, D.H.; and GREENE, L.S. (1985): Lysozyme-mediated Aggregation and Lysis of the Periodontal Microorganism *Capnocytophaga gingivalis* 2010, *Infect Immun* 47:457-464.

JONES, P.C.; COHEN, R.E.; and LEVINE, M.J. (1987): Streptococcal Agglutination by Human Submandibular-Sublingual Saliva Depleted of Mucin Glycoproteins, *J Dent Res* 66:Abst. No. 1431.

KAPSIMILIS, P.; ROSENTHAL, S.L.; UPDEGRAVE, W.; EVANS, R.; HURLEY, B.; and COBE, H.M. (1966): The Relationship between Caries Activity, Flow Rate, Total Nitrogen and the Mucin Content of Saliva, *J Oral Med* 21:107-110.

KASINATHAN, C.; GRZELINSKA, E.; OKAZAKI, K.; SLOMIANY, B.L.; and SLOMIANY, A. (1990): Purification of Protein Fatty Acyltransferase and Determination of its Distribution and Topology, *Biol Chem* 265:5139-5144.

KIRK, E.C. (1910): A Consideration of the Question of Susceptibility and Immunity to Dental Caries, *Dent Cosmos* 52:729-739.

KOLENBRANDER, P.E. (1988): Intergeneric Coaggregation Among Human Oral Bacteria and Ecology of Dental Plaque, *Ann Rev Microbiol* 42:627-656.

KOLENBRANDER, P.E. and PHUCAS, C.S. (1984): Effect of Saliva on Coaggregation of Oral *Actinomyces* and *Streptococcus* species, *Infect Immun* 44:228-236.

KOMIYAMA, K. and GIBBONS, R.J. (1984): Inhibition of Lactose-reversible Adherence between *Actinomyces viscosus* and Oral Streptococci by Salivary Components, *Caries Res* 18:193-201.

KONDO, W.; SATO, M.; and SATO, N. (1978): Properties of the Human Salivary Aggregating Factor for *Leptotrichia buccalis*, *Arch Oral Biol* 23:453-458.

KOOP, H.M.; VALENTIJN-BENZ, M.; NIEW AMERONGEN, A.V.; ROUKEMA, P.A.; and DE GRAAFF, J. (1990): Involvement of Human Mucous Saliva and Salivary Mucins in the Aggregation of the Oral Bacteria *Streptococcus sanguis, Streptococcus oralis* and *Streptococcus rattus*, *Anton van Leeuw* 57:245-252.

LAMONT, R.J.; ROSAN, B.; MURPHY, G.M.; and BAKER, C.T. (1988): *Streptococcus sanguis* Surface Antigens and Their Interactions with Saliva, *Infect Immun* 56:64-70.

LAN, M.S.; BATRA, S.K.; QI, W-N.; METZGAR, R.S.; and HOLLINGSWORTH, M.A. (1990): Cloning and Sequencing of a Human Pancreatic Tumor Mucin cDNA, *J Biol Chem* 265:15294-15299.

LEVINE, M.J.; HERZBERG, M.C.; LEVINE, M.S.; ELLISON, S.A.; STINSON, M.W.; LI, H.C.; and VAN DYKE, T. (1978): Specificity of Salivary-bacterial Interactions: Role of Terminal Sialic Acid Residues in the Interaction of Salivary Glycoprotein with *Streptococcus sanguis* and *Streptococcus mutans*, *Infect. Immun* 19:107-115.

LEVINE, M.J.; L.A.TABAK; REDDY, M.S.; and MANDEL, I.D. (1985): Nature of Salivary Pellicles in Microbial Adherence: Role of Salivary Mucins. In: *Molecular Basis of Oral Microbial Adhesion*, S.E. Mergenhagen and B. Rosan, Eds. Washington: American Society for Microbiology, pp. 125-130.

LEVINE, M.J.; REDDY, M.S.; TABAK, L.A.; LOOMIS, R.E.; BERGEY, E.J.; JONES, P.C.; COHEN, R. E.; STINSON, M. W.; and AL-HASHIMI, I. (1987): Structural Aspects of Salivary Glycoproteins, *J Dent Res* 66:436-441.

LIGTENBERG, A.J.M.; CAMP, P.J.M.; VAN DER HOEVEN, J.S.; VEERMAN, E.C.I.; and NIEW AMERONGEN, A.V. (1991): Aggregation of Oral Streptococci Selected by Growth on Human Saliva from Different Glands, *Microbial Ecol Health Dis* 4:29-37.

LIGTENBERG, M.J.L.; VOS, H.L.; GENNISSEN, A.M.C.; and HILKENS, J. (1990): Episialin, a Carcinoma-associated Mucin, is Generated by a Polymorphic Gene encoding Splice Variants with Alternative Amino Termini, *J Biol Chem* 265:5573-5578.

LILJEMARK, W.F.; BLOOMQUIST, C.G.; FENNER, L.J.; ANTONELLI, P.J.; and COULTER, M.C. (1989): Effect of Neuraminidase on the Adherence to Salivary Pellicle of *Streptococcus sanguis* and *Streptococcus mitis*, *Caries Res* 23:141-145.

LILJEMARK, W.F.; BLOOMQUIST, C.G.; and OFSTEHAGE, J.C. (1979): Aggregation and Adherence of *Streptococcus sanguis*: Role of Human Salivary Immunoglobulin A, *Infect Immun* 26:1104-1110.

LOOMIS, R.E.; PRAKOBPHOL, A.; LEVINE, M.J.; REDDY, M.S.; and JONES, P.C. (1987): Biochemical and Biophysical Comparison of Two Mucins from Human Submandibular-Sublingual Saliva, *Arch Biochem Biophys* 258:452-464.

MAGNUSSON, I. and ERICSON, T. (1976): Effect of Salivary Agglutinins on Reactions Between Hydroxyapatite and a Serotype c Strain of *Streptococcus mutans*, *Caries Res* 10:273-286.

MALAMUD, D.; BROWN, C.; and GOLDMAN, R. (1984): Inhibition of Bacterial Aggregation by Serum and Blood-derived Proteins, *Infect Immun* 43:386-390.

MANDEL, I.D. (1974): Relation of Saliva and Plaque to Caries, *J Dent Res* 53 (Suppl):246-266.

MANDEL, I.D. (1980): Sialochemistry in Diseases and Clinical Situations affecting Salivary Glands, *CRC Crit Rev Clin Lab Sci* 12:321-366.

MANDEL, I.D. (1987): The Functions of Saliva, *J Dent Res* 66 (Spec Iss):623-633.

MAYHALL, C.W. (1970): Concerning the Composition and Source of the Acquired Enamel Pellicle of Human Teeth, *Arch Oral Biol* 15:1327-1341.

MAYHALL, C.W. and BUTLER, W.T. (1976): The Carbohydrate Composition of Experimental Salivary Pellicles, *J Oral Pathol* 5:358-370.

MCBRIDE, B.C. and GISSLOW, M.T. (1977): Role of Sialic Acid in Saliva-induced Aggregation of *Streptococcus sanguis*, *Infect Immun* 18:35-40.

MCDOUGALL, W.A. (1963): Studies on the Dental Plaque. I. The Histology of the Dental Plaque and its Attachment, *Austral Dent J* 8:261-273.

MCGAUGHEY, C. and STOWELL, E.C. (1967): The Adsorption of Human Salivary Proteins and Porcine Submaxillary Mucin by Hydroxyapatite, *Arch Oral Biol* 12:815-828.

MORRIS, E.J. and MCBRIDE, B.C. (1984): Adherence of *Streptococcus sanguis* to Saliva-coated Hydroxyapatite: Evidence for Two Binding Sites, *Infect Immun* 43:656-663.

MURRAY, P.A.; LEVINE, M.J.; REDDY, M.S.; TABAK, L.A.; and BERGEY, E.J. (1986): Preparation of a Sialic-binding Protein from *Streptococcus mitis* KS32AR, *Infect Immun* 53: 359-365.

MURRAY, P.A.; LEVINE, M.J.; TABAK, L.A.; and REDDY, M.S. (1982): Specificity of Salivary-bacterial Interactions: II. Evidence for a Lectin on *Streptococcus sanguis* with Specificity for a NeuAcα2, 3Galβ1, 3GalNAc Sequence, *Biochem Biophys Res Comm* 106:390-396.

MURRAY, P.A.; LEVINE, M.J.; TABAK, L.A.; and REDDY, M.S. (1984): Neuraminidase Activity: A Biochemical Marker to Distinguish *Streptococcus mitis* from *Streptococcus sanguis*, *J Dent Res* 63: 111-113.

NAGATA, H.; MORAKAMI, Y.; INOSHITA, E.; SHIZUJUISKI, S.; and TSUNEMITSU, A. (1990): Inhibitory Effect of Human Plasma and Saliva on Coaggregation Between *Bacteroides gingivalis* and *Streptococcus mitis*, *J Dent Res* 69:1476-1479.

NIEUW AMERONGEN, A.V.; ODERKERK, C.H.; and DRIESSEN, A.A. (1987): Role of Mucins from Human Whole Saliva in the Protection of Tooth Enamel Against Demineralization *in vitro*, *Caries Res* 21:297-309.

POLLOCK, J.J.; IACONO, V.J.; BICKER, H.G.; MACKAY, B.J.; KATONA, L.I.; TAICHMAN, L.B.; and THOMAS, E. (1976): The Binding, Aggregation and Lytic Properties of Lysozyme. In: *Microbial Aspects of Dental Caries*, Vol 1, H.M. Stiles, W.J. Loesche and T.C. O'Brien, Eds. Washington: Information Retrival, pp. 325-352.

PRAKOBPHOL, A.; LEVINE, M.J.; TABAK, L.A.; and REDDY, M.S. (1982): Purification of a Low-molecular Weight, Mucin-type Glycoprotein from Human Submandibular-Sublinguai Saliva, *Carbohydr Res* 108:111-122.

RAMASUBBU, N.; REDDY, M.S.; BERGEY, E.J.; HARASZTHY, G.H.; SONI, S.; and LEVINE, M.J. (1991): Large-scale Purification and Characterization of the Major Phosphoproteins and Mucins of Human Submandibular-Sublingual Saliva, *Biochem J*, 280:341-352.

RATHMAN, W. M.; KEYBUS, P.A.M.; VAN ZEYL, M.J.; VEERMAN, E.C.I.; and NIEW AMERONGEN, A. V. (1990): Characterization of Monoclonal Antibodies to

Human Salivary (Glyco)proteins. Cellular Localization of Mucin, Cystatin-like 14 kD protein and 29 kD Glycoprotein in the Human Submandibular Gland, *J Biol Buc* 18:19-27.

REDDY, M.S.; BOBEK, L.A.; HARASZTHY, G.G.; BIESBROCK, A.R.; and LEVINE, M.J. (1992): Structural Features of the Low Molecular Weight Salivary Mucin, *Biochem J* 287:639-643.

REDDY, M.S.; LEVINE, M.J.; PRAKOBPHOL, A.; and AL-HASHIMI, I. (1984): Oligosaccharides of Salivary Mucin from Caries Resistant and Susceptible Subjects, *J Dent Res* 63: Abst. No. 652.

REEH, E.S.; AGUIRRE, A.; SAKAGUCHI, R.L.; RUDNEY, J.D.; LEVINE, M.J.; and DOUGLAS, W.H. (1990): Hard Tissue Lubrication by Salivary Fluids, *Clin Mater* 6:151-161.

RØLLA, G. and JONSEN, J. (1968): A Glycoprotein Component from Human Sublingual-Submaxillary Saliva, *Caries Res* 2:306-316.

RUNDEGREN, J. (1986): Calcium-dependent Salivary Agglutinin with Reactivity to Various Oral Bacterial Species, *Infect Immun* 53:173-178.

RUSSELL, M.W. and RAHEMTULLA, B.M. (1989): Interaction between Surface Protein Antigens of *Streptococcus mutans* and Human Salivary Components, *Oral Microbiol Immun* of 4:106-111.

SAJJAN, S. and FORSTNER, J. F. (1990): Role of the Putative "Link" Glycopeptide of Intestinal Mucin in Binding of Piliated *Escherichia coli* Serotype 0157:H7 Strain CL-49, *Infect Immun* 58:868-873.

SCANNAPIECO, F.A.; LEVINE, M.J.; BERGEY, E.J.; and COHEN, R.E. (1987): Composition of Human Submandibular-Sublingual Saliva Pellicle of *Streptococcus sanguis*, *J Dent Res* 66:Abst. No. 1432.

SHIP, J.A.; FOX, P.C.; and BAUM, B.J. (1991): How Much Saliva is Enough?, *J Amer Dent Assoc* 122:63-69.

SLOMIANY, B.L.; MURTY, V.L.N.; AONO, M.; SLOMIANY, A.; and MANDEL, I.D. (1982): Lipid Composition of Human Parotid and Submandibular Saliva from Caries-resistant and Caries-susceptible adults, *Arch Oral Biol* 27:803-808.

SLOMIANY, B.L.; MURTY, V.L.N.; MANDEL, I.D.; ZALESNA, G.; and SLOMIANY, A. (1989a): Physico-chemical Characteristics of Mucus Glycoproteins and Lipids of the Human Oral Mucus Coat in Relation to Caries Susceptibility, *Arch Oral Biol* 34:229-237.

SLOMIANY, B.L.; MURTY, V.L.N.; SLOMIANY, A.; ZIELENSKI, J.; and MANDEL, I.D. (1986): Mucus Glycoprotein of Human Saliva: Differences in the Associated and Covalently Bound Lipids with Caries, *Biochim Biophys Acta* 882:18-28.

SLOMIANY, B.L., MURTY, V.L.N., MANDEL, I.D., SENGUPTA, S.; and SLOMIANY, A. (1990): Effect of Lipids on the Lactic Acid Retardation Capacity of Tooth Enamel and Cementum Pellicles Formed *In Vitro* from Saliva of Caries-resistant and Caries-susceptible Human Adults, *Arch Oral Biol* 35:175-180.

SLOMIANY, B.L.; SLOMIANY, A.; and MANDEL, I.D. (1989b). Lipids of Saliva and Salivary Concretions. In: *Human Saliva: Clinical Chemistry and Microbiology*, Vol. II, J.O. Tenouvo, Ed., Boca Raton: CRC Press, pp.101-130.

SØNJU, T.; CHRISTENSEN, T.B.; KORNSTAD, L.; and RØLLA, G. (1974): Electron Microscopy, Carbohydrate Analysis and Biological Activities of the Proteins Adsorbed in Two Hours to Tooth Surfaces *In Vivo*, *Caries Res* 8:113-122.

STINSON, M.W.; LEVINE, M.J.; CAVESE, J.M.; PRAKOBPHOL, A.; MURRAY, P.A.; TABAK, L.A.; and REDDY, M.S. (1982): Adherence of *Streptococcus sanguis* to Salivary Mucins Bound to Glass, *J Dent Res* 61:1390-1393.

STINSON, M.W.; SAFULKO, K.; and LEVINE, M.J. (1991): Adherence of *Porphyromonas (Bacteroides) gingivalis* to *Streptococcus sanguis In Vitro*, *Infect Immun* 59:102-108.

TABAK, L.A.; LEVINE, M.J.; JAIN, N.K.; BRYAN, A.R.; COHEN, R.E.; MONTE, L.D.; ZAWACKI, S.; NANCOLLAS, G.H.; SLOMIANY, A.; and SLOMIANY, B.L. (1985): Adsorption of Human Salivary Mucins to Hydroxyapatite, *Arch Oral Biol* 30:423-427.

TABAK, L.A.; LEVINE, M.J.; MANDEL, I.D.; and ELLISON, S.A. (1982): Role of Salivary Mucins in the Protection of the Oral Cavity, *J Oral Pathol* 11:1-17.

TIMPTE, C.S.; ECKHARDT, A.E.; ABERNETHY, J.L.; and HILL, R.L. (1988): Porcine Submaxillary Gland Apomucin Contains Tandemly Repeated, Identical Sequences of 81 Residues, *J Biol Chem* 263:1081-1088.

VAN DER HOEVEN, J.S. and CAMP, P.J.M. (1991): Synergistic Degradation of Mucin by *Streptococcus oralis* and *Streptococcus sanguis* in Mixed Chemostat Cultures, *J Dent Res* 70:1041-1044.

VAN DER HOEVEN, J.S.; VAN DER KIEBOOM, C.W.A.; and CAMP, P.J.M. (1990): Utilization of Mucin by Oral Streptococcus species, *Anton van Leeuw* 57:165-172.

VAN HALBEEK, H. (1990): NMR of Complex Carbohydrates. In: *Frontiers of NMR in Molecular Biology*, Vol 109, D. Live, I.M. Armitage and D. Patel, Eds., Wiley-Liss, New York, pp. 195-213.

VAN HOUTE, J. (1980): Bacterial Specificity in the Etiology of Dental Caries, *Int Dent J* 30:305-326.

VLIEGENTHART, J.F.G.; DORLAND, L.; AND VAN HALBEEK, H. (1983): High-resolution ^{1}H-Nuclear Magnetic Resonance Spectroscopy as a Tool in the Structural Analysis of Carbohydrates Related to Glycoproteins. In: *Advances in Carbohydrate Chemistry and Biochemistry*, Vol 41, R.S. Tipson and D. Horton, Eds., Academic Press, New York, pp. 209-375.

WEIS, W.; BROWN, J.H.; CUSACK, S.; PAULSON, J.C.; SKEHEL, J.J.; and WILEY, D.C. (1988): Structure of the Influenza Virus Haemagglutinin Complexed with its Receptor, Sialic Acid, *Nature* 333: 426-431.

WILLIAMS, R.C. and GIBBONS, R.J. (1972): Inhibition of Bacterial Adherence by Secretory Immunoglobulin A: A Mechanism of Antigen Disposal, *Science* 177:697-699.

WOLD, A.E.; MESTECKY, J.; TOMANA, M.; KOBATA, A.; OHBAYASHI, H.; ENDO, T.; and EDEN, C.S. (1990): Secretory Immunoglobulin A Caries Oligosaccharide Receptors for *Escherichia coli* Type 1 Fimbrial Lectin, *Infect Immun* 58: 3073-3077.

WRIGHT, C.S. (1990): 2.2 Å Resolution Structure Analysis of Two Refined *N*-acetylneuraminyl-lactose-Wheat Germ Agglutinin Isolectin Complexes, *J Mol Biol* 215:635-651.

Human Salivary Pellicle Glycoproteins: Identification and Bacterial Receptor Activity

AKRAPORN PRAKOBPHOL AND SUSAN J. FISHER

Two types of adhesive interactions involving salivary glycoproteins are critical determinants of bacterial adherence within the oral cavity. In the first, salivary glycoproteins either adhere to oral surfaces, producing a thin film termed pellicle, or remain in the solution phase. In the second, bacteria interact with a specific subset of these salivary glycoproteins and, depending on whether or not these receptors are pellicle constituents, are targeted for either adherence or clearance. Thus, an important factor controlling bacterial adherence is the potentially bivalent nature of salivary glycoprotein adhesive interactions.

The role of glycosylated salivary proteins in both pellicle formation and adherence of oral bacteria is of particular interest since bacterial adhesion is often the result of specific interactions between the carbohydrate portions of receptors and protein complexes (termed adhesins) on bacterial cell surfaces (Ofek and Perry, 1985). With regard to the contribution of glycosylated salivary components to pellicle, external radiolabeling techniques showed that the high and low molecular weight salivary mucins, MG1 and MG2, respectively, are the major constituents of short term (1 h) human enamel and cementum pellicles formed both *in vivo* and *in vitro* (Fisher *et al.*, 1987; Kajisa *et al.*, 1990). Other studies using specific antibodies showed that α-amylase and sIgA are also important components of short term (2 h) human pellicle formed *in vivo* (Al-Hashimi and Levine, 1989). Significantly, other carbohydrate-containing salivary components such as the highly glycosylated proline-rich glycoprotein are not major pellicle constituents (Fisher *et al.*, 1987; Kajisa *et al.*, 1990), suggesting the highly selective nature of the interactions that govern the adsorption of pellicle to enamel and cementum surfaces.

Equally important in the functional analysis of salivary glycoprotein adhesive interactions is determining which of these molecules can serve as bacterial

This work was supported by NIH grant DE-07244.

receptors. A variety of indirect techniques (e.g., inhibition of agglutination by simple saccharides, production of monoclonal antibodies against receptors) have been used to determine the structural requirements of these interactions (Beachy, 1981; Jones and Isaacson, 1983). These methods can elucidate the structural basis of receptor specificity, but usually cannot identify specific salivary components as receptors for particular bacteria. Such studies normally require purified salivary components. Extremely useful techniques that eliminate the requirement for purifying receptor molecules involve overlaying thin-layer chromatograms of glycolipids (Hansson *et al.*, 1985) and neoglycolipids (Stoll *et al.*, 1988) or nitrocellulose transfers of SDS-PAGE-separated proteins (Prakobphol *et al.*, 1987) with radiolabeled bacteria, which then bind to the immobilized receptors. The relative ease of these techniques offers the possibility of rapid identification of bacteria-receptor interactions. For example, we combined data from all three overlay methods to show the structural basis for the adherence of *F. nucleatum* to the carbohydrate residues of the highly glycosylated proline-rich glycoprotein (Gillece-Castro *et al.*, in press).

Taken together, information concerning the role of salivary components in pellicle formation and as receptors for particular organisms can be used to make predictions about factors governing the adherence or clearance of bacteria from the oral cavity. The data described here represent our continuing efforts to apply this strategy more effectively by gaining additional information about the adhesive functions of salivary glycoproteins. With regard to pellicle formation we now demonstrate, by periodic acid-Schiff (PAS) staining, that MG1 and MG2 are the major glycosylated constituents of pellicles formed *in vitro* and *in vivo*. We then quantified the adsorption of the mucins under both conditions. With regard to receptor function, we also show an example of a bacterium (*S. sanguis* 804) that interacts specifically with MG2 and which we would predict would adhere to pellicle *in vivo*.

Material and Methods

Formation, collection and analysis of pellicles.—In vitro pellicles were formed by incubating cleaned human enamel and cementum slabs in a 1:1 mixture of parotid and submandibular/sublingual (SM/SL) saliva for 0-60 min essentially as described by Fisher *et al.* (1987). Binding of salivary components at time 0 was assessed by placing the slabs in the saliva mixture and immediately removing them. For each time point, the pellicle was removed from two enamel and two cementum slabs by extraction with SDS-PAGE sample buffer. *In vivo* pellicles were formed on enamel surfaces that had been cleaned by scraping with a sterile scaler followed by application of a coarse pumice. After 30 min, during which the subjects neither ate nor drank, the newly formed pellicle was collected by scraping with a sterile scaler and was transferred directly into sample buffer. Pellicles collected from four subjects were pooled for further analysis. The *in vitro* and the *in vivo* pellicles were electrophoretically separated on 7.5% SDS-PAGE gels (Laemmli, 1970) and the glycosylated proteins were demonstrated by PAS staining (Wada *et al.*, 1979). The adsorption of MG1 and MG2 per cm^2 of enamel and cementum was quantified by scanning densitometry, with purified MG1 and MG2 (2-100 μg) as the reference standards.

Bacterial overlay of electrophoretically separated salivary components.—Parotid and SM/SL salivas were collected separately from ten individuals of known blood type. The adherence patterns of two subjects represented the variations that were observed among the ten members of this group. Subject 1 was blood type B+, Le (a−b−), and was a secretor. Subject 2 was blood type O+, Le (a−b+), and was also a secretor. The samples were collected as the ductal secretions into an equal volume of SDS-PAGE loading buffer. After separation on 7% slab gels, the electrophoretically separated components were transferred to nitrocellulose membranes according to the procedure of Towbin *et al.* (1979). After blotting, gels were routinely stained with silver (Morrissey, 1981) or with PAS (Wada *et al.*, 1979) to estimate the efficiency of transfer.

The bacterial strain that was used to overlay the blots (*S. sanguis* 804) was from the culture collection of the Division of Oral Biology, University of California San Francisco. This strain was stored at −70°C in trypticase yeast extract medium with 15% glycerol. To metabolically label bacteria, batch cultures of the organism were grown at 37°C to late log phase (16-18 h) in trypticase soy broth containing 0.25% yeast extract and 10 μCi/ml [^{35}S]methionine. Radiolabel incorporation was routinely 2-6 × 10^3 bacteria/cpm. Bacteria were harvested by centrifugation and washed three times in 0.01 M phosphate buffer (pH 7.0) containing 0.154 M sodium chloride. Cells were resuspended in 0.05 M Tris-HCl, 0.15 M NaCl, pH 7.4 containing 5% bovine serum albumin and briefly sonicated on ice (< 10 sec) to disperse aggregates. Bacteria were then adjusted to a final concentration of 5 × 10^8/ml by A_{620} determinations previously related to cell number by direct counting in a Petroff Hauser chamber. Labeled bacteria were allowed to adhere to blots of electrophoretically separated salivary glycoproteins as described previously (Prakobphol *et al.*, 1987), after which the blots were air dried and exposed to Hyperfilm.

Results

PAS staining of electrophoretically separated components was used to demonstrate the glycosylated proteins of human parotid and SM/SL salivas and of pellicles formed *in vitro* and *in vivo*. This chemical approach was chosen as a means of eliminating any possible bias inherent in the external radiolabeling

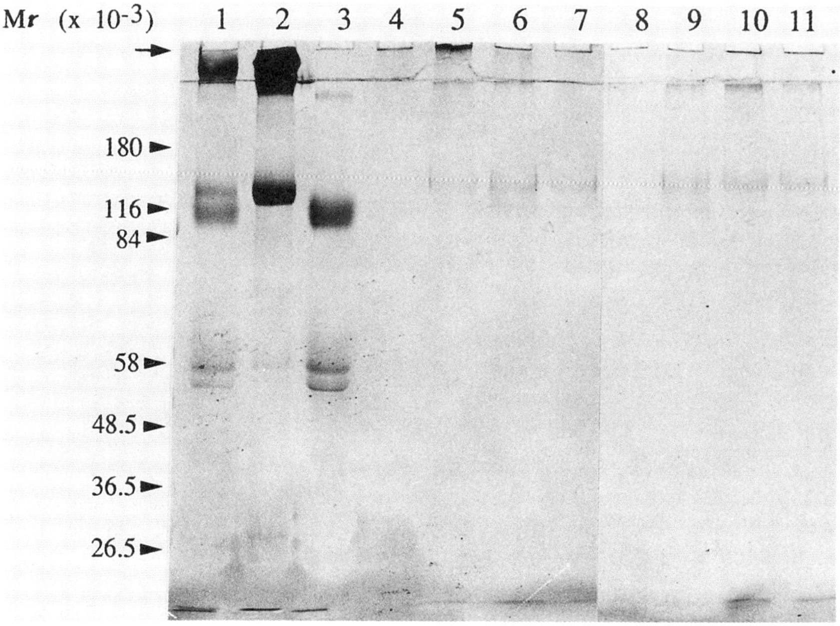

Figure 1. PAS staining of electrophoretically separated cementum and enamel pellicles formed *in vitro*. Lane 1, salivary incubation medium (1:1 [v/v] mixture of human parotid and SM/SL salivas collected as the ductal secretions); Lane 2, SM/SL saliva; Lane 3, parotid saliva; Lanes 4-7, enamel pellicles formed at 0, 10, 30 and 60 min; Lanes 8-11, cementum pellicles formed at 0, 10, 30 and 60 min; → = top of the stacking gel.

techniques we had used previously to identify pellicle components (Fisher *et al.*, 1987). This method also allowed quantification of glycoproteins bound to the tooth surface.

With regard to PAS-reactive salivary constituents, our experiments showed that MG1 (M_r > 1,000,000) and MG2 (M_r 120,000) were the major glycosylated components of human submandibular/sublingual saliva (Fig. 1, lane 2). A high molecular weight variant of the glycosylated proline-rich glycoprotein (M_r 89,000; Gillece-Castro *et al.*, 1991) and α-amylase (M_r 50,000-60,000) were the major PAS-reactive components in parotid saliva (Fig. 1, lane 3). The 1:1 (v/v) mixture of the two salivas that was used to form the *in vitro* pellicles contained all of the aforementioned components (Fig. 1, lane 1).

Staining of electrophoretically separated pellicle components showed that only a subset of the PAS-reactive components in saliva are adsorbed to the tooth surface. The major glycosylated component of pellicles formed *in vitro* that entered the running gel had the same electrophoretic mobility as MG2. This glycoprotein was absent at time 0 and present on both enamel (lanes 4-7) and cementum slabs (lanes 8-11) from the 10-min incubation onward. We used scan-

TABLE 1 *Quantification of MG2 and MG1 in Salivary Pellicles.*

Time	Amount adsorbed (μg/cm²)		
	In Vitro Pellicle		*In Vivo* Pellicle
(min)	*enamel*	*cementum*	*enamel*
		MG2	
0	0	0	0
10	2.0	2.6	ND*
30	2.9	2.8	0.48
60	2.3	2.6	ND
		MG1	
0	0	0	0
10	2.3	2.7	ND
30	2.5	3.4	0.45
60	0	2.0	ND

*Not determined

ning densitometry to quantify MG2 adsorbed per cm^2 of enamel and cementum, with purified MG2 (2-100 μg) as the reference standard (Table I). For both surfaces maximum adsorption (2.9 and 2.8 μg/cm^2, respectively) occurred at 30 min. The glycosylated components of the 30-min *in vivo* pellicle were quantified by the same method (gel not shown). Again, the only component that entered the running gel had the same electrophoretic mobility as MG2. *In vivo* enamel pellicles, collected at 30 min, contained 0.48 μg MG2/cm^2.

Both the *in vitro* and the *in vivo* pellicles also contained a high molecular weight component that was PAS-reactive. This component, which was found at the interface between the stacking gel and the running gel, had the same electrophoretic characteristics as MG1. Maximum adsorption of MG1 to the enamel and the cementum surfaces *in vitro* (2.5 and 3.4 μg/cm^2, respectively) again occurred at 30 min. *In vivo* enamel pellicles collected at 30 min contained 0.45 μg MG1/cm^2.

Next, we investigated whether any of the bacteria that colonize the oral cavity could interact preferentially with the mucins, which would suggest that these bacteria are targeted for adherence to the tooth surface. To date we have studied the adherence of 16 strains of streptococci by overlaying electrophoretically separated samples of submandibular/sublingual and parotid saliva with radiolabeled bacteria and identifying potential bacterial receptors by autoradiography (Murray *et al.*, submitted for publication). The results of these experiments showed that certain of the streptococci, including *S. sanguis* 804 (Fig. 2), bound only to the low molecular weight mucin found in submandibular/sublingual saliva. No binding to the molecular weight markers (data not shown), to the high molecular weight mucin (MG1) or to any other submandibular/sublingual

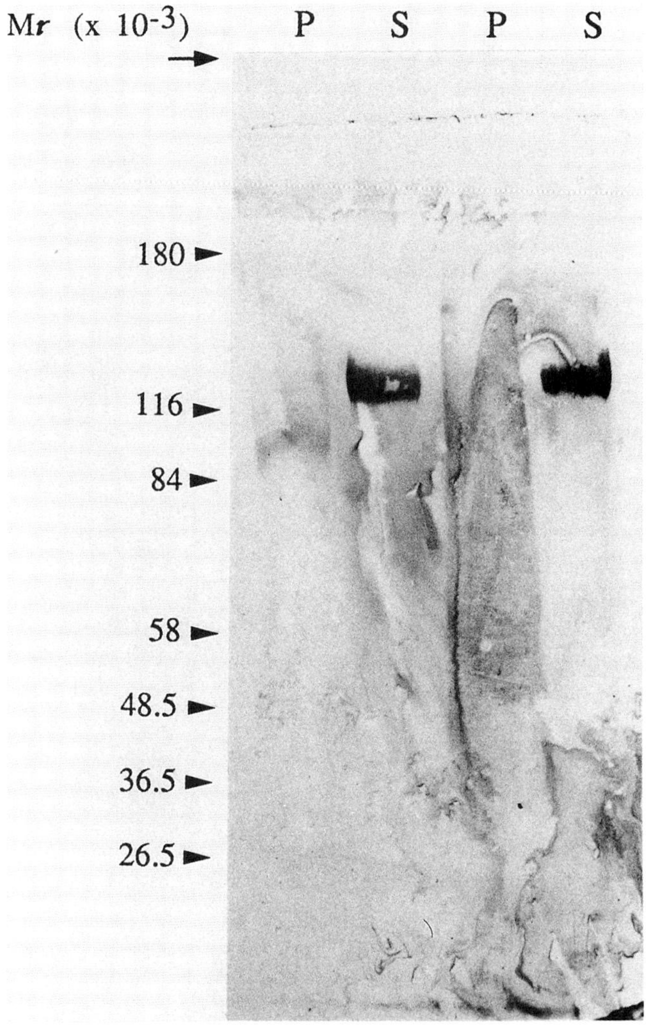

Figure 2. Binding of ^{35}S-labeled *S. sanguis* 804 to MG2. The salivary glycoproteins were separated by SDS-PAGE, transferred to nitrocellulose and overlaid with the metabolically labeled bacterium. P, parotid; S, submandibular/sublingual; → = top of the stacking gel.

salivary components was observed. Occasionally, a very weak interaction with the highly glycosylated proline-rich glycoproteins was also detected. Since staining showed that none of the salivary glycoproteins remained in the original gel, the highly selective interaction with MG2 was not the result of differential transfer of only a subset of salivary glycoproteins.

Discussion

This study of glycosylated pellicle components showed that the composition of pellicles formed *in vitro* and *in vivo* is identical, and that the salivary mucins are the major carbohydrate-containing components of both. Thus, PAS staining of pellicle constituents confirmed the results of our previous study of pellicle composition that used external radiolabeling techniques (Fisher *et al.*, 1987, Kajisa *et al.*, 1990). Interestingly, quantification of mucin adsorption showed that significantly less (approximately 20%) MG1 and MG2 were adsorbed to the tooth surface after 30 min *in vivo* than *in vitro*. The explanation for this finding is unknown. However, it is possible that the kinetics of mucin adsorption are different under the two conditions and that the times at which maximal adsorption occurs *in vitro* (30 min) and *in vivo* are different.

We extended this study of pellicle composition to determine if any of the bacteria that colonize the oral cavity adhere preferentially to the major glycosylated pellicle components, the salivary mucins. These studies showed that MG2 is a potential receptor for *S. sanguis* 804. Thus, we would suggest that interactions with the low molecular weight mucin in pellicle is one important mechanism by which this organism colonizes the oral cavity. In recently completed studies we showed that several strains of streptococci that colonize the oral cavity interact with specific salivary components (Murray *et al.*, submitted for publication). In certain cases, interactions with a single component of submandibular/sublingual and/or parotid saliva were detected. For example, *S. sanguis* 72-40, like *S. sanguis* 804, interacted only with MG2 and *S. sobrinus* OMZ 176 only with a component of M_r 45,000 whose identity is unknown. In other cases (*S. gordonii* G9B and 10558, *S. sanguis* 10556, and *S. oralis* 10557 and 72-41), interactions with multiple salivary components, including the low molecular weight salivary mucin, highly glycosylated proline-rich glycoproteins, and α-amylase, were detected. These results suggest that bacteria interact with a specific subset of salivary glycoproteins and that these interactions play an important role in governing their subsequent adherence or clearance.

The structural basis of the bi-functional adhesive properties of salivary glycoproteins is largely unknown. Much of the existing information concerning pellicle formation has been obtained from the study of adsorption of salivary components onto hydroxyapatite (Bennick *et al.*, 1983; Kousvelari *et al.*, 1980), which is amphoteric and binds both acidic and basic macromolecules (Bernardi *et al.*, 1972). However, factors other than electrostatic interactions are also involved. Moreno and co-workers have shown that adsorption of acidic proline-rich glycoproteins to hydroxyapatite and fluorapatite is an endothermic process related to the secondary structure of the adsorbed proteins (Moreno *et al.*, 1982; Moreno *et al.*, 1984). Whether similar or different factors promote mucin adsorption is unknown.

As to the structural basis of salivary glycoprotein bacterial receptor activity, interesting data is emerging. For example, *A. naeslundii* has a high-affinity binding site for glycolipids with the sequence GalNAcβ (Stromberg and Karlsson, 1990) and also binds to desialylated MG2, whose *O*-linked oligosaccharides contain a high proportion of *N*-acetylgalactosamine (Prakobphol and Fisher, unpublished observations). Other work from this laboratory has shown that *F. nucleatum* adherence to a highly glycosylated proline-rich glycoprotein is mediated by a biantennary oligosaccharide with an unusual structure: one antenna is substituted with two fucose residues, whereas the other antenna is not fucosylated (Gillece-Castro *et al.*, 1991). However, the bacterial-receptor interactions that actually occur *in vivo* are likely to be complicated by many other factors. For example, the tertiary structure of salivary molecules can change upon adsorption, exposing previously buried sequences that can now serve as bacterial receptors (Gibbons *et al.*, 1990). Nevertheless, the fact that specific interactions are being identified for two important functions of salivary glycoproteins, pellicle formation and bacterial receptor activity, offers the exciting possibility that a better understanding of the structural bases of these interactions will be forthcoming.

REFERENCES

AL-HASHIMI, I. and LEVINE, M.J. (1989): Characterization of *In Vivo* Salivary-Derived Enamel Pellicle, *Arch Oral Biol* 34:289-295.

BEACHEY, E.H. (1981): Bacterial Adherence: Adhesin-Receptor Interactions Mediating the Attachment of Bacteria to Mucosal Surface, *J Infect Dis* 143:325-345.

BENNICK, A.; CHAU, G.; GOODLIN, R.; ABRAMS, S.; TUSTIAN, D.; and MADAPALLIMATTAM, G. (1983): The Role of Human Acidic Proline-Rich Proteins in the Formation of Acquired Dental Pellicle *In Vitro* and Their Fate After Adsorption to the Human Enamel Surface, *Arch Oral Biol* 28:19-27.

BERNARDI, G.; GIRO, M.-G.; and GAILLARD, C. (1972): Chromatography of Polypeptides and Proteins on Hydroxyapatite Columns: Some New Developments, *Biochim Biophys Acta* 78:409-420.

FISHER, S.J.; PRAKOBPHOL, A.; KAJISA, L.; and MURRAY, P.A. (1987): External Radiolabelling of Components of Pellicle on Human Enamel and Cementum, *Arch Oral Biol* 32:509-517.

GIBBONS, R.J.; HAY, D.I.; CHILDS, W.C.; and DAVIS, G. (1990): Role of Cryptic Receptors (Crytitopes) in Bacterial Adhesion to Oral Surfaces, *Arch Oral Biol* 35:107-114.

GILLECE-CASTRO, B.L.; PRAKOBPHOL, A.; BURLINGAME, A.L.; LEFFLER, H.; and FISHER S. J. (1991): Structure and Bacterial Receptor Activity of a Human Salivary Proline-Rich Glycoprotein, *J Biol Chem.* 266:17358-17368.

HANSSON, G.C.; KARLSSON, K.-A.; LARSON, G.; STROMBERG, N.; and THURIN, J. (1985): Carbohydrate-Specific Adhesion of Bacteria to Thin-Layer Chromatograms: A Rationalized Approach to the Study of Host Cell Glycolipid Receptors. *Anal Biochem* 146:158-163.

JONES, G.W. and ISAACSON, R.E. (1983): Proteinaceous Bacterial Adhesins and Their Receptors, *CRC Crit Rev Microbiol* 10:229-260.

KAJISA, L.; PRAKOBPHOL, A.; SCHIØDT, M; and FISHER, S.J. (1990): Effect of plasma on composition of human enamel and cementum pellicle, *Scand J Dent Res* 98:461-471.

KOUSVELARI, E.E.; BARATZ, R.S.; BURKE, B.; and OPPENHEIM, F.G. (1980): Immunochemical Identification and Determination of Proline-Rich Proteins in Salivary Secretions, Enamel Pellicle, and Glandular Tissue, *J Dent Res* 59:1430-1438.

LAEMMLI, U.K. (1970): Cleavage of Structural Proteins During the Assembly of the Head of Bacteriophage T4, *Nature* 277:680-685.

MORENO, E.C.; KRESAK, M.; and HAY, D.I. (1982): Adsorption Thermodynamics of Acidic Proline-Rich Salivary Proteins onto Calcium Apatites, *J Biol Chem* 257:2981-2989.

MORENO, E.C.; KRESAK, M.; and HAY, D.I. (1984): Adsorption of Molecules of Biological Interest onto Hydroxyapatite, *Calcif Tissue Int* 36:48-59.

MORRISSEY, J.H. (1981): Silver Stain for Proteins in Polyacrylamide Gels: Modified Procedure with Enhanced Uniform Sensitivity, *Anal Biochem* 117:307-310.

MURRAY, P.A.; PRAKOBPHOL, A.; LEE, T.; HOOVER, C.I.; and FISHER, S.J. (1992): Adherence of Oral Streptococci to Salivary Glycoproteins. *Infect Immun:* 60:31-38.

OFEK, I. and PERRY, A. 1985: Molecular Basis of Bacterial Adherence to Tissues. In *Molecular Basis of Oral Microbial Adhesion*. E. Mergenhagen and B. Rosen (eds.) American Society for Microbiology, Washington, D.C. pp. 7-13.

PRAKOBPHOL, A.; MURRAY, P.A.; and FISHER, S.J. (1987): Bacterial Adherence to Replicas of SDS-PAGE Gels., *Anal Biochem* 164:5-11.

STOLL, M.S.; MIZUOCHI, T.; CHILDS, R.A.; and FEIZI, T. (1988): Improved Procedure for the Construction of Neoglycolipids Having Antigenic and Lectin-Binding Activities, From Reducing Oligosaccharides. *Biochem J* 256:661-664.

STROMBERG, N. and KARLSSON, K.-A. (1990): Characterization of the Binding of *Actinomyces naeslundii* (ATCC 12104) and *Actinomyces viscosus* (ATCC 19246) to Glycosphingolipids, Using a Solid-Phase Overlay Approach, *J Biol Chem* 265:11251-11258.

TOWBIN, H.; STAEHELIN, T.; and GORDON, J. (1979): Electrophoretic Transfer of Proteins from Polyacrylamide Gels to Nitrocellulose Sheets: Procedure and Some Applications, *Proc Natl Acad Sci USA* 76:4350-4354.

WADA, H.G.; HAAS, P.E.; and SUSSMAN, H.H. (1979): Transferrin Receptor in Human Placental Brush Border Membranes, *J Biol Chem* 254:12629-12635.

Salivary Antimicrobials: Where Are We?

T. Xu and F.G. Oppenheim*

The antimicrobial qualities of saliva have been the focus of many investigations over the last 20 years (Mandel and Ellison, 1985; Mandel, 1987; Tenovuo *et al.*, 1987). Since the oral cavity functions as the port of entry to the gastrointestinal system, a balanced microbiological ecology is important not just for the maintenance of oral health but for the entire organism. The functional significance of saliva in maintaining a healthy environment for protecting oral tissues has been recognized from patients suffering from salivary disfunction. In such patients the microbiological balance is clearly lost leading to pathological disorders affecting both hard and soft tissues. Even in subjects with normal salivary function, salivary access to oral hard and soft tissues can become limiting or restricted at specific sites by the formation of bacterial plaques. The benefits of the most widely used and accepted clinical measures of oral hygiene and oral prophylaxis treatment for the prevention of caries and periodontal diseases are related to both the physical removal of oral microbial plaques and the reestablishment of a salivary environment at these sites. The beneficial effects of the salivary environment have only recently gained more recognition in the clinical world in light of advances made in salivary research. These demonstrably protective properties of saliva are of course related to its constituents. This has stimulated interest in identifying and characterizing salivary components exhibiting antimicrobial activities with the ultimate goal of exploiting such knowledge for preventive and therapeutic purposes.

Physical Parameters

Physical parameters provide the initial physiological protection of the oral cavity. Among all physical parameters, flow rate and buffer capacity may be the

* To whom correspondence and reprint requests should be addressed.

This work was supported by the National Institutes of Health Grants DE07652, DE05672, and DE08649.

most important. Lubrication of oral surfaces and removal of dietary, bacterial, and cellular substrates are dependent on salivary flow. Replenishment of antimicrobial components, such as lactoferrin, peroxidase, lysozyme, histatins, and immunoglobulins is related to the salivary flow rate (McNabb and Tomasi, 1981; Mandel, 1987).

The buffer capacity of saliva is important for maintaining thc pH and mineral dynamics of the enamel surface, counteracting dietary induced pH changes and neutralizing acids produced by oral bacteria. It is important to note that the oral cavity represents an open system where the salivary pool is constantly renewed. Therefore components rendered inactive after interacting with the oral environment are constantly replaced by active components entering as salivary flow is stimulated. A decrease in salivary flow rate has been related to changes in buffer capacity, a reduction of salivary defense components, as well as alteration in both the amount and the composition of bacterial plaque and the progression of caries (Bratthall and Carlsson, 1986).

Host Immune and Non-Immune Defense System

Besides the physical parameters of saliva protection mentioned above, salivary characteristics such as the concentrations of lysozyme, lactoferrin, salivary peroxidase, myeloperoxidase, thiocyanate, hypothiocyanite, histatin, and the major classes of immunoglobulins as well as total protein concentration have been considered relevant to salivary antimicrobial activities (Mandel, 1987; Grahn *et al.*, 1988; Oppenheim, 1989). Functionally, these salivary components are usually divided into two categories, comprising immune and non-immune host defense factors. Each of these components or factors has been shown *in vitro* to exhibit various antimicrobial activities. It is impossible to review here the extensive literature which exists on some of these factors. Emphasis will be given to the more recent information on salivary components with antimicrobial activities.

Oral Immune Defense

Secretory immunoglobulin A (sIgA) is the predominant immunoglobulin class in oral secretions and is considered to be the pivotal functional element of the oral immune defense system. sIgA has been shown to aggregate oral microorganisms, prevent their adherence to mucosal surfaces, and neutralize viruses (Boackle and Suddick, 1980; and Camling *et al.*, 1987). Recent studies have focused on qualitative and quantitative differences in the secretory immune system which occur over a life span. Infants at ages under 12 months have been shown to exhibit a relatively high proportion of monomeric IgA and fragments of IgA which suggest that the secretory immune system undergoes a maturation process

(Tenovuo *et al.*, 1986; Cripps *et al.*, 1989; Hyyppa *et al.*, 1989). Smith and co-workers (1987) studied salivary IgA levels over an age span from early infancy to senescence. Total sIgA concentrations in infants age 2 to 5 months old were about half of those found in adults. In adults (ages 18 to 91) no significant changes were observed. Specific antibody levels to glucosyltransferase (GTF) from serotypes c and d of the mutans streptococci were highest in adults (ages 30 to 65), were reduced in the elderly (ages 66 to 91), and practically absent in infants due to the absence of *Streptococcus mutans* prior to tooth eruption. On the other hand, antibody levels to poliovirus resulting from early immunization were high in infants and in adults 30 to 40 years of age but showed a steady decline after age 40. There are clear indications that the oral immune response can be triggered in infancy and remains functional even at late stages of life. Critical for effective immune responses are apparently quantitative and qualitative differences in the antigenic challenge and antigenic processing which seem to change with progressing age.

Salivary IgG levels show a different pattern than those of sIgA. IgG decreases from a high level at birth to a low level after several months of birth, and this low level is maintained until the first year of life (Gleeson *et al.*, 1982). The only increase of IgG levels occurs between childhood and teenage years. About 10% of all individuals have no detectable IgG in saliva (Grundbacher, 1988). The presence of IgG, as well as IgM, in saliva is considered to be the result of a local immune response (Gleeson, 1991).

There are many studies aimed at finding correlations between total salivary immunoglobulin levels and/or specific antibody levels and clinical parameters. Most of such published data, however, show conflicting results with regard to antibody levels and caries incidence (Burgio *et al.*, 1980; Gleenson *et al.*, 1982; Finkelstein *et al.*, 1984; Widerstrom *et al.*, 1984; Ganguly, 1986; Aaltonen *et al.*, 1988; and Grundacher, 1988).

Oral Non-Immune Defense

The classical salivary non-immune defense system includes several proteins which are also present in cells, organs or body fluids not restricted to the oral cavity. The major proteins in this category are lysozyme, myeloperoxidase, lactoperoxidase and lactoferrin.

Lysozyme, a cationic protein, is well known for its muramidase activity, cleaving the beta-1,4 glucosidic linkage between N-acetyl muramic acid and N-acetylglucosamine of bacterial peptidoglycans. The salivary enzyme differs compositionally only slightly from hen egg-white lysozyme but its specific activity is 3.5 times greater. Submandibular/sublingual secretions contain about 2 mg% lysozyme, three times the concentration found in parotid secretion. Salivary concentrations of lysozyme are inversely related to flow rate which may be due to the fact that most salivary lysozyme is derived from ductal and not acinar cells (Rudney, 1989). Earlier work indicated that many microorganisms present in the oral cavity are resistant to the muramidase action of lysozyme (Gibbons *et al.*, 1966). More recent work of several investigators indicates that lysozyme can exhibit several antimicrobial effects not necessarily related to its muramidase activity. Such antimicrobial mechanisms include bacterial aggregation or adherence, interaction and/or disruption of cell membranes in the presence of anions and the activation of autolysins (Iacono *et al.*, 1980, 1985; Golub *et al.*, 1985; Tellefson and Germaine, 1986). Studies carried out by Pollock and coworkers (1987) demonstrated synergistic effects on cell lysis of *S. mutans* and lactobacilli when lysozyme was added to cells pre-treated with proteases or whole saliva. The lytic activity was particularly activated in the presence of monovalent anions such as bicarbonate. The effect observed could be related to disruption of the cell membrane in response to autolysin activation. While the mechanism of this synergistic cell lysis system is not understood, the interplay of lysozyme with other constituents of saliva may broaden the significance of lysozyme in the antimicrobial spectrum of saliva. Clinical correlations with salivary lysozyme concentrations are inconclusive. Stuchill and Mandel (1983) have shown similar salivary lysozyme levels in caries-active and caries-resistant individuals. In a study comprising 13 to 15 year-old children with high lactobacilli counts, however, salivary lysozyme levels were found to be negatively correlated with glucose triggered acid production (Twetman *et al.*, 1987).

Human salivary peroxidase (SPO) has been recently purified to homogeneity by Mansson-Rahemtulla and coworkers (1988). SPO occurs in parotid secretion as three active fractions with different apparent molecular weights. The enzyme has a characteristic heme spectrum and is inhibited by cyanide and azide. Its amino acid composition is similar to that of lactoperoxidase but SPO contains more proline. SPO contains 7% and LPO 4.6% neutral sugars, with each enzyme exhibiting different ratios of glucosamine, galactosamine, mannose, fucose and galactose. Furthermore the specific activity of SPO is five times that of LPO. It is well established that SPO catalyzes the oxidation of thiocyanate (SCN-) in the presence of hydrogen peroxide generating the hypothiocyanite anion (OSCN-) and hypothiocyanous acid (HOSCN) (Pruitt, 1987). Both of these enzymatic products inhibit bacterial growth and metabolism. In addition, hydrogen peroxide is consumed in the enzymatic reaction which leads to a reduction of hydrogen peroxide toxicity. The antimicrobial effects appear to be related to the oxidation of protein sulfhydryl groups. For instance glycolysis is inhibited by the oxidation of the enzyme glyceraldehyde-phosphate dehydrogenase. Glucose metabolism studies have shown that *S. mutans* is more affected by the SCN-peroxidation reaction than *S. sanguis* and *S. mitior* since the latter strains may possess an oxido-reductase capable of reducing OSCN-/HOSCN to thiocyanate and water. The inhibition of glucose metabolism in *S. mutans* is pH dependent. It is of interest to note that as pH values drop below six and as the cariogenic threat increases, the OSCN-/HOSCN mediated inhibition of glucose metabolism becomes more efficient. This feature suggests that the SPO system is uniquely suited for optimal host protection (Tenovuo *et al.*, 1981; Carlsson, 1987).

Lactoferrin is a basic iron binding glycoprotein with a M_r of 76,000 (Tenovuo, 1985). It is present in both parotid and submandibular/sublingual secretions at a concentration ranging from 0.5 to 1.0 mg% (Dipaola and Mandel, 1980). It can bind two ferric ions concomitant with two carbonate or bicarbonate anions but is usually secreted in the apo or iron-free state. In earlier studies the bacteriostatic effects of lactoferrin have been related to the sequestration of iron leading to nutritional deprivation. Arnold and coworkers have shown that apo LF can exhibit bacteriocidal activity against a variety of oral strains including *S. mutans* at pH 5-6. LF saturated with iron on the other hand failed to be bacteriocidal (Arnold *et al.*,1980; Lassiter *et al.*, 1987). They made the interesting observation that anions play a critical role in the bacteriocidal mechanism of LF. Since various anions could impede the bacteriocidal effect, apo LF appears to have specific anionic binding sites on its surface which can interact with anionic groups present on streptococcal surfaces. It is feasible that the affinity for anionic binding sites on bacterial surfaces exceeds the affinity for exogenous or free anions. Once the bacterial binding to LF has occurred the addition of iron does not inhibit bacteriocidal activity. Furthermore, bacteriocidal activity by LF may be related to radical formation since this activity is inhibited by the presence of the oxygen scavenging enzymes, catalase or peroxidase, or under strictly anaerobic conditions. The data demonstrate that given the appropriate microenvironment LF can be effective against *S. mutans* and other cariogenic bacteria.

Considerable efforts have been made by many investigators to relate antimicrobial qualities of saliva to the prevalence of caries and more recently to clinical measures of gingivitis or periodontitis (Brandtzaeg, 1983; Grahn *et al.*, 1988; Emilson *et al.*, 1989; and Saxen *et al.*, 1990). The majority of such studies fail to show significant correlations between specific salivary antimicrobial factors and caries scores, caries increments or gingival health parameters. Grahn and coworkers (1988) conducted such a study with a homogeneous population of 50 naval recruits. None of the salivary non-immune factors showed any correlation with past or present caries status or gingival bleeding. Even among the immune factors correlations were only found between total IgA and salivary counts of *S. mutans* and lactobacilli. Specific antibodies to *S. mutans* showed no relationship to dental caries or *S. mutans* counts. Only buffer capacity and flow rate values are frequently found to show an inverse relationship with past caries experience and counts of *S. mutans* and lactobacilli. The absence of clear correlations between salivary antibacterial components and clinical or microbiological parameters may be due to several factors. Salivary proteins can vary widely in concentrations between subjects. Some of the salivary proteins interact with each other in functionally synergistic or antagonistic ways. For example, SPO can enhance the effect of sIgA and lactoferrin while sIgA can lower the bacteriocidal activity of lactoferrin (Tenovuo *et al.*, 1982, Rudney and Smith

1985). Mucins can form complexes with sIgA, lysozyme and cystatins (Tabak *et al.*, 1982; Schachter and Williams, 1982). The cellular origins of all salivary defense proteins are not identical. While most proteins in saliva originate from acinar cells, some originate from ductal cells and others enter the oral cavity via gingival fluid. This may give rise to short and long term variations in the concentrations of individual components. In specific cases, such as enzymes and immunoglobulins, the concentration levels are not directly related to activity in saliva. The question whether the levels of salivary antimicrobial proteins are correlated with each other or vary independently has been addressed by Rudney (1985, 1989). He utilized multivariate statistical methods to probe for patterns of common variations and clusters of similar concentration profiles. Such patterns and clusters could be identified in two separate studies measuring the same salivary parameters using populations of 44 and 198 subjects, respectively, but the patterns and clusters identified in the first study did not coincide with those of the second study. It is therefore not surprising that such cross-sectional investigations of salivary defense factors have not provided much insight into the salivary defense system. It is feasible that longitudinal studies of salivary defense factors with concomitant monitoring of clinical and microbiological parameters could identify a clearer relationship between the classical salivary defense system and oral disease.

Since existing data on the classical salivary defense components has not yielded striking revelations regarding their effectiveness, it is important to consider that other constituents of saliva may be more important. Proteins such as proline-rich proteins, cystatins, mucins and histatins are truly major constituents of salivary secretions which might play important roles in the bacterial ecology of the oral cavity. Some of these proteins are not only specific for salivary secretions but are present at concentrations much higher than those of lysozyme, lactoferrin and salivary peroxidase. While direct comparisons of antimicrobial activities among salivary proteins are currently not feasible considering the differences of assay conditions and test organisms used by investigators, efforts will have to be made to determine specific activities. The structural and functional characterization of major salivary proteins has generated information which suggests that these proteins may be significant players of the host's non-immune defense armamentarium. Among these proteins, the antimicrobial properties of histatins have generated considerable interests since histatin was shown to be antifungal and to be 50 to 200 times more active than lysozyme in the inhibition of germination of *Candida albicans* (Oppenheim *et al.* 1986).

Histatins are a group of small molecular weight proteins present in both parotid and submandibular secretions (Oppenheim *et al.*, 1986, 1988; Troxler *et al.*, 1990). Cationic electrophoresis of proteins in glandular secretions separates histatins into three major protein pairs and several more cathodically migrating components. Histatin 1, histatin 3, and histatin 5 are the major histatins representing between 70-80% of this protein family (Oppenheim *et al.*, 1988).

The amino acid sequences of histatins show that histatin 1, histatin 3, and histatin 5 comprise 38, 32, 24 amino acid residues, respectively (Figure 1). Each major histatin contains seven histidine residues but only histatin 1 is phosphorylated. There is considerable sequence homology between histatin 1 and histatin 3. Twenty of the 22 amino-terminal amino acid residues are identical. The seven carboxyl-terminal residues are also identical. Unique to histatin 1 is the nonapeptide Glu_{23}-Gly_{31} and to histatin 3 the tripeptide Gly_{23}-Arg_{25}. Histatin 1 and histatin 3 are derived from separate genes, while histatin 5 is a proteolytic product of histatin 3 (Oppenheim *et al.*, 1988; Sabatini and Azen, 1989; vanderSpek *et al.*, 1990). The molecular weights of histatins 1, 3, and 5 are 4,929, 4,063, and 3,037, respectively. Only histatins 3 and 5 are basic proteins with a net charge of +5 at neutral pH. Immunological determinations of histatin concentrations in 15 subjects showed a range between 2 and 40 nmol/ml assuming an average M_r of 4,000 (Atkinson *et al.*, 1990).

Several investigations have shown that histatins exhibit antibacterial activities. These include inhibition of hemagglutination of *Porphyromonas gingivalis* (Murakami *et al.*, 1990), inhibition of protease activity of *P. gingivalis* (Nishikata *et al.*, 1991) and bacteriocidal and bacteriostatic activity with several strains of the mutans group of streptococci (MacKay *et al.*, 1984; Xu and Oppenheim, 1990).

We have studied the bacteriocidal effects of histatins on seven serotypes of the mutans group of streptococci (Xu and Oppenheim, 1990). The LD_{50} values indicated that all of these serotypes were susceptible to histatins (Table 1). A comparison among histatins revealed that histatin 5 was the most and histatin 1 the least bacteriocidal histatin. To measure the inhibition of growth by histatins, streptococci were spread uniformly on brain heart infusion agar. Ten ml aliquots of histatins were applied at different concentrations to sterilized filter disks. The disks were placed directly onto the agar plates containing the test strain. After incubation at 37°C for 48 h, growth inhibition areas were determined. Table 2 shows the results obtained with *S. mutans*, strain JBP, indicating that the three major histatins inhibited growth in a histatin-dependent manner and that histatin 5 was the most effective growth inhibitor.

Histatins also exhibit antifungal effects, which have been studied specifically with respect to effects on *C. albicans* (Pollock *et al.*, 1984; Oppenheim *et al.*, 1986, 1988; Xu *et al.*, 1991). To evaluate the anticandidal activity of histatins, three different assays were developed to characterize the effects of histatins on the dimorphic fungus *C. albicans* (Xu *et al.*, 1990). The first two assays were designed to measure the killing of blastoconidia or germinated *C. albicans*, respectively, whereas the third assay was designed to measure the inhibition of germination, i.e. the transition from blastospore to germ tube. Of the two candidal strains tested, one was an oral isolate (Odds, 1980) whereas the other one was obtained from a patient with systemic candidiasis (Hasenclever and Mitchell, 1962). The data obtained with these assays showed that major human

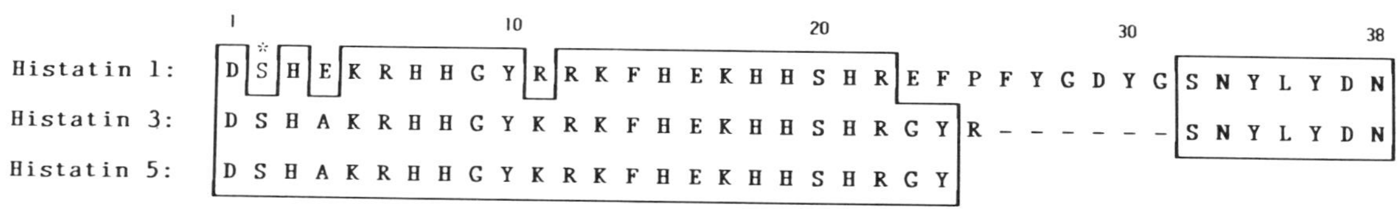

Figure 1 Sequence homology of human salivary histatins 1, 3 and 5. Boxes indicate identical amino acid residues. Dashes indicate gaps introduced to align the sequences. Abbreviations: A, alanine; D, aspartic acid; E, glutamic acid; F, phenylalanine; G, glycine; H, histidine; K, lysine; L, leucine; N, asparagine; P, proline; R, arginine; S, serine; Y, tyrosine (Oppenheim et al., 1988). * serine-2 in histatin 1 is phosphorylated.

TABLE 1 *Microbicidal Effects of Salivary Histatins*

Microbe (strain)	*Serotype*	*Histatin 1*	*Histatin 3*	*Histatin 5*
		LD_{50}(nmol/ml)		
Mutans of streptococci				
S. cricetus (AHT)	a	107.7	47.1	21.4
S. rattus (BHT)	b	48.5	16.3	9.3
S. mutans (JBP)	c	42.4	15.8	8.9
S. sobrinus (MB2R)	d	67.8	25.3	15.7
S. mutans (LM7)	e	55.3	18.2	7.9
S. mutans (OMZ175)	f	39.6	7.5	5.3
S. sobrinus (6715)	g	84.2	33.4	16.3
C. albicans strains*				
yeast form				
ATCC32354 (B311)	a	5.8	4.6	2.2
ATCC44505		6.3	4.2	2.0
mycelial form				
ATCC32354 (B311)	a	74.2	13.5	8.5
ATCC44505		72.0	11.6	9.7

* Data from Xu *et al.*, 1991.

histatins killed blastoconidia of *C. albicans* effectively with LD_{50} values of 5.8, 4.6, and 2.2 nmol/ml for histatins 1, 3, and 5, respectively. For germinated cell killing, the LD_{50} values for histatins 1, 3, and 5 were 74.2, 13.5, and 8.5 nmol/ml, respectively (Table 1). The results obtained with the inhibition of germination assay indicated that 100% inhibition was reached at a histatin concentration of 108 nmol/ml. The ID_{50} values for all three histatins were in the range of 37 to 55 nmol/ml (Table 3). The LD_{50} and ID_{50} values revealed that all three histatins exhibited anticandidal activities. It is evident that histatins are most effective in killing blastoconidia, somewhat less effective in killing germinated cells and least effective in inhibiting germination. Comparisons between the three major histatins show that in both killing assays histatin 5 exhibits LD_{50} values

TABLE 2 *Growth Inhibition of* Streptococcus mutans *by Salivary Histatins**

Proteins (nmol/ml)	*1.0*	*2.0*	*4.0*
		Inhibition areas (mm^2)	
Histatin 1	8.7	14.5	50.3
Histatin 3	24.5	86.9	153.0
Histatin 5	36.7	95.7	201.6

* The degree of inhibition of *S. mutans* (strain JBP) by histatins was measured using a disk agar diffusion assay. Ten μl of histatin solution was added to each disk.

TABLE 3 *Inhibition of Germination of* Candida albicans *by Salivary Histatins**

Proteins	*Strains* ATCC32354 (B311)	ATCC44505
	ID_{50}(nmol/ml)	
Histatin 1	52.8	52.2
Histatin 3	41.3	38.9
Histatin 5	46.3	49.2

* Data from Xu *et al.*, 1991.

which are lower than those of histatin 3, and the LD_{50} values of histatin 3 are lower than those of histatin 1. For the inhibition of germination, however, histatin 3 is more effective than histatin 1 or histatin 5. The comparisons of the data obtained with both candidal strains show that the effectiveness of histatins was very similar whether the fungus was an oral isolate or derived from systemic candidiasis.

One of the strategies for identifying the functional domains of a biologically active protein is to use *in vitro* techniques to synthesize portions of the protein and test these for activity. The small size of histatins makes this approach feasible. In the case of histatin 1, three peptides were synthesized representing the amino-terminal, the middle, and the carboxyl-terminal with the exception that residue 2 in the amino-terminal peptide was not phosphorylated (Xu and Oppenheim, 1989). Candidacidal assays with each of these peptides demonstrated that only the middle peptide exhibited distinct activity but less activity than the native protein (Fig. 2). When the same approach was taken with histatin 3 (Xu and Oppenheim, 1991), synthesizing three peptides representing the amino-terminal, the middle, and the carboxyl-terminal domains once again only the middle region of histatin 3 exhibited fungicidal activity (Fig. 2). Activity was lost when this middle peptide was further divided into two separate segments. These results not only identified the region in the protein which is functionally important, but also indicated that the middle peptide of histatin 3 was at least 10 times more effective than the native protein in killing candidal blastospores.

The studies presented here with histatins do not give insights into their functional importance *in vivo*. These studies do demonstrate a strategy, however, for showing how the combination of structural and functional characterization of antimicrobial proteins might be clinically exploited. Information gained in this fashion may lead to the preventive or therapeutic utilization of an oral host defense system. The feasibility of the approach is clearly dependent on the level of molecular characterization achieved for such salivary macromolecules. Advances in molecular biology provide additional tools to synthesize *in vitro* functional domains or modifications of functional domains. The molecular mapping of functional, binding, catalytic and other sites within salivary antimicrobial proteins

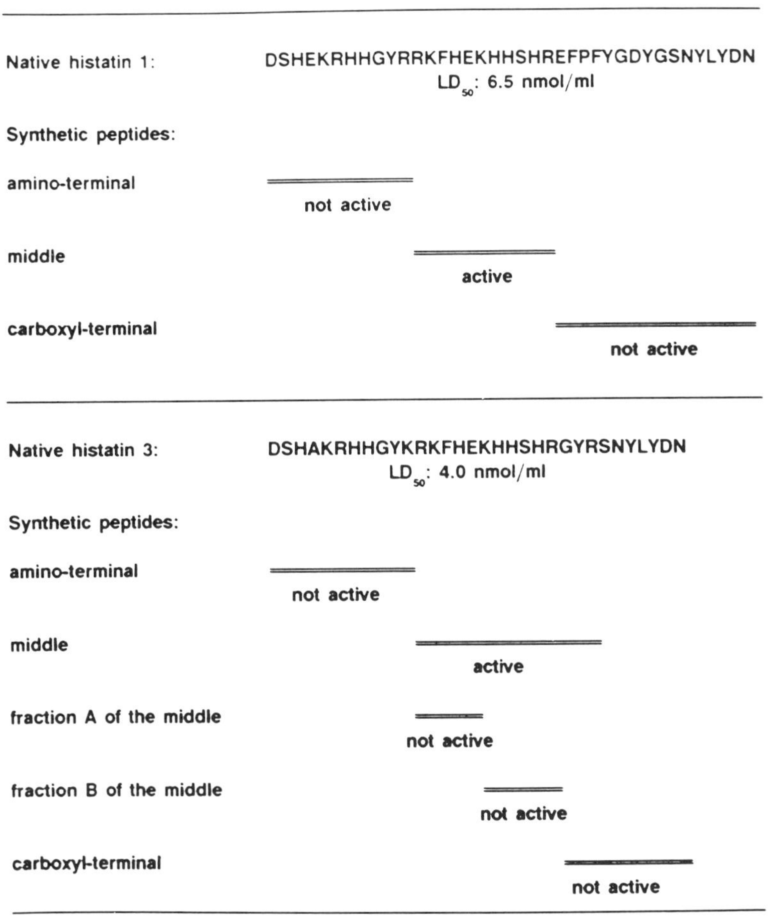

Figure 2 Functional analysis of histatin 1 and histatin 3 using synthetic peptides. The killing of candidal blastospores was only affected by the middle peptides of both histatins.

may be utilized to design chimeric molecules. The effectiveness of such constructs in the oral cavity may be optimized by combining native domains from different molecules, by duplicating domains, or by modifying native sequences.

REFERENCES

AALTONEN, A.S.; TENOUVO, J.; and LEHTONEN, O.-P. (1988): Antibodies to the oral bacterium *Streptococcus mutans* and development of caries in children in relation to maternal dental treatment during pregnancy. *Arch Oral Biol* 33:33-39.

ARNOLD, R.R.; BREWER, M.; and GAUTHIER, J.J. (1980): Bactericidal activity of human lactoferrin: sensitivity of a variety of microorganism. *Infect Immun* 28:893-898.

ATKINSON, J.C.; YEH, C.; OPPENHEIM; F.G.; BERMUDEZ, D.; BAUM, B.J.; and FOX, P.C. (1990): Elevation of salivary antimicrobial proteins following HIV-1 infection. *J Acquired Immune Defic Syndr* 3:41-48.

BRANDTZAEG, P. (1983): The oral secretory immune system with special emphasis on its relation to dental caries. *Proc Finn Dent Soc* 79:71-84.

BRATTHALL, D. and CARLSSON, J. (1986): Current status of caries activity tests. In: *Textbook of cariology* Thylstrup, A and Fejerskov, O. Eds., Copenhagen: Munksgaard, pp.249-265.

BOACKLE, R.J. and SUDDICK, R.P. (1980): Salivary proteins and oral health. In: *Biological basis of dental caries: an oral biology textbook*. Manalen, L. Ed., Maryland: Harper & Row Publishers, Inc., pp.113-131.

BURGIO, G.R.; LANZAVECCHIA, A.; PLEBANI, A.; JAYAKAR, S.; and UGAZIO, A.G. (1980): Ontogeny of secretory IgA and natural antibodies in saliva. *Pediatr Res* 14:1111-1114.

CAMLING, E.; GAHNBERG, L.; and KRASSE, B. (1987): The relationship between IgA antibodies to *Streptococcus mutans* antigens in human saliva and breast milk and the numbers of indigenous oral *Streptococcus mutans*. *Arch Oral Biol* 32:21-25.

CARLSSON, J. (1987): Salivary peroxidase: an important part of our defense against oxygen toxicity. *J Oral Pathol* 16:412-416.

CRIPPS, A.W.; GLEESON, M.; and CLANCY, R.L. (1989): Molecular characteristics of IgA in infant saliva. *Scand J Immunol* 29:317-324.

DIPAOLA, C. and MANDEL, I.D. (1980): Lactoferrin concentration in human parotid saliva as measured by an enzyme-linked immunosorbent assay (ELISA). *J Dent Res* 59:1463-1465.

EMILSON, C.G.; CIARDI, J.E.; OLSSON, J.; and BOWEN, W.H. (1989): The influence of saliva on infection of the human mouth by mutans streptococci. *Arch Oral Biol* 34:335-340.

FINKELSTEIN, M.S.; TANNER, M.; and FREEDMAN, M.L. (1984): Salivary and serum IgA levels in a geriatric outpatient population. *J Clin Immun* 4:85-91.

GANGULY, R.; STABLEIN, J.; LOCKEY, R.F.; SHAMBLIN, P.; and VARGAS, L. (1986): Defective antimicrobial functions of oral secretions in the elderly. *J Infect Dis* 153:163-164.

GERMAINE, G.R. and TELLEFSON, L.M. (1986): Potential role of lysozyme in bactericidal activity of *in vitro*-acquired salivary pellicle against *Streptococcus faecium* 9790. *Infect Immun* 51:846-854.

GIBBONS, R.J.; DE STOPPELAAR, J.D.; and HARDEN, L. (1966): Lysozyme insensitivity of bacteria to the oral cavity of man. *J Dent Res* 45:877-881.

GLEESON, M.; CRIPPS, A.W.; CLANCY, R.L.; HUSBAND, A.J.; HENSLEY, M.J.; and LEEDER, S.R. (1982): Ontogeny of the secretory immune system in man. *Aust N Z J Med* 12:255-258.

GLEESON, M.; DOBSON, A.J.; FIRMAN, D.W.; CRIPPS, A.W.; CLANCY, R.L.; WLODARCZYK, J.H,; and HENSLEY, M.J. (1991): The variability of immunoglobulins and albumin in salivary secretions of children. *Scand J Immunol* 33:533-541.

GOLUB, E.E.; CHERUKA, J.; BOOSZ, B.; DAVIS, C.; and MALAMUD, D. (1985): A comparison of bacterial aggregation induced by saliva, lysozyme, and zinc. *Infect Immun* 48:204-210.

GRAHN, E.; TENOVUO, J.; LEHTONEN, O.-P.; EROLA, E.; and VILJA, P. (1988): Antimicrobial systems of human whole saliva in relation to dental caries, cariogenic bacteria, and gingival inflammation in young adults. *Acta Odontol Scan* 46:67-74.

GRUNDBACHER, F.J. (1988): Variation in levels of immunoglobulins A, G and E in human saliva. *Arch Oral Biol* 33:121-126.

HASENCLEVER, H.F. and MITCHELL, W.O. (1962): Production in mice of tolerance to the toxic manifestations of *Candida albicans*. *J Bacteriol* 84:402-409.

HYYPPA, T.; KARHUVAARA, L.; TENOVUO, J.; LUMIKARI, M.; and VILJA, P. (1989): Antimicrobial factors in whole saliva of human infants: a longitudinal study. *Pediatr Dent* 11:30-36.

IACONO, V.J.; MACKAY, B.J.; DIRIENZO, S.; and POLLOCK, J.J. (1980): Selective antibacterial properties of lysozyme for oral microorganisms. *Infect Immun* 29:623-632.

IACONO, V.J.; ZOVE, S.M.; GROSSBARD, B.L.; POLLOCK, J.J; FINE, D.H.; and GREENE, S.L. (1985): Lysozyme-mediated aggregation and lysis of the periodontal microorganism *Capnocytophaga gingivalis* 2010. *Infect Immun* 31:457-464.

LASSITER, M.O.; NEWSOME, A.L.; SAMS, L.D.; and ARNOLD, R.R. (1987): Characterization of lactoferrin interaction with *Streptococcus mutans*. *J Dent Res* 66:480-485.

MACKAY, B.J.; DENEPITIYA, L.; IACONO, V.J.; KROST, S.B.; and POLLOCK, J.J. (1984): Growth-inhibitory and bactericidal effects of human parotid salivary histidine-rich polypeptides on *Streptococcus mutans*. *Infect Immun* 44:695-701.

MANSSON-RAHEMTULLA, B.; RAHEMTULLA, F.; BALDONE, D.C.; PRUITT, K.M.; and HJERPE, A. (1988): Purification and characterization of human salivary peroxidase. *Biochemistry* 27:233-239.

MANDEL, I.D. (1987): The functions of saliva. *J Dent Res* 66(Spec. Iss.), 623-627.

MANDEL, I.D. and ELLISON, S.A. (1985): The biological significance of the nonimmunoglobulin defense factor. In: *The lactoperoxidase system: chemistry and biological significance*. Pruitt, K.M.; and Tenovuo, J. Eds. New York: Marcel Dekker, pp.1-14.

MCNABB, P.C. and TOMASI, T.B. (1981): Host defense mechanisms at mucosal surfaces. *Ann Rev Microbiol* 35:477-496.

MURAKAMI, Y.; AMANO, A.; TAKAGAKI, M; SHIZUKUISHI, S.; TSUNEMITSU, A.; and AIMOTO, S. (1990): Purification and characterization from human parotid secretion of a peptide which inhibits hemagglutination of *Bacteroides gingivalis* 381. *FEBS Microbiol Lett* 72:275-280.

NISHIKATA, M.; KANEHIRA; TAKASHI; OH, H.; TANI, H.; TAZAKI, M.; and KUBOKI, Y. (1991): Salivary histatin as an inhibitor of a protease produced by the oral bacterium *Bacteroides gingivalis*. *Biochem Biophys Res Comm* 174:625-630.

ODDS, F.C. (1980): A simple system for the presumptive identification of *C. albicans* and differentiation of strains within the species. *Sabouraudia* 18:301-317.

OPPENHEIM, F.G. (1989): Salivary histidine-rich proteins. In: *Human salivary:clinical chemistry and microbiology*, Vol.1, Tenovuo, J.O., Ed., Florida: CRC Press, Incs., pp.151-160.

OPPENHEIM, F.G.; XU, T.; MCMILLIAN, F.M.; LEVITZ, S.M.; DIAMOND, R.D.; OFFNER, G.D.; and TROXLER, R.F. (1988): Histatins, a novel family of histidine-rich proteins in human parotid secretion. Isolation, characterization, primary structure and fungistatic effects on *Candida albicans*. *J Biol Chem* 263:7472-7477.

OPPENHEIM, F.G.; YANG, Y.; DIAMOND, R.D.; HYSLOP, D.; OFFNER, G.D.; and TROXLER, R.F. (1986): The primary structure and functional characterization of the neutral histidine-rich polypeptide from human parotid saliva. *J Biol Chem* 261:1177-1182.

POLLOCK, J.J.; LOTARDO, S.; GAVAI, R.; and GROSSBARD, B.L. (1987): Lysozyme-protease-inorganic monovalent anion lysis of oral bacterial strains in buffers and stimulated whole saliva. *J Dent Res* 66:467-474.

POLLOCK, J.J.; DENEPITIYA, L.; MACKAY, B.J.; and IACONO, V.J. (1984): Fungistatic and fungicidal activity of human parotid saliva histidine-rich polypeptides on *Candida albicans*. *Infect Immun* 44:702-707.

PRUITT, K.M. (1987): The salivary peroxidase system: thermodynamic, kinetic and antibacterial properties. *J Oral Pathol* 16:417-420.

RUDNEY, J.D. (1989): Relationship between human parotid saliva lysozyme, lactoferrin, salivary peroxidase and secretory immunoglobulin A in a large sample population. *Arch Oral Biol* 34:499-506.

RUDNEY, J.D.; KAJANDER, K.C.; and SMITH, Q.T. (1985): Correction between human salivary levels of lysozyme, lactoferrin, salivary peroxidase and secretory immunoglobulin A with different stimulatory studies and over time. *Arch Oral Biol* 30:765-771.

RUDNEY, J.D. and SMITH, Q.T. (1985): Relationships between levels of lysozyme, lactoferrin, salivary peroxidase, and secretory immunoglobulin A in stimulated parotid saliva. *Infect Immun* 49:469-475.

SABATINI, L.M. and AZEN, E.A. (1989): Histatins, a family of salivary histidine-rich proteins, are encoded by at least two loci (His1 and His2). *Biochem Biophys Res Comm* 160:495-502.

SAXEN, L.; TENOVUO, J.; and VILJA, P. (1990): Salivary defense mechanisms in juvenile periodontitis. *Acta Odontol Scand* 48:399-407.

SCHACHTER, H. and WILLIAMS, D. (1982): Biosynthesis of mucus glycoproteins. In: *Mucus in health and disease II*. Chantler, E.N.; Elder, J.B.; and Elstein, M. Eds., New York: Plenum Press, pp.3-28.

SMITH, D.I.; TAUBMAN, M.A.; and EBERSOLE, J.L. (1987): Ontogeny and senescence of salivary immunity. *J Dent Res* 66:451-456.

STUCHILL, R.N. and MANDEL, I.D. (1983): A comparative study of salivary lysozyme in caries-resistant and caries-susceptible adults. *J Dent Res* 62:552-554.

TABAK, L.A.; LEVINE, M.J.; MANDEL, I.D.; and ELLISON, S.A. (1982): Role of salivary mucins in the protection of the oral cavity. *J Oral Pathal* 11:175-189.

TELLEFSON, L.M. and GERMAINE, G.R. (1986): Adherence of *Streptococcus sanguis* to hydroxyapatite coated with lysozyme and lysozyme-supplemented saliva. *Infect Immun* 51:750-759.

TENOVUO, J. (1985): The lactoperoxidase system: chemistry and biological significance. In: *The lactoperoxidase system: chemistry and biological significance*, Pruitt, K.M.; and Tenovuo, J. Eds., New York: Marcel Dekker, pp.102-122.

TENOVUO, J.; GRAHN, E.; LEHTONEN, O.-P.; HYYPPA, T.; KARHUVAARA, L.; and VILJA, P. (1987): Antimicrobial factors in saliva: ontogeny and relation to oral health. *J Dent Res* 66:475-479.

TENOVUO, J.; LEHTONEN, O.-P.; AALTONEN, A.S.; VILJA, P.; and TUOHIMAA, P. (1986): Antimicrobial factors in whole saliva of human infants. *Infect Immun* 51:49-53.

TENOVUO, J.; MANSSON-RAHEMTULLA, B.; PRUITT, K.M.; and ARNOLD, A. (1981): Inhibition of dental plaque acid production by the salivary lactoperoxidase antimicrobial system. *Infect Immun* 34:208-215.

TENOVUO, J.; MOLDOVEANU, Z.; MESTECKY, J.; PRUITT, K.; and RAHEMTULLA, B. (1982): Interaction of specific and innate factors of immunity: IgA enhances the antimicrobial effect of the lactoperoxidase system against *Streptococcus mutans*. *J Immunol* 128:726-731.

TROXLER, R.F.; OFFNER, G.D.; XU, T.; VANDERSPEK, J.C.; and OPPENHEIM, F.G. (1990): Structure relationship between human salivary histatins. *J Dent Res* 69:2-6.

TWETMAN, S.; DAHLLOF, G.; and WIKNER, S. (1987): Lysozyme activity and L(+)-lactic acid production in saliva in school children with high lactobacillus counts. *Scan J Dent Res* 95:128-131.

VANDERSPEK, J.C.; OFFNER, G.D.; TROXLER, R.F.; and OPPENHEIM, F.G. (1990): Molecular cloning of human submandibular histatins. *Arch Oral Biol* 35:137-143.

WIDERSTROM, L. and BRATTHALL, D. (1984): Increased IgA levels in saliva during pregnancy. *Scand J Dent Res* 92:33-39.

XU, T.; LEVITZ, S.M; DIAMOND, R.D.; and OPPENHEIM, F.G. (1991): Anticandidal activity of major human salivary histatins. *Infect Immun* 59:2549-2554.

XU, T. and OPPENHEIM, F.G. (1989): Structural/functional analysis of anti-Candida activities of histatin 1. *J Dent Res* 68(Spec. Iss.):973.

XU, T. and OPPENHEIM, F.G. (1990): Antibacterial effects of histatins on different mutans streptococci serotypes, *J Dent Res* 69(Spec. Iss.):239.

XU, T. and OPPENHEIM, F.G. (1991): Anti-fungal functional domain of histatin 3. *J Dent Res* 70(Spec. Iss.):1852.

XU, T.; TELSER, E.; TROXLER, R.F.; and OPPENHEIM, F.G. (1990): Primary structure and anticandidal activity of the major histatin from parotid secretion of the subhuman primate, *Macaca fascicularis*. *J Dent Res* 69:1717-1723.

The Ebb and Flow of the Salivary Tide

C. DAWES

In this article I will summarize mostly the work from my own laboratory which relates to the title given to me by the organizers of the conference. In particular, I will discuss four common but incorrect assumptions about saliva which derive from the concept of a salivary tide.

The "ebb and flow of the salivary tide" immediately conjures up the vision of saliva as a large ocean which moves restlessly backwards and forwards; whose volume, in relation to its area of contact with plaque, is immense; whose composition is relatively uniform; and which can absorb considerable amounts of environmental pollutants without a significant effect on its composition. This vision does not in fact accord with reality.

1. *There is no tide* - The assumption that salivary flow rate is constant is made by those who characterize flow rate on the basis of one measurement made at some arbitrary time point. Fig. 1 illustrates the circadian rhythm of high amplitude in the unstimulated salivary flow rate (Dawes, 1972). Peak flow rate occurs in the late afternoon with the lowest flow rate in the early morning. Similar rhythms have also been described by Ferguson and Fort (1974) and others. The dashed line in Fig. 1 also illustrates the clinically very important finding of Schneyer *et al.* (1956), that salivary flow rate is greatly decreased during sleep. Thus sleep would seem to be a period of increased caries susceptibility in those consuming fermentable carbohydrates just prior to sleep.

   Studies are needed on patients with xerostomia to determine whether they also show such rhythms, but with a lower mean flow rate.

My own studies summarized in this article were supported by the Medical Research Council of Canada.

I thank Munksgaard and the Journal of Periodontal Research for permission to reproduce Fig. 5, and the Journal of Dental Research for permission to reproduce Figs. 2, 3, 4, 6 and 7.

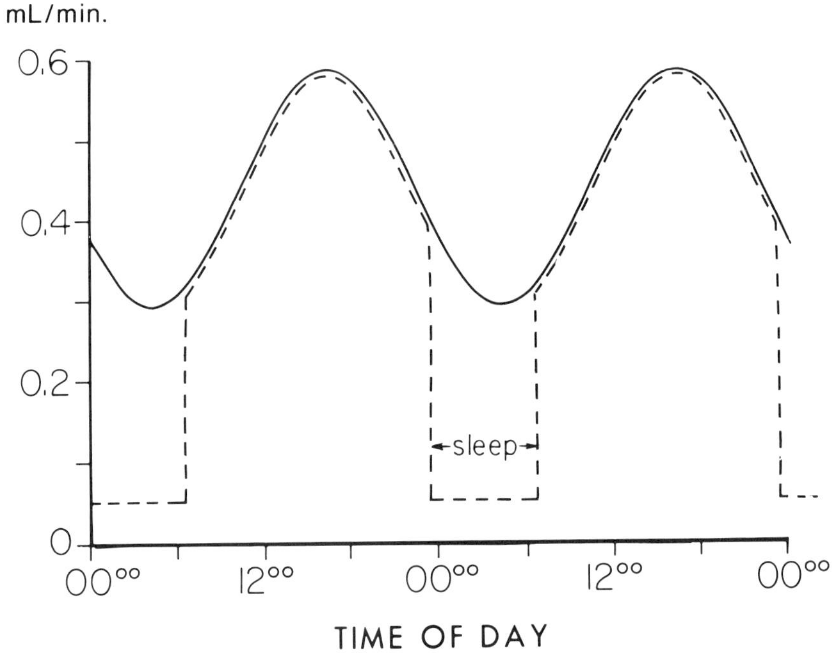

Figure 1. The circadian rhythm in unstimulated salivary flow rate (continuous line) and the idealized effect of sleep (dashed line) from 23:00 to 07:00 h.

Clearly though, this predictable variability in flow rate throughout the 24-hour day makes it inappropriate to take one measurement of salivary flow rate at some arbitrary time point.

Salivary protein and electrolyte concentrations also show circadian rhythms of high amplitude (Dawes, 1974) and thus, unlike the ocean's, the composition of saliva is certainly not almost constant. Although some of the rhythms in salivary electrolyte content are caused by rhythms in secretion of hormones such as aldosterone, very little is known of the factors responsible for the rhythms in flow rate and protein content (Dawes, 1974).

2. *Saliva is present in the mouth as a large volume.* - This assumption is implicit in the title I was given for this paper, which compares the saliva in the mouth to an ocean, the composition of which is not changed when diffusants pass into it from dental plaque. I believe that this assumption has been a major error.

Lagerlöf and Dawes (1984) estimated the volumes of saliva present in the adult mouth before and after swallowing to be 1.07 mL (range, 0.52 - 2.14 mL) and 0.77 mL (range, 0.38 - 1.73 mL), respectively.

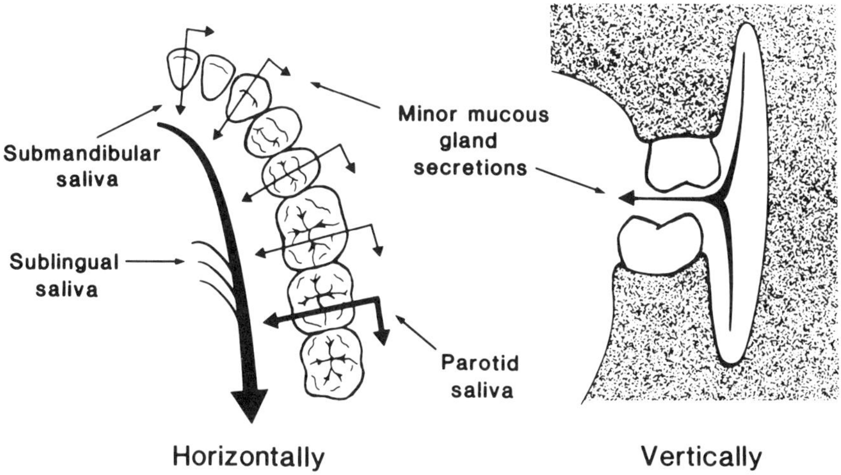

Figure 2. Diagrammatic representation of the anticipated directions and volumes of salivary flow in different locations in the mouth.

Collins and Dawes (1987) measured the surface area of the mouth and found a mean value of 215 ± 13 cm^2. A simple calculation shows that if the saliva were spread uniformly around the mouth, it would be present as a thin film only 0.1 mm or less in thickness. Watanabe and Dawes (1990), in a study on five-year-old children, reported a similar salivary film thickness, despite lower values for the oral surface area and the volumes of saliva in the mouth before and after swallowing.

When flow rate is unstimulated, the velocity of the salivary film appears to be extremely low and Dawes *et al.* (1989) estimated this to vary between 0.8 mm/min in the upper anterior buccal sulcus and 8 mm/min lingual to the lower anterior teeth.

Clearly then, saliva is not present as a large volume but as a slowly moving film. As will be seen later, this has important clinical implications.

3. *Saliva is well mixed in the mouth.* - Fig. 2 illustrates, for unstimulated saliva, our best estimates of the directions of movement of the salivary film at different locations in the mouth (Lecomte and Dawes, 1987). The widths of the arrows represent the estimated volumes of saliva. Studies by Weatherell *et al.* (1984) and Jenkins and Krebsbach (1985) have shown that there is very little migration of saliva from one side of the mouth to the other, except when materials are placed in the midline below the tongue. Weatherell *et al.* (1984) have also shown that when a fluoride tablet is placed in the buccal sulcus, there is very little increase in fluoride concentration anteriorly or posteriorly to the tablet, which implies

TABLE *A Comparison of Some Properties of Unstimulated Parotid, Submandibular/Sublingual and Minor Mucous Gland Secretions of Particular Relevance to Caries.*

	Parotid	*Submandibular/ Sublingual*	*Minor Mucous Glands*
% contribution to whole saliva	25	67	8
Viscosity	very low	medium	very high
Ca (mmol/L)	1.05	1.56	2.29
Inorg. P (mmol/L)	10.8	3.6	0.6
HCO_3 (mmol/L)	1.0	2.2	0.0

that the main direction of salivary flow in the buccal sulcus is occlusally, over the teeth, to the lingual region. Fluoride introduced into the mouth is also cleared at very different rates from different locations (Dawes and Weatherell, 1990).

Thus there is very little evidence that unstimulated saliva is well mixed in the mouth or that its direction of movement varies (ebbs and flows). This is important because the compositions of parotid, submandibular/sublingual, and minor mucous gland secretions are so different in many respects. Some of these differences relevant to caries are shown in the Table. Fig. 2 suggests that plaque on the buccal surfaces of the teeth will mainly be in contact with the minor mucous gland secretions rather than with secretions from the major glands.

4. *Only the microbiology of plaque is important for its cariogenicity.* - This assumption, which is perhaps the most mischievous of all, suggests that it is the proportion of mutans streptococci in plaque which determines its cariogenicity.

Virtually all plaques from people on a normal Western diet are able to produce acid by metabolism of fermentable carbohydrate. Removal of the acid occurs mainly by its diffusion into the overlying film of saliva. When the film velocity is low, diffusant tends to accumulate in the salivary film, and particularly at the distal end, as illustrated in Fig. 3. This reduces the concentration gradient for clearance, which is prolonged, especially at the distal edge. This process of acid clearance can be modelled by use of the two-dimensional form of Fick's second law of diffusion.

On the basis of the techniques described by Dawes and Dibdin (1986), we produced a computer model of a Stephan curve by modelling the normal salivary clearance of sucrose, the diffusion of sucrose into plaque after a sucrose rinse, the production of acid by the plaque bacteria, and the outward diffusion of the acid into the moving salivary film.

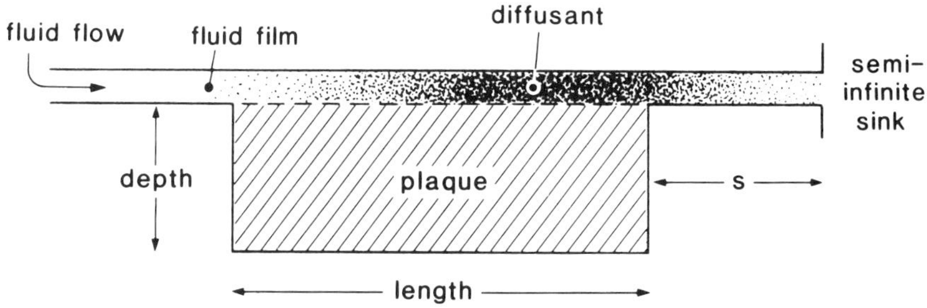

Figure 3. Diagrammatic representation of the accumulation of diffusant in the thin film of saliva passing slowly over a dental plaque.

Fig. 4 shows the results, which suggest that, other things being equal, the lower the salivary film velocity, the deeper and more prolonged will be the Stephan curve, particularly at the distal edge of the plaque (Dawes, 1989).

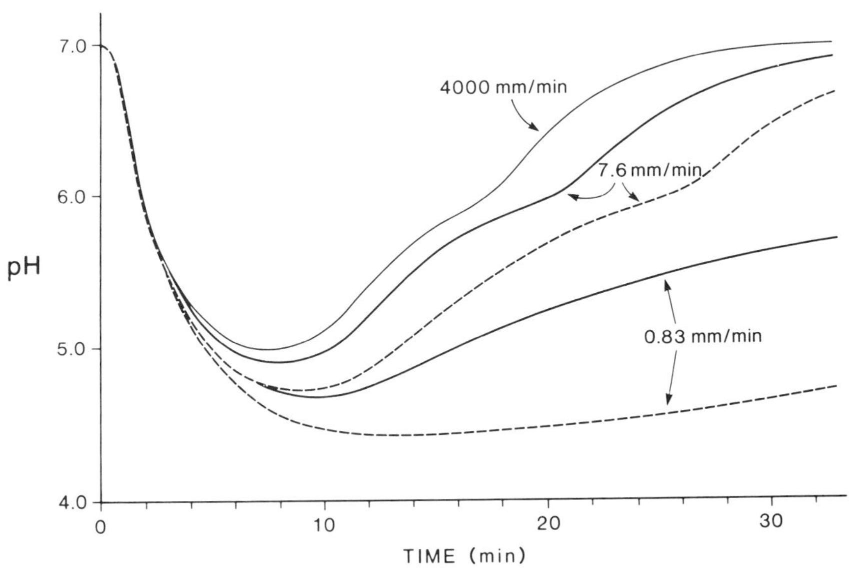

Figure 4. The predicted effects of three different salivary film velocities on Stephan curves for plaque 0.5 mm thick and 6 mm wide, after an initial exposure to a saturated sucrose solution, followed by normal salivary clearance. The solid lines give the predicted pH values at the enamel surface under the proximal side of the plaque that comes into contact with the fluid film first, whereas the dashed lines are for the exit or distal side of the plaque. At the high salivary film velocity, these two lines are identical.

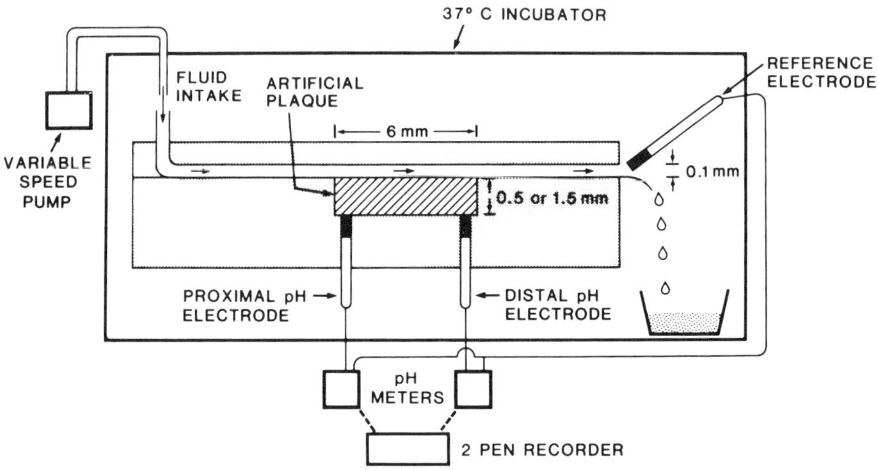

Figure 5. The design of the apparatus used for pH measurements at the proximal and distal undersurfaces of artificial plaques during passage of fluid over the surface at different velocities.

It is very hard to test this concept *in vivo* because of the difficulty of obtaining physically and microbiologically identical plaques in different regions of the mouth. Thus we have developed an *in vitro* model (Macpherson and Dawes, 1991a, b) which is illustrated in Fig. 5.

The well contained 10% of the acidogenic microorganism *Streptococcus oralis* in a 1% agarose gel. We found that including about 10% *S. oralis* in the agarose gel would give a maximum velocity of acid production which was equivalent to that in natural dental plaque. In some studies we also incorporated up to 57% dead bacteria to simulate the buffer capacity of the bacteria in plaque. Saliva was passed over the surface at different velocities and the pH measured proximally and distally under the plaque.

Fig. 6 shows the effect of fluid film velocity on the types of Stephan curves generated (Macpherson and Dawes, 1991b). As with the computer model, the slower the fluid film velocity, the deeper and more prolonged were the Stephan curves, especially in the well-buffered plaques containing 57% dead bacteria as well as the 10% live *S. oralis*.

These results are of great significance with respect to the site-specificity of caries. They imply that given two plaques of identical area, depth and microbial composition, the one which is located in a region of the mouth where salivary film velocity is lower, will be more cariogenic. However, when caries-preventive agents such as fluoride are put into the mouth, the model suggests that these will be retained longer at the sites which are more caries susceptible.

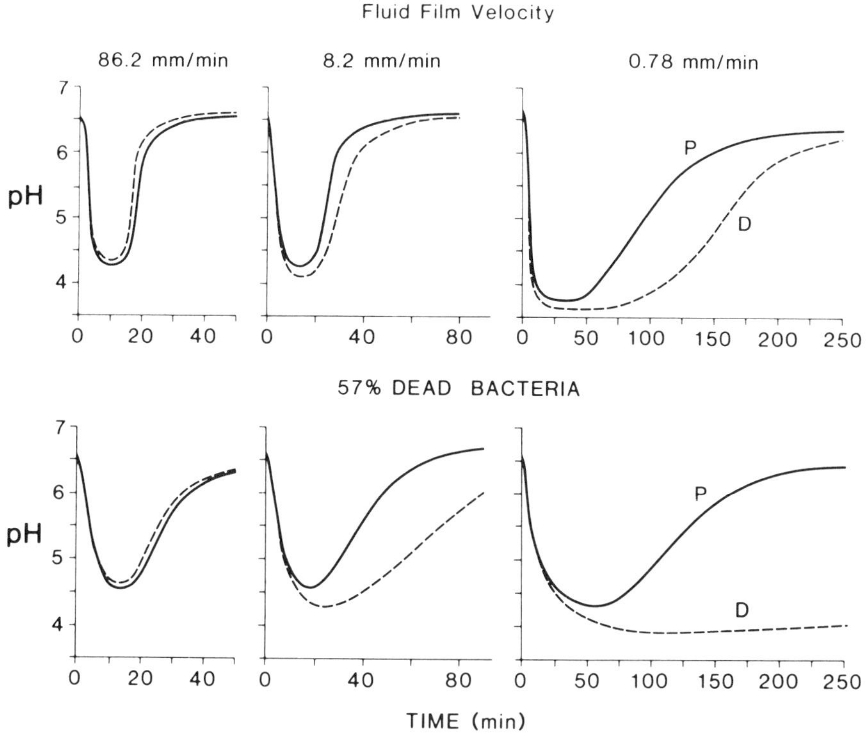

Figure 6. The effect of fluid film velocity and percentage dead bacteria on the pH proximally (P) and distally (D) under an artificial plaque 0.5-mm deep after exposure to a 10% sucrose solution for 1 min.

Our studies on salivary film velocity showed that the velocity was much lower buccally than lingually. Thus one would expect that if the model is valid, buccal smooth surfaces should be more caries-susceptible than lingual smooth surfaces. Fig. 7 shows some results, from the 1986 Dutch National Dental Survey, on caries prevalence on the buccal and lingual surfaces of the upper canines and premolars. These teeth were chosen because they typically do not have developmental pits or fissures. The higher prevalence of caries on the buccal smooth surfaces certainly fits with the predictions of the model.

There are, of course, other possible factors involved, one being that the minor mucous gland secretions, which are the main fluids in contact with the buccal surfaces of the teeth, have a composition which is quite different from that of the major salivary gland secretions (Table). Nevertheless, the role of salivary film velocity would seem to be an unrecognized but important factor in the site-specificity of caries.

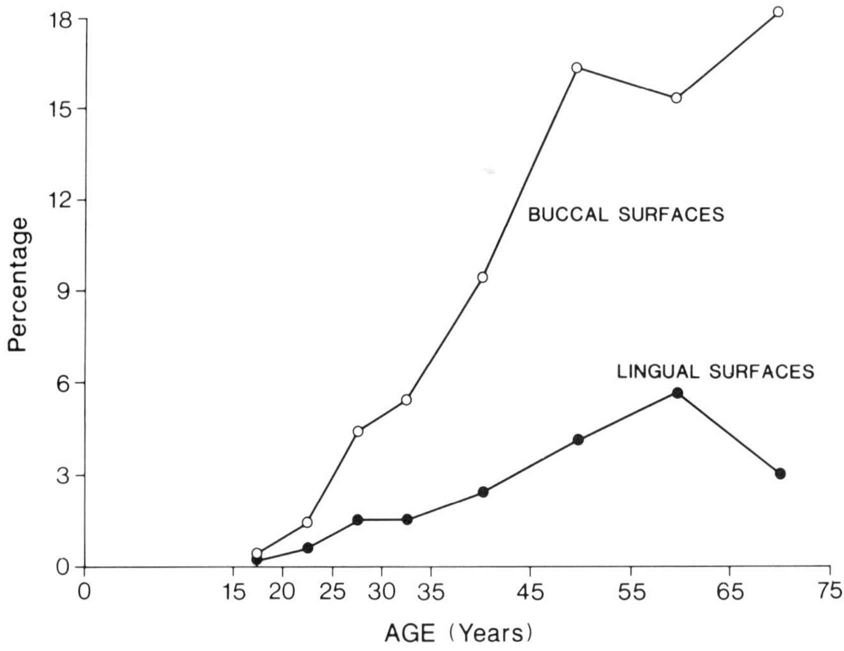

Figure 7. The change with age in the prevalence of smooth surface caries, buccally and lingually, on the upper canines and premolars (Data from Dutch National Dental Survey, 1986, courtesy of Dr. H.J.P. Kroeze).

Areas for Further Research

I suggest that a major need is for epidemiologists to give us more information on the site-specificity of oral disease. This would include not only caries, but also gingivitis, calculus, periodontal disease, and mucosal lesions of various types. If we are ever to explain the site-specificity of oral disease, we need much more information than summary statistics for the mouth as a whole, which are provided by most epidemiological surveys. I think that the time has long gone when we should consider the mouth to be a uniform environment. The mouth is in fact a collection of microenvironments. We also need much more information about the properties of the minor mucous gland secretions, with respect to their composition and rheology.

I think that we need to explore in much greater depth the implications of the concept that saliva is present in the mouth as a thin, slowly moving film. There will, of course, be localized variations in film thickness, velocity, and composition throughout the mouth and throughout the day and we presently have very little understanding of these.

REFERENCES

COLLINS, L.M.C. and DAWES, C. (1987): The Surface Area of the Adult Human Mouth and Thickness of the Salivary Film Covering the Teeth and Oral Mucosa, *J Dent Res* 66: 1300-1302.

DAWES, C. (1972): Circadian Rhythms in Human Salivary Flow Rate and Composition, *J Physiol* (Lond) 220: 529-545.

DAWES, C. (1974): Rhythms in Salivary Flow Rate and Composition, *Int J Chronobiol* 2: 253-279.

DAWES, C. (1989): An Analysis of Factors Influencing Diffusion from Dental Plaque into a Moving Film of Saliva and the Implications for Caries, *J Dent Res* 68: 1483-1488.

DAWES, C. and DIBDIN, G.H. (1986): A Theoretical Analysis of the Effects of Plaque Thickness and Initial Salivary Sucrose Concentration on Diffusion of Sucrose into Dental Plaque and its Conversion to Acid During Salivary Clearance, *J Dent Res* 65: 89-94.

DAWES, C.; WATANABE, S.; BIGLOW-LECOMTE, P.; and DIBDIN, G.H. (1989): Estimation of the Velocity of the Salivary Film at Some Different Locations in the Mouth, *J Dent Res* 68: 1479-1482.

DAWES, C. and WEATHERELL, J.A. (1990): Kinetics of Fluoride in the Oral Fluids, *J Dent Res* 69 (Spec Iss): 638-644.

FERGUSON, D.B. and FORT, A. (1974): Circadian Variations in Human Resting Submandibular Saliva Flow Rate and Composition, *Arch Oral Biol* 19: 47-55.

JENKINS, G.N. and KREBSBACH, P.H. (1985): Experimental Study of the Migration of Charcoal Particles in the Human Mouth, *Arch Oral Biol* 30: 697-699.

LAGERLÖF, F. and DAWES, C. (1984): The Volume of Saliva in the Mouth Before and After Swallowing, *J Dent Res* 63: 618-621.

LECOMTE, P. and DAWES, C. (1987): The Influence of Salivary Flow Rate on Diffusion of Potassium Chloride from Artificial Plaque at Different Sites in the Mouth, *J Dent Res* 66: 1614-1618.

MACPHERSON, L.M.D. and DAWES, C. (1991a): Urea Concentration in Minor Mucous Gland Secretions and the Effect of Salivary Film Velocity on Urea Metabolism by *Streptococcus vestibularis* in an Artificial Plaque, *J Periodont Res* 26:395-401.

MACPHERSON, L.M.D. and DAWES, C. (1991b): Effects of Salivary Film Velocity on pH Changes in an Artificial Plaque Containing *Streptococcus oralis*, After Exposure to Sucrose, *J Dent Res* 70:1230-1234.

SCHNEYER, L.H.; PIGMAN, W.; HANAHAN, L.; and GILMORE, R.W. (1956): Rate of Flow of Human Parotid, Sublingual, and Submaxillary Secretions During Sleep, *J Dent Res* 35: 109-114.

WATANABE, S. and DAWES, C. (1990): Salivary Flow Rates and Salivary Film Thickness in Five-year-old Children, *J Dent Res* 69: 1150-1153.

WEATHERELL, J.A.; ROBINSON, C.; RALPH, J.P.; and BEST, J.S. (1984): Migration of Fluoride in the Mouth, *Caries Res* 18: 348-353.

TEETH

Enamel and Dentine Gene Expression and Caries Resistance

HAROLD C. SLAVKIN

Calcium phosphate formation resulting in calcium hydroxyapatite crystal (HAP) in bone, dentine, cementum and enamel are associated with heterogeneous nucleation processes, controlled by specific regulatory and structural gene products within temporally- and positionally-restricted extracellular microenvironments (Weiner, 1986). It is assumed that extracellular matrix organic components [ECM] (e.g. type I collagen, phosphoproteins, anionic enamel glycoproteins, phospholipids) function as nucleators or substrates; chemical groups (e.g. amino acid side chains in the case of proteins) produce intermolecular three dimensional stereochemical geometry with attendant electrical charge distribution which replicates specific crystal planes of the HAP crystal to be nucleated. The nucleation substrate for HAP crystal formation is assumed to be a solid state aggregate.

Therefore, the specific physiochemical properties of the solid state aggregate, such as structural details of each of the dental tissue ECM proteins, provides tissue-specific biomineralization (e.g. number of crystals, size of crystals and pattern of crystal growth) (see reviews Deutsch, 1989; Linde, 1989; Slavkin *et al.*, 1988b; Veis, 1985). The challenge is to determine how these solid state aggregates induce and control tissue-specific patterns of HAP crystal growth, and how these patterns confer relative resistance to dental caries.

Specific protein domains are crucial components in the regulatory system that coordinates tissue-specific HAP crystal formation and growth. Domains within proteins such as type I collagen, dentine phosphoprotein (DPP), and amelogenin proteins may mediate their pleiotropic actions by binding to

The author would like to especially thank my colleagues Drs. Alan Fincham, Ed Lau, Mary MacDougall, Masanori Nakamura, Tony Nanci, Mal Snead and Maggie Zeichner-David from whom so much as been learned. These studies were supported by the United States Public Health Service, the National Institutes of Health, the National Institute For Dental Research, research grants DE-02848 and DE-06988.

calcium, interacting with one another and/or specific enzymes. These multiple functional regions possess physiochemical properties which may define when, where and to what size HAP crystals will form. The following discussion attempts to highlight selected advances which provide molecular explanations for tissue-specific biomineralization patterns which characterize dentine and enamel. It is suggested that this information can be used to augment clinical efforts to enhance resistance to dental caries.

The Role of the Extracellular Matrix in Biomineralization

Enamel and dentine ECM biomineralization provide two curiously different and unique examples of ECM protein-mediated biomineralizations (see reviews Slavkin, 1990a,b). Ectodermally-derived epithelia synthesize and secrete enamel proteins to form an ECM in juxtaposition and coordinated with ectomesenchymally-derived odontoblast which synthesize and secrete proteins to form the dentine ECM. Hole zone regions formed within type I collagen fibrils, and odontoblast-derived matrix vesicles appear to provide de novo nucleation sites for initial HAP crystal formation to form the putative dentino-enamel junction (DEJ) (Arsenault and Robinson, 1989). From the putative DEJ, relatively small and randomly arranged HAP crystals increase in number (multiplication) but not size and form dentine. In juxtaposition, HAP crystals at the DEJ grow in length along their c-axis and become highly-ordered enamel-specific HAP crystals — two different tissue-specific patterns of biomineralization appear to be initiated at the same interface yet grow to different sizes and patterns in opposite directions, regulated by two very different cell phenotypes.

Enamel Gene Products

Two major groups of proteins participate in the formation of the enamel ECM: (i) the anionic enamel glycoproteins (enamelins, circa 58 - 72 kDA) rich in glutamic acid, aspartic acid, serine and glycine, and (ii) the hydrophobic amelogenins (26 kDa) rich in proline, histidine and glutamine (Eastoe, 1979; Eggert *et al.*, 1973; Fearnhead, 1979; Fincham *et al.*, 1989a,b; 1990; 1991a,b; Limeback and Simic, 1989; Robinson *et al.*, 1989; Sasaki and Shimakowa, 1979; Slavkin *et al.*, 1988a; Termine *et al.*, 1981). The enamelins are synthesized and secreted by the enamel organ epithelia in tandem with the initial formation of the DEJ (Deutsch, 1989; Deutsch *et al.*, in press; Slavkin *et al.*, 1988a; Snead *et al.*, 1988), whereas the amelogenins are expressed after the initiation of enamel biomineralization (Slavkin *et al.*, 1988a; Snead *et al.*, 1988). Enamelins represent approximately 10% and are localized on the surfaces of enamel HAP, whereas amelogenins represent 90% of the total organic enamel ECM and are localized to the intercrystalline spaces between forming enamel HAP (Termine *et al.*, 1981; Deutsch, 1989; Deutsch *et al.*, in press).

The suggested functions for these two groups of enamel proteins include enamelins as the candidates for the nucleation of HAP crystals (Deutsch, 1989), and amelogenins regulate the rates, size and patterns of HAP crystal growth (Aoba and Moreno, 1989; Aoba *et al.*, 1987). The anionic enamelins and type I collagen forming the putative dentino-enamel junction may serve to nucleate HAP crystal formation (Arsenault and Robinson, 1989; Deutsch, 1989; Deutsch *et al.*, in press; Slavkin *et al.*, 1988a,b). The hydrophobic amelogenin proteins form aggregates at physiological temperatures and pH, and these properties may indicate their putative role in the regulation of enamel HAP crystal growth patterns (Nikiforuk and Simmons, 1965; Fincham *et al.*, 1991). During the progression of enamel biomineralization, amelogenins are essentially removed by proteolysis from the forming enamel along with water (DenBesten *et al.*, 1989; Fincham *et al.*, 1991b; Nanci *et al.*, 1987; Shimizu *et al.*, 1979; Smith *et al.*, 1989; Strawich and Glimcher, 1985; Suga, 1970), whereas enamelins appear to be retained and bound to the HAP crystal surfaces (see review by Deutsch,1989).

Recently, an enamelin protein primary structure was deduced from the nucleic acid sequence found within a 2674 base pair cDNA constructed and sequenced from a bovine ameloblast expression library (Deutsch *et al.*, in press). The deduced primary structure contains 389 amino acids and has a predicted molecular mass of 43,814 kDa (Deutsch *et al.*, in press). Southern hybridization studies of the cloned enamelin cDNA with genomic bovine DNA suggested a single gene with one or more introns (Deutsch *et al.*, in press).

Earlier, a cDNA for mouse amelogenin (pMa5-5) corresponding to a 26 kDa amelogenin protein was successfully constructed in our laboratory from mRNA extracted from young postnatal mouse molar tooth organs (Snead, *et al.*, 1983). In 1985 the nucleotide sequence for pMa5-5 was determined in our laboratory and the amino acid sequence was deduced from the nucleotide sequence (Snead *et al.*, 1985). The primary structure of bovine AMEL was reported (Tagaki *et al.*, 1984), as well as characterization of bovine AMEL transcripts (Shimokawa *et al.*, 1987; Young *et al.*, 1987) and gene (Gibson *et al.*, 1991).

In the mouse genome there is one AMEL loci located on the most distal locus in the genetic map of the X-chromosome and positioned proximal to the X:Y pairing region (Chapman *et al.*, 1991). The mouse AMEL locus is located in the region of Hyp (hypophophstemia) and Gy (Gyro) loci on the X-chromosome (Chapman *et al.*, 1991). In the human genome there are two AMEL loci with one copy of the gene on each of the sex chromosomes (AMELX and AMELY) (Lau *et al.*, 1989). Moreover, in support of the postulate that both the X and Y AMEL sequences are expressed during enamel formation, Fincham and his colleagues have recently reported that human developing enamel proteins exhibit a sex-linked polymorphism (1991a). Further support for this interpretation is also derived from the recent evidence from Gibson and colleagues which indicated that AMEL is also localized to both the X and Y chromosomes (1991). The AMELX structural gene has been mapped to the distal short arm in the p22.1 — p22.3 region of the X-chromosome; the AMELY is near the centromere in the q11 region of the Y chromosome (Lau *et al.*, 1989; 1990). This region is associated with the X-Y pair region and is subject to frequent recombinations which could contribute towards inherited diseases of enamel such as AI. Our results and those from other laboratories (Nakahori and Nakagome, 1989; Shimokawa *et al.*, 1987a.b; 1989) provide evidence that X-linked amelogenesis imperfecta (AI) is mapped to the same region as the AMELX structural gene (see Lau *et al.*, 1989; 1990; Backman and Holmgren, 1988; Witkop, 1989).

Dentine Gene Products

During the initial formation of dentine, odontoblasts express and secrete a fibrillar ECM, primarily consisting of Type I collagen. Whereas collagen represents approximately 90% of the organic ECM, odontoblasts also express and secrete an intriguing array of non-collagenous proteins including *dentine phosphoproteins* (i.e. *phosphoryns*) (see reviews by Butler *et al.*, in press; Linde, 1989; MacDougall, *et al.*, 1985a; Veis, 1985), *dentine sialoprotein (DSP)* (Butler *et al.*, 1989a,b; Fisher *et al.*, 1990), *osteocalcin (GLA protein)* (see reviews by Hauschka *et al.*, 1989; Price, 1988), *matrix GLA protein* (Price, 1988), *osteonectin* (Bolander *et al.*, 1988), *proteoglycans* and a number of growth factors and serum-derived glycoproteins.

Of these non-collagenous proteins, both dentine phosphoprotein (DPP) and dentine sialoprotein (DSP) are unique as dentine gene products (Butler *et al.*, in press; MacDougall *et al.*, 1985a,b; 1989; in press). DPP molecules consist of approximately 45% phosphoserine and 35% aspartic acid residues. DPPs demonstrate an isoelectric point of 1.1. This highly anionic macromolecule has high avidity for calcium ions and possibly functions in the regulation of biomineralization (see Linde, 1989; Stetler and Veis, 1983). DPP is unique to dentine; it is not found in other mineralizing ECM systems such as bone, cementum or enamel.

Mouse and human dentine phosphoproteins (DPP) have been isolated and partially characterized (MacDougall *et al.*, in press). The mouse ECM DPP has a molecular weight of 72 kDa and migrates in SDS/PAGE as a single band not detectable with Coomassie Blue but only with Stains All (phosphorylated and glycosylated proteins). DPPmRNA has been isolated and characterized. Cell-free translation studies indicated that the nascent DPP is synthesized as a molecule of 43 kDa. These studies confirm the result obtained by desphosphorylation of DPP. The size of the mouse DPP mRNA has been shown to be the same in several other mammalian species (MacDougall, personal communication).

The RNA extracted has been used to produce a lamda gtll mouse tooth organ cDNA library. The cDNA library has been screened utilizing both the DPP antibody and a synthetic oligonucleotide containing a unique sequence for DPP determined for the N-terminal sequence of rat DPP by Butler and his colleagues (1983). Positive cDNA clones for both probes were isolated and partially characterized. The DPP oligonucleotide probe was used to determine the human chromosomal localization of DPP. Results clearly show that DPP is not encoded within chromosome 4. Since linkage analysis has mapped the locus of DGI-II and III to chromosome 4 (see Boughman *et al.*, 1986), the new evidence indicates that the DPP structural gene is not directly involved in this genetic defect. The DPP gene is localized to human chromosome 1 (MacDougall *et al.*, in press). A human chromosome 1 library was screened and several positive clones isolated.

Prospectus

The last decade has produced a significant increase in the database describing many structural and regulatory genes and their suggested functions in human diseases. Human chromosomes contain 3.5 x 109 nucleotide base pairs within each parental strand of DNA or 7 billion bits of information within the human genome. Within the genome there are approximately 100,000 different structural and regulatory genes. Approximately 4,000 inherited human diseases have been identified.

The recent advances in molecular genetic studies of dental genes and their gene products provides new strategies to pursue studies of diagnosis, treatment, prognosis, and prevention, as well as studies to develop new biomaterials. Methods are now available to characterize the molecular genetics for enamel, dentine, cementum, bone, periodontal tissues, saliva, oral microoganisms and the host immune system. For example, the human amelogenin structural gene has been mapped to both the human X chromosome as well as the human Y chromosome. The human dentine phosphoprotein structural gene appears to be located on chromosomes 1 and 16. Therefore, the structural gene for DPP is not located on human chromosome 4 and, therefore, a mutation in the DPP gene is unlikely to be the molecular lesion in dentinogenesis inperfecta (DI) which has previously been linked to chromosome 4 (see Ball *et al.*, 1984). The molecular genetic studies regarding the structure and chromosome localizations for human dental genes serves as a paradigm for future studies, and also provides a rationale and strategy to investigate susceptibility and resistance to dental diseases.

REFERENCES

AOBA, T. and MORENO, E.C. (1989): Mechanism of amelogenitic mineralization in minipig secretory enamel. In: *Tooth Enamel V*, R.W. Fearnhead, Ed., Florence Publishers, Yokohama, pp. 163-167.

AOBA, T.; TAMABE, T.; and MORENO, E.C. (1987): Function of amelogenins in porcine enamel mineralization during the secretory stage of amelogenesis. *Adv Dent Res* 1:252-260.

ARSENAULT, L.R. and ROBINSON, B.W. (1989): The dentino-enamel junction: a structural and microanalytical study of early mineralization. *Calcif Tiss Inter* 45:111-121.

BACKMAN, B. and HOLMGREN, G. (1988): Amelogenesis imperfecta: a genetic study. *Hum Hered* 38:189-206.

BOLANDER, M.E.; YOUNG, M.F.; FISHER, L.W.; YAMADA, Y.; and TERMINE, J.D. (1988): Osteonectin cDNA sequence reveals potential binding regions for calcium and hydroxyapatite and shows homologies with both a basement membrane protein (SPARC) and a serine proteinase (ovomucoid). *Proc Natl Acad Sci (USA)* 85:2919-2923.

BOUGHMAN, J.A.; HALLORAN, S.L.; and ROULSTON, D. (1986): An autosomal dominant form of juvenile periodontitis: Its localization to chromosome 4 and linkage to dentinogenesis imperfecta and Gc. *J Craniofac Genet & Develop Biol* 6:341-350.

BUTLER, W.T. (1989a): The nature and significance of osteopontin. *Connective Tiss Res* 23:123-136.

BUTLER, W.T. (1989b): Sialoproteins of bone and dentin. *J Biol Buccale* 19:83-89.

BUTLER, W.T.; BROWN, M.; DIMUZIO, M.T.; and COTHRAN, W.C. (1983): Multiple forms of rat dentin phosphoproteins. *Arch Biochem Biophys* 225:178-186.

BUTLER, W.T.; D'SOUZA, R.N.; BRONCKERS, A.L.J.J.; HAPPONEN, R.P.; and SOMERMAN, M.J. (1992): Recent advances on dentine specific proteins. *Finnish Dental Soc Journal*. 88:369-376.

CHAPMAN, V.M.; KEITZ, B.T.; DISTECHE, C.M.; LAU, E.C.; and SNEAD, M.L. (1991): Linkage of amelogenin (Amel) to the distal portion of the mouse X chromosome. *Genomics* 10:23-28.

DENBESTEN, P.K.; AWBREY, B.J.; and TREADWELL, B.V. (1989): Similarities between proteinase in secretory enamel matrix and a neutral metalloproteinase found in cartilage. In: *Tooth Enamel V*, R.W. Fearnhead, Ed., Florence Publishers, Yokohama, pp. 278-282.

DEUTSCH, D. (1989): Structure and function of enamel gene products. *Anat Rec* 224:189-210.

DEUTSCH, D.; PALMON, A.; FISHER, L.W.; KOLODNY, N.; TERMINE, J.D.; and YOUNG, M.F. (1991): Sequencing of bovine enamelin ("Tuftelin"): A novel acidic enamel protein. *J Biol Chem* 266:16021-16028.

EASTOE, J.E. (1979): Enamel protein chemistry—past, present and future. *J Dent Res* 58(B):753-764.

EGGERT, G.M.; ALLEN, G.A.; and BURGESS, R.C. (1973): Amelogenins: purification and partial characterization of proteins from developing bovine enamel. *Biochem J* 131:471-484.

FEARNHEAD, R.W. (1979): Matrix-mineral relationships in enamel tissues. *J Dent Res* 58(B):909-916.

FINCHAM, A.G.; BESSEM, C.; BRINGAS, P.; HU, Y.; SNEAD, M.L.; and SLAVKIN, H.C. (1989a): Amelogenesis in vitro: a model for studies of epithelial postsecretory processing during tissue-specific extracellular matrix biomineralization. *Differentiation* 41:62-71.

FINCHAM, A.G.; HU, Y.; PAVLOVA, Z.; SLAVKIN, H.C.; and SNEAD, M.L. (1989b): Human amelogenins: Sequences of "TRAP" molecules. *Calcif Tissue Int* 45:243-250.

FINCHAM, A.G.; HU, Y.; LAU, E.; PAVLOVA, Z.; SLAVKIN, H.C.; and SNEAD, M.L. (1990): Isolation and partial characterization of a human amelogenin from a single fetal dentition using HPLC techniques. *Calcif Tissue Int* 47:105-111.

FINCHAM, A.G.; BESSEM, C.C.; LAU, E.C.; PAVLOVA, Z.; SHULER, C.; SLAVKIN, H.C.; and SNEAD, M.L. (1991a): Human developing enamel proteins exhibit a sex-linked dimorphism. *Calcif Tissue Int* 48:288-290.

FINCHAM, A.G.; BESSEM, C.C.; SLAVKIN, H.; and SNEAD, M.L. (1991b): Amelogenin post-secretory processing during biomineralization in the postnatal mouse molar tooth. *Arch Oral Biol* 36:305-317.

FISHER, L.W.; MCBRIDE, O.W.; TERMINE, J.D.; and YOUNG, M.F. (1990): Human bone sialoprotein. *J Biol Chem* 265:2347-2351.

GIBSON, C.W.; DING, W.; RISSER, M.; DIXON, M.; TERMINE, J.D.; YOUNG, M.F.; and ROSENBLOOM, J. (1991): The structure and expression of the bovine amelogenin gene. *Proceedings of The Third International Conference on Molecular Biology and Pathology of Matrix*, pp. 12.

HAUSCHKA, P.V.; LIAN, J.B.; COLE, D.E.C.; and GUNDBERG, C.M. (1989): Osteocalcin and matrix GLA protein: Vitamin K-dependent proteins in bone. *Physiol Rev* 69:990-1047.

LAU, E.C.; MOHANDAS, T.K.; SHAPIRO, L.J.; SLAVKIN, H.C.; and SNEAD, M.L. (1989): Human and mouse amelogenin gene loci are on the sex chromosomes. *Genomics* 4:162-168.

LAU, E.C.; SLAVKIN, H.C.; and SNEAD, M.L. (1990): Analysis of human enamel genes: insights into genetic disorders of enamel. *Cleft Palate J* 27:121-130.

LIMEBACK, H. and SIMIC, A. (1990): Biochemical characterization of stable high molecular weight aggregates of amelogenins formed during porcine enamel development. *Arch Oral Biol* 35:459-468.

LINDE, A. (1989): Dentin matrix proteins: Composition and possible functions in calcification. *Anat Rec* 224:154-166.

MACDOUGALL, M.; ZEICHNER-DAVID, M.; BRINGAS, P.; and SLAVKIN, H.C. (1985a): Dentine phosphoprotein expression during in vitro mouse tooth organ culture. In: *The Chemistry and Biology of Mineralized Tissues* W. Butler, Ed., Ebsco Media, Inc., Birmingham, AL., pp. 177-181.

MACDOUGALL, M.; ZEICHNER-DAVID, M.; and SLAVKIN, H.C. (1985b): Production and characterziation of antibodies against murine dentine phosphoprotein. *Biochem J* 232:493-500.

MACDOUGALL, M.; ZEICHNER-DAVID, M.; and SLAVKIN, H.C. (1989): Characterization of extracellular and nascent dentin phosphoproteins. *Connect Tissue Res* 22:71-77.

MACDOUGALL, M.; ZEICHNER-DAVID, M.; DAVIS, A.; SNEAD, M.L.; and SLAVKIN, H.C. (in press): Characterization of mouse dentine phosphoprotein mRNA. *Calcif Tissue Int*

MACDOUGALL M.; ZEICHNER-DAVID M.; MURRAY J.; CRALL M.; DAVIS A.; and SLAVKIN H.C. (1992): Dentine phosphoprotein gene locus is not associated with Dentinogenesis Imperfecta Types II and III. *Am J Hum Genet* 50:190-194.

NAKAHORI, Y. and NAKAGOME, Y. (1989): Xp - Yq homologous region encodes open reading frames corresponding to "amelogenin." *Cytogenetics & Cell Genet* 51:1050.

NANCI, A.; SLAVKIN, H.C.; and SMITH, C.E. (1987): Immunocytochemical and radioautographic evidence for secretion and intracellular degradation of enamel proteins by ameloblasts during the maturation stage of amelogenesis in rat incisors. *Anat Rec* 217:107-123.

NIKIFORUK, G. and SIMMONS, N.S. (1965): Purification and properties of enamel proteins. *J Dent Res* 44:229-248.

PRICE, P.A. (1988): Role of vitamin K-dependent proteins in bone metabolism. *Ann Rev Nutr* 8:565-583.

ROBINSON, D.; KIRKHAM, J.; and FINCHAM, A.G. (1989): The enamelin/non-amelogenin problem: A brief review. *Conn Tissue Res* 22:93-100.

SASAKI, S. and SHIMOKAWA, H. (1979): Enamel protein: biosynthesis and chemistry. *J Dent Res* 58(B):765-771.

SHIMOKAWA, H.; SOBEL, M.E.; SASAKI, M.; TERMINE, J.D.; and YOUNG, M.F. (1987): Heterogeneity of amelogenin mRNA in the bovine tooth. *J Biol Chem* 262:4042-4047.

SHIMIZU, M.; TANABE, T.; and FUKAE, M. (1979): Proteolytic enzyme in porcine immature enamel. *J Dent Res* 58(B):782-788.

SLAVKIN, H.C.; BESSEM, C.; BRINGAS, P. JR.; ZEICHNER-DAVID, M.; NANCI, A.; and SNEAD, M.L. (1988a): Sequential expression and differential function of multiple enamel proteins during fetal neonatal and early postnatal stages of mouse molar organogenesis. *Differentiation* 37:26-39.

SLAVKIN, H.C.; SNEAD, M.L.; ZEICHNER-DAVID, M.; MACDOUGALL, M.; FINCHAM, A.G.; LAU, E.C.; LUO, W.; NAKAMURA, M.; OLIVER, P.; and EVANS, J. (1988b): Factors influencing expression of dental ECM biomineralization. In: *Cell and Molecular Biology of Hard Tissues* D. Evered and S. Harnett, Eds., John Wiley & Sons, Chichester, England, pp. 22-35.

SLAVKIN, H.C. (1990): Molecular determinants of tooth development: A review. *Critical Reviews In Oral Biology and Medicine* 1:1-16.

SLAVKIN, H.C.; SNEAD, M.L.; ZEICHNER-DAVID, M.; LAU, E.C.; and FINCHAM, A.G. (1990): Dental enamel biomineralization: A prospectus. In: *MRS Proceedings* P. Rieke, P. Calvert, and M. Alper, Eds., pp. 3-8.

SMITH, C.E.; BORENSTEIN, S.; FAZEL, A.; and NANCI, A. (1989): In vitro studies of the proteinases which degrade amelogenins in developing rat incisor enamel. In: *Tooth Enamel V* R.W. Fearnhead, Ed. Florence Publishers, Yokohama, pp. 286-290.

SNEAD, M.L.; ZEICHNER-DAVID, M.; CHANDRA, T.; ROBSON, K.J.H.; WOO, S.; and SLAVKIN, H.C. (1983): Construction and identification of mouse amelogenin cDNA clones. *Proc Natl Acad Sci (USA)* 80:7254-7258.

SNEAD, M.L.; LAU, E.C.; ZEICHNER-DAVID, M.; FINCHAM, A.G.; WOO, S.L.C.; and SLAVKIN, H.C. (1985): DNA sequence for cloned cDNA for murine amelogenin reveal the amino acid sequence for enamel-sepcific protein. *Biochem Biophys Res Commun* 129:812-818.

SNEAD, M.; LUO, W.; LAU, E.; and SLAVKIN, H.C. (1988): Spatial- and temporal-restricted pattern of amelogenin gene expression during mouse molar tooth organogenesis. *Development* 104:77-85.

STETLER-STEVENSON, W.G. and VEIS, A. (1983): Bovine dentin phosphophoryn: composition and molecular weight. *Biochemistry* 22:4326-4335.

STRAWICH, E. and GLIMCHER, M.J. (1985): Synthesis and degradation in vivo of a phosphoprotein from rat dental enamel. *Biochem J* 230:423-433.

SUGA, S. (1970): Histochemical observations of proteolytic enzyme activity in the developing dental hard tissues of the rat. *Arch Oral Biol* 5:555-558.

TAGAKI, T.; SUSUKI, M.; BABA, T.; MINIGESHI, K.; and SASAKI, S. (1984): Complete amino acid sequence of amelogenin in developing bovine enamel. *Biochem Biophys Res Commun* 121:592-597.

TERMINE, J.D.; BELCOURT, A.B.; CHRISTNER, P.J.; CONN, K.M.; and NYLEM, M.U. (1981): Properties of dissociatively extracted fetal tooth matrix proteins. Principal molecular species in developing bovine enamel. *J Biol Chem* 255:9760-9768.

VEIS, A. (1985): Phosphoproteins of dentin and bone. Do they have a role in matrix biomineralization? In: *The Chemistry and Biology of Mineralized Tissues* W.T. Butler, Ed., EBSCO Media, Birmingham, Al., pp. 170-176.

WEINER, S. (1986): Organization of extracellularly mineralized tissues: A comparative study of biological crystal growth. *CRC Critical Rev Biochem* 20:365-408.

WITKOP, C.J. (1989): Amelogenesis imperfecta, dentinogenesis imperfecta and dentin dyspasia revisited: problems in classification. *J Oral Pathol* 17:547-553.

YOUNG, M.F.; SHIMOKAWA, H.S.; SOBEL, M.E.; and TERMINE, J. D. (1987): A characterization of amelogenin messenger RNA in the bovine tooth germ. *Adv Dent Res* 1:289-292.

Structure and Composition of Cementum

M. J. SOMERMAN, G. M. MORRISON, M. B. ALEXANDER, AND
R. A. FOSTER

The name cementum has been ascribed to the mineralized tissue on the root surface of teeth, but it also has been used to describe the mineralized tissue associated with the enamel surface in some species (Heritier 1982; Listgarten, 1967, and 1968; Listgarten and Shapiro, 1975). Its main function in health is to attach periodontal ligament fibers to the root surface. Prior to the awareness of the importance of non-collagenous proteins in the regulation of mineralized tissues, it was generally thought that bone and cementum were identical in composition (Sicher and Bhasker, 1972).

The growing appreciation of the importance of cementum for maintaining and regenerating periodontal tissues, for controlling root surface caries and for determining appropriate orthodontic procedures, has resulted in increased research directed at understanding its structure, function and regenerative capability. As early as 1946, studies indicated that an abnormality in cementum deposition, "cementopathia", is strongly correlated with formation of periodontitis (Gottlieb, 1946). More recently Page and Baab (1986) reported that several patients with prepubertal periodontitis had no cementum or hypoplastic cementum, a finding which led to the suggestion that aberrant or lack of cementum results in abnormal connective tissue attachment which makes teeth susceptible to invasion by periodontal pathogens. Similar findings were reported a few years earlier by Lindskog and Blomlöf (1983) in their scanning electron microscopic study of roots of teeth extracted from patients with juvenile periodontitis, i.e., aplastic or hypoplastic cementum was evident. Many of these patients had diagnostic features of hypophosphatasia, e.g., low levels of alkaline phosphatase, and presence of phosphoethanolamine in the urine. However, in some cases no medical

The authors would like to thank the skillful assistance of Ms. Sandra Phillips, Ms. Sue Duncan and Mr. Norman Schiff. The studies presented here were funded in part by NIDR, NIH grants DE-09532, and DE-00262.

abnormalities were noted. These studies indicate that cementum has properties that are required specifically for the maintenance of a healthy periodontium.

This report is an attempt to review the developments in the understanding of structure and composition cementum. While significant progress has been made, additional critical information on the properties of cementum clearly is required before therapies for treatment of root associated diseases can be developed.

Structure and Composition

Excellent descriptions of the histology of cementum during health and disease, have been reviewed in detail previously (Selvig, 1963, 1964, 1965, 1977; Sicher and Bhaskar, 1972; Stahl, 1975; Owens, 1979; Schroeder, 1986; Yamasaki *et al.*, 1987; Cho and Garant, 1988, 1989), and thus the information and discussion provided here focus more on the composition of the extracellular matrix of cementum during development, regeneration and in the mature healthy state.

a) Developmental - Current evidence suggests that cells derived from the dental follicle and dental papillae are capable, when appropriately stimulated of forming cementum, periodontal ligament and bone (Ten Cate *et al.*, 1978; Schroeder, 1986; Palmer and Lumsden, 1987; Osborn and Price, 1988). However, the factors triggering such cells to migrate and attach to the root surface and subsequently secrete a cementum matrix are largely unknown. Some researchers report that the initial event in cementum formation is the secretion of an extracellular matrix (ECM) called intermediate cementum possibly by epithelial cells of Hertwig's epithelial root sheath (HERS), onto the dentin surface (Owens, 1979; Lindskog, 1982; Thomas and Kollar, 1989; MacNeil and Thomas, 1989; and Slavkin *et al.*, 1976, 1990).

Studies by Slavkin *et al.* (1989a, b) support a role for enamel-related proteins in inducing formation of cementum. Using a mouse molar model system, *in vivo* and *in vitro,* their results suggest that HERS synthesizes and secretes polypeptides similar, although distinct from crown enamel proteins and are involved in the process of acellular cementum formation. Additional reports by Heritier (1982) also support this concept. He demonstrated that during root development exposure of follicular tissues to the crown enamel resulted in the stimulation of cementogenesis, *in vivo.* In contrast, Cho and Garant (1989), in their histological studies, did not observe such an ECM. Other studies, examining the development of cementum have suggested that adhesion proteins including fibronectin, laminin, osteopontin (OPN), and tenascin, play a role in regulation of cementum formation (Thesleff *et al.* 1981; Andujar *et al.* 1985; Vaino *et al.*, 1989; MacNeil and Thomas, 1989; Somerman *et al.*, 1990).

The next event, the disruption and migration of cells of HERS away from the dentinal surface has been confirmed by many groups (review, Ten Cate, 1989). However, the exact mechanisms involved in regulating the disruption of HERS is yet to be determined. Ultrastructural studies in the rat, by Cho and Garant (1988, 1989) directed at determining the stages involved in formation of initial, acellular cementum indicated that coincident with the disruption of HERS directed migration of precementoblasts occurs from the region of the dental follicle toward the dentin matrix. Such cells appear to adhere to the dentin surface for a short period where they express a cementoblast-like phenotype secreting an extracellular matrix. Subsequently, they detach from the root surface and are incorporated into the periodontal ligament where they act as a fibroblast-like cell.

If it is true that epithelial - mesenchymal interactions are required for cementum formation, then one must wonder how 'reparative' cementum is formed subsequent to disease and what events allow for new cementum formation during the normal history of a tooth? Ultrastructurally, Philipson, *et al.* (1990) noted that reparative cementum was the same as original cementum; however, the events/factors triggering cementum formation were not examined. In a similar tissue, dentin, it is known that reparative dentin is not induced through epithelial-mesenchymal interactions, as is the initial formed dentin. In this situation it is thought that the odontoblasts have been programmed during development and thus do not need the epithelial interaction. Studies by Aukhil *et al.* (1990) suggest that induction of 'reparative' cementum formation requires an interaction of cells with dentin. In addition, Cho and Garant (1988) indicated, that follicular cells contact dentin matrix prior to the formation of acellular cementum. Dentin is known to have osteoinductive capacity (Urist, 1971; Butler *et al.*, 1977; Inoue *et al.*, 1986, Somerman *et al.*, 1987; Veis *et al.*, 1990; Bessho *et al.*, 1991), and this property may be important for formation, as well as regeneration of the periodontium.

b) Mature Cementum - Mature cementum contains two major cell types. Cementoblasts that line the root surfaces and cementocytes, defined by location as cells within lacunae of the cementum matrix (Selvig, 1974, 1975). Studies by Lindskog *et al.* (1987) indicate that the cells lining the root surface do not respond to parathyroid hormone as do cells lining bone, and thus reinforce previous studies suggesting a protective function for these cells as a barrier against root resorption (Lindskog and Hammarström, 1980). Indeed, such protection against root resorption is important in clinical situations including the application of orthodontic techniques. Cementum does not remodel, but, instead is subject to a slow process of material deposition (Zander & Hürzeler, 1958). Thus, 'clastic' cells are only observed in certain pathological conditions, in resorption of deciduous teeth and where excessive orthodontic force is present. Our understanding of the properties of cementum, at the cellular and molecular level has been limited largely because of two handicaps. One, the limited number of cementoblasts present on a root surface and the difficulty in separating such cells from the large population of periodontal ligament fibroblasts in the area and two, unlike osteoblasts, which have been isolated from bone for *in vitro* studies, cementoblasts have not successfully been isolated in culture. As discussed below studies directed at identifying unique cemental proteins will provide markers for cementoblasts so that such a cell type can be identified and their properties established *in vitro*.

The inorganic matrix which is approximately 50% of cementum content, is composed of hydroxyapatite. In contrast, in the other mineralized tissue, the inorganic matrix makes up more of the tissues content; i.e., enamel ≅ 95%, bone ≅ 60%, dentin ≅ 70%. Approximately 90% of the organic matrix of cementum is collagen. The predominant collagen of this matrix is type I collagen, with less than 5% of type III collagen (Birkedal-Hansen *et al.*, 1977; Tung *et al.*, 1985).

The realization that non-collageneous proteins associated with mineralized tissues may be utilized to remedy mineralized tissue defects caused by injury and disease has stimulated considerable research activities directed at purifying and characterizing these matrix constituents (see symposia by Butler, 1985; Glimcher and Lian, 1988). Indeed, several of these proteins from bone, enamel and dentin have been purified and biochemically characterized. However, until recently, few studies have focused on the purification and characterization of the non-collagenous proteins of cementum. This work has progressed slowly due to the difficulty in obtaining significant quantities of cementum (Chovelon *et al.*, 1975; Smith *et al.*, 1983; Miki *et al.*, 1987; Craig *et al.*, 1989;, McAllister *et al.*, 1990; and Somerman *et al.*, 1991). Recently, however, with the utilization of improved techniques, including nucleic acid probes, more sophisticated extraction procedures and histochemical methods, information on the properties of cementum is evolving more rapidly, so that hopefully we can now address some issues that are critical to our understanding and to improved treatment of root caries and periodontal diseases.

Recent evidence indicates that proteins of cementum influence the behavior of periodontal cells (Table 1). For example, studies have shown that protein extracts of cementum promote cell attachment (Somerman *et al.*, 1987c, 1991; McAllister *et al.*, 1990), stimulate cell migration (Nishimura *et al.*, 1989), enhance cell synthetic activity (Somerman *et al.* 1987a, b) and have mitogenic activity (Miki *et al.*, 1987). Most recently, investigations have shown that mature cementum contains at least three RGD-associated adhesion proteins, bone sialoprotein (BSP) (Somerman *et al.*, 1991), a bone-associated adhesion protein, tenascin, an adhesion protein considered to have a role in cell differentiation (Lukinmaa *et al.*, 1990) and fibronectin, a universal adhesion protein enhancing attachment of many cell types, including bacteria (Yamada, 1985, Lukinmaa *et al.*, 1990). BSP which prior to being identified in cementum, was considered selective to bone and dentin (Fisher *et al.*, 1983, 1987, 1990; Chen *et al.*, 1991) may prove to be a marker for osteoblast and cementoblast-like cells. Other proteins factors identified in cementum include osteonectin (Tung *et al.*, 1985) a bone associated protein (Termine *et al.*, 1981), although found in other tissues as well (Nomura *et al.*, 1988; and Wasi *et al.*, 1984), proteoglycans (Alexander *et al.*, 1991; Bartold *et al.*, 1988, 1990) and γ-carboxyglutamic acid, probably associated with osteocalcin (Glimcher *et al.*, 1979, Alexander, *et al.*, 1991).

Clinical Concerns

a) Regeneration of cementum - There is general agreement that tissues of the periodontium harbor cells with the capacity to regenerate the periodontium (McCulloch *et al.*, 1987; see review, Aukhil *et al.* 1990). *In vitro* evidence supports the theory that periodontal cells can form acellular cementum on a dentinal surface (Beerstein and Vanden Bos, 1991). Also, studies in monkeys have shown that cells from the peridontium can form cementum around titanium implants (Buser *et al.*, 1990). This has fostered an interest in developing clinical methodologies to restore periodontal support by stimulating such cells to function in a regenerative capacity. Initial research efforts have focused on development of reliable procedures to restore connective tissue attachment to previously diseased root surfaces. Results indicate that cemental regeneration is possible and that this is best achieved at sites that received a combination treatment of epithelial exclusion, via root submersion, and osseous grafting (Bowers *et al.*, 1989; review, Becker and Becker, 1991). In addition, there is some indication that both cell and fiber attachment can be enhanced with root surface preparations, such as demineralization and the coating of root surfaces with adhesive factors (Register and Burdick, 1976; Smith *et al.*, 1987; Terranova and Wikesjo, 1987).

While showing some success in regenerating periodontal tissues the above procedures have not been predictable in the clinical environment. Key information is missing on exactly which cells play a role in stimulating periodontal regeneration and which factors are involved in triggering the appropriate cells to function in a regenerative capacity. To improve the success of clinical procedures, research efforts must succeed in understanding, at the cellular and molecular levels, the conditions necessary for cells to function in a regenerative capacity, i.e., as a fibroblast, cementoblast or osteoblast.

b) Root Planing - Root planing defined as 'a definitive treatment procedure designed to remove cementum or surface dentin that is rough, impregnated with calculus or contaminated with toxins or microorganisms' (O'Leary and Hurt, 1986), has been advocated for removal of "diseased" cementum. Riffle (1953) recommended complete removal of cementum to eliminate surface irritation to the periodontal pocket. Support for this procedure came from Hatfield and Bauhammers (1971) who noted that diseased root surfaces retained materials that were inhibitory to cell growth, *in vitro*. Subsequently, Aleo *et al.* (1974, 1975, 1980) identified this material as microbial endotoxin, thus, providing a biological rationale for root planing. Aleo's studies (1974, 1975) as well as others' (Register and Burdick, 1976; Jones and O'Leary, 1978; and Hughes and Caffesse, 1978) showed that root planing and/or chemical modification of root

TABLE 1 *Factors/Proteins Associated With Cementum*

Protein/Factor	*Location and Suggested Function**	*Reference*
Attachment Factors/ Proteins		
Tenascin Fibronectin	Identified in mature cementum and also associated with root formation. May regulate selective adhesion and subsequent differentiation of cells during development and regeneration of cementum. Fibronectin also promotes cell migration.	Thesleff *et al.* 1981 Vaino *et al.* 1989 Lukinmaa *et al.* 1991
Bone sialoprotein (BSP)	Bone sialoprotein (BSP), formerly called BSP II, has been isolated from mature cementum. In addition to a role in regulation of development and regeneration of cementum, BSP may serve as a marker for cementoblasts.	Fisher *et al.* 1987,1990 Butler *et al.* 1991 Somerman *et al.* 1991
OPN**	OPN has been associated with root formation and may control adhesion and differentation of precementoblasts.	Butler 1989 (review) Somerman *et al.* 1990
Laminin	An adhesion protein associated with basement membranes and with root development. Laminin may have a role in initiation of cementum formation based on its localization on the root surface prior to cementogenesis.	Thesleff *et al.* 1981 Andujar *et al.* 1985 MacNeil, Thomas 1989
Other adhesion factors	Several additional adhesion factors have been identified during root formation and in mature cementum, but have not been characterized.	McAllister *et al.* 1990 Somerman *et al.* 1991

Other Factors/Proteins		
Osteonectin/Sparc	Associated with the developing root surfaces and mature cementum. While present in many tissues its role in mineralized tissues may be related to its high affinity for calcium, hydroxyapatite and type I collagen.	Termine *et al*. 1981 Wasi *et al*. 1984 Nomura *et al*. 1988
Enamel-related proteins	Identified in region of HERS and considered to have a role in stimulating cementogenesis.	Slavkin *et al*. 1989a, 1989b
'Gla'-containing proteins	γ-carboxyglutamic acid, probably attached to osteocalcin, has been identified in mature cementum. The role of mineral 'gla' proteins in cementum has not been established.	Glimcher *et al*. 1979 Alexander *et al*. 1991 (reviews: Butler 1985; Glimcher, Lian, 1988; Hauschka *et al*. 1989)
Mitogenic (growth) factor	Identified in mature cementum and may stimulate cell proliferation, an important event for wound healing.	Miki *et al*. 1987
Chemotactic factor	Associated with mature cementum and may serve to recruit appropriate cells to a healing site.	Nishimura *et al*. 1989
Proteoglycans/ Glycosaminoglycans		
Biglycan	Small proteoglycan identified in bone and other tissues; appears to be present in mature cementum.	Fisher *et al*. 1987 Alexander *et al*. 1991

(*continued*)

TABLE 1 *Factors/Proteins Associated With Cementum (continued)*

Protein/Factor	*Location and Suggested Function**	*Reference*
Proteoglycans/ Glycosaminoglycans cont'd.		
Chondroitin sulfate	The predominant glycosaminoglycan identified in mature cementum; located in lacunae and ECM.	Bartold *et al.* 1988, 1990
Dermatan sulfate Heparan sulfate Hyaluronate	These other glycosaminoglycans have also been isolated from mature cementum. Proteoglycans interact with several ECM proteins and may be associated with initiation of mineralization.	
Collagens		
Collagen I, III	Located in developing and mature cementum. The major form in mature tissue is type I collagen, with type III collagen representing less than 5%. Collagens may act as a matrix for mineralization and for insertion of PDL.	Birkedal-Hansen *et al.* 1977 Tung *et al.* 1985

* Suggested function only as related to cementum.

** OPN has been given several names which include: [1] 44 kilodalton bone phosphoprotein (44kDaBPP), based on molecular weight determined by sedimentation equilibrium (Prince *et al.*, 1987), [2] osteopontin, suggesting a bridging potential between cells and mineral in bone (Oldberg *et al.*, 1986), [3] 2ar, a tumor promoter-inducible protein secreted by mouse JB6 epidermal cells (Smith & Denhardt, 1987), [4] mouse secreted phosphoprotein I (Spp I) (Fet *et al.*, 1989), [5] tumor secreted phosphoprotein, secreted by spontaneously transformed cells is related if not identical to OPN (Senger, 1985, 1988), [6] BSP-I, bone sialoprotein I (Fisher *et al.*, 1987) and [7] Eta-1 (early T-lymphocyte activation gene), based on its expression in activated T-lymphocytes (Patarca *et al.*, 1989; Singh *et al.*, 1990). At an Osteopontin Workshop, May 1990 it was decided, for consistency among researchers, that this attachment protein should be named OPN.

surfaces removed endotoxin, providing a surface that allows for formation of connective tissue attachment and new cementum formation. Thus the importance of detoxifying the cemental surface was established in the 1970's. However, at that time (Nabers *et al.*, 1970) and still ongoing, is the controversy as to the degree of cementum removal and chemical treatment of root surfaces necessary for achieving clinical success. Studies by several groups, including Schallhorn (1972), Hildebrand and Morse (1980), Nyman *et al.* (1982), and Blomlöf *et al.*, (1987), emphasize the importance of retaining some root cementum for regenerative therapy, as well as preventing exposure of the dentin surface which may increase caries susceptibility and endodontic complications. In addition, *in vitro* studies suggest that cementum, but not dentin, has adhesive properties required to achieve connective tissue attachment (Somerman *et al.*, 1987c)

Aleo, in a review article on cementum in 1980, predicted that the debate on the degree of root planing would go on for the next twenty years. Eleven years later this issue remains unsettled. Questions still unresolved include: How much cementum should be removed? Are ultrasonic instruments adequate for root detoxification? Are any chemical procedures helpful in achieving new attachment? Can cementum predictably be regenerated with connective tissue attachment? In the 1970's the finding of toxins on the root surface provided a biological rationale for detoxifying root surfaces. The studies of the 1980's and 1990's are focusing on understanding the composition of healthy cementum and on factors/proteins required during the development and regeneration of cementum. Their results should provide the biological information needed to establish a rational basis for procedures that will regenerate tooth structure without compromising the remaining tissues.

c) Root Surface Caries - Improved procedures for maintaining teeth has resulted in an increased population of people with root surface caries and their associated consequences. Thus, there is an increasing demand to understand the process of root caries development, so that consistent treatment modalities, including preventive, restorative and regenerative procedures can be established. An initial concern was the determination of similarities or differences between carious-mediated destruction of cementum and that of enamel and dentin. Studies indicate that, in fact, caries formation in enamel and dentin is different from that in cementum (Frank *et al.*, 1989; Frank, 1990). Histologically, in enamel and dentin prior to bacterial invasion, a gradient of demineralization occurs, while in cementum there is a simultaneous destruction of mineral and organic components. Furthermore, bacterial invasion in cementum occurs at an earlier stage than in coronal enamel. The predominant bacteria noted in these areas are gram-positive rods, cocci and filamentous organisms (Andriens *et al.*, 1988; Frank *et al.*, 1989; Bowden, 1990; Nyvad and Fejerskov, 1990).

Other research has focused on preventive measures such as the use of fluorides and other agents prophylactically, including application of antibiotics

(Johansen *et al.*, 1987; Jensen *et al.*, 1988; Demirel *et al.*, 1991) and on clinical treatments such as procedures to remineralize carious cementum and appropriate restorations, that protect against future lesions. In this regard, Schüpback, Guggenheim and Lutz (1989, 1990) reported that remineralization of active root lesions does occur and that non-invasive treatments for root caries should be considered. Indeed, it is possible that procedures used in the future to stimulate periodontal regeneration including cementum, may also prove beneficial for the treatment of root surface caries.

Another area of clinical importance to the topics discussed under this section is the composition of saliva. Slomiany *et al.* (1990) suggested that lipids in the saliva determine the susceptibility of the tooth surface to caries. In terms of treatment of periodontal diseases, studies indicate that saliva inhibits attachment of fibroblasts to root surfaces, *in vitro* (Heaney, 1986). However, Wikesjo *et al.* (1990) reported that exposure of root surfaces to saliva during surgery did not affect normal wound healing in dogs. The question remains as to whether demineralization of root surfaces, protects against saliva by increasing removal of absorbed saliva from the root surface (Heaney, 1986) or, in fact, result in a structure that is more susceptible to caries?

Future Directions

Knowledge of the fundamental properties of cementum and of the capacity, factors and cells required during development and regeneration of this tissue is critical to designing appropriate modalities for the treatment of root caries and periodontal diseases. Such information is not only important to dental related diseases, but will also enhance knowledge with regard to mineralized tissues in general. Major questions that must be addressed is what is cementum, i.e., is it a ''unique'' mineralized tissue? Are the alterations in cementum caused by disease, e.g., caries, periodontal diseases, correctable? Evidence to date indicate that cementum can be regenerated; however, in clinical studies this regeneration is not predictable. Similarly, studies indicate that prophylactic use of fluoride rinses may have a preventive role in the control of root caries; however, here, as well, results are not predictable. In addition, there is evidence that incipient root caries can be halted by specific treatments, and the site remineralized. Again, these results are not consistent.

Additional research is needed in several other areas including determining the specific bacteria involved in root caries formation, the role of saliva and chemotherapeutic agents in regulating root lesions, the regenerative capacity of cementum and genetic versus dietary aspects of root caries formation.

Information in these areas is required to establish treatment modalities that will successfully regenerate the periodontium and provide the necessary information to develop prophylactic treatments that will decrease the incidence of root caries.

REFERENCES

ADRIENS, P.A.; EDWARDS, C.A.; DEBOEVER, J.A.; and LOESCHE, W.J. (1988): Ultrastructural Observations on Bacterial Invasion in Cementum and Radicular Dentin of Periodontally Diseased Human Teeth, *J Periodontol* 59:493-503.

ALEO, J.J.; DE RENZIS, F.A.; FARBER P.A. and VARBONCOER, A.P. (1974): The Presence and Biologic Activity of Cementum Bound Endotoxin, *J Periodontol* 45:672-675.

ALEO, J.J.; DE RENZIS, F.A.; and FARBER, P.A. (1975): *In Vitro* Attachment of Human Gingival Fibroblasts to Root Surfaces, *J Periodontol* 46: 639-645.

ALEO, J.J. and VANDERSALL, D.C. (1980): Recent Concepts Related to Periodontal Disease Therapy, *Dental Clinics of North America* 24:627-650.

ALEXANDER, M.; SAUK, J.; ARGRAVES, W.; MORRISON, G.; NORRIS, K.; FOTER, R.; and SOMERMAN, M. (1991): Non-Collagenous Proteins of Cementum *IADR Abstr* 70: No. 1395.

ANDUJAR, M.B.; MAGLOIRE, H.; HARTMANN, D.J.; VILLE, G. and GRIMAUD, J.A. (1985): Early Mouse Molar Root Development: Cellular Changes and Distribution of Fibronectin, Laminin and Type -IV Collagen, *Differentiation* 30:111-122.

AUKHIL, I.; NISHIRMURA, K.; and FERNYHOUGH W. (1990): Experimental Regeneration of the Periodontium, *Critical Review in Oral Biol and Med* 1:101-116.

BARTOLD, P.M.; REINBOTH, B.; NAKAE, H.; NARAYANAN, A.S.; and PAGE, R.C. (1990): Proteoglycans of Bovine Cementum: Isolation and Characterization, *Matrix* 10:10-19.

BARTOLD, P.M.; MIKI, Y.; NARAYANAN, A.S.; and PAGE, R.C. (1988): Glycosaminoglycans of Human Cementum, *J Periodont Res* 23: 13-17.

BECKER, B.E. and BECKER, W. (1991): Regeneration Procedures: Grafting, Materials, Guided Tissue Regeneration and Growth Factors, *Current Opinion in Dent* 1:93-97.

BEERTSEN, W. and VAN DEN BOS, T. (1991): Alkaline Phosphatase Induces the Deposition of Calcified Layers in Relation to Dentin: An *In Vitro* Study to Mimic the Formation of Afibrillar Acellular Cementum, *J Dent Res* 70:176-181.

BESSHO, K.; TANAKA, N.; MATSUMOTO, J.; TAGAWA, T.; and MURATA, M. (1991): Human Dentin-Matrix-Derived Bone Morphogenetic Protein, *J Dent Res* 70:171-175.

BIRKEDAL-HANSEN, H.; BUTLER, W.T., and TAYLOR, R.E. (1977): Proteins of the Periodontium: Characterization of the Insoluble Collagens of Bovine Dental Cementum, *Calc Tiss Res* 23: 39-44.

BLOMLÖF, L.; LINDSKOG, S.; APPELGREN, R.; JONSSON, B.; WEINTRAUB, A.; and HAMARSTROM, L. (1987): New Attachment in Monkeys with Experimental Periodontitis With and Without Removal of the Cementum, *J Clin Periodontol* 14:136-143.

BOWDEN, G.H.W. (1990): Microbiology of Root Surface Caries in Humans, *J Dent Res* 69:1205-1210.

BOWERS, G.; CHADROFF, B., CARNEVALE, R.; MELLONIG, J.; CORIO, R.; and EMERSON, J. (1989): Histological Evaluation of New Human Attachment Apparatus Formation in Humans, Part I, *J Periodontol* 60: 664-674.

BUSER, D.; WARRER, K.; and KARRING, T. (1990): Formation of a Periodontal Ligament Around Titanium Implants. *J Periodontol* 61: 597-601.

BUTLER, W.T. Ed. (1985): *The Chemistry and Biology of Mineralized Tissues*. Birmingham, EBSCO Media.

BUTLER, W.T. (1989): The Nature and Significance of Osteopontin, *Connective Tiss Res* 23: 123-126.

BUTLER, W.T. (1991): Sialoproteins of Bone and Dentin, *J Biol Buccale* 19: 83-89.

BUTLER, W.T.; MIKULSKI, A.; and URIST, M.R. (1977): Non-collagenous Proteins of a Rat Dentin Matrix Possessing Bone Morphogenetic Activity, *J Dent Res* 56:228-232.

CHEN, J.; SHAPIRO, H.S.; WRANA, J.L.; ZHANG, Q.; McCULLOCH, C.A.G.; REIMERS, S.; HEERSCHE, J.N.M.; and SODEK, J. (1991): Expression and Distribution of Bone Sialoprotein (BSP) in Mineralized Tissues *IADR Abst* 70: No. 1579.

CHO, M. and GARANT, P. (1988): Ultrastructural Evidence of Directed Cell Migration During Initial Cementoblast Differentiation in Root Formation, *J Periodont Res* 23:268-276.

CHO, M. and GARANT, P (1989): Radiographic Study of Mannose Utilization during Cementoblast Differentiation, Formation of Acellular Cementum, and Development of Periodontal Ligament Principal Fibers, *Anat Rec* 223:209-222.

CHOVELON, A.; CARMICHAEL, D.J.; and PEARSON, C.H. (1975): The Composition of the Organic Matrix of Bovine Cementum, *Arch Oral Biol* 20:537-541.

CRAIG, R.; McCANN, J.; and LALLY, E. (1989): Generation of Monoclonal Antibodies to Bovine Cementum Matrix, *IADR Abst* 68: No. 1239.

DEMIREL, K.; BAER, P.N.; and McNAMARA, T.F. (1991): Topical Application of Doxycycline on Periodontally Involved Root Surfaces *In Vitro:* Comparative Analysis of Substantivity on Cementum and Dentin, *J Periodontol* 62:312-316.

FET, V.; DICKINSON, M.E.; and HOGAN, B.L.M. (1989): Localization of the Mouse Gene for Secreted Phosphoprotein I (SppI) (2ar, Osteopontin, Bone Sialoprotein 1, 44-kDa Bone Phosphoprotein, Tumor-Secreted Phosphoprotein) to Chromosome 5, Closely Linked to Ric (Rickettsia resistance), *Genomics* 5: 375-377.

FISHER, L.W.; HAWKIN, G.R.; TUROSS, N.; TERMINE, J.D. (1987): Purification and Partial Characterization of Small Proteoglycans I and II, Bone Sialoproteins I and II, and Osteonectin from the Mineral Compartment of Developing Human Bone, *J Biol Chem* 262: 9702-9708.

FISHER, L.W.; McBRIDE, O.W.; TERMINE, J.D.; and YOUNG, M.F. (1990): Human Bone Sialoprotein, Deduced Protein Sequence and Chromosomal Localization, *J Biol Chem* 265:2347-2351.

FISHER, L.W.; WHITSON, S.W. AVIOLI, L.V.; and TERMINE J.D. (1983): Matrix Sialoprotein of Developing Bone, *J Biol Chem* 285:12723-12727.

FRANK, R.M. (1990): Structural Events in the Caries Process in Enamel, Cementum, and Dentin. *J Dent Res* 69:559-566.

FRANK, R.M.; STEUER, P.; and HEMMERLE, J.(1989): Ultrastructural on Human Root Caries, *Caries Research* 23:209-217.

GLIMCHER, M.J.; LEFTERIOU, B.; and KOSSIVA, D. (1979): Identification of O-phosphoserine, O-phosphothreonine and γ-carboxyglutamic Acid in the Non-Collagenous Proteins of Bovine Cementum; Comparison with Dentin, Enamel and Bone. *Calc Tiss Int* 28:83-86.

GLIMCHER, M.J. and LIAN, J.B.; Eds. (1988): *The Chemistry and Biology of Mineralized Tissues*. Proceedings of the Third International Conference on the Chemistry & Biology of Mineralized Tissues, Gordon & Breach Science Publishers.

GOTTLIEB, B (1946): The New Concept of Periodontoclasia. *J Periodontol* 17: 7-13.

HATFIELD, C.G.; and BAUMHAMMERS, A. (1971): Cytotoxic Effects of Periodontally Involved Surfaces of Human Teeth, *Arch Oral Biol* 16: 465-468.

HAUSHKA, P.V.; LIAN, J.B.; COLE, D E.; and GUNDBERG, C.M. (1989): Osteocalcin and Matrix Gla Protein: Vitamin K-Dependent Proteins in Bone, *Physiol Rev* 69:990-1047.

HEANEY, T.G. (1986): Inhibition of Fibroblast Attachment. *J Clin Periodontol* 13:987-997.

HERITIER, M. (1982): Experimental Induction of Cementogenesis on the Enamel of Transplanted Mouse Tooth Germs, *Arch Oral Biol* 27:87-97.

HILDEBRAND, C.N. and MORSE, D.R. (1980): Periodontic-Endodontic Inter-Relationships, *Dent Clin North Am* 24:797-812.

HUGHES, T.P. and CAFFESSEE, R.G. (1978): Gingival Changes Following Scaling, Root Planing and Oral Hygiene, *J Periodontol* 49:245-252.

INOUE, T.; DEPORTER, D.A.; and MELCHER, A.H. (1986): Induction of Chondrogenesis in Muscle, Skin, Bone Marrow, and Periodontal Ligament by Demineralized Dentin and Bone Matrix *In Vivo* and *In Vitro, J Dent Res* 65: 12-22.

JENSEN, M.E. and KOHOUT, F. (1988): The Effect of a Fluoridated Dentifrice on Root and Coronal Caries in an Older Adult Population, *JADA* 17:829-832.

JOHANSEN, E.; PAPAS, A.; FONG, W.; and OLSEN, T.O. (1987): Remineralization of Carious Lesions in Elderly Patients. *Gerodontics* 3:47-50.

JONES, W.A. and O'LEARY, T.J.(1978): The Effectiveness of *In Vivo* Root Planing in Removing Bacterial Endotoxin from the Roots of Periodontally Involved Teeth, *J Periodontol* 48:337- 342.

LINDSKOG, S (1982): Formation of Intermediate Cementum. II: A Scanning Electron Microscopic Study of the Epithelial Root Sheath of Hertwig in Monkey, *J Craniofac Genet Dev Biol* 2: 161-169.

LINDSKOG, S. and BLOMLÖF, L. (1983): Cementum Hypoplasia in Teeth Affected by Juvenile Periodontitis, *J Clin Periodontol* 10: 443-450.

LINDSKOG, S.; BLOMLÖF, L. and HAMMARSTRÖM, L. (1987): Comparative Effect of Parathyroid Hormone on Osteoblasts and Cementoblasts, *J Clin Periodontol* 14:386-389.

LINDSKOG, S. and HAMMARSTRÖM, L. (1980): Evidence in Favor of an Anti-Invasion Factor in Cementum or Periodontal Membrane of Human Teeth, *Scand J Dent Res* 88:161-163.

LINDSKOG, S.; HAMMARSTRÖM, L.; and BLOMLÖF, L. (1983): Repair of Periodontal Tissues *In Vivo* and *In Vitro, J Clin Periodontol* 10:188-205.

LISTGARTEN, M.A. (1967): A Mineralized Cuticular Structure with Connective Tissue Characteristics on the Crowns of Human Unerupted Teeth in Amelogenesis Imperfecta, *Arch Oral Biol* 12: 877-889.

LISTGARTEN, M.A. (1968): A Light and Electron Microscopic Study of Coronal Cementogenesis, *Arch Oral Biol* 13: 93-114.

LISTGARTEN, M.A. and SHAPIRO, I.M. (1974): Fine Structure and Composition of Coronal Cementum in Guinea-pig Molars, *Arch Oral Biol* 19:679-696.

LUKINMAA, P.L.; MACKIE, E.J.; and THESLEFF, I. (1991): Immuno-Histochemical Localization of the Matrix Glycoproteins - Tenascin and the ED-Sequence Form of Cellular Fibronectin, *J Dent Res* 70:19-26.

McALLISTER, A.S.; NARAYANAN, A.S.; MIKI, Y.; and PAGE, R.I. (1990): Isolation of a Fibroblast Attachment Protein from Cementum, *J Periodont Res* 25: 99-105.

McCULLOCH, C.A.;, NEMENTH, E.; LOWENBERG, B. and MELCHER, A.H. (1987): Paravascular Cells in Endosteal Spaces of Alveolar Bone Contribute to Periodontal Ligament Cell Populations, *Anat Rec* 219: 233-242.

MacNEIL, R.L. and THOMAS, H.F. (1989): The Role of Basement Membrane in Murine Cementogenesis, *IADR Abst* 68: No. 791.

MIKI, Y.; NARAYANAN, A.S.; and PAGE, R.C. (1987): Mitogenic Activity of Cementum Components to Gingival Fibroblasts, *J Dental Res* 66:1399-1403.

NABERS, C.L.; PRICHARD, J.F.; ROBINSON, R.E. and SCHALLHORN, R.G. (1970): In Order to Secure "Fill" in Osseous Defects, Is It Necessary or Desirable to "Plane" the Exposed Root Surfaces Until They are Hard to the Touch? *J Periodontol* 41: 419-423.

NISHIMURA, K.; HAYASHI, M.; MATSUDAK; SHIGEYAMA, Y.; YAMASAKI, A.; and YAMAOKA, A. (1989): The Chemoattractive Potency of Periodontal Ligament, Cementum and Dentin for Human Gingival Fibroblasts, *J Periodont Res* 24:146-148.

NOMURA, S.; WILLS, A.J.; EDWARDS, D.R.; HEATH, J.K.; and HOGAN, B.L.M. (1988): Developmental Expression of 2ar (Osteopontin) and Sparc (Osteonectin) RNA as Revealed by *In Situ* Hybridization, *J Cell Biol* 106:441-450.

NYMAN S.; LINDHE, J.; KARRING, T.; and RYLANDER, H. (1982): New Attachment Following Surgical Treatment of Human Periodontal Disease, *J Clin Periodontol* 9:290-296.

NYVAD, B. and FEJERSKOV, O. (1990): An Ultrastructural Study of Bacterial Invasion and Tissue Breakdown in Human Experimental Root-Surface Caries, *J Dent Res* 69:1118-1125.

OSBORN, J.W. and PRICE, D.G. (1988): An Autoradiographic Study of Periodontal Development in the Mouse, *J Dent Res* 67:455-461.

OWENS, P.D.A. (1979): A Light and Electron Microscopic Study of the Early Stages of Root Surface Formation in Molar Teeth in the Rat, *Arch Oral Biol* 24:901-907.

PAGE, R.C. and BAAB, D.A. (1986): A New Look at the Etiology and Pathogenesis of Early-Onset Periodontitis. Cementopathia Revisited, *J Periodontol* 56:748-751.

PALMER, R.M. and LUMSDEN, A.S. (1987): Development of the Periodontal Ligament and Alveolar Bone in Homografted Recombinations of Enamel Organs and Papillary, Pulpal and Follicular Mesenchyme in the Mouse, *Arch Oral Biol* 32:281-289.

PATARCA, R.; FREEMAN, G.J.; SINGH, R.P.; WEI, F.X.; DURFEE, T.; BLATTNER, F.; REGNIER, D.C.; KOZAK, C.A.; MOCK, B.A.; MORSE, III, H.C.; JERRELLS, T.R.; CANTOR, H. (1989): Structural and Functional Studies of the Early T-lymphocyte Activation 1 (Eta-1) Gene. Definition of a Novel T Cell-Dependent Response Associated with Genetic Resistance to Bacterial Infection, *J Exp Med* 170: 145-161.

PHILIPSON, S.; LINDSKOG, S; and FLOCK, A. (1990): Mineralization of and Cementoblast Attachment to Original and Reparative Cementum, *J Dent Res* 98:295-300.

PRINCE, C.W.; OOSAWA, T.; BUTLER, W.T.; TOMAMA, M.; BHOWN, A.S.; BHOWN, M. and SCHROHENLOHER, R.E. (1987): Isolation, Characterization and Biosynthesis of a Phosphorylated Glycoprotein from Rat Bone, *J Biol Chem* 262: 259-265.

REGISTER, A.A. and BURDICK, F. (1976): Accelerated Attachment and Cementogenesis to Dentin, Demineralized *In Situ* (II) Defect Repair. *J Periodontol* 47:497-504.

RIFFLE, A.B. (1953): Dentin; Its Physical Characteristics during Curettage, *J Periodontol* 24:232-241.

SCHALLHORN, R.G. and McCLAIN, P.R. (1988): Combined Osseous Composite Grafting, Root Conditioning, and Guided Tissue Regeneration, *Int J Periodontics Restorative Dent* 3:9-32.

SCHÜPBACK, P.; GUGGENHEIM, B.; and LUTZ, F. (1989): Human Root Caries: Histopathology of Initial Lesions in Cementum and Dentin, *J Oral Pathol Med* 18:146-156.

SCHÜPBACK, P.; GUGGENHEIM, B.; and LUTZ, F. (1990): Histopathology of Root Surface Caries, *J Dent Res* 26: 1195-1204.

SELVIG, K.A. (1964): An Ultrastructural Study of Cementum Formation, *Acta Odont Scand* 23:423-441.

SELVIG, K.A. (1965): The Fine Structure of Human Cementum, *Acta Odont Scand* 23:423-441.

SELVIG, K.A. (1963): Electron Microscopy of Hertwig's Epithelial Sheath and of Early Dentin and Cementum Formation in the Mouse Incisor, *Acta Odontol Scand* 21:175-186.

SELVIG, K.A. and HALS, E, (1977): Periodontally Diseased Cementum Studied by Correlated Microradiography, Electron Probe Analysis, and Electron Microscopy, *J Periodontol Res* 12:419-429.

SENGER, D.R. and PERRUZZI, C.A. (1985): Secreted Phosphoprotein Markers for Neoplastic Transformation of Human Epithelial and Fibroblastic Cells, *Cancer Res* 45: 5818-5823.

SCHROEDER, H.E. (1986): The Periodontium. In: *Handbook of Microscopic Anatomy*, New York-Tokyo, Springer-Verlag Berlin Heidelberg. 5:23-128.

SICHER, H. and BHASKAR, S.N. Eds (1972): *Orban's Oral Histology and Embryology*. CV Mosby Co. Chapter 6, pp. 160-181.

SINGH, R.P.; PATARCA, R.; SCHWARTZ, J.; SINGH, P.; and CANTOR, H. (1990): Definition of a Specific Interaction Between the Early T Lymphocyte Activation 1 (Eta-1) Protein and Murine Macrophages *In Vitro* and Its Effect upon Macrophages *In Vivo, J Exp Med* 171: 1931-1942.

SLAVKIN, H.C. (1976): Towards a Cellular and Molecular Understanding of Periodontics: Cementogenesis Revisited, *J Periodontol* 47:249-255.

SLAVKIN, H.C. (1990): Molecular Determinants of Tooth Development: A Review. *Critical Review in Oral Biol and Med* 1:1-16.

SLAVKIN, H.C.; BESSEM, C.; FINCHAM, A.G.; BRINGAS, P.Jr.; SANTOS, V.; SNEAD, M.L.; and ZEICHNER-DAVID, M. (1989a): Human and Mouse Cementum Proteins Immunologically Related to Enamel Proteins, *Biochem Biophys Acta* 991:12-18.

SLAVKIN, H.C.; BRINGAS, P.Jr.; BESSEM, C.; SANTOS, V.; NAKAMURA, M.; HSU, M.Y.; SNEAD, M.L.; ZEICHNER-DAVID, M.; and FINCHAM, A.G.

(1989b): Hertwig's Epithelial Root Sheath Differentiation and Initial Cementum and Bone Formation During Long-Term Organ Culture of Mouse Mandibular First Molars Using Serumless, Chemically-Defined Medium, *J Periodont Res* 24:28-40.

SMITH, A.J.; LEAVER, A.G.; and SMITH, G. (1983): The Amino-Acid Composition of the Non-Collagenous Organic Matrix of Human Cementum, *Arch Oral Biol* 28:1047-1054.

SMITH, B.; CAFFESSE, R.; NASJLETI, C.; KON, S.; and CASTELLI, W. (1987): Effects of Citric Acid and Fibronectin and Laminin Application in Treating Periodontitis, *J Clin Periodontol* 44:396-402.

SMITH, J.H. and DENHARDT, D.T. (1987): Molecular Cloning of a Tumor Promoter-Inducible mRNA Found in JB6 Mouse Epidermal Cells: Induction is Stable at High, But Not at Low, Cell Densities. *J Cell Biochem* 34: 13-22.

SOLMIANY, B.L.; MURTY, V.L.; MANDEL, I.D.; SENGUPTA, S.; and SOLMIANY, A. (1990): Effect of Lipids on the Lactic Acid Retardation Capacity of Tooth Enamel and Cementum Pellicles Formed *In Vitro* from Saliva of Caries-Resistant and Caries-Susceptible Human Adults, *Arch Oral Biol* 35:175-180.

SOMERMAN, M.J.; ARCHER, S.Y.; SHTEYER, A.; and FOSTER, R.A. (1987a): Protein Production by Human Gingival Fibroblast Is Enhanced by Guanidine EDTA Extracts of Cementum, *In Vitro, J Periodont Res* 22:75-77.

SOMERMAN, M.J.; ARGRAVES, W.S.; FOSTER, R.A.; DICKERSON, K.; NORRIS, K.; and SAUK, J.J.(1991): Cell Attachment Activity of Cementum: Bone Sialoprotein II Identified in Cementum. *J Periodont Res* 26:10-16.

SOMERMAN, M.J.; HASSELL, T.M.; ARCHER, S.Y. and FOSTER, R.A. (1987b): Enhancement by Extracts of Mineralized Tissues of Protein Productivity By Human Gingival Fibroblasts, *Arch Oral Biol* 32:879-883.

SOMERMAN, M.J.; MERKHOFER, R.M.; PEREZ-MERA, M.; and FOSTER, R.A. (1987c): *In Vitro* Evaluation of Extracts of Mineralized Tissues for their Application in Fibrous Tissue Attachment, *J Periodontol* 58: 349-351.

SOMERMAN, M.J.; NATHANSON, M. SAUK, J.J.; and MANSON, B. (1987d): Dentin Matrix Induces Cartilage Formation by Mesenchymal Cells, *In Vitro, J Dent Res* 66: 1551-1558.

SOMERMAN, M.J.; SHROFF, B.; ARGRAVES, W.S.; MORRISON, G.; CRAIG A.M.; DENHARDT, D.T.; FOSTER, R.A.; and SAUK, J.J. (1990): Expression of Attachment Proteins During Cementogenesis, *J Biol Buccale* 18:207-14.

STAHL, S.S. (1975):The Nature of Healthy and Diseased Root Surfaces, *J Periodontol* 46:157-161.

TEN CATE, A.R. Ed. (1989): *Oral Histology Development, Structure and Function.* The C.V. Mosby Company, St. Louis, Baltimore, Toronto.

TERMINE, J.D.; KLEINMAN, H.K.; WHITSON, S.W.; CONN, K.W.; McGARVEY, M.L.; and MARTIN G.R. (1981): Osteonectin, a Bone Specific Protein Linking Mineral to Collagen, *Cell* 26:99-105.

THESLEFF, I., BARRACH, H.J.; FOIDART, M.J.; VAHERI, A.; PRATT, R.M.; and MARTIN, G.R. (1981): Changes in the Distribution of Type IV Collagen, Laminin, Proteoglycan and Fibronectin During Mouse Tooth Development, *Dev Biol* 81:182-192.

THOMAS, H.F. and KOLLAR, E.J. (1989): Tissue Interactions in Normal Murine Root Development, In: *Biological Mechanisms of Tooth Eruption and Root Resorption,* Z. Davidovitch, Ed., EBSCO Media, Alabama, pp 107-116.

TUNG, P.S.; DOMENICUCCI, C.; WASI, S., and SODEK, J. (1985): Specific Immunohistochemical Localization of Osteonectin and Collagen Types I and III in Fetal and Adult Porcine Dental Tissues, *J Histochem Cytochem* 33:531-540.

URIST, M.R. (1971): Bone Histogenesis and Morphogenesis in Implants of Demineralized Enamel and Dentin, *J Oral Surg* 29:88-102.

VAINO, S.; JALKANEN, M.; and THESLEFF, I. (1989): Syndecan and Tenascin Expression Is Induced by Epithelial-Mesenchymal Interactions in Embryonic Tooth Mesenchyme, *J Cell Biol* 108:1945-1954.

VEIS, A.; SIRES, B.; CLOHISY, J.; SABSAY, B.; and AMAR, S. (1990): Rat Incisor Dentine Contains a Factor which Alters the Phenotypic Expression and Stimulates Chondrogenesis in Fibroblast-Like Cell *In Vitro, Biomaterials* 11:35-37.

WASI, S.; OTSUKA, K.; YAO, K-L; TUNG, P.S.; AUBIN, J.E.; SODEK, J.; and TERMINE, J.D. (1984): An Osteonectin-Like Protein in Porcine Periodontal Ligament and Its Synthesis by Periodontal Ligament Fibroblasts, *Can J Biochem Cell Biol* 62:470-478.

WIKESJO, U.M.; HAGEN, K.; and NIELSEN, D.D. (1990): Periodontal Repair in Dogs: Effect of Saliva Contamination of the Root Surface, *J Periodontol* 61:559-563.

YAMADA, K.M. (1983): Cell Surface Interactions with Extracellular Matrix, *Ann Rev Biochem* 52:761-799.

YAMASAKI, A.; ROSE, G.G.; PINERO, G.J.; and MAHAN, C.J. (1987): Ultrastructural and Morphometric Analyses of Human Cementoblasts and Periodontal Fibroblasts, *J Periodontol* 58:192-201.

ZANDER, H. and HÜRZELER, (1958): Continuous Cementum Apposition, *J Dent Res* 2:1035-1044.

Enamel - Plaque Fluid Interactions

H.C. MARGOLIS

An extremely limited amount of data has been obtained on the chemical composition of dental plaque, despite the fact that it is generally accepted that the caries process is initiated by chemical events which take place within plaque, following exposure to fermentable carbohydrates. Thus, the cariogenic conditions in plaque have not been well defined and, as will become evident below, such information is crucial to our understanding of the caries process and to the development of anti-caries procedures.

Importantly, the cariogenic conditions generated by plaque microorganisms are reflected in changes in the ionic composition of the extracellular aqueous phase of dental plaque, referred to as plaque fluid. The key to the importance of plaque fluid is that it is in intimate contact with the enamel surface and that it is accessible for chemical and biochemical analyses. Studies of plaque fluid, however, are complicated by the fact that caries is a localized disease and, thus, limited amounts of relevant plaque are available. The development (Rankine *et al.*, 1985; Margolis *et al.*, 1988a; Vogel *et al.*, 1990) of isolation and analytical procedures for the study of micro- and nanoliter volumes of dental plaque fluid has led to several important investigations of its composition and has provided a means by which the cariogenic potential of dental plaque can be assessed. The use of pooled plaque samples, however, is still required for many studies. Much work remains to be done, including the development of more sensitive analytical procedures.

The purposes of this paper are 1) to discuss the significance of what is presently known about the chemical conditions generated within dental plaque, in light of appropriate physicochemical considerations and knowledge obtained through *in vitro* studies of enamel demineralization, and 2) to identify new areas of research needed to elucidate other key factors involved in cariogenesis.

This study was supported by grants (DE-07493 and DE-07009) from the National Institute of Dental Research.

The author wishes to thank Drs. E.C. Moreno and J. van Houte for their helpful comments.

Enamel Demineralization *In vitro*

Laboratory studies have demonstrated that the rates of enamel demineralization *in vitro* are dependent on solution pH (Theuns *et al.*, 1984a) as well as on the concentration of undissociated organic acid (Gray, 1962; Featherstone and Rodgers, 1981; Theuns *et al.*, 1984b). In addition, several *in vitro* studies (Moreno and Zahradnik, 1974; Margolis *et al.*, 1985; Theuns *et al.*, 1983) have shown that the rates of enamel demineralization are affected tremendously by the degree of saturation (DS) of the demineralizing medium with respect to enamel. Recently, these parameters have been incorporated into a single model which shows that the kinetics of dissolution of hydroxyapatite (a prototype for enamel mineral) can be described (Margolis and Moreno, 1992a) as a function of the DS with respect to the dissolving phase (*i.e.* hydroxyapatite) and the total activity of the acid species (*i.e.* organic and phosphoric) in solution:

[1] $$R = K\,(1 - DS)^m(\Sigma(B_iH))^n$$

Here, R is the dissolution rate expressed in terms of mols of Ca appearing per liter of solution per unit of time and surface area and (B_iH) stands for the activity of the i-th neutral undissociated acid. Individual undissociated acid activities can be calculated (Moreno and Margolis, 1988) from solution compositions and are equal to $(B_i^-)(H^+)/K_i$, where (B_i^-) is the activity of the acid anion and K_i is the dissociation constant for the given acid. Accordingly, equation [1] represents an empirical relationship and does not imply necessarily a unique and specific role for undissociated acid species in the dissolution process. The exponents *m* and *n* reflect the contribution of DS and the sum of acid activities, respectively, to the overall order of the dissolution reaction. In the study of the dissolution of hydroxyapatite, *m* and *n* were found to have values of 2.8 and 0.3, respectively. Lower values of DS and higher activities of acid species accelerate rates of dissolution.

In the above study, DS was defined as the ratio of the mean ionic activity product for hydroxyapatite ($Ca_5OH(PO_4)_3$) in solution to its solubility product constant, K,

$$DS = \left[\frac{(Ca^{++})^5\,(OH^-)\,(PO_4^{3-})^3}{K}\right]^{1/9}$$

$$K = (Ca^{++})_0^5\,(OH^-)_0\,(PO^{3-})_0^3$$

where, parentheses represent the activities of the enclosed ions, K is equal to 7.36×10^{-60} (Moreno *et al.*, 1977), and $(\ )_o$ represents activities of the enclosed ions determined at saturation. DS values greater than, less than, or equal to one correspond to conditions of supersaturation, undersaturation, or saturation with respect to the mineral in question, respectively.

Consequently, in order for the mineral to dissolve, the solution in question must be undersaturated with respect to the dissolving phase (DS < 1). Thus, equation [1] requires that the rate of dissolution approach zero as DS approaches 1 (saturation). Interestingly, preliminary studies suggest (Lee *et al.*, 1990) that this function also describes adequately the kinetics of enamel demineralization *in vitro,* when enamel is assumed to have the same stoichiometry as hydroxyapatite with, however, a larger solubility product constant, K_{En}, equal to 5.5×10^{-55} (Moreno and Zahradnik, 1974).

Although dental enamel is apatitic in nature, it contains significant quantities of constituents such as Na^+ and CO_3^{2-}. Thus, in principle, these constituents should be taken into account in the definition of its solubility product. In fact, as will be discussed later, there are possible limitations to assuming the stoichiometry of hydroxyapatite for enamel. Nevertheless, from these *in vitro* studies using hydroxyapatite and enamel it is apparent that the onset of caries and the rate of caries progression is highly dependent on the chemical properties of *both* the enamel mineral and the solution (plaque fluid) with which it is in contact at the enamel-plaque interface. Thus, the influence of both the properties of plaque fluid and enamel must be explored with regard to caries formation. Again, however, it should be recalled that the chemical changes observed in plaque fluid are a reflection of microbial activity; thus, the cariogenic potential of plaque depends on both the whole plaque and plaque fluid components (Margolis, 1990).

Plaque Fluid

Plaque fluid has been shown (Tatevossian and Gould, 1976; Moreno and Margolis, 1988) to be a distinct entity within the oral cavity having a composition different from that of either saliva or crevicular fluid. Although these findings suggest that plaque fluid is compartmentalized, the influence of these latter two biological fluids on the composition of plaque fluid has not been thoroughly investigated. The effect of saliva on dental plaque and caries has been discussed (Edgar, 1976; Jenkins, 1979; Abelson and Mandel, 1981) in considerable detail, but its precise influence on plaque fluid composition and subsequent influence on its cariogenic potential has not been elucidated. Moreover, it is quite reasonable to assume that saliva can influence significantly plaque chemistry since it has been shown, for example, that elevated levels of salivary urea and ammonia (De Stoppelaar, 1982; Peterson *et al.*, 1985) are associated with lower levels of caries incidence, presumably as a result of increasing plaque (fluid) pH. Interestingly, if one examines (Margolis and Moreno, 1992b) the composition of starved plaque fluid (obtained from plaque following overnight fasting) from caries-free (CF) and caries-positive (CP) individuals, as given in Table 1, one observes a tremendous similarity in ionic composition with the particular exception of plaque pH values; carbonate concentrations in these samples,

TABLE 1 *Composition of Starved Plaque Fluid from Caries-Free and Caries-Positive Individuals*[a]

	CF	*CP*		*CF*	*CP*
pH	7.02 ± 0.05*	6.79 ± 0.12	Succinic	4.4 ± 1.5	4.6 ± 1.0
Na^+	14.2 ± 3.5	16.5 ± 5.4	Lactic	1.8 ± 0.7	2.6 ± 1.2
NH_4^+	26.3 ± 3.9	22.6 ± 3.9	Acetic	19.9 ± 3.5	20.3 ± 4.6
K^+	59.9 ± 4.9	71.4 ± 11.3	Propionic	5.8 ± 1.5	9.2 ± 3.6
Mg^{2+}	2.0 ± 0.4	2.6 ± 0.4			
Ca^{2+}	2.8 ± 0.2	2.7 ± 0.5			
P	13.9 ± 1.9	15.6 ± 3.6			
Cl^-	23.8 ± 3.6	27.2 ± 2.9			

a. all concentrations in mmol/L; mean baseline data from Margolis and Moreno, 1992b ; formic and butyric acid concentrations were low (0 - 5 mmol/L) and not consistently detected in all samples.

* CF and CP values significantly different at $p < 0.001$ (n = 12 or 13)

however, were not determined. Plaque pH values were found to be significantly lower in plaque fluid obtained from CP subjects as compared to that observed in CF subjects. Similar findings in whole plaque were reported (Stephan, 1944) years ago. In addition (Margolis and Moreno, 1992b), starved plaque fluid from white-spot surfaces had measurably lower pH values than starved plaque fluid isolated from plaque associated with sound surfaces from the same CP individuals. The overall similarity of results in Table 1 may suggest that observed differences in plaque and plaque fluid pH result from differences in buffer capacity in plaque fluid associated with CF and CP individuals. This is not known and the influence of saliva (*e.g.*, via its carbonate content) on plaque fluid buffering in starved samples has not been explored. Differences in the buffer capacity of whole plaque (cells, extracellular matrix, etc.) from CF and CP individuals may also explain (van Houte *et al.*, 1989) the results shown in Table 1; studies in this area are badly needed, but have not been carried out.

The significance of the differences in plaque fluid pH in starved samples becomes evident when saturation levels within plaque are considered. For example, as shown in Table 2, starved plaque fluid (Margolis and Moreno, 1992b) is supersaturated with respect to enamel mineral and calcium phosphate phases, such as dicalcium phosphate dihydrate (DCPD). These results suggest that, in principle, starved plaque fluids can promote the remineralization of partially demineralized enamel mineral. Importantly, as seen in Table 2, starved plaque fluid from CF individuals is more highly supersaturated with respect to enamel than comparable samples from CP individuals; this difference is primarily related to differences in the corresponding plaque fluid pH values. Higher DS values were also found (Margolis and Moreno, 1992b) in samples of plaque fluid from sound surfaces as compared to samples from white-spot surfaces from CP individuals; differences in DS were again primarily associated with differences

TABLE 2 *Degrees of Saturation of Plaque Fluid from Caries-Free and Caries-Positive Individuals*[a]

	DS(Enamel)	*DS(DCPD)*
CF	7.11 ± 0.66*	2.56 ± 0.20
CP	5.42 ± 0.68	2.37 ± 0.30

a. from Margolis and Moreno, 1992b.
* CF and CP values significantly different at $p < 0.001$ (Student's t-test)

in plaque fluid pH. One study (Margolis *et al.*, 1988b), however, showed similar pH and DS values in starved plaque fluid samples from CF and CP individuals. Significantly higher DS values were also found (Margolis *et al.*, 1988a) in resting (obtained one to several hours after eating) plaque fluid samples from CF individuals as compared to that found for CP samples. These latter results, however, appear to be related to both higher pH values and concentrations of ammonium ion in the CF samples. The influence of base production on the overall cariogenic potential of dental plaque deserves further study and is addressed elsewhere (Marquis, 1992) within this text.

Based on the results discussed in the preceding paragraph, one can generally characterize plaque fluid from CF individuals under starved conditions as having a greater remineralization potential than that from CP individuals. Since observed enamel demineralization *in vivo* is the net result of periods of demineralization and remineralization, the suggested differences in remineralization potential may contribute significantly to the difference in the caries experience of these subjects. In fact, it is reasonable to assume that a potential for remineralization exists in plaque for greater periods of time than periods when enamel is at risk. The relative influence of periods of remineralization on caries progression *in vivo* has not been determined.

Following exposure to fermentable carbohydrate (sucrose) pH values in plaque (*e.g.*, Stephan, 1944; Abelson and Mandel, 1981) and plaque fluid (*e.g.*, Edgar *et al.*, 1986; Margolis and Moreno, 1992b) decrease rapidly. This decrease in pH corresponds primarily to the rapid production of lactic acid. Notably, a greater decrease in plaque fluid pH values and a greater increase in lactic acid concentrations were observed (Margolis and Moreno, 1992b) following sucrose exposure in samples from CP subjects as compared to those changes observed in samples from CF subjects. In addition, the DS_{En} of plaque fluid also decreased rapidly and to a greater degree in samples from CP individuals. Concomitantly, total activities of acid species in plaque fluid increase, following sucrose exposure and, also, to a greater degree in plaque fluid from CP subjects. Thus both factors, lower values of DS and larger activities of acid species, which were found to accelerate rates of hydroxyapatite and enamel dissolution *in vitro*, have been found to be associated with increased caries activity. Further *in vitro* studies are required to test this model (described by equation [1]) for

TABLE 3 *Total Concentration of Calcium in Whole Plaque From Caries-Free and Caries-Positive Individual*[a]

	CF	*CP*
Margolis & Moreno, 1992b	16.2 ± 5.2 *	6.9 ± 0.4
	12.8 ± 1.5 *	7.9 ± 3.0
Shaw *et al., 1983*		
posterior	3.6 ± 3.2	1.6 ± 1.2
anterior	11.6 ± 12.4	2.6 ± 1.8

a. expressed as mg Ca per gram dry weight of plaque
* CF and CP values significantly different at $p < 0.05$

enamel demineralization over a wide range of conditions reflecting the ionic composition of dental plaque fluid. In this fashion, it should be possible to determine the dependency of the overall rate of enamel demineralization on the DS and the total activity of acid species in plaque fluid-like media.

Following sucrose exposure and coinciding with lactic acid production, several studies (Edgar *et al.*, 1981, Rankine, *et al.*, 1985) have observed an increase in calcium concentrations in plaque fluid. Contradictory results have been observed, however, for phosphate. Significantly, it has been observed (Margolis and Moreno, 1992b) that calcium concentrations increase to similar levels in plaque fluid from CF and CP individuals (at 7-minutes following sucrose exposure), despite the production of less lactic acid in the CF samples. These results suggested that whole plaque may contain a pool of mineral ions that become available with increasing acidity in plaque. As can be seen in Table 3, whole plaque from the CF subjects contained significantly more calcium than did plaque from the CP subjects. As it turns out, several studies (Ashley, 1975; Shaw *et al.*, 1983) have also found this to be the case (Table 3). A release of calcium ions into plaque fluid at low pH will increase the DS of this important medium and, thus, lower the driving force for enamel dissolution. This effect of increased calcium concentration in plaque fluid on DS_{En}, following acid production, is illustrated in Figure 1. Here DS_{En} is calculated using mean data (Margolis and Moreno, 1992b) obtained from CF and CP individuals obtained at 7 minutes following a 10% sucrose rinse. The abscissa represents the hypothetical change in the calcium concentration in plaque fluid relative to the mean concentrations of calcium found in plaque fluid prior to sucrose exposure (*i.e.*, CF: 2.8 mmol/L; CP: 2.7 mmol/L). In both cases, the DS_{En} increases significantly with increasing concentrations of calcium, illustrating the potential reduction in the driving force for demineralization with increasing calcium concentration in plaque fluid. In this study, actual mean calcium concentrations (denoted in Figure 1) in plaque fluid increased by 6.8 mmol/L in the CF samples and by 5.5 mmol/L in the CP samples, following sucrose exposure; the observed difference between CF and CP samples was not significant. The association of

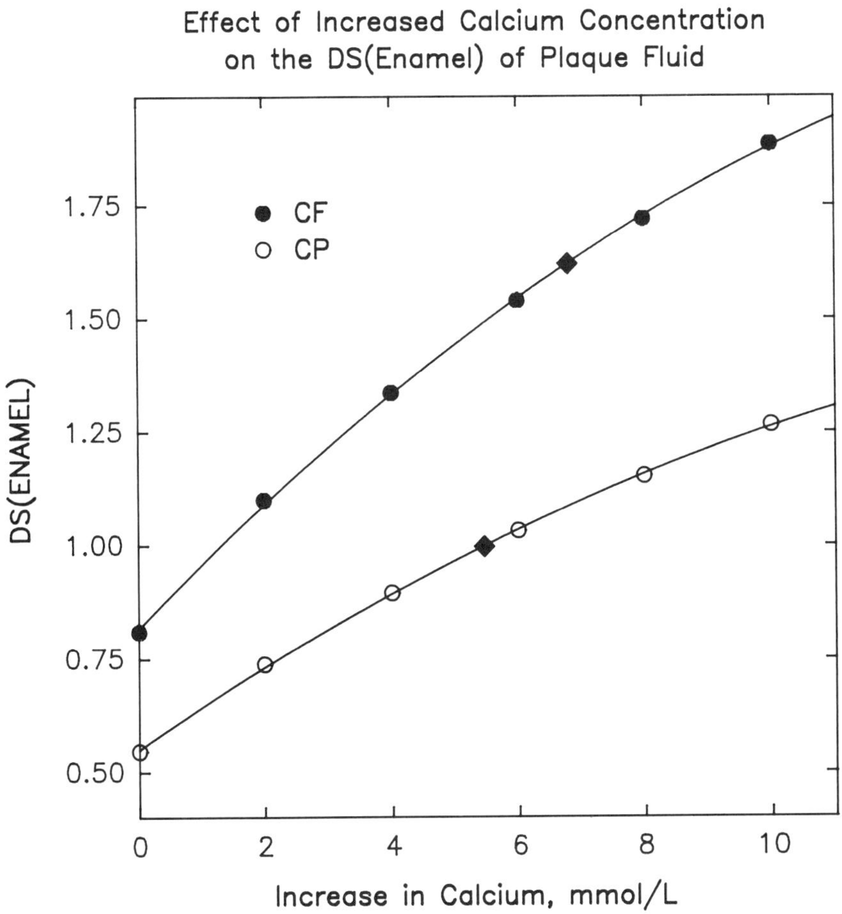

Figure 1. The influence of an increase in the concentration of calcium in plaque fluid on its degree of saturation with respect to enamel mineral (DS_{En}). DS_{En} is calculated using mean data (Margolis and Moreno, 1992b) obtained from caries-free (CF) and caries-positive (CP) individuals at 7 minutes following a 10% sucrose rinse. Initial calcium concentrations in the CF and CP plaque fluid were 2.8 mmol/L and 2.7 mmol/L, respectively. Filled diamonds represent the actual mean increase in calcium concentrations (and calculated DS_{En}) observed in these plaque fluids, 7-minutes following sucrose exposure.

greater concentrations of calcium in plaque in samples from CF individuals may indeed suggest that the observed pool of calcium ions provides an important cariostatic effect. Certainly, it has been demonstrated (Pearce, 1982) that the induced formation of soluble mineral phases (fluoridated hydroxyapatite) within dental plaque results in a cariostatic effect. The manner by which calcium is concentrated in natural whole plaque is not fully understood, although mineral phases in young plaque have been identified (Kaufman and Kleinberg, 1973; Leach and Appleton, 1981) by X-ray examination; however, since plaque samples were dried for these studies, these results may be inconclusive. Nevertheless, it is interesting to point out that since starved plaque fluid from CF subjects is more highly supersaturated with respect to calcium phosphate phases, as compared to plaque fluid from CP subjects, these samples also have a greater potential to precipitate calcium phosphates within plaque. It is also possible that calcium-rich plaque may be associated with specific microorganisms, but no information on this important point is presently available.

In vitro models related to enamel demineralization have, thus, proven to be extremely valuable in identifying appropriate driving forces for mineral dissolution and describing those factors which influence the kinetics of this process. Such models, however, do not consider the potential role that specific proteins, present in plaque fluid, may play in modifying rates of demineralization or remineralization at the enamel-plaque interface. No studies have attempted to identify potential inhibitors of mineralization processes in plaque, although plaque fluid has been shown to have a high protein content (Tatevossian and Gould, 1976). Salivary proteins (Moreno *et al.*, 1979), as well as fragments (Aoba *et al.*, 1984; Hay *et al.*, 1987) of these proteins, have been shown to inhibit mineralization processes *in vitro*. Degraded salivary proteins within dental plaque may, therefore, play a role in controlling such events. It has also been suggested (Edgar *et al.*, 1981; Carey *et al.*, 1986; Tatevossian, 1987) that macromolecules bind a portion of the total calcium ion in plaque fluid. The nature of these ligands and their influence on free calcium ion activities as a function of pH may have important implications with regard to DS values in plaque fluid. Studies of this type are essential to assessing the cariogenic potential of plaque.

Fluoride ion concentrations in plaque fluid are extremely low and have been reported (Tatevossian and Gould, 1976; Carey *et al.*, 1986; Moreno and Margolis, 1988) to be in the range of 0.04 to 0.1 ppm in resting samples. However, it has been suggested (Birkeland and Charlton, 1976) that fluoride ion activity in plaque increases as plaque pH values decrease. Whole plaque actually can accumulate relatively large concentrations of fluoride, and it appears that the percentage of "tightly-bound" fluoride is not as great as once thought (Ophaug *et al.*, 1987). Despite the fact that low levels of fluoride ion in solution have been shown (Ten Cate and Duijsters, 1983a,b; Margolis *et al.*, 1986) to inhibit enamel demineralization *in vitro,* the significance of such low levels of fluoride ion found in plaque fluid on enamel demineralization has been ignored. In the latter noted study, 1 ppm fluoride in solution was shown to inhibit enamel demineralization in a partially saturated lactic acid buffer with a DS_{En} value equal to about 0.12. We have noted (Margolis and Moreno, 1990) that the concentration of fluoride required to reduce (or inhibit) rates of enamel demineralization is dependent upon the driving force for enamel demineralization present in solution, *i.e.* DS_{En}. The results from a study (Nakashima and Moreno, 1991) designed to examine this important point in greater detail indeed suggest that concentrations of fluoride less than 1 ppm can effectively inhibit enamel demineralization *in vitro* when the driving force (DSEn) for demineralization is small. Importantly, current estimates (Margolis and Moreno, 1992b) of the minimum DS_{En} values in plaque fluid, following sucrose exposure, appear to be significantly greater than 0.12. Therefore, it is reasonable to suggest that fluoride concentrations found in plaque fluid may be in a range which can influence significantly rates of enamel demineralization *in vivo*. In fact, appreciably lower concentrations of fluoride than that found in plaque fluid may be effective in controlling demineralization barring, of course, the influence of protein inhibitors of remineralization (the mechanism by which fluoride appears to inhibit net demineralization under these conditions). Further *in vitro* studies are required to more precisely define the relationship between fluoride ion concentrations in solution and the onset of enamel demineralization. Through such studies, carried out under *in vivo*-like conditions, we can address the key question as to how much fluoride within plaque fluid is required to inhibit enamel demineralization *in vivo*.

Enamel Mineral

Equating driving forces for enamel demineralization to the DS with respect to enamel, when enamel is considered to be a more soluble hydroxyapatite, has been extremely useful in *in vitro* studies. In such studies, however, rates of enamel demineralization in a single solution can be extremely variable in different teeth and even at different areas of the same tooth. Such differences may reflect, in part, the inadequacy of considering enamel to be a hydroxyapatite and/or variations in mineral composition. In particular, the influence of fluoride and carbonate incorporated in the enamel mineral structure should be considered with regard to enamel demineralization.

Fluoride Incorporation

It is clear from considerations presented in the preceding sections that any factor which reduces enamel solubility will reduce its rate of demineralization and, thus, provide a cariostatic effect. For example, it has been demonstrated (Moreno *et al.*, 1974) that, by increasing the fluoride content in hydroxyapatite, the solubility of the resulting fluoridated hydroxyapatites ($Ca_5(OH)_{1-x}F_x(PO_4)_3$), in general, decreases. Such findings suggest that the cariostatic effects of systemic fluorides result, in part, by increasing the fluoride content of the enamel surface. Interestingly, the effectiveness of increasing enamel fluoride content as a cariostatic measure is still debated. Recently, however, it has been demonstrated (Tanaka *et al.*, 1992) that by increasing the fluoride content of the enamel surface to 6,000 ppm (via a topical procedure), enamel demineralization *in vitro* can be essentially inhibited during a 5-day exposure of the fluoride-enriched enamel surface to a given demineralizing solution. Significantly, this remarkable inhibition results despite the fact that the fluoride content of the enamel decreases rapidly from the surface (6,000 ppm) to about 200 ppm at a depth of about 5 μm below the surface. The amount of fluoride in the enamel mineral surface required to prevent enamel demineralization will depend upon the driving force for demineralization in solution. Perhaps, therefore, a more appropriate driving force for enamel demineralization should consider enamel as a fluoridated mineral and appropriately include F^- in the definition of DS_{En}. Further studies in this area are required to clarify this important point. Again, these results point to the importance of being able to define and determine the appropriate driving force for enamel demineralization in plaque fluid. Through further *in vitro* enamel demineralization studies, the relative importance of fluoride ion in solution and in the mineral must also be assessed under conditions similar to that found in dental plaque fluid. Such information may greatly assist in assessing the relative efficacy of systemic and topical fluoride agents in the preventative treatment of dental caries.

Enamel as a Carbonated Phase

Enamel mineral contains about 3% carbonate on a weight basis. Recently, a solubility product for human enamel was determined (Moreno and Aoba, 1991), based on the following (experimentally determined) stoichiometry considering both its acid phosphate and carbonate content:

$$(Ca)_{4.62}(HPO_4)_{0.07}(CO_3)_{0.31}(PO_4)_{2.62}(OH)_{0.62}$$

$$DS_{H.E.} = [(Ca^{++})^{4.62}(HPO_4^{--})^{0.07}(CO_3^{--})^{0.31}(PO_4^{3-})^{2.62}(OH^-)^{0.62}/K_{H.E.}]^{1/8.24}$$

The solubility product constant, $K_{H.E.}$, defined as the activity product of this mineral phase at saturation, was found to be equal to 4.57×10^{-49}. The stability of enamel mineral within the oral cavity, when considered to be a carbonated phase, will depend on the carbonate content of plaque fluid. In turn, the carbonate content in plaque fluid will be a function of its pH and partial pressure of CO_2 (P_{CO2}). Variations in the P_{CO2} within dental plaque can be expected to result from the presence of different bacterial species as well as from variations in salivary carbonate levels and salivary exposure. The potential influence of variations in carbonate concentrations in plaque fluid is illustrated by the results presented in Table 4. Here, the DS with respect to human enamel (H.E.), as

TABLE 4 *Degrees of Saturation With respect to Human Enamel as a Function of Partial Pressure of CO_2*[a]

P_{CO2}, %	*Total Carbonate*[b]	*DS (H.E.)*[c]
0.03	0.023	0.719
0.5	0.383	0.799
1.0	0.767	0.820
3.0	2.302	0.854
5.0	3.836	0.870

a. calculated using data from Margolis and Moreno, 1992b; mean values for CP subjects at 7 minutes following a 10% sucrose rinse

b. mmol/L

c. as defined in text

defined above, was calculated in a solution having a composition similar to that found (Margolis and Moreno, 1992b) in plaque fluid following (7 minutes) sucrose exposure and assuming various levels of P_{CO2}. Results presented in Table 4 show that by increasing P_{CO2} the total concentration of carbonate (CO_3^{--} + HCO_3^- + H_2CO_3) in solution increases and results in an increase in $DS_{H.E.}$. These results suggest that the driving force for demineralization should decrease with increased carbonate concentrations in solution. The variations in carbonate concentrations used in these calculations appear to influence $DS_{H.E.}$ to a small degree. However, the influence of such small changes in $DS_{H.E.}$ on rates of enamel demineralization is not precisely known but expected from studies on the dissolution of hydroxyapatite (Margolis and Moreno, 1992a) to vary proportionally to (1-$DS_{H.E.}$) raised at least to about the third power, according to equation [1]. Thus, these calculated differences in $DS_{H.E.}$ may alter significantly the rates of enamel demineralization. The noted variations in P_{CO2} have essentially no influence on DS_{En}, when enamel is consider to be a hydroxyapatite; the calculated DS_{En} is 0.99 for all systems shown in Table 4. Accordingly, the driving force for enamel demineralization in a solution like plaque fluid would be assessed to be significantly less if enamel is assumed to be a hydroxyapatite rather than a carbonated-hydroxyapatite. Furthermore, its solubility would be unaffected by varying concentrations of carbonate in solution. The overall significance of considering enamel as a carbonated phase must be explored by determining carbonate levels in plaque fluid and assessing the effects of such carbonate levels on enamel demineralization *in vitro*.

Conclusions

In order to assess the cariogenic potential of dental plaque, properties of both the enamel tissue and plaque fluid must be properly considered. Such studies lend themselves to the establishment of a much-needed link between plaque composition, microbiological factors, and the onset of dental caries. The establishment of more relevant *in vitro* enamel demineralization models will greatly improve our understanding of the mechanism of the caries process and facilitate the development of preventative procedures.

REFERENCES

ABELSON, D.C. and MANDEL, I.D. (1981): The Effect of Saliva on Plaque pH *in vivo*, *J Dent Res* 60:1634-1638.

AOBA, T.; MORENO, E.C.; and HAY, D.I. (1984): Inhibition of Apatite Crystal Growth by the Amino-Terminal Segment of Human Salivary Acidic Proline-Rich Proteins, *Calcif Tissue Int* 36:651-658.

ASHLEY, F.P. (1975): Calcium and Phosphorus Concentrations of Dental Plaque Related to Dental Caries in 11- to 14-year old Male Subjects, *Caries Res* 9:351-362.

BIRKELAND, J.M. and CHARLTON, G. (1976): Effect of pH on the Fluoride Activity of Plaque, *Caries Res* 10:72-80.

CAREY, C.; GREGORY, T.; RUPP, W.; TATEVOSSIAN, A.; and VOGEL, G.L. (1986): The Driving Forces in Human Dental Plaque Fluid for Demineralisation and Remineralisation of Enamel Mineral. In: *Factors Relating to Demineralisation and Remineralisation of the Teeth*, S.A. Leach, Ed., Oxford: IRL Press Ltd., pp 163-173.

DE STOPPELAAR, J. (1982): Urea and Ammonia in Saliva of Caries Inactive Children with Renal Disease, *J Dent Res* 61:225, Abstract No. 424.

EDGAR, W.M. (1976): The Role of Saliva in the Control of pH Changes in Human Dental Plaque, *Caries Res* 10:241-254.

EDGAR, W.M.; BOWEN, W.H.; and COLE, M.F. (1981): Development of Rampant Dental Caries, and Composition of Plaque Fluid and Saliva in Irradiated Primates, *J Oral Path* 10:284-295.

EDGAR, W.M.; DODDS, M.W.J.; and HIGHAM, S.M. (1986): Changes in Carboxylic Acid and Free Amino Acid Profiles in Human Dental Plaque After a Carbohydrate Challenge *in situ*, *Biochem Soc Trans* 14:977.

FEATHERSTONE, J.D.B. and RODGERS, B.E. (1981): Effect of Acetic, Lactic and Other Organic Acids on the Formation of Artificial Carious Lesions, *Caries Res* 15:377-385.

GRAY, J.A. (1962): Kinetics of Dissolution of Human Dental Enamel in Acid, *J Dent Res* 41:633-645.

HAY, D.I.; CARLSON, E.R.; SCHLUCKEBIER, S.K.; MORENO, E.C.; and SCHLESINGER, D.H. (1987): Inhibition of Calcium Phosphate Precipitation by Human Salivary Acidic Proline-Rich Proteins: Structure-Activity Relationships, *Calcif Tissue Int* 40:126-132.

JENKINS, G.N. (1979): Salivary Effects on Plaque pH, In: *Saliva and Dental Caries*, I. Kleinberg, S.A. Ellison, I.D. Mandel, Eds., New York, Information Rctricval, Inc. pp. 307-322.

KAUFMAN, H.W. and KLEINBERG, I. (1975): X-ray Diffraction Examination of Calcium Phosphate in Dental Plaque, *Calcif Tiss Res* 11:97-104.

LEACH S.A. and APPLETON, J. (1981): Ultrastructural Investigations by Energy Dispersive X-ray Microanalysis of Some of the Elements Involved in the Formation of Dental Plaque and Pellicle. In: *Tooth Surface Interactions and Preventative Dentistry*, G. Rolla, T. Sonju and G. Emberry, Eds.,IRL Press Ltd., London, pp. 65-79.

LEE, C.Y.; MARGOLIS, H.C.; and MORENO, E.C. (1990): Factors Influencing the Rate of Enamel Demineralization *in vitro*, *J Dent Res* 69 (special issue):302, Abstract No. 1547.

MARGOLIS, H.C. (1990): An Assessment of Recent Advances In the Study of the Chemistry and Biochemistry of Dental Plaque Fluid, *J Dent Res* 69:1337-1342.

MARGOLIS, H.C.; DUCKWORTH, J.H.; and MORENO, E.C. (1988a): Composition of Pooled Resting Plaque Fluid from Caries-Free and Caries-Susceptible Individuals, *J Dent Res* 67:1468-1475.

MARGOLIS, H.C.; DUCKWORTH, J.H.; MORENO, E.C. (1988b): Composition and Buffer Capacity of Pooled Starved Plaque Fluid from Caries-Free and Caries-Susceptible Individuals, *J Dent Res* 67:1476-1482.

MARGOLIS, H.C. and MORENO, E.C. (1990): Physicochemical Perspectives on the Cariostatic Mechanisms of Systemic and Topical Fluorides. *J Dent Res* 69:606-613.

MARGOLIS, H.C. and MORENO, E.C. (1992a): Kinetics of Hydroxyapatite Dissolution in Acetic, Lactic, and Phosphoric Acid Solutions, *Calcif Tissue Int* 50:137-143.

MARGOLIS, H.C. and MORENO, E.C. (1992b): Composition of Pooled Plaque Fluid from Caries-Free and Caries-Positive Individuals Following Sucrose Exposure, *J Dent Res* 71:1776-1784.

MARGOLIS, H.C.; MORENO, E.C.; and MURPHY, B.J. (1986): Effect of Low Levels of Fluoride in Solution on Enamel Demineralization, *in vitro*, *J Dent Res* 65:23-29.

MARGOLIS, H.C.; MURPHY, B.J.; and MORENO, E.C. (1985): Development of Carious-Like Lesions in Partially Saturated Lactate Buffers, *Caries Res* 19:36-45.

MARQUIS, R. (1992): Arginine Deaminase and Alkali Generation in dental Plaque, *this text*.

MORENO, E.C.; KRESAK, M.; and ZAHRADNIK, R.T. (1977): Physicochemical Aspects of Fluoride-Apatite Systems Relevant to the Study of Dental Caries, *Caries Res* [Suppl. 1] 11:142-177.

MORENO, E.C. and MARGOLIS, H.C. (1988): Composition of Human Plaque Fluid, *J Dent Res* 67:1181-1189.

MORENO, E.C. and ZAHRADNIK, R.T. (1974): Chemistry of Enamel Subsurface Demineralization, *J Dent Res* 53:226-235.

MORENO, E.C.; VARUGHESE, K.; and HAY, D.I. (1979): Effect of Human Salivary Proteins on the Precipitation Kinetics of Calcium Phosphate, *Calcif Tissue Int* 28:7-16.

MORENO, E.C. and AOBA, T (1991): Formation and Solubility of Carbonated Tooth Minerals, In: *Mechanisms and Phylogeny of Mineralization in Biological Systems*, S. Suga and H. Nakahara, Eds., Springer-Verlag, Tokyo, pp. 179-186.

MORENO, E.C.; KRESAK, M.; and ZAHRADNIK, R.T. (1974): Fluoridated Hydroxyapatite Solubility and Caries Formation, *Nature (Lond.)* 247:64-65.

NAKASHIMA, S. and MORENO, E.C. (1991): Effect of Degree of Saturation and Fluoride Concentration on Demineralization of Human Enamel by Lactate Buffer - A Study by Single Thin Section Technique, *J Dental Health (Japan)* 41:596-606.

OPHAUG, R.H.; JENKINS, G.N.; SINGER, L.; and KREBSBACH, K. (1987): Acid Diffusion Analysis of Different Forms of Fluoride in Human Dental Plaque, *Arch Oral Biol* 32:459-461.

PEARCE, E.I.F. (1982): Effect of Plaque Mineralization on Experimental Dental Caries, *Caries Res* 16:460-471.

PETERSON, S; WOODHEAD, J.; and CRALL, J. (1985): Caries Resistance in Children with Chronic Renal Failure: Plaque pH, Salivary pH, and Salivary Composition. *Pediatr Res* 19:796-799.

RANKINE, C.A.N.; MORENO, E.C.; VOGEL, G.L.; and MARGOLIS, H.C., (1985): Micro- analytical Determination of pH, Calcium, and Phosphate in Plaque Fluid, *J Dent Res* 64:1275-1280.

SHAW, L.; MURRAY, J.J.; BURCHELL, C.K.; and BEST, J.S. (1983): Calcium and Phosphorus Content of Plaque and Saliva in Relation to Dental Caries, *Caries Res* 17:543-548.

STEPHAN, R.M. (1944): Intra-oral Hydrogen-Ion Concentrations Associated with Dental Caries Activity, *J Dent Res* 23:257-266.

TATEVOSSIAN, A. and GOULD, C.T. (1976): The Composition of the Aqueous Phase in Human Dental Plaque, *Arch Oral Biol* 21:319-323.

TATEVOSSIAN, A. (1987): Calcium and Phosphate in Human Dental Plaque and their Concentrations after Overnight Fasting and After Ingestion of a Boiled Sweet, *Arch Oral Biol* 32:201-205.

TANAKA, M; MORENO, E.C.; and MARGOLIS, H.C. (1992): Effect of Fluoride Incorporation into Enamel on Its Demineralization *In Vitro*, (submitted).

TEN CATE, J.M. and DUIJSTERS, P.P.E. (1983a): Influence of Fluoride in Solution on Tooth Demineralization. I. Chemical Data, *Caries Res* 17:193-199.

TEN CATE, J.M. and DUIJSTERS, P.P.E. (1983b): Influence of Fluoride in Solution on Tooth Demineralization. I. Microradiographic Data, *Caries Res* 17:513-519.

THEUNS, H.M.; VAN DIJK, J.W.E.; DRIESSENS, F.C.M.; and GROENEVELD, A. (1983): Effect of Time and Degree of Saturation of Buffer Solutions on Artificial Carious Lesion Formation in Human Tooth Enamel, *Caries Res* 17:503-512.

THEUNS, H.M.; VAN DIJK, J.W.E.; DRIESSENS, F.C.M.; and GROENEVELD, A. (1984a): Effect of the pH of Buffer Solutions on Artificial Carious Lesion Formation in Human Tooth Enamel, *Caries Res* 18:7-11.

THEUNS, H.M.; VAN DIJK, J.W.E.; DRIESSENS, F.C.M.; and GROENEVELD, A. (1984b): Effect of Undissociated Acetic-Acid Concentration of Buffer Solutions on Artificial Carious Lesion Formation in Human Tooth Enamel, *Arch Oral Biol* 29:759-763.

VAN HOUTE, J.; RUSSO, J.; and PROSTAK, K.S. (1989): Increased pH-lowering Ability of *Streptococcus mutans* Cell Masses Associated with Extracellular Glucan-rich Matrix Material and the Mechanisms Involved, *J Dent Res* 68:451-459.

VOGEL, G.L.; CAREY, C.M.; CHOW, L.C.; and TATEVOSSIAN, A. (1990): Microanalysis of Plaque Fluid from Single-site Fasted Plaque, *J Dent Res* 69:1316-1323.

Physical Chemical Aspects of the Mineralization and Demineralization of Tooth Components

BRUCE ELDER AND GEORGE H. NANCOLLAS

Interest in the mechanism of demineralization and remineralization of enamel and other tooth components stems from the need to elucidate the mechanism of caries formation. Tooth enamel is degraded in the oral environment by acidic species, usually of bacterial origin and three main types of attack have been distinguished (a) Surface softening or short term exposure to low pH such as enamel dissolution that occurs as a result of the ingestion of food or beverages, (b) Subsurface demineralization or lesion formation which is thought to occur due to the protecting properties of adsorbed macromolecules (pellicle and plaque) during long term exposure under mildly acidic conditions, (c) Surface etching involving strong acid exposure for relatively short periods of time. Although numerous *in vitro* studies have been made of enamel re- and demineralization kinetics by exposing it to solutions either super- or undersaturated with respect to calcium phosphate phases, it is now well established that the nature of the deposited and dissolving phases may change during reactions. Nevertheless, the rates of reaction, J, are usually expressed in terms of the relative supersaturation, σ = (S-1) or undersaturation, σ = (1-S) of a particular calcium phosphate phase where S is the saturation ratio (equation 1)

[1] $$S = (IP/K_{SO})^{1/\nu}$$

IP is the ionic activity product written in the same form as the solubility product, K_{SO}, and ν is the number of ions in a formula unit. The rates of reaction are usually expressed in terms of an expression such as in equation 2

We acknowledge the Procter & Gamble Company and the National Institutes of Dental Research (Grant #DEO3223) for financial support of this work and Dr. D. G. A. Nelson for MAS-NMR measurements.

[2] $$J = k\,F(m/m_o)\sigma^n$$

where k is the rate constant, F is a function of the ratio of mass of solid phase at time t to the initial value, and n is the effective order of reaction.

A significant problem in applying such simple kinetics that have been established for synthetic systems to tooth components, is the difficulty of estimating the solubility of the solid phases. In earlier studies, Patel and Brown (1975) obtained values ranging from 7.2×10^{-53} to 6.4×10^{-58} $(\text{mol L}^{-1})^9$ while two other studies reported values ranging from 5.4×10^{-54} to 3.9×10^{-55} $(\text{mol L}^{-1})^9$ (Chen and Nancollas, 1986) and 5.5×10^{-55} (Moreno and Zahradnik, 1974). The appropriateness of any of these values may be questioned since they were all calculated assuming a hydroxyapatite $Ca_5(PO_4)_3OH$ model whereas it is well known that tooth minerals contain appreciable amounts of carbonate as well as other lattice substituted ions. Thus although the solubility behavior of synthetic phases such as HAP is in good agreement with theory, the results for tooth components show inconsistencies that are more marked for dentin than for enamel (Moreno and Aoba, 1991). Recent studies have therefore been concerned with solution speciation during mineralization and demineralization experiments attempting to base the relative supersaturation upon solubility values for carbonated apatite (CAP) having 2-5% CO_3^{2-} and relating the concentration data to calculated stoichiometries for the solid phases. This has led to a proposed formula for porcine enamel $[Ca]_{5-x}\ [HPO_4]_v\ [CO_3]_w\ [PO_4]_{3-x}\ [OH]_{1-x}$.

Although it is important to characterize bioapatites in terms of accepted phase equilibria, it should be noted that kinetic events may be even more important than considerations based purely upon equilibrium solubility studies. Thus the most recent solubility studies of Moreno and Aoba (Moreno and Aoba, 1991, Aoba and Moreno, 1991) were made by equilibrating enamel samples with dilute phosphoric acid. It was shown that during the reaction, the precipitation of another carbonate-containing apatitic phase took place. This observation underlines the importance of taking into account intermediate phases that may form and subsequently dissolve during mineralization and demineralization reactions. It was for this reason that the Constant Composition (CC) and Dual Constant Composition (DCC) techniques, to be discussed in this paper, were developed.

The preferential loss of carbonate from enamel during acid dissolution has been suggested by several workers (Little, 1961, Hallsworth *et al.*, 1973). However, more recently (Mayer *et al.*, 1988) an infrared study indicated that at moderate carbonate content (below about 4%) no preferential loss of carbonate was observed whereas at higher carbonate content, the carbonate ions were released preferentially. In general, CAP is considered to be the most soluble fraction of enamel due to its lower crystallinity and increased reactivity. Carbonate loss has also been linked to the existence of preferential sites for acid attack (Arends, 1982) such as the central core of apatite crystallites. The origin of the strained area and its vulnerability might be traced to the presence of dislocations created by the carbonate ions suggesting a surface controlled dissolution. This mechanism has now been quite well established from kinetics studies as discussed later in this chapter.

In the creation of subsurface lesions at enamel surfaces, models have been proposed based on dissolution/precipitation mechanisms (Margolis and Moreno, 1985) involving the dissolution of CAP and subsequent precipitation of dicalcium phosphate dihydrate (DCPD), fluorapatite (FAP) and HAP. These phases were assumed to be in quasiequilibrium with aqueous phases in the enamel pores. In terms of this mechanism, the partially dissolved surface layer plays an important role in that it can be continuously regenerated. Arends and Christoffersen (1986) developed a model predicting a third root dependence of lesion depth upon demineralization time. They were able to satisfactorily interpret the progress of lesions in both bovine and human enamel at pH 4-5 in terms of this model. These results suggest that inhibitor action and penetration are the most important events in white spot formation.

In contrast to the free-drift experiments in which equilibration is allowed to proceed to equilibrium without ion replenishment, a number of studies have been made in which the pH was held constant but the calcium and phosphate ion concentrations were allowed to relax to equilibrium (Gramain *et al.*, 1989). The results revealed interesting effects of stirring with apparent changes in mechanism from a diffusive process at low stirring to a solid or surface controlled process at higher stirring speeds. Moreover, the results suggested an accumulation of calcium ions at the surface resulting in a reduction in dissolution rate during the reactions. These studies suggested an interfacial calcium /phosphate rich layer at the solid surfaces that influenced the subsequent rates of reaction. Here, again, research points to the formation of intermediate phases during the reactions suggesting the importance of kinetics events.

Methods

Although *in vitro* seeded crystallization and dissolution experiments yield highly reproducible results and, in the case of pH-stat techniques, the hydrogen ion activity can be held constant during the reaction, they all suffer from the disadvantage that the lattice ion concentrations change as the reactions proceed towards equilibrium. In contrast, the CC method enables experiments to be made at relatively low driving forces to large extents of reaction, allowing detailed kinetic analysis on both solution and solid phases. In this method, upon seeding the reaction, the concentrations of lattice ions are maintained constant through the addition of titrant solutions of appropriate stoichiometry for the growing phase of interest. Since its development, CC has been used extensively to investigate the mechanisms of many different mineral systems. However, it allows studies to be made of only single growing or dissolving phases.

In vivo, simultaneous processes at solid surfaces are not rare. Thus mineralization has frequently been suggested as proceeding through precursor phases such as amorphous calcium phosphate (ACP) or octacalcium phosphate (OCP) before transforming to the thermodynamically more stable HAP. In the presence of fluoride ion, HAP can transform to FAP or hydroxyfluorapatite (FHAP) with or without calcium fluoride (CaF_2) formation. During such transformations, the nucleation and subsequent growth of the new phase may occur at the expense of the original phase. For these reasons, the DCC method was developed incorporating two CC instrumentations each controlled by its own sensor electrode in order to monitor the individual reactions. The method is invaluable for investigating the initial events that occur during de- or re-mineralization of tooth components that might otherwise go unnoticed in conventional free-drift and CC methods. It has recently been demonstrated, theoretically, that two distinct processes can be monitored even if the solid phases contain a common ion (Ebrahimpour, 1990). In a typical DCC reaction, stable supersaturated or undersaturated solutions are prepared and the reaction is initiated by the addition of seed crystals. Separate sets of titrant solutions are automatically added in order to control each of the reactions. For example for HAP growth, typical titrant concentrations would be given by equations 3-6

[3] $$T_1 = (2[\mathrm{Ca}]_s + 5\ C_{eff}) + (2[\mathrm{Na}]_s - 10\ C_{eff})$$

[4] $$T_2 = 2[\mathrm{PO_4}]_s + 2[\mathrm{OH}]_s$$

[5] $$T_3 = (2[\mathrm{PO_4}]_s + 3\ C_{eff}) + (2[\mathrm{OH}]_s + 7\ C_{eff})$$

[6] $$T_4 = 2[\mathrm{Ca}]_s + (2[\mathrm{Na}]_s - 10\ C_{eff})$$

In these equations, subscript s refers to concentrations in the reaction medium while C_{eff} is the effective concentration for HAP growth, denoting the number of mols of HAP formed per unit volume of titrant addition. Titrants 1 and 2 would be controlled by a calcium ion selective electrode while titrants 3 and 4 would be controlled by a pH electrode.

Dissolution Kinetics

The CC method has been used to investigate the dissolution kinetics of HAP, CAP and both human and bovine enamel in the presence and absence of inhibitors. Interpreting the kinetics in terms of equation 2, the rate of dissolution of HAP in the pH range 5-7.2 in 30-90% undersaturated solution gave a value $n > 4$, with a rate less than that calculated on the basis of pure diffusion (Fick's law) by a factor of almost 10^4 (Christoffersen 1978) suggesting a polynucleation mechanism. It was also shown that hydrogen ions played an important role in the dissolution process not only as a complexing agent for hydroxyl ions in solution, but also as a catalyst for the exchange of phosphate ions between the crystal surface and the solution (Tomazic *et al.*, 1989). For OCP dissolution, the value of n showed a change from 2 to 1 at $\sigma \approx 0.5$ as the driving force increased. This suggests that desorption and/or volume diffusion may be important at higher driving forces while surface diffusion and/or detachment may offer the dominating resistance at lower undersaturation (Zhang and Nancollas, 1988). Typical CC plots of titrant volume as a function of time following the addition of seed materials to undersaturated solutions of calcium phosphate are shown for HAP, human and bovine enamel in Fig. 1.

In the CC experiments (Fig. 1) only the overall dissolution rate can be calculated directly from the record of titrant consumption as a function of time. Given the constancy of composition, the last term in Equation 2 remains constant and the rate can therefore be expressed in terms of $F(m/m_0)$. Even after making generous correction for the reduction of surface area during dissolution, it can be seen that the rates of reaction, a function of the slopes of the curves in Fig. 1, decreased markedly as the reactions proceeded. Thus the dissolution of HAP crystals at pH 4.5 and $\sigma = 0.5$ virtually stopped after 40-70% reaction despite the maintenance of constant undersaturation. For the proposed surface dissolution processes controlled by spiral dislocation or polynucleation mechanisms, J should be constant if the properties of the crystal surface remain unchanged. It was shown that the decrease in rate cannot be attributed to the adsorption of impurities in the solutions (Zhang and Nancollas, 1991, Budz and Nancollas, 1988) suggesting that other factors might be responsible. For the dissolution of phases controlled by spiral dislocation mechanisms, the decrease in the number of dislocations emerging at the crystal surface might be responsible for the rate reduction (Zhang, 1990). A similar mechanism might be involved in the dissolution of the bioapatites.

Mineralization Kinetics

The principal advantage of the CC method is the ability to study crystallization reactions at specified driving forces with respect to each of the calcium phosphate phases. Thus in the pH range 6-7 following the addition of OCP seed crystals, OCP has been shown to grow exclusively by a spiral growth mechanism at low supersaturation changing to polynucleation participation at higher driving forces (Heughebaert and Nancollas, 1984, Lundager Madsen, 1987). The ability to obtain reliable rate data at very low supersaturation has also enabled the growth of HAP seed crystals to be investigated. Careful analysis of the kinetics data has revealed the formation of defect apatites ranging in composition from OCP to HAP depending upon the pH of the solution and the relative supersaturation. Thus apatites with calcium/phosphate molar ratios ranging from

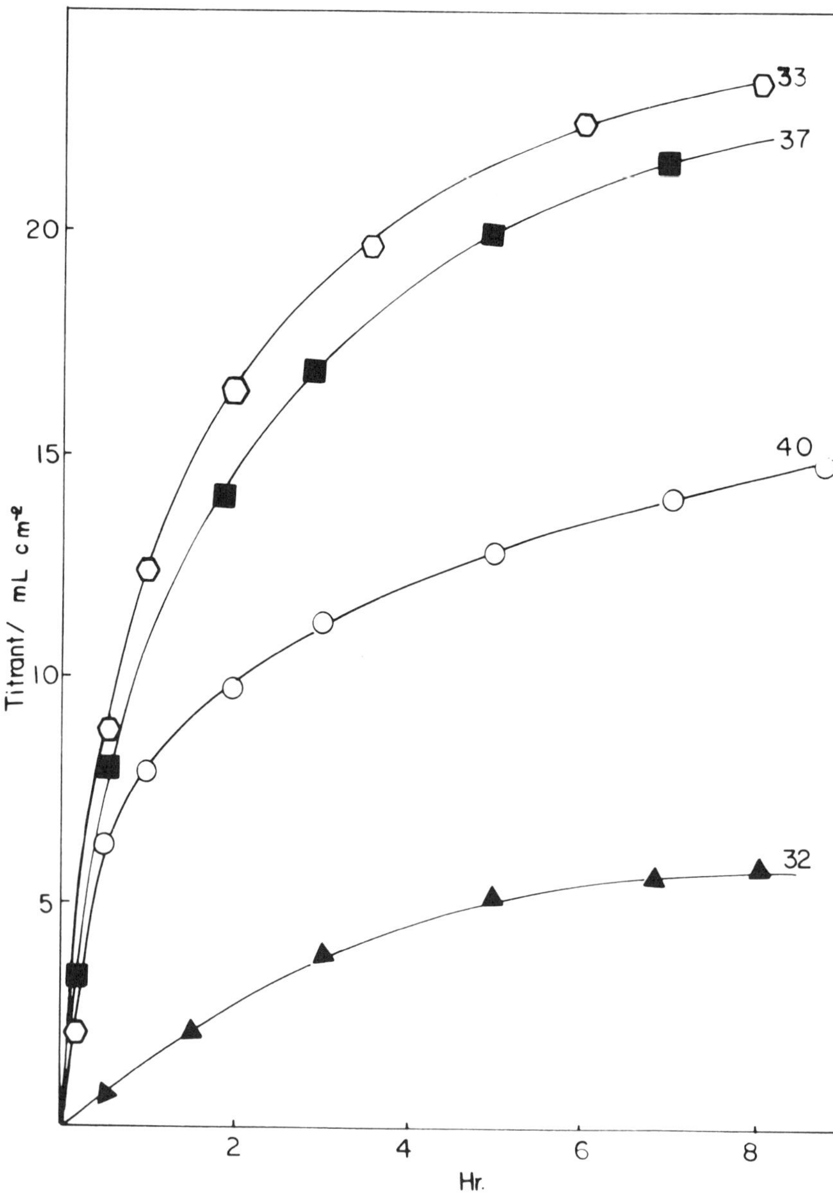

Figure 1. Dissolution of powdered enamel and HAP. Plots of titrant volume against time. T_{Ca} = 5mM, T_{PO4} = 3mM, T_{HCl} = 7mM, 37° C, pH = 4.50. 32-HAP, 37-Human enamel, 33-bovine enamel, 40-bovine enamel in the presence of 0.5ppm F^-.

1.49 to 1.65 were formed as the pH was changed from 6.0 to 9.0 (Heughebaert *et al.*, 1990, Zawacki *et al.*, 1990).

For the bioapatites, the CC remineralization rate of shallow lesions in enamel surfaces was shown to be faster than in deep lesions and in all cases there was a linear correlation between the extent of remineralization and surface hardness. During the reactions, the Ca/P ratio increased suggesting that more acidic precursor calcium phosphate phases were involved (Christoffersen *et al.*, 1978). Studies of the influence of fluoride ions on *in vitro* de- and re-mineralization rates were supportive of the efficacy of fluoride ion in preventing caries. The introduction of this ion into dental tissues is of interest since there has been much debate over the designations "firmly" and "loosely" bound fluoride. Historically, the former has referred to FAP formation while the latter is usually attributed to CaF_2-like phases. However, it should be noted that when comparisons are made of the rates of these reactions, the data refer to quite different phases rather than modifications of the same phase. There is little doubt that surface softened enamel can be remineralized more extensively in the presence of fluoride ion (Arends and Gelhard, 1983) and that lesions formed in the presence of fluoride ion are more resistant to secondary acid attack.

Application of Dual Constant Composition

The preceding brief discussion of de- and re-mineralization processes involving both synthetic and natural apatitic phases clearly points to the participation of multiple mineral phases. As discussed above, the DCC technique is ideally suited for studying the individual kinetic events involved in such reactions. The results of a typical experiment involving simultaneous dissolution of DCPD and growth of OCP in solutions undersaturated with respect to the former and supersaturated with respect to the latter phase is shown in Fig. 2. The first titrant, controlled by means of a calcium electrode was designed for DCPD dissolution, while the second set of titrants, having OCP stoichiometry was controlled by means of a pH electrode (Ebrahimpour, 1990). It can be seen that upon the introduction of mixed DCPD and OCP seed crystals, both dissolution and growth reactions commenced immediately and the DCPD was completely dissolved after about 65 min. This was confirmed by X-ray powder diffraction. By seeding such solutions only with DCPD crystals it is possible to investigate the nucleation kinetics of OCP accompanying the transformation reaction, which has been shown to be strongly dependent upon solution pH and supporting electrolyte (Tomazic, 1989). The DCC method has also been used to investigate the simultaneous growth HAP and FAP. Here, it has been possible to investigate, by both chemical analysis and F^{19} MAS-NMR, the nature of the fluoridated phases

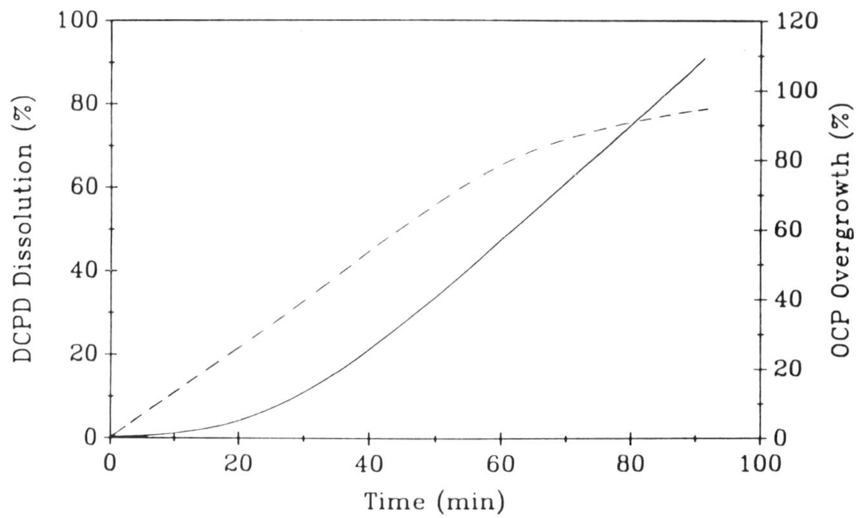

Figure 2. Simultaneous DCPD seeded dissolution (-----) and OCP seeded growth (——) at pH = 7.00, T_{Ca} = T_{PO4} = 1.80mM and ionic strength = 0.150 M (NaCl).

formed during mineralization of calcium phosphate surfaces in the presence of fluoride ion (Elder, unpublished results). This is of especial interest for enamel surfaces where different kinds of fluoride interaction have been postulated.

Preliminary studies of enamel and dentin dissolution using the DCC method also provide information about important initial kinetics events. These are reflected by changes in calcium, phosphate or base requirements during the reactions. Analysis of such data will provide new kinetics information about the de- and re-mineralization of these natural surfaces without simply having to rely on the results of equilibrium ''solubility'' studies.

REFERENCES

AOBA, T. and MORENO, E.C. (1991): Changes in the Solubility of Enamel Mineral at Various Stages of Porcine Amelogenesis, *Calcif Tissue Int* in press.

ARENDS, J. (1982): Mechanism of Dental Caries. In: *Biological Mineralization and Demineralization*, G.H. Nancollas, Ed., New York: Springer Verlag pp 303-324.

ARENDS, J. and CHRISTOFFERSEN, J. (1986): The Nature of Early Caries Lesions in Enamel, *J Dent Res* 65:2-11.

ARENDS, J. and GELHARD, T.B.F.M. (1983): *In Vivo* Remineralization of Human Enamel. In: Leach, Edgar, *Remineralization and Demineralization of Teeth*, Oxford. IRL Press pp 1-16.

BUDZ, J. and NANCOLLAS, G.H. (1988): The Mechanism of Dissolution of Hydroxyapatite and Carbonated Apatite in Acidic Solutions, *J Cryst Growth* 91:490-496.

CHEN, W.C. and NANCOLLAS, G.H. (1986): The Kinetics of Dissolution of Tooth Enamel-A Constant Composition Study, *J Dent Res* 65:663-668.

CHRISTOFFERSEN, J.; CHRISTOFFERSEN, M.R.; and KJAERGAARD, N. (1978): The Kinetics of Dissolution of Calcium Hydroxyapatite in Water at Constant pH, *J Cryst Growth* 43:501-511.

EBRAHIMPOUR, A.; ZHANG, J.; and NANCOLLAS, G.H. (1990): Dual Constant Composition Method and Its Application to Studies of Phase Transformation and Crystallization of Mixed Phases, in press.

GRAMAIN, PH.H.; THOMANN, J.M.; GUMPPER, M.; and VOEGEL, J.C. (1989): Dissolution Kinetics of Human Enamel Powder. I. Stirring Effects and Surface Calcium Accumulation, *J Colloid Int Sci* 128:370-381.

HALLSWORTH, A.S.; WEATHERELL, J.A.; and ROBINSON, C. (1973): Loss of Carbonate During the First Stages of Enamel Cries, *Caries Res* 7:345-348.

HEUGHEBAERT, J.C. and NANCOLLAS, G.H. (1984): Kinetics of Crystallization of Octacalcium Phosphate, *J Phys Chem* 88:2478-2481.

HEUGHEBAERT, J.C.; ZAWACKI, S.J.; and NANCOLLAS, G.H. (1990): The Growth of Nonstoichiometric Apatite from Aqueous Solution at 37°C. I. Methodology and Growth at pH 7.4, *J Colloid Int Sci* 135:20-32.

LITTLE, M.F. (1961): Studies of the Inorganic Carbon Dioxide Component of Human Enamel. II. The Effect of Acid on Enamel Co_2, *J Dent Res* 40:903-914.

LUNDAGER MADSEN, H.E. (1987): Comment on "The Growth of Dicalcium Phosphate Dihyderate on Octacalcium Phosphate at 25°C." by J.C. Heughebaert, J.F. Rooj and G.H. Nancollas, *J Cryst Growth* 80:450-452.

MARGOLIS, H.C. and MORENO, E.C.(1985): Kinetic and Thermodynamic Aspects of Enamel Demineralization, *Caries Res* 19:22-35

MAYER, I.; VOEGAL, J.C.; BRES, E.F.; and FRANK, R.M. (1988): The Release of Carbonate During the Dissolution of Synthetic Apatites and Dental Enamel, *J Cryst Growth* 87:129-136.

MORENO, E.C. and AOBA, T. (1991): Comparative Solubility Study of Human Dental Enamel, Dentin and Hydroxyapatite, *Calcif Tissue Int*, in press.

MORENO, E.C. and ZAHRADNIK (1974): Chemistry of Enamel Subsurface Demineralization *in vitro*, *J Dent Res* 53:226-235.

NANCOLLAS, G.H. (1991): Kinetics of Crystal Growth and Dissolution Using Constant Composition and Dual Constant Composition Methods. In: *Challenges and Opportunities in Crystallization Research*, M. Larson Ed., NSF publication in press.

PATEL, P.R. and BROWN, W.E. (1975): Thermodynamic Solubility Product of Human Enamel: Powdered Sample, *J Dent Res* 54:728-736.

TOMAZIC, B.B.; TUNG, T.S.; GREGORY, T.M.; and BROWN, W.E. (1989): Mechanism of Hydrolysis of Octacalcium Phosphate, *Scanning Mic* 3:119-

WHITE, D.J.; CHEN, W.C.; and NANCOLLAS, G.H. (1988): Kinetic and Physical Aspects of Enamel Remineralization - A Constant Composition Study, *Caries Res* 22:11-19.

ZAWACKI, S.J.; HEUGHEBAERT, J.C.; and NANCOLLAS, G.H. (1990): The Growth of Nonstoichiometric Apatite from Aqueous Solution at 37°C. II. Effects of pH Upon the Precipitated Phase, *J Colloid Int Sci* 135:33-44.

ZHANG, J. (1990): PhD Thesis, State University of New York at Buffalo.

ZHANG, J. and NANCOLLAS, G.H. (1988): Dissolution of Octacalcium Phosphate, *J Dent Res* 67:122-

ZHANG, J. and NANCOLLAS, G.H. (1991): Dissolution Kinetics of Calcium Phosphates Involved in Biomineralization. In: *Advances in Industrial Crystallization*, J. Garside, R.J. Davey, A.G. Sones Eds., Oxford: Butterworth-Heinemann Ltd. pp 47-62.

Relationship of *In Vitro* Studies to Clinical Problems

DOROTHY A M GEDDES

This article is concerned with two issues in cariology research, firstly the role of *in vitro* studies and secondly the clinical problems which urgently require investigation in this decade if we are to further improve the dental health of patients.

In a 19th century *in vitro* study quoted by Bibby (1990) which was carried out in France by Magitot, "caries" was produced after incubating teeth in flasks containing saliva and sucrose for several months. By the end of the 19th century Miller had cultivated oral microorganisms and shown that the incubation of sugar in saliva gave rise to lactic acid which could be found in decayed areas of teeth. The methodology of these early *in vitro* experiments included the main factors used in modern test systems (Table 1) and the results from these studies laid the foundations of our understanding of dental caries. Further elucidation of the nature of the disease process, of its aetiological factors and of modern preventative measures has come from interpretation of evidence from epidemiological studies, *in vivo* experiments with human volunteers and animal studies in addition to *in vitro* systems. In cariology, no less than in the study of other diseases, the strength of the association of aetiological or preventative factors is enhanced by the accumulation of evidence for a temporal relationship, a dose response and a plausible biological explanation, and from experimental verification. In the important area of biological plausibility *in vitro* tests have had much to offer. Dental caries is a multifactorial disease and the use of *in vitro* systems permits the selection of specific variables for testing while others are controlled. Such systems are normally comparatively cheap compared to epidemiological and animal studies and create no ethical dilemmas. In cariology *in vitro* systems range in complexity from single strain or mixed microbial cultures for the study of the metabolic capabilities of various cariogenic bacteria to complex cycling demineralisation/remineralisation "artificial mouths". In the last decade computer modelling has been increasingly used and should now be included under the heading of *in vitro* tests. By using existing data derived from *in*

TABLE 1 *In Vitro* Studies in Cariology

System	*Tests*
Mineralised Tooth Tissues	
enamel, dentine ± cementum	Preventive Agents
Microflora	
plaque or cultures	Sugar Substances
Substrate	
dietary components	remineralisation enhancers
Saliva	
or substitute	

vitro and *in vivo* studies computer programmes have been devised to investigate, for instance, salivary clearance of sugars and plaque - saliva interactions (see Dawes this Conference). The exponents of these model systems conclude that they may be used to study the effect of the many variables important in the oral cavity, for instance the clearance of fluoride (Lagerlöf and Oliveby, 1990). Data produced from such programmes may be helpful in designing future laboratory experiments and clinical trials with the aim of designing more effective preventative agents and regimens.

An early type of laboratory "artificial mouth", the Orafax (Bibby, 1978), used thawed fresh - frozen human saliva as the nutrient and plaque collected from the same saliva donor as a bacterial innoculum. When used in that closed chamber system with a heavy innoculum of plaque bacteria the selective antimicrobial activity of the saliva kept bacterial contamination from the air under control. Bacterial deposits grew on pieces of enamel surface in two or three days and produced caries-like lesions after a week or so if carbohydrate foods were introduced several times each day. Microscopic measurement of the size of the enamel lesions produced was used to compare the potential cariogenicity of test foods. Results from the Orafax (Bibby *et al.*, 1983) ranked the cariogenicity of foods in essentially the same order as that given for the same foods by caries tests in rats (Navia and Lopez, 1983) and in human plaque pH studies (Dodds and Edgar, 1988). Systems devised more recently, especially those investigating the use of topical fluorides, employ pre-programmed cycles of conditions conducive to demineralisation and remineralisation (Cate and Duijsters, 1982). Koulourides and his co-workers (1976) developed a new method for testing the potential cariogenicity of foods, the system consisted of pieces of bovine enamel attached to acrylic flanges on the right and left buccal flanges of lower dentures or specially made appliances worn in the human mouth for a period of a week during which time plaque formed on the enamel slabs. Several times a day the dentures or appliances were removed from the mouth and the enamel slabs immersed for several minutes in either a solution of the test food substance or a sucrose solution as the cariogenic control. Thus although the bacterial deposit on the bovine enamel developed within and under the influence of the oral cavity the cariogenic challenge was administered *in vitro*. After a brief period of *in vitro* exposure to the substrate the appliance was replaced in the mouth to again be influenced by the oral environment. This system has an ethical advantage in that it does not require exposure of the subject's natural teeth to the test or sucrose control or other cariogenic challenges. However, it underestimates the effect of saliva which would normally be stimulated by taste, texture and the chewing of the cariogenic challenge. When remimeralisation rather than demineralisation is being tested enamel slabs carrying pre-formed lesions can be used and the whole study carried out intra-orally (Koulourides and Cameron, 1980; Creanor *et al.*, 1986) Such tests using these *in situ* models are then classified as a type of *in vivo* test.

At first sight it could be thought that investigation into a particular aetiological factor or preventive measure would normally start with *in vitro* tests and, should these results look promising, be taken through *in vivo* studies and then to clinical trials. This, of course, is often the case. For example, the use of acidulated topical fluoride agents was first suggested by Bibby following *in vitro* tests in 1947. Some years later, Brudevold and his co-workers (1963) followed their own laboratory studies with clinical tests (Wellock and Brudevold, 1963) and over the following 25 years very many laboratory and clinical studies have led to the development and method of use of the acidulated gels employed today (See DePaola, this Conference). A similar history can be seen for the development of acid-etched fissure sealants. Following the early work of Buonocore's *in vitro* study in 1955 and his group's clinical trial in 1967 (Cueto and Buonocore) innumerable *in vitro* and clinical studies have led to the development of the modern generation of fissure sealants. These later studies have investigated improvements in the fissure sealant material and the criteria for successful clinical use and have led to a fuller understanding of the mechanism of etching and bonding (Strang *et al.*, 1985). From these historical examples of the development of two major modern preventative procedures it can be seen that not only did the *in vitro* studies form the basis of the line of research but *in vitro* experiments were also employed in further testing and development of the preventive clinical regimens. These examples also illustrate that progress towards the applications of new scientific knowledge to patient care requires collaboration between laboratory workers and clinicians.

A somewhat different history can be seen from the literature on the caries protective properties of cheese in the diet. It would seem that the first cariology experiment was conducted in rats by König (1967) followed some years later by human *in vivo* pH studies (Rugg-Gunn *et al.*, 1975). The results suggested that the flow of saliva, stimulated by eating cheese after a sugar challenge, reduced plaque acidogenicity and by inference caries susceptibility. At that time it was assumed that the protective effect was mainly due to the washing and buffering effect of stimulated saliva. Further animal experiments lent weight to the

TABLE 2

Prevention	——————?? ?——————		*Treatment*
loss of calcium and phosphate ions	surface softening and porosity	sub surface demineralisation	bacterial invasion
			CAVITATION

salivary anti caries effect (Edgar *et al.*, 1982; Rosen *et al.*, 1983; Harper *et al.*, 1986). *In vitro* studies (Silva *et al.*, 1984) some 20 years after the initial rat experiment indicated that the release of calcium and possibly phosphates from the cheese provided a further beneficial preventive factor. This was supported by further evidence from *in situ* and *in vivo* studies (Silva *et al.*, 1986; Silva *et al.*, 1987; Jenkins and Hargreaves, 1989). A further rat experiment, this time using de-salivated animals, confirmed the protective effect of cheese even in the absence of saliva (Krobicka *et al.*, 1987). This example illustrates how researchers choose from a battery of tests the system which is most appropriate to the study of the specific hypothesis which they wish to test. The accumulation of evidence from the various tests strengthens the theory of the mode of action, in this case of the anti caries effect of cheese.

Despite the deep understanding of the process of dental caries which has emerged in this century and the success of preventive measures such as topical fluorides, fissure sealants, sugar substitutes and the use of 'safe for teeth' foods there are important clinical problems awaiting resolution. These can be grouped under the four headings of diagnosis, treatment, prevention and assessment of the risk. Dental caries occurs on tooth surfaces in individual human beings, thus as the level of caries in the general population declines it becomes imperative that the dentist can tailor preventative measures and treatment to the individual patient who seeks professional advice and care. Before discussing the clinical problems surrounding diagnosis, the term dental caries must be defined. Research has now established beyond doubt that dental caries is a dynamic process with an imprecise beginning which takes place within the microbial plaque deposit covering the tooth surface and if a more favourable environment is not created the outcome of this process results in a disturbance of the equilibrium between the hard tissue (enamel, dentine or cementum) and the immediately surrounding plaque fluid such that net loss of mineral and eventually cavitation occurs. However, the very fact that this is a process which may be halted and reversed and may then progress again creates a dilemma for the clinician. At what point in the process (Table 2) will preventive therapy no longer be successful? To date there are no criteria to guide the clinician to identify that point and thus make the important decision to excise the lesion and restore the tooth. The situation is further confused by the fact that the term dental caries is used for all stages of the process from the loss of the first calcium ion to frank cavitation! The epidemiologist counting cavities and the laboratory worker measuring calcium release or early surface softening and sub-surface demineralisation in enamel samples both use the same term, "dental caries", for these extreme stages in the carious process. Research in the 90's must provide the clinician with more precise guidelines and *in vitro* studies have a role to play in such research.

The clinician will also have to make a decision as to whether areas of altered enamel are undergoing active decay or are arrested caries. The use of bite wing radiographs show mineral loss but the technique, even if repeated at intervals, is imprecise. Patients are increasingly reluctant to have regular radiographic examinations, but other clinical methods of assessing mineral loss such as electrical conductivity (Rock and Kidd, 1988; Stephen *et al.*, 1987) and fibre optic transillumination (Flaitz *et al.*, 1986) have not yet fulfilled their early promise and require further evaluation (Verdondchot *et al.*, 1991). The clinician seeing a questionable fissure would traditionally use a sharp probe to assess the quality of the hard tissue. However, a sharp probe pressed onto a softened or undermined surface may precipitate the very cavitation which preventive measures are designed to arrest and reverse.

If cavitation is established and operative procedures are necessary the diseased tooth tissue is customarily removed by a rotary drill. The air turbine was revolutionary in the 1950s but such mechanical removal is at best unpleasant. Little research effort however has been applied to more "patient - friendly" methods for the removal of diseased tissue although chemical removal has been suggested (Schutzbank *et al.*, 1978) and studied (Yip *et al.*, 1991). There is currently much interest by the dental profession in the use of lasers for the diagnosis and in the treatment of dental caries. However, the mode of action requires to be elucidated and efficacy established. Much research has gone into the development of new filling materials. Toxicity testing is well established but a recent review casts doubt on the validity of many of the *in vitro* systems used in these tests (Hensten-Pettersen, 1988). Even when a biocompatible material is available and the decayed tooth has been restored subsequent leakage between restoration and tooth tissue and the development of secondary caries (Goldberg *et al.*, 1981) present further clinical problems in diagnosis and management (Kidd, 1991). This would seem to be another area where *in vitro* testing in modern demineralisation/remineralisation cycling systems could be employed.

Because of the multifactorial nature of the disease practical prevention in the individual patient normally requires a number of preventive measures. This being so, the patient's co-operation is essential. It normally will be necessary for the patient to adopt new patterns of dental care within his or her habitual lifestyle. This is best achieved if the patient can be given knowledge and taught skills appropriate to his or her own problem and a behavioural change is more readily brought about if the patient can see early positive results for the effort expended. Applying this basic psychological principle is particularly difficult in the management of caries. The patient will be able to assess the success of the preventive programme only if, over the ensuing years, no further restorations are required. This long time lag for positive reinforcement is a distinct disadvantage. The acquisition of knowledge about their oral health can help motivation. However, as patients acquire knowledge of the carious process they ask questions specific to their preventive regime. For instance, "How frequently should I clean my teeth with a fluoride toothpaste?", "How often and when, in relation to eating, should the tooth cleaning be carried out?", "Is there a threshold of frequency of consumption and amount of sucrose I can take below which my teeth will not decay?" These are the obvious, simple questions that patients ask and the easy way out for the clinician is to advise an excessive preventative regime with which it is difficult for the patient to comply and which tends to be non-specific. Under the controlled regime of animal experiments the threshold of frequency and amount of fermentable carbohydrate consumption can be definitively established but no tests have yet been devised for the individual human patient. The use of chairside *in vitro* tests such as Lactobacillus and *S. mutans* counts to assess increased carbohydrate consumption requires wider evaluation in general dental practice (Krasse, 1985).

A consideration of these clinical problems faced daily by the dentist who attempts to motivate his patient to healthy behaviour leads naturally to the area of individual patient risk assessment. Despite much recent research in this area no single or indeed multifactorial *in vitro* caries-activity test has been devised which is sufficiently reliable and valid. Despite the considerable research effort over the past 20 years to develop microbial-based caries activity tests those currently available are insufficiently precise to identify individual patients who are at risk. This failure may, in part, be due to the fact that not all mutans streptococci are equally virulent and also that other species contribute to the cariogenic process. Is this an area for gene probes and DNA finger-printing (Russell, 1991) to identify cariogenic strains from a patient's plaque flora? If such tests could be developed and prove to be reliable they could be used in conjunction with assessments of the individual patient's habitual plaque control, salivary factors, dietary habits and social background (Blinkhorn and Geddes, 1987) to aid the clinician to identify and appropriately counsel individual high risk patients?

This, par excellence, is an area where it is imperative that *in vitro* tests are developed. The practising dentist needs chairside tests which are acceptable, applicable, reliable, and valid and whose outcome is specific to the needs of the individual patient.

In summary *in vitro* tests have had and continue to play an essential role in cariology research. Well tested *in vitro* models have been developed and are used as part of a cascade of studies to explain the biological processes involved and help to refine treatment and preventative regimes. There is an urgent need for improved caries diagnostic criteria and a redefinition of the terminology used to identify the various important stages of the caries process. New diagnostic tests must be developed, validated and passed to the practising dentists.

REFERENCES

BIBBY, B.G. (1947): A consideration of the effectiveness of various fluoride mixtures, *JADA* 34:26-32.

BIBBY, B.G. (1978): The Orafax In: *Methods of Caries Prediction*, B.G. Bibby and R.J. Shern, Eds., Sp. Supp. Microbiology Abstracts, Washington, D.C.: Information Retrieval Inc., pp.237-240.

BIBBY, B.G. (1990): *Food and the Teeth*. Vantage Press, Inc. New York, p.28.

BIBBY, B.G.; MUNDORF, S.A. and HAUNG, C.T. (1983): Enamel demineralisation tests with some standard foods and candies. *J Dent Res* 62:885-888.

BLINKHORN, A.S. and GEDDES, D.A.M. (1987): "Assessment of Caries Risk and the potential for preventive management. In: *Positive Dental Prevention* Ed. Elderton, R.J. William Heinemann Medical Books, London.

BRUDEVOLD, F.; SAVORY, A.; GARDNER, D.E.; SPINELLI, M. and SPEIRS, R. (1963): A study of acidulated fluoride solutions I. *in vitro* effects on enamel. *Arch Oral Biol* 8:167-177.

BUONOCORE, M.G. (1955): A simple method of increasing the adhesion of acrylic filling materials to enamel surfaces. *J Dent Res* 34:849-853.

CATE, ten J.M. and DUIJSTERS, P.P.E. (1982): Alternating demineralisation and remineralisation of artificial enamel lesions. *Caries Res* 16:201-210.

CREANOR, S.L.; STRANG, R.; TELFER, S.; MacDONALD, I.; SMITH, M.J. and STEPHEN, K.W. (1986): *In situ* appliance for the investigation of enamel de- and remineralisation. *Caries Res* 20:385-391.

CUETO, E.I. and BUONOCORE, M.G. (1967): Sealing of pits and fissures with an adhesive resin: its use in caries prevention. *JADA* 75:121-128.

DODDS, M.W.J. and EDGAR, W.M. (1988): The relationship between plaque pH, plaque acid anion profiles and oral carbohydrate retention after ingestion of several "reference foods" by human subjects. *J Dent Res* 67:861-865.

EDGAR, W. M.; BOWEN, W. H.; AMSBAUGH, S.; MONELL-TORRENS, E. and BRUNELLE, J. (1982): Effects of different eating patterns on dental caries in the rat. *Caries Res* 16:384-389.

FLAITZ, C. M.; HICKS, M.J.and SILVERSTONE, L.M. (1986): Radiographic, histologic and electronic comparison of occlusal caries: an *in vitro* study. *Pediatric Dent* 8:24-28.

GOLDBERG, J.; TANZER, J.; MUNSTER, E.; AMARA, J.; THAL, F. and BIRKHED, D. (1981): Cross-sectional clinical evaluation of recurrent enamel caries, restoration of marginal integrity and oral hygiene status. *JADA* 102:635-641.

HARPER, D.S.; OSBORN, J.C.; HEFFERREN, J.J. and CLAYTON, R. (1986): Cariostatic evaluation of cheese with diverse physical and compositional characteristics. *Caries Res* 20:123-130.

HENSTEN-PETTERSEN, A. (1988): Comparison of the methods available for assessing cytotoxicity. *Int Endodontic Journal* 21:89-99.

JENKINS, G.N. and HARGREAVES, J.A. (1989): Effect of eating cheese on Ca and P concentrations of whole mouth saliva and plaque. *Caries Res* 23:159-164.

KIDD, E.A.M. (1991): A critical evaluation of caries diagnostic methods and epidemiological methods. Can we trust the available data? In: *Risk Markers for Oral Disease* Vol.1. *Dental Caries* Ed. Johnston, N.W. Cambridge University Press, Cambridge, U.K.

KÖNIG, K.G. (1967): Caries induced in laboratory rats. *Br Dent J* 123:585-589.

KOULOURIDES, T.; BODDEN, R.; KELLER, S.; MANSON-HING, L.; LASTRA, J. and HOUSCH, T. (1976): Cariogenicity of nine sugars tested with an intraoral device in man. *Caries Res* 10:427-441.

KOULOURIDES, T. and CAMERON, B. (1980): Enamel remineralisation as a factor in the pathogenesis of dental caries. *J Oral Path* 9:255-269.

KRASSE, B. (1985): In: *Caries Risk* chapter 7, p.53-57. Quintessence Publishing Co., Inc., Chicago, London, Dublin, Rio de Janeiro and Tokyo.

KROBICKA, A.; BOWEN, W.H.; PEARSON, S. and YOUNG, D.A., (1987): The effects of cheese snacks on caries in desalivated rats. *J Dent Res* 66:1116-1119.

LAGERLÖF, F. and OLIVEBY, A. (1990): Computer simulation of oral fluoride clearance. *Computer Methods and Programs in Biomedicine* 31:97-104.

MILLER, W.D. (1890): *The Microorganisms of the Human Mouth* (Philadelphia: SS White).

NAVIA, J.M. and LOPEZ, H. (1983): Rat caries assay of reference foods and sugar containing snacks. *J Dent Res* 62:893-898.

ROCK, W.P. and KIDD, E.A.M. (1988): The electronic detection of demineralisation in occlusal fissures. *Br Dent J* 164:243-247.

ROSEN, S.; MIN, D.B.; HARPER, D.S.; HARPER, W.J.; BECK, E.X. and BECK, F.M. (1984): Effect of cheese, with and without sucrose, on dental caries and recovery of *Streptococcus mutans* in rats. *J Dent Res* 63:894-896.

RUGG-GUNN, A.J.; EDGAR, W.M.; GEDDES, D.A.M. and JENKINS, G.N. (1975): The effect of different meal patterns upon plaque pH in human subjects. *Br Dent J* 139:351-356.

RUSSELL, R.R.B. (1991): New Methods for Microbial Screening In: *Risk Markers for Oral Disease* Vol.1. *Dental Caries* Ed. Johnston, N.W. Cambridge University Press, Cambridge, U.K.

SCHUTZBANK, S.G.; GALAINI, J.; KRONMAN, J.H.; GOLDMAN, M. and CLARK, R.E. (1978): A comparative *in vitro* study of GK-101 and GK-101E in caries removal. *J Dent Res* 57:861-864.

SILVA, M.F.A.; BURGESS, R.C. and SANDHAM, H.J. (1987): Effects of cheese extract and its fractions on enamel demineralisation *in vitro* and *in vivo* in humans. *J Dent Res* 66:1527-1532.

SILVA, M.F.A.; JENKINS, G.N.; BURGESS, R.C. and SANDHAM, H. J. (1986): Effects of cheese on experimental caries in human subjects. *Caries Res* 20:263-269.

SILVA, M.F.A.; BURGESS, R.C.; SANDHAM, H.J. and JENKINS, G.N. (1987): Effects of water-soluble components of cheese on experimental caries in humans. *J Dent Res* 66:38-41.

STEPHEN, K.W.; RUSSELL, J.I.; CREANOR, S.L.; and BURCHELL, C.K. (1987): Comparison of fibre optic transillumination with clinical and radiographic caries diagnosis. *Community Dent Oral Epidemiol* 15:90-94.

STRANG. R.; CUMMINGS, A. and STEPHEN, K.W. (1986): Laboratory studies of visible light cured fissure sealants; setting times and depth of polymerisation. *J Oral Rehabil* 13:305-310.

VERDONCHOT, E.H.; BURGERSDIJK, R.C.W.; KÖNIG, K.G.; SCHAEKEN, M.J.M. and TRUIN, G.J. (1991): Performance of some diagnostic systems in examinations for small occlusal caries lesions. *Caries Res* 25:217.

WELLOCK, W.D. and BRUDEVOLD, F. (1963): A study of acidulated fluoride solutions II. The caries inhibiting effect of single annual topical applications of an acidic fluoride and phosphate solution. A 2 year experience. *Arch Oral Biol* 8:179-182.

YIP, H.K.; BEELEY, J.A. and STEVENSON, A.G (1991): The interface between carious and sound dentine - an SEM study. *Med Sci Res* 19:187-188.

CLINICAL STUDIES

The University of North Carolina Caries Risk Assessment Study: Final Results and Some Alternative Modelling Approaches

JOHN W. STAMM
JUDY A. DISNEY
JAMES D. BECK
JANE A. WEINTRAUB
PAUL W. STEWART

During the 1980s, risk assessment and its application to oral diseases has marched to the front of the dental health care policy field. With respect to dental caries, the drive for this advance comes from two sources. First, with the unrelenting rise in health care costs, the combining of health risk assessment with the "appropriate care" movement is seen as a potentially powerful strategy for cost containment. With national dental care expenditures estimated at 31 billion dollars in 1989, risk assessment for oral diseases, particularly dental caries, and the resultant impact on dental treatment provision is thought to offer significant efficiencies in the future U.S. dental care market (ADA News, 1990).

The second impetus for risk assessment in dentistry derives from the substantial decrease in caries incidence and severity in western industrialized countries (Leclercq *et al.*, 1987; WHO, 1989; Downer, 1991). Dramatic evidence has been accumulated showing that approximately 60 to 70 percent of the caries burden falls on approximately 20 - 25 percent of schoolchildren (Bohannan *et al.*, 1985). Recently examined evidence confirms that this trend is similarly affecting the young adult population (Graves *et al.*, 1986). Anecdotally, United States dental educators and clinical researchers know that fewer patients are available for the teaching of stainless steel crown techniques or for the placement of experimental multisurface posterior restorations in clinical trials. These developments have made it obvious that extensive dental caries is not the ubiquitous oral

---

This study was supported by a grant from the Robert Wood Johnson Foundation

health problem among the younger population as was once the case. In turn, that reality has lead to the recognition that individualized or targeted approaches to prevention and treatment, alongside universal water fluoridation or its substitutes, may represent a more effective and efficient strategy for the management of dental caries.

The desirability of identifying individuals highly susceptible to dental caries is not new to the dental profession. Attempts to develop predictive tests began even before 1900 (Miller, 1890; Black, 1899). Since that time, many investigators have studied a wide variety of demographic, dietary, physical, chemical, electrical, and microbiological factors in searching for methods to predict caries occurrence. Most caries prediction work up to 1976 was summarized in a publication (Bibby and Shern, 1978) reporting the proceedings of an international symposium, "Methods of Caries Prediction," held in October of 1977. In short, no method reviewed was sufficiently valid or reliable to warrant a recommendation for use at that time.

The acknowledged lack of success with caries prediction reported in 1977 dampened the enthusiasm of funding agencies for further prediction research, particularly in the United States. Nevertheless, several investigators continued caries prediction efforts through a series of small studies, principally investigating single risk factors, or limited combinations thereof (Crossner and Holm, 1977; Holm, 1978; Rundegren and Ericson, 1978; Klock and Krasse, 1979). Interest in caries prediction in the United States reawakened in the early 1980s when a sizable secular decline in caries among children was reported (National Caries Program, 1981; Glass, 1982; Epidemiology and Oral Disease Prevention Program, 1989). The National Dental Caries Prevalence Survey and the National Survey of Dental Caries in U.S. Schoolchildren reported both a significant decrease in permanent tooth caries experience and an increase in the proportion of children aged 5-17 free of caries in the permanent dentition. Those surveys also revealed a strongly skewed distribution of dental caries, with high caries experience exhibited mainly in 20 percent of the children.

This chapter seeks to achieve five goals. First, it lays out a rationale and conceptual framework for caries risk assessment. Second, it reports key three-year results of the University of North Carolina Caries Risk Assessment Study (UNCCRAS). Third, it compares caries risk models based on dichotomization of the caries increment gradient into the "high" versus "low and no" increment groups to the results from models based on dichotomization into "any caries" increment versus "no caries" increment. Fourth, it examines the distinction between models whose sole purpose is accurate patient caries risk *prediction* and those that strive to identify direct or indirect biological relationships in what may be called *etiologic* models of caries risk. Fifth, it presents preliminary information evaluating the performance of caries risk models in children who are completely *caries free* at baseline and contrasts these results with those obtained from samples of children who had already experienced, at baseline, caries in either the primary or permanent dentition. The chapter concludes with a discussion that emphasizes data and technical limitations, speculates on future applications and suggests new avenues for research.

Rationale for Caries Risk Assessment

At the conceptual level, the epidemiologic work to develop an accurate and practical caries prediction model can provide fundamental knowledge about four related goals (Stamm *et al.*, 1988).

1. Targeting those in need. Accurate and practical caries prediction will successfully identify children at high risk to disease. Such a result would permit preventive dental services to be targeted to those individuals who need them most.
2. Greater effectiveness of preventive procedures. By targeting those children most susceptible to caries, more intensive preventive services can be employed that may have a significantly greater impact in preventing tooth decay.
3. Appropriate levels of care. By successfully identifying the high-risk group, the larger low caries risk group is also defined. Analogous to the more intensive care for the high-risk group, preventive care for the low-risk group can be scaled down to a level commensurate with the lower expected disease pattern.
4. Economic efficiency. By appropriately matching preventive care to the assessed risk status of each individual, it may be possible to achieve economic benefits in private and/or public health care settings. For high-risk individuals the major impact would be to increase the net benefit from preventive services. For the low caries risk individuals, the major outcome would be savings in expenditures by avoiding preventive dental services that would demonstrate only marginal effects.

Health risk assessment draws from two intellectual roots, each of which has provided a particular view on how risk assessment may be used to improve health (Jeffery, 1989). The first and most common of these is the population perspective, an approach developed almost entirely within the field of epidemiology and public health. The second view is the individual perspective, a system that employs epidemiological findings but owes its real origins to clinical preventive medicine and the science of clinical decision theory.

The *population perspective* does not attempt to predict which individuals in society are most likely to develop disease. Rather, the population perspective is concerned with the identification and quantification of risk factors that significantly compromise the whole population's health. This approach is also known as hazard appraisal, and besides its epidemiological roots, owes its development to occupational and environmental medicine (Gordis, 1988).

Turning to the *individual perspective,* this approach is based on Robbin's early work in the 1930s and 1940s in which he developed methods to aid the physician in measuring and recording patient health risk factors, leading then to the selection and application of appropriate counter measures that would be effective in preventing the otherwise anticipated future health problems (Robbins and Hall, 1970). The objective was to create a prospective (preventive) rather than a retrospective (treatment) orientation for the physician.

A distinctive characteristic of this perspective is its use of epidemiologic data to generate quantitative risk predictions based on the presence or absence of identified risk indicators in the individual (Schoenbach, 1987). Information describing an individual's biological characteristics, personal and family medical history, habits, lifestyle and health-related practices was inserted into statistical decision models, developed from epidemiological data and vital statistics, to project that person's risk of mortality over some future period. These projections were then used to reinforce educational and motivational techniques to encourage the patient to adopt a healthier, prevention-oriented lifestyle. Historically, one of this system's most notable contributions to preventive medicine has been its application to the prediction and prevention of coronary heart disease in individuals where stress, smoking, obesity, alcohol use and lack of exercise were identified as strong predictors of heart disease.

Dentistry, too, has been experimenting with efforts to predict the occurrence of future disease. Most of these past attempts have focussed on linear regression and correlation methods to predict dental caries in individual subjects, usually schoolchildren (Bibby and Shern, 1978). An evolution from these earlier caries prediction approaches will be examined in the next section.

Key Three-Year Results of UNCCRAS

The University of North Carolina Caries Risk Assessment study was conducted on 5,233 grade 1 and grade 5 children in low fluoride communities surrounding Aiken, South Carolina and Portland, Maine. These sites were selected because: (1) both represent regions of historically high caries experience in the United States; (2) both were without topical fluoride programs in schools; (3) both had relatively low dentist to population ratios; and (4), both had interested and cooperative school systems. The two sites also represented cultural and ethnic diversity that would permit more robust testing of caries prediction models and would tend to strengthen the generality of inferences from the study (Stamm *et al.*, 1988).

Sample sizes were determined after consideration of the desired accuracy of the estimates to be calculated from the sample, the probable variances associated with the estimates, expected differences in the estimates between groups to be compared, and anticipated attrition rates. For the purpose of sample size determination, the proportion of children in the observed (true) high risk group was defined arbitrarily as the 25 percent most severely affected children in the total group. The desired accuracy of the predicted three year DMFS increments, i.e. the acceptable limit from the true mean increment, was set at 0.4 DMFS for grade 1 and 0.8 DMFS for grade 5 cohorts. Data from the National Preventive Dentistry Demonstration Program (NPDDP) provided an estimate of the variance in DMFS increments and the annual attrition rate (Klein and Bohannan, 1979; Bohannan *et al.*, 1981; Foch, 1981). With this information, plus the decision to accept a 0.95 probability of obtaining estimated means with the specified accuracy, sample sizes at the outset of the study were calculated as approximately 325 high risk children in each grade. This number was considered adequate to yield 215 high risk children in each grade and site cohort at the end of the study. Total sample size was four times the number of high risk children of 1,300 children in each grade at each site. Sample sizes were calculated such that analyses could be done separately for all four site/grade cohorts.

The field work for this study got underway in the fall of 1986 and was completed in the fall of 1989. Table 1 shows the children participating by site and grade cohort. Since many potential caries risk indicators could only be determined from a questionnaire completed by the head of household, only those children whose parent(s) completed a questionnaire became eligible for continuation in the study. Furthermore, since this study was focussed on the 3-year caries increment in the permanent dentition as the outcome measure, only children who completed the baseline and the final clinical examination were incorporated into the statistical analyses of caries risk assessment. Table 1 gives the final analyses sample participation rates, with the denominator being the number of children for whom informed consent was obtained and who received an initial clinical examination.

The information used for analysis can be grouped into four categories. In the first group are largely the standard clinical variables determined from the intraoral examination. White spot lesions were recorded because they represent the earliest clinically detectable evidence of enamel demineralization and are clearly the antecedents to cavitation of the smooth surfaces. Klock and Krasse

TABLE 1 *Children Participating by Site and Grade*

	Aiken SC		*Portland ME*	
	Grade 1	*Grade 5*	*Grade 1*	*Grade 5*
Baseline Examination	1406	1206	1404	1217
Returned Questionnaire	1332	1126	1381	1173
Baseline and 3 Year Examination	1102	977	1100	979
Participation Rate (%)	78	81	78	80

(1979) found that high, two year caries increments related well to initial white spot lesions on the smooth surfaces. Caries in the primary dentition was recorded because the literature indicates a generally positive, but weak, relationship between primary tooth caries and future permanent tooth decay (Bruszt, 1959; Klein *et al.*, 1985). Oral hygiene was recorded as the Silness and Löe (1964) Plaque Index. This measure was included in spite of equivocal epidemiological findings relating dental plaque scores and future caries development.

A relatively novel clinical measure in this study was pit and fissure morphology. With the continuing decline of smooth surface caries, pit and fissure lesions are forming an increasing proportion of the total caries experience among young children. A recent preliminary study has suggested that quantifying pit and fissure morphology could lead to the establishment of a relationship between pit and fissure anatomy, particularly depth, and future caries increment (Bader *et al.*, 1986).

The second broad category of information comprised two microbiological variables generated from an evaluation of salivary Mutans streptococci and Lactobacilli. To obtain the relevant data from 5,233 children at baseline required the reliance on the dip slide methods pioneered by Larmas (1975), Köhler and Bratthal (1979) and Jordan *et al.* (1987). Stimulated saliva samples were collected from all children at baseline and were used to inoculate culture media for the Mutans streptococci (Cariescreen®, J.O. Butler Co., Chicago) and lactobacilli (Bactotest®, APO Diagnostics, Toronto) test kits. Culturing, incubation, slide reading and reporting were performed according to the manufacturer's instructions.

Sociodemographic data, the third category of information, were obtained from a questionnaire designed and tested for this purpose. A variety of social, demographic, family and personal history data was acquired through an instrument that was sent home with the children and returned by mail. The fourth information category comprised a short list of questions to elicit data on health behaviors that were thought to have a possible bearing on caries increment susceptibility or its appropriate analysis in risk models. Some of these behavioral variables have potentially obvious relationships to caries development. Frequent between meal snacks, fluoride dentifrice use, tooth brushing frequency, fluoride supplements and mouthrinses might be relevant examples. In contrast, modelling the relationship of the number of dental visits made by the child during the past 12 months would be more problematical. Thus, a 6-year old child who didn't see the dentist at all may be a non-user and may exhibit a relatively high dmfs, composed mainly of d and m. The child who has made 1 or 2 visits may be attending for routine prevention, may also come from an upper SES family, and may present with little or no caries experience. The child with 3 or more visits could be one experiencing considerable dental decay that has required a fair amount of treatment resulting in a potentially high dmfs score, primarily f. Antibiotic use presents a second example of potential modelling problems.

Errata

There are a number of errata in the Table of Contents for which the University of Rochester Press apologizes.

Page v

"DENNIS O'MULLANE"
should read
"DENIS O'MULLANE"

Page vi

"J. HANS von HOUTE"
should read
"J. HANS VAN HOUTE"

"Alternatives for Conventional Clinical Caries Trials"
should read
"Alternatives to Conventional Clinical Caries Trials"

"Adhesion and Cohesion in Plaque Microflora"
should read
"Adhesion and Cohesion of Plaque Microflora"

Page vii

"Ecological Determinants in Dental Root Surface Caries"
should read
"Ecological Determinants of Dental Root Surface Caries"

"DOROTHEA JOHNSON"
should read
"DORTHEA JOHNSON"

Thus, frequent antibiotic use may be associated with depressed levels of carcinogenic microflora with a concomitant impact on the caries status (Littleton and White, 1964). On the other hand, infrequent but recent antibiotic use will not have influenced the caries index, but may have affected the presence of salivary microorganisms, which in turn could influence the dip slide test, thereby throwing off expected relationships in the data analysis.

Among the four calibrated examiners in this study, extensive interexaminer reliability testing was conducted, using embedded single-blind reexaminations, for many of the clinical measures as well as for the scoring of microbiological results. For the caries determinations, replicate examinations resulted in intraclass correlation coefficients that were 0.90 or higher in 34 of 36 samples evaluated.

The data analysis for the UNCCRAS was carried out on the variable set listed in Table 2. A total of 47 independent variables were included, with "examiner codes" accounting for four dummy variables (i.e. variables 44-47). The definitions for all independent variables are provided in the table. A number of cross-product terms were included to test for interactions of potential interest. The outcome measure for this study was the three-year DMFS increment experienced by children in the four site/grade cohorts. Between baseline and the final examination, many children received sealants on their permanent teeth, particularly in Portland. When sealants had been applied to a surface previously diagnosed as carious, the sealant was considered as a treatment intervention and the surface was recoded as "filled" on the final examination for purposes of calculating the DMFS.

Table 3 provides a frequency distribution of the three-year DMFS increment for the four site/grade cohorts. The table shows, first, that a significant number of children developed no DMFS increment at all during a three-year period when children in both age groups are generally considered to be highly susceptible to caries. Second, the tendency to develop no or only low DMFS increments was particularly pronounced in Portland where 69 and 54 percent of the grade 1 and 5 children, respectively, exhibited 0 DMFS increment. Third, relatively elevated DMFS increments tended to concentrate in the Aiken cohorts where 9 and 18 percent of grade 1 and 5 children developed 6 or more new DMF surfaces. [The overall mean DMFS increments, with standard deviations in parentheses were, Aiken G1 1.9 (2.4), Aiken G5 3.1 (4.3), Portland G1 0.8 (1.5) and Portland G5 1.5 (2.7)].

Following appropriate data editing and recoding, the first step in the caries risk prediction model development was the reduction of the independent variables into a useable, parsimonious subset. This procedure was carried out in stages. First, in Portland, race and four interaction terms involving race were removed because the analysis sample consisted exclusively of white children. Second, to reduce the impact of multicollinearity, pairwise correlations were examined for all independent variables. Where correlations were $\geq .70$, one

TABLE 2 *Logistic Regression Full Model Independent Variables*

1. DMFS (baseline)
2. dmfs (baseline)
3. Mean plaque score: mean of 6 surfaces scored; none = 0, some = 1, moderate = 2, thick = 3
4. White spot lesions: sum of lesions on primary and permanent tooth surfaces
5. Sealants: sum of permanent tooth surfaces sealed
6. Sound permanent tooth surfaces:
7. Fluorosis: absent = 0, present in primary or permanent or both dentitions = 1
8. Referral caries score: urgency for care; none = 0, low = 1, moderate = 2, high = 3
9. Other referral score: no need = 0, orthodontic or periodontal or fracture = 1
10. Predicted 3 year DMFS increment score: none = 0, low = 1, moderate = 2, high = 3
11. Morphology score: sum of 8 surfaces tested; shallow = 0, moderate = 1, deep = 2, or NA
12. S. mutans score: bacteria/ml saliva; none = 0, 10^4 = 1, 5×10^4 = 2, 10^5 = 3, 2.5×10^5 = 4, 5×10^5 = 5
13. Lactobacillus score: bacteria/ml saliva; none = 0, 10^4 = 1, 5×10^4 = 2, 10^6 = 3
14. Mean Plaque × Morphology
15. Mean Plaque × S. mutans
16. Mean Plaque × Lactobacillus
17. S. mutans × White spot lesions
18. Lactobacillus × White spot lesions
19. S. mutans × Morphology
20. Lactobacillus × Morphology
21. Fluorosis × White spot lesions
22. Gender: male = 0, female = 1
23. Age: in years to two decimals
24. Race: black = 0, white = 1
25. Brush A: toothbrushing frequency, 2/day = 0, 1/day = 1, < 1/day = 0
26. Brush B: toothbrushing frequency; 1/day = 0, 2/day = 1, < 1/day = 0
27. Time Dentist A: number of child's dental visits in past year; 1-2 = 0, 0 = 1, ≥ 3 = 0
28. Time Dentist B: number of child's dental visits in past year; 0 = 0, 1-2 = 1, ≥ 3 = 0
29. Type visit A: reason for dental visit; filled/pulled = 1, other reasons = 0, no visit = 0
30. Type visit B: reason for dental visit; other reasons = 1, filled/pulled = 0, no visit = 0
31. Ear infection history: yes = 0, no = 1
32. Strep throat history: yes = 0, no = 1
33. Antibiotics in past 60 days: yes = 0, no = 1
34. Flutabs use of fluoride drops, tablets or vitamins: yes = 0, no = 1

(continued)

TABLE 2 *Logistic Regression Full Model Independent Variables (continued)*

35. FMR rinse: use of fluoride mouth rinse; yes = 0, no = 1
36. Between-meal snack: sugar, chips, or cereal = 0; all other = 1
37. Education HHH: years of school for household head
38. Dentist HHH: household head number of dental visits in past year
39. Other children: number of other children living in the household
40. Race × Education HHH
41. Race × Age
42. Race × Other children
43. Race × Sex
44. Examiner codes:

Examiners	*Z1*	*Z2*	*Z3*	*Z4*
AA	1	0	0	0
BB	0	1	0	0
CC	0	0	1	0
DD	0	0	0	1
Other	0	0	0	0

NOTE: AA = children examined by Examiner A at year 1 and year 4; BB = children examined by Examiner B at year 1 and 4, etc. Other = children not examined by same examiner at year 1 and year 4.

member of the pair was removed. This procedure eliminated 11 variables in Aiken and 9 in Portland, primarily interaction terms.

The third step began with defining the high caries risk criteria. For Aiken this was DMFS increment ≥ 4 for the grade 1 cohort and ≥ 5 for the grade 5 cohort; for Portland this was DMFS increment ≥ 2 for the grade 1 cohort and ≥ 3 for the grade 5 cohort. These high caries risk criteria placed 21 and 25 percent of Aiken grade 1 and grade 5 children respectively into the high risk group, coded as "1". The equivalent figures for Portland were 20 and 20 percent. The remaining children at both sites were classified as low risk, with low risk being coded as "0". The four site/grade cohorts were then independently analyzed using unconditional, stepwise logistic regression. A liberal .50 significance level for variable entry into the model was employed. If an independent variable failed to enter into any of the four site/grade models under this condition, it was dropped from the analysis at this stage. Fourteen of the remaining 32 variables in Aiken and 12 of the remaining 29 variables in Portland were eliminated by this procedure. Four dummy variables were then created to assess the effect of maintaining examiner/child pairings over the baseline and final examination.

Excessive reliance on stepwise regression procedures can result in model misspecification by forcing sample dependency on the variable selection process. To overcome this potential problem, all deleted variables were examined for their biological relevance, regardless of their statistical significance in the

TABLE 3 *Frequency Distribution of Three-year DMFS Increment by Site and Grade*

	Aiken SC				*Portland ME*			
DMFS	*Grade 1*		*Grade 5*		*Grade 1*		*Grade 5*	
Increment	*No.*	*%*	*No.*	*%*	*No.*	*%*	*No.*	*%*
≤ 0	463	42	325	34	748	69	522	54
1	175	16	155	16	118	11	144	15
2	136	13	104	11	87	8	95	10
3	91	8	76	8	35	3	69	7
4	81	7	73	7	42	4	49	5
5	54	5	57	6	23	2	27	3
≥ 6	99	9	177	18	33	3	59	6
Total	1099	100	967	100	1085	100	965	100

models generated. This step resulted in the reinsertion of the mutans streptococci score variable into the risk assessment models in light of its putative importance in caries initiation. The final models contained 23 independent variables for Aiken and 22 variables for Portland.

The key results for the four site/cohort caries risk prediction models are shown in Table 4. At the bottom of the table the observed mean DMFS increments are given for high and low risk groups. In Aiken, the 79 percent of children constituting the observed low risk group of the grade 1 cohort had a three-year DMS increment of 0.8 versus 5.8 for their high risk colleagues. In the grade 5 cohort the equivalent DMFS means were 1.2 and 9.0 respectively. For both Aiken cohorts, the caries attack level was 7 times higher in the high risk than the low risk group. For Portland, the 80 percent of children making up the observed low risk group of the grade 1 cohort experienced a three-year DMFS increment of only 0.1 versus 3.6 for their high risk counterparts. In the Portland grade 5 cohort the equivalent figures were 0.4 and 5.5 DMFS respectively. The ratio of observed DMFS increment in Portland high to low risk groups exceeded 10 for both grade cohorts.

The logistic regression caries risk prediction model for the Aiken grade 1 cohort, shown in Table 4, includes only four statistically significant predictors. These are baseline DMFS and dmfs, pit fissure morphology score and the clinician's subjectively determined predicted caries increment. For the Aiken grade 5 cohort, six predictor variables achieve statistical significance, specifically: DMFS, morphology score, the number of sound permanent tooth surfaces at risk, the mean plaque score, the dentists referral score relative to the patient's caries condition, and the lactobacillus score.

For Portland, significant predictors for the grade 1 cohort were pit and fissure morphology score and the clinician's prediction of caries increment. Maintenance of examiner/child pairing influenced caries risk classification for children seen by examiners A and B. For the grade 5 cohort, significant predictors included DMFS, sound permanent tooth surfaces at risk, the mean plaque index

TABLE 4 *High Caries Risk Prediction Models Using Logistic Regression for Three-year DMFS Increment: Grade Cohorts 1 and 5, Aiken SC and Portland ME*

	Betas for Aiken SC		*Betas for Portland ME*	
Variables	*Grade 1 Cohort, N = 1000*	*Grade 5 Cohort, N = 877*	*Grade 1 Cohort, N = 1023*	*Grade 5 Cohort, N = 912*
Clinical				
DMFS Baseline	.19*	.15**	.00	.16**
dmfs Baseline	.03**	.02	.03	.02
Morphology score	.09**	.10**	.08*	.07
Sealants		-.67	.10	-.02
White Spot (WS) Lesions	-.02	.08	.11	.11
Fluorosis Score	-.24	.28	.08	.03
Sound Surfaces (Perm.)	.01	.02**	-.00	.02**
Mean Plaque Score	.03	.37*	.17	.34*
Referral Caries Score	.04	.24*	-.07	.12
Predicted Caries Score	.43**	.14	.75**	.60**
Fluorosis × WS Lesions	.18	.15	.00	.40
Microbiological				
Mutans Streptococci Score	.11	.14	-.07	-.00
Lactobacillus Score	.02	.18*	.15	.26**
Socio-demographic				
Race	.11	.14		
Age	-.06	.01	-.16	-.03
Health Behavior				
Brush A (1/day vs. < daily)	.16	.12	-.26	-.08
Brush B (2/day vs. < daily)	.27	.25	-.33	-.33
Between Meal Snacks	-.23	-.15	-.55	-.29
FMR (ever vs. never used)	.32	.00	.15	-.03
Examiner Scores				
Examiner AA vs. other	.35	-.52	.78**	.42
Examiner BB vs. other	.08	.17	.65*	.68*
Examiner CC vs. other	.06	-.33	.30	-.56
Examiner DD vs. other	-.02	-.27	.20	.64*
R	.37	.41	.32	.47
*p < .05 **p < .01				
Predicted High Risk DMFS Criterion	4	5	2	3
Mean DMFS increment observed				
High Risk Children	5.8	9.0	3.6	5.5
Low Risk Children	0.8	1.2	0.1	0.4

and the clinicians's prediction of likely caries increment. Two examiner child pairing variables influenced risk prediction. For all four caries risk models, the R statistic, similar to the multiple correlation coefficient in least squares regression analysis, was moderately high and ranged from .32 to .47.

High Caries Risk versus Any Caries Risk

The caries risk models, as developed above, have been criticized on two grounds, the first of which is that the definition of what constitutes significant or high caries is variable, and in fact seems to be population dependent. Taking the Portland grade 5 cohort for example, by choosing a DMFS score of ≥ 3, children with three-year DMFS increments of 3 or 4 are defined as high risk in Portland, but would not be so defined in Aiken where, for the grade 5 cohort, the high risk criterion is ≥ 5. Evidently, by arbitrarily moving the criterion up or down on the caries increment gradient, one is able to assign 20-25 percent of children to the high risk group, but the meaning of high risk becomes somewhat obfuscated. The second criticism is that the models as a whole do not correspond well with medically determined risk models. In medicine the typical risk distinction is between those that experience the disease and those that don't. The medical model therefore would place all children who develop any non-negative caries increment during a given time period into a high risk category and would reserve the low risk classification for those developing no or negative caries increments. Development of caries models on the dichotomization between "0" and "1 or more" DMFS increment would address both of the above concerns simultaneously.

Tables 5 and 6, for Aiken and Portland respectively, lay out the essential contrast between the proposed "any caries risk" model and the standard "high caries risk" model. For the Aiken grade 1 cohort the similarity of the two models is evident, except that the "any caries risk" model enters four additional predictive factors into the model, namely the mutans streptococci score, race, toothbrushing habit and the number of dental visits made by the parent during the previous 12 months. For Aiken grade 5, the "any caries risk" model is also similar to the standard model, except that it eliminates mean plaque score as a variable, while picking up education of the head of household and examiner A as significant predictors. The R values are very similar among the two model types. The comparability between these two modelling approaches appears to be maintained for the two Portland grade cohorts in Table 6.

Etiological Modelling Versus Risk Prediction Modelling

An occasionally voiced criticism of all the preceding caries risk prediction models is that they appear to contain variables relatively remote from the

TABLE 5 *Comparison of "High Caries" with "Any Caries" Logistic Regression Risk Prediction Models for Three-year DMFS Increments: Grade Cohorts 1 and 5, Aiken SC*

	Betas for Grade 1 Cohort		*Betas for Grade 5 Cohort*	
Variables	*High Risk* $\Delta \geq 4$ *DMFS*	*Any Risk* $\Delta \geq 1$ *DMFS*	*High Risk* $\Delta \geq 5$ *DMFS*	*Any Risk* $\Delta \geq 1$ *DMFS*
Clinical				
DMFS Baseline	.19*	.41*	.15**	.20**
dmfs Baseline	.03**	.04**	.02	.01
Morphology score	.09**	.06*	.10**	.13**
Sealants			-.67	
White Spot (WS) Lesions		-.01	.21*	.31*
Fluorosis Score	-.24		.18	
Sound Surfaces (Perm.)	.01	.00	.02**	.01**
Mean Plaque Score	.03		.37**	
Referral Caries Score	.04	.14	.24*	.29*
Predicted Caries Score	.43**	.47**	.14	.20
Fluorosis × WS Lesions	.18		.15	
Microbiological				
Mutans Streptococci Score	.11	.14*	.08	.05
Lactobacillus Score	.02	.12	.18*	.26**
Socio-demographic				
Race	.11	.39*	.14	.17
Age	-.06		.01	
Education, Parent[a]		.06		-.02**
Health Behavior				
Brush A (1/day vs. < daily)	.16	-.07*	.12	-.04
Brush B (2/day vs. < daily)	.27		.25	
Between Meal Snacks	-.23		-.15	
FMR (ever vs. never used)	.32		.00	
No. Dent. Visits, Parent		.40*		-.26
Child's Dent. Visits (1+ vs. 0)		.02		-.54
Child's Visits (0 & 3+ vs. 1 & 2)		.04		-.13
Fluoride Tablet Use		.03		-.31
Examiner Scores				
Examiner AA vs. other	.35	-.03	-.52	-.89**
Examiner BB vs. other	.08	.02	.17	-.08
Examiner CC vs. other	.06	-.31	-.33	-.51
Examiner DD vs. other	-.02	.23	-.27	-.22
R	.37	.40	.41	.39

*p < .05 **p < .01
[a]Parent reflects head of household

TABLE 6 *Comparison of "High Caries" with "Any Caries" Logistic Regression Risk Prediction Models for Three-year DMFS Increments: Grade Cohorts 1 and 5, Portland ME*

	Betas for Grade 1 Cohort		*Betas for Grade 5 Cohort*	
Variables	*High Risk* $\Delta \geq 2$ *DMFS*	*Any Risk* $\Delta \geq 1$ *DMFS*	*High Risk* $\Delta \geq 3$ *DMFS*	*Any Risk* $\Delta \geq 1$ *DMFS*
Clinical				
DMFS Baseline	.00	.18	.16**	.13**
dmfs Baseline	.03	.01	.02	.01
Morphology score	.08*	.05	.07	.03
Sealants	.10		-.02	
White Spot (WS) Lesions	.11	.14	.11	.20*
Fluorosis Score	.08	.33	.03	-.11
Sound Surfaces (Perm.)	-.00	-.00	.02**	.02**
Mean Plaque Score	.17		.34**	
Referral Caries Score	-.07	-.03	.12	.39
Predicted Caries Score	.75**	.75**	.60**	.60**
Fluorosis × WS Lesions	.00		.40	
Microbiological				
Mutans Streptococci Score	-.07	-.02	-.00	-.00
Lactobacillus Score	.15	.20*	.26**	.29**
Socio-demographic				
Race				
Age	-.16		-.03	
Education, Parent[a]		-.12**		.05
Health Behavior				
Brush A (1/day vs. < daily)	-.26	-.20	-.08	.71*
Brush B (2/day vs. < daily)	-.33		-.33	
Between Meal Snacks	-.55		-.29	
FMR (ever vs. never used)	.15		-.03	
No. Dent. Visits, Parent		.12		-.09
Child's Dent. Visits (1+ vs. 0)		-.08		-.69*
Child's Visits (0 & 3+ vs. 1 & 2)		-.49		-.64*
Fluoride Tablet Use		.44*		.26
Examiner Scores				
Examiner AA vs. other	.78**	.59*	.42	-.21
Examiner BB vs. other	.65*	.25	.68*	-.20
Examiner CC vs. other	.30	-.07	-.56	-.13
Examiner DD vs. other	.20	-.09	.64	.39
R	.32	.38	.47	.44

*p < .05 **p < .01

[a]Parent reflects head of household

biological caries process. In the eyes of the critics, this argument gains force because the multivariate caries risk prediction models frequently result in statistical nonsignificance for variables believed to have high biological relevance. This has already been noted for the high caries risk prediction models discussed earlier. In order to determine the characteristics of a caries model that emphasizes etiologic factors, it is necessary to relate the outcome variable, in this case caries increment dichotomized into "none" or "any caries", to only those independent variables that have direct or near indirect etiological relevance. As shown in Table 7, this approach excludes variables such as baseline DMFS, baseline dmfs, white spot lesions, referral caries score, predicted caries score, race and parental dental visits from the equation. The effect of that step generates an *etiological* model that, for the Aiken grade 1 cohort, causes three biologically relevant variables to enter the model equation, namely sealants, fluorosis score and mean plaque score. For this *etiological* model the plaque score is statistically highly significant; the morphology and lactobacillus scores become significant at the $p < .01$ level; and two health behavior variables also reach statistical significance in the model. A standard *prediction* model, based on "any caries risk", is shown for comparison. In the Aiken grade 5 cohort, the etiologic model shows a strong effect for sealants, a greater effect due to lactobacillus and stronger influence for the child dental visit variables. The pattern can be readily compared with the standard *prediction* model. While these *etiologic* models might make more sense, it should be noted that the multiple R values are substantially lower than for the *prediction* models. In general terms, the etiologic models for Portland exhibit analogous differences from the Portland predictive models, and the multiple R values are also lower for etiologic models. The reader can examine Table 8 for the details.

Caries Risk Assessment in Children Caries Free at Baseline

A further complaint with previous caries risk models is that by using baseline dmfs and DMFS as predictors, one is approaching the problem too late—after the horse is out of the stable so to speak. To investigate whether analytical insights can be gained from confronting this issue, Tables 9 and 10 display analyses that compare "any caries risk" prediction models in children whose dmfs and DMFS at baseline summed to zero with models based on children with nonzero caries levels at baseline. Before looking at the actual coefficients in Tables 9 and 10, several general observations should be considered. First, the grouping of children by baseline caries experience created multicollinearity between the White Spot Lesions variable and the Fluorosis x WS Lesions interaction term, causing the latter to be dropped from the analyses. Second, for the groups with zero baseline caries scores, the Referral Caries Score contained virtually no

TABLE 7 *Comparison of "Etiologic" with "Prediction" Logistic Regression Models Based on "Any Caries" Risk Criterion for Three-year DMFS Increment: Grade Cohorts 1 and 5, Aiken SC*

	Betas for Grade 1 Cohort		*Betas for Grade 5 Cohort*	
Variables	*Etiologic Model*	*Prediction Model*	*Etiologic Model*	*Prediction Model*
Clinical				
DMFS Baseline	—[a]	.41*	—	.20**
dmfs Baseline	—	.04**	—	.01
Morphology score	.09**	.06*	.06**	.13**
Sealants	-.14		-.25**	
White Spot (WS) Lesions	—	-.01	—	.31*
Fluorosis Score	-.15		.06	
Sound Surfaces (Perm.)	-.00	.00	.01**	.01**
Mean Plaque Score	.51**		.17	
Referral Caries Score	—	.14	—	.29*
Predicted Caries Score	—	.47**	—	.20
Microbiological				
Mutans Streptococci Score	.18*	.14*	.06	.05
Lactobacillus Score	.35**	.12	.47**	.26**
Socio-demographic				
Race	—	.39*	—	.17
Education, Parent[b]		.06		-.02**
Health Behavior				
Brush A (1/day vs. < daily)		-.07*		-.04
No. Dent. Visits, Parent	—	.40*	—	-.26
Child's Dent. Visits (1+ vs. 0)	-.52*	.02	-.74*	-.54
Child's Visits (0 & 3+ vs. 1 & 2)	-.56*	.04	-.41	-.13
Fluoride Tablet Use		.03		-.31
Examiner Scores				
Examiner AA vs. other	-.08	-.03	-.54*	-.89**
Examiner BB vs. other	-.02	.02	.17	-.08
Examiner CC vs. other	-.10	-.31	-.43	-.51
Examiner DD vs. other	.47*	.23	.11	-.22
R	.29	.40	.27	.39

*p < .05 **p < .01

[a]—indicates variable excluded from etiologic model

[b]Parent reflects head of household

TABLE 8 *Comparison of "Etiologic" with "Prediction" Logistic Regression Models Based on "Any Caries" Risk Criterion for Three-year DMFS Increment: Grade Cohorts 1 and 5, Portland ME*

	Betas for Grade 1 Cohort		*Betas for Grade 5 Cohort*	
Variables	*Etiologic Model*	*Prediction Model*	*Etiologic Model*	*Prediction Model*
Clinical				
DMFS Baseline	—[a]	.18	—	.13**
dmfs Baseline	—	.01	—	.01
Morphology score	.15**	.13**	.04	.03
Sealants	.09		-.07	
White Spot (WS) Lesions	—	.14	—	.20*
Fluorosis Score	.09		-.43*	
Sound Surfaces (Perm.)	-.01	-.00	.02**	.02**
Mean Plaque Score	.47**		.34**	
Referral Caries Score	—	-.03	—	.39*
Predicted Caries Score	—	.75**	—	.60**
Microbiological				
Mutans Streptococci Score	.11	-.02	.10	-.00
Lactobacillus Score	.35**	.20*	.39**	.29**
Socio-demographic				
Race	—		—	
Education, Parent[b]	—	-.12**	—	.05
Health Behavior				
Brush A (1/day vs. < daily)		-.20		.71*
No. Dent. Visits, Parent	—	.12	—	-.09
Child's Dent. Visits (1+ vs. 0)	-.43	-.08	-.74*	-.69
Child's Visits (0 & 3+ vs. 1 & 2)	-1.00**	-.49	-.90**	-.64*
Fluoride Tablet Use		.44*		.26
Examiner Scores				
Examiner AA vs. other	.45	.59*	-.31	-.21
Examiner BB vs. other	.06	.25	.08	-.20
Examiner CC vs. other	-.06	-.07	-.08	-.13
Examiner DD vs. other	-.11	-.09	.35	.39
R	.32	.38	.30	.44

*p < .05 **p < .01

[a]—indicates variable excluded from etiologic model

[b]Parent reflects head of household

TABLE 9 *Three-year "Any Caries" (Δ_3DMFS > 0) Logistic Regression Risk Models Comparing Baseline Caries Free Group with Group Presenting Caries Experience: Grade Cohorts 1 and 5, Aiken SC*

Variables	*Betas for Aiken Grade 1 Cohort*		*Betas for Aiken Grade 5 Cohort*	
	Caries=0 o	*Caries=≥1 o*	*Caries=0 o*	*Caries=≥1 o*
Clinical				
DMFS Baseline	—	.29*	—	.25**
dmfs Baseline	—	.03*	—	.02
Morphology Score	-.02	.10**	.18**	.13**
Sealants	.22	-.32	-.31	-.07
White Spot (WS) Lesions	-.63	.01	.27	.35**
Fluorosis Score	.42	-.12	.41	.35
Sound Surfaces (Perm.)	.01	-.01	-.00	.02**
Mean Plaque Score	.56	.07	-.14	.13
Referral Caries Score	—	.04	—	.29*
Predicted Caries Score	1.29**	.30*	-.18	.15
Microbiological				
Mutans Streptococci Score	-.10	.12	.13	-.03
Lactobacillus Score	.17	.10	.46	.30**
Socio-demographic				
Race	-.52	-.41*	.23	-.22
Age	.03	.09	-.27	-.19
Health Behavior				
Brush A (1/day vs. < daily)	-.18	-.17	.15	-.13
Brush B (2/day vs. < daily)	-1.08*	-.26	.20	-.01
Between Meal Snacks	-.27	.04	.25	.87**
FMR (ever vs. never used)	.09	.03	.24	.22
Examiner Scores				
Examiner AA vs. other	.37	-.06	-1.95**	-.63*
Examiner BB vs. other	.25	-.16	-.10	.21
Examiner CC vs. other	-.13	-.37	-1.55**	-.24
Examiner DD vs. other	1.23*	-.22	-.89	-.28
R	.00	.29	.00	.34
N	262	738	178	699

*p < .05 **p < .01

variance, which forced exclusion of this variable from the regression. Third, it may be noted that the R index for goodness of fit in the logistic regressions displayed in Tables 9 and 10 are lower again than previous models presented. Specifically for models based on the baseline caries free children in Aiken, the index of model fit dropped to virtually zero, presumably due to little variation in caries

TABLE 10 *Three year "Any Caries" ($\Delta_3DMFS > 0$) Logistic Regression Risk Models Comparing Baseline Caries Free Group with Group Presenting Caries Experience: Grade Cohorts 1 and 5, Portland ME*

	Betas for Portland Grade 1 Cohort		*Betas for Portland Grade 5 Cohort*	
Variables	*Caries=0* *o*	*Caries=≥1* *o*	*Caries=0* *o*	*Caries=≥1* *o*
Clinical				
DMFS Baseline	—	.08	—	.14*
dmfs Baseline	—	-.01	—	-.02
Morphology score	.01	.12**	.02	.05
Sealants	-.07	.17*	.09	.08
White Spot (WS) Lesions	.26	.07	.15	.21*
Fluorosis Score	.55*	.35	-.62	.35
Sound Surfaces (Perm.)	-.02	-.01	.02**	.01*
Mean Plaque Score	.57	.18	.17	.09
Referral Caries Score	—	-.01	—	.41*
Predicted Caries Score	1.02**	.73**	.75*	.61**
Microbiological				
Mutans Streptococci Score	-.02	-.03	.11	-.04
Lactobacillus Score	-.20	.26*	.32*	.25**
Socio-demographic				
Race	—	—	—	—
Age	.19	.15	-.46	.16
Health Behavior				
Brush A (1/day vs. < daily)	-.43	-.38	.49	.46
Brush B (2/day vs. < daily)	-.82*	-.36	.25	.06
Between Meal Snacks	.01	-.35	.01	.29
FMR (ever vs. never used)	-.02	.12	-.19	-.25
Examiner Scores				
Examiner AA vs. other	.46	1.11**	-.64	.21
Examiner BB vs. other	-.02	.46	-.22	.70*
Examiner CC vs. other	-.06	-.12	-.05	.05
Examiner DD vs. other	.07	-.24	.24	.65*
R	.19	.28	.22	.34
N	624	399	344	568

*p < .05 **p < .01

increment to explain. This result does not, however, eliminate the model's usefulness in caries prediction.

Turning to the examination of the coefficients for baseline caries free children in Tables 9 and 10, it is evident that very few variables retain statistical significance. On the one hand, this suggests that it may be very difficult for clinicians to employ clinical, microbiological or other objective criteria for predicting which caries free six-year olds will develop one or more caries lesions in the subsequent three years. On the other hand, this difficulty occurs mainly because relatively little caries develops in these children. Lack of a generous sample size may be a problem for the models focussing on caries free children in Aiken. In contrast, for children with prior caries experience at baseline, the quantity of caries experience, several other clinical variables and the salivary lactobacillus status become effective predictors for children's susceptibility to more caries in the three years following examination.

The examination of alternative caries risk modelling approaches is not complete unless one compares their performance by the indices of sensitivity and specificity. *Sensitivity,* it will be recalled, is the ratio of true positives over the sum of true positives and false negatives. *Specificity* is the ratio of true negatives over the sum of true negatives and false positives. Table 11 displays these two criteria for a number of the models presented in Tables 4 through 8. The results in Table 11 are quite revealing. The "high caries risk" prediction models from Table 4 are the current standard, and produce sensitivities around 0.60 and the specificities between .81 and .84. These results are below the target sensitivity of .75 but almost meet the target specificity of .85. The sum of the sensitivities and specificities for the high risk models consistently exceeds 1.40.

TABLE 11 *Sensitivity and Specificity Values for High Caries Risk Prediction Models, Any Caries Risk Prediction Models and Any Risk Etiologic Models*

Group/Model	*Sensitivity*	*Specificity*
Aiken, Grade 1		
High Caries Risk	.59	.83
Any Caries Risk	.80	.61
Etiologic	.74	.55
Aiken, Grade 5		
High Caries Risk	.62	.81
Any Caries Risk	.84	.54
Etiologic	.81	.50
Portland, Grade 1		
High Caries Risk	.59	.84
Any Caries Risk	.66	.78
Etiologic	.59	.74
Portland, Grade 5		
High Caries Risk	.62	.84
Any Caries Risk	.76	.71
Etiologic	.69	.65

The "any caries risk" prediction models, based on dichotomizing outcomes between 0 DMFS increment and 1 or more DMFS increment, achieve superior sensitivities ranging between .66 and .84. Although these sensitivities are more variable, on average they well exceed the target criterion of .75. Unfortunately, the specificities fluctuate quite a bit and fall consistently short of the .85 criterion. Specificity for these four models ranges from .54 to .78. The sum of sensitivity and specificity lies near 1.40 and compares favorably with the standard high risk prediction models. For the "etiologic" caries risk models, sensitivities and specificities were yet more volatile, and in the case of specificity, even lower than for the "any caries risk" models. It would be premature, however, to conclude from this that the etiologic models were poor performers.

Discussion

A number of issues arise out of the various analyses presented above. The first essential is that researchers must be more specific in defining the purpose of modelling caries risk assessment. Is the objective to identify susceptible children falling above varying high caries increment levels along the caries gradient curve? Does one want to identify the most severely affected 20 percent of children, regardless how clinically significant the caries increment criterion is? Alternatively, is it the purpose to identify *a priori* the children who develop an absolute high caries increment level, regardless of how relatively large or small the high risk group is? Or is the objective to predict reliably those children who will develop any caries increment at all over a given time period? Finally, is one seeking to establish caries risk predicated on known or etiological factors only?

The analyses in Tables 5 and 6 have shown that the time may be approaching when it will be appropriate to model whether patients develop any new caries in a given time interval. This arises because the distribution of caries increment is becoming increasingly asymmetrical as demonstrated by the Portland data. With more children falling into the 0 DMFS increment category, the time may have arrived where diagnosing and classifying children into predicted caries free and caries-prone groups, over defined future time periods, may be practical.

Evaluated by the indices of sensitivity and specificity, models that emphasize one or other of these two choice criteria are beginning to appear, though more work is still required. Thus for public prevention programs that operate on scarce resources, standard caries risk prediction with high specificity will be very effective in sorting out the low risk children, thereby helping to ensure the program's financial integrity by focussing expensive resources, eg. sealant programs, only on the most at risk children. On the other hand, in private practice where the risk of *a priori* misclassifying a true caries positive may be unacceptable, the "any caries risk" model may be preferable since it results in substantially higher prediction sensitivity.

Turning to the etiological models, the lower sensitivity and disappointing specificity may not be tremendously relevant. The purpose of etiological models is not to predict an individual's caries risk at all, but rather is intended to identify factors that may be linked to the biological process of caries. By identifying relevant factors, such models may lead to better understanding about the conditions promoting or retarding caries or may suggest avenues for preventive or therapeutic interventions that could reduce caries occurrence. The etiologic models proposed in this chapter were more effective in accounting for microbiological and health behavior factors than were the pure prediction models. Again, it is the objective of the modelling that is most important.

In theory, the ultimate etiological model might be those developed from children who have 0 dmfs and 0 DMFS at baseline. In this connection, preliminary results obtained from the UNC Caries Risk Assessment study are disappointing. Because too few children were baseline caries free in Aiken, the sample sizes were too small to provide powerful tests of various potential etiological factors. In Portland, where caries-free samples in both grade 1 and grade 5 cohorts were larger, some encouragement can be derived from the identification of variables such as mean plaque index and sugary snack foods. Nevertheless, these models show signs of instability and need revision before they can be accepted with confidence.

Turning back to the key results from the UNC Caries Risk Assessment study, a number of important findings emerged. The sensitivity of .60 and specificities of .81 - .84 have already been commented on. A second result of major interest was the predominance of clinical measures from the intraoral examination as significant predictors of future high caries increment occurrence. Third, the significance of the pit and fissure morphology score and the clinicians' subjective prediction of the future three-year caries increment were surprising for both their strength and relative consistency across the models. The observation pertaining to pit and fissure morphology as a predictor is fairly novel, and confirms in this large study an earlier preliminary finding by Bader *et al.*, (1986).

The examiner's subjective prediction of the child's future three-year caries increment was a powerful predictor with a difficult underlying logic. This variable, which was designed into the study from the start and on which no calibration was attempted, had two conceptual purposes. One, the predicted caries score attempted to determine whether, after all relevant variables had been measured and recorded, there was an overarching synthesis of clinical information by a skilled examiner that somehow contained predictive information overlooked by the variables included in the study. Two, it was hoped that some among the four clinical examiners might prove to be more skilled at predicting which children were at high risk for large caries increments. If so, the strategy was to determine what specific information the superior prognosticator employed to arrive at the decision. Unfortunately, no difference emerged among the examiners' ability to predict, so that that particular aspiration of the study could not be fulfilled. Nevertheless, the general results concerning predictive caries score suggest that experience clinical examiners have a collective ability to predict future caries occurrence that goes beyond the information base acquired through the more discrete, objective variables employed in the study.

The relative weakness of the microbiological variables to predict high caries increment in this study was disappointing. A great deal of expense, careful work and commitment had gone into this phase of the work. In preliminary bivariate analyses of caries increment on mutans streptococci and lactobacilli scores, impressive relationships were exhibited. Yet when combined into the multivariate analyses, neither Mutans streptococci nor lactobacilli, singly or combined in an additive or multiplicative manner, showed strong or consistent predictive ability. At least three possibilities exist for this failure. One, salivary microorganisms simply may not be the relevant measure, and one would need to consider plaque organisms as a better alternative. Two, it is possible that the dip slide kits were not functioning optimally or that inoculation, culturing and scoring were not well done in the field. This possibility might be discounted because of the positive results obtained from the bivariate analyses involving caries increments. Three, it is also possible that the microbiological dip slide test employed, especially for Mutans streptococci, was too general. Specifically, the Cariescreen® may have grown many strains of Mutans streptococci whereas only a subset of the genetically diverse strains of MS may be related to significant caries initiation (Kuramitsu, 1987).

The ineffectiveness of sociodemographic and dental behavioral variables to predict high caries risk in this study may have many causes. Among the most important may be the limit of large scale field studies to accurately determine or measure the type of information being sought. Thus, for variables such as education of the head of household, toothbrushing frequency, fluoride supplement use and the like, it is probable that considerable response error exists. This would have the effect of attenuating the respective variable's relationship with the outcome measure. In the case of diet determination, it is almost certain that the one time, one question, self-reporting mechanism was inadequate to elicit the minimum amount and quality of information needed for a meaningful analysis.

Finally, it may be supposed that methods other than logistic regression analysis might generate superior caries risk assessment models. Several methods, including linear discriminant function analyses and classification analysis and regression trees (CART) have been applied to the UNC Caries Risk Assessment study (Stewart and Stamm, 1991). These alternative approaches do generate different models, though they frequently retain similar key predictor variables. When examined by predictive sensitivity and specificity indices, these alternative statistical methods have developed models that performed similarly to those generated through logistic regression.

Conclusions

1. The UNC Caries Risk Assessment Study obtained three-year predictive specificity values of nearly .83, close to the criterion established *a priori*. In this study approximately 83 percent of children with low susceptibility to caries over a three-year period were correctly classified as *low risk* at baseline.
2. The variables included in the UNC Caries Risk Assessment Study were able to achieve a caries prediction sensitivity of approximately .60, lower that the .75 criterion level.
3. Using logistic regression in standard high caries risk prediction models, clinical variables, such as pit and fissure morphology, baseline primary and permanent caries and clinician's caries risk prediction were the most powerful predictors.
4. In the presence of pertinent clinical predictor variable information, sociodemographic, dental behavior and salivary bacterial variables contributed little additional three-year caries prediction power in the UNC Caries Risk Assessment Study.
5. Because many children remained caries free over the three-year duration of this study, caries prediction models based on the medical convention of "any disease" versus "no disease" performed nearly as well as the "high caries" increment versus "low and no caries" increment models. Conceptually, the any caries versus no caries increment models may have more application in private than public dental practice.
6. Reducing model predictor variables to the set believed to have etiologic relevance resulted in equations that better modelled disease process. In the UNC data set, etiologic models raised the microbiologic and dietary variables to statistical significance, though this did not occur in all models and invariable resulted in reduced sensitivity and specificity performance.
7. Prediction of caries susceptibility in children who have no caries experience at baseline is difficult and will lead to inconsistent models across different populations. Putative etiologic variables may still not enter such prediction models at levels of statistical significance. Further, clinical variables such a clinician's subjective prediction of caries increment remained as the most potent predictors in such models.
8. The failure of etiological variables to play a larger role in predicting caries susceptibility among children in Aiken, South Carolina and Portland,

Maine suggests that more refined methods than those employed in large scale epidemiological field studies must be employed to search for etiological relationships that almost certainly must exist.

REFERENCES

BADER, J.D.; GRAVES, R.C.; DISNEY, J.A.; BOHANNAN, H.M.; STAMM, J.W.; ABERNATHY, J.R.; and LINDAHL, R.L. (1986): Identifying children who will experience high caries increments. *Comm Dent Oral Epid* 14(4):198-201.

BIBBY, B.C. and SHERN, R.J. (1978): Methods of caries prediction. *Microbiol Abstr—Bacteriol* (Supp).

BLACK, G.V. (1899): Susceptibility and immunity to dental caries. *Dental Cosmos* 41:826.

BOHANNAN, H.M.; GRAVES, R.C.; DISNEY, J.A.; STAMM, J.W.; ABERNATHY, J.R.; and BADER, J.D. (1985): Effect of secular decline in caries on the evaluation of preventive dentistry interventions. *J Public Health Dent* 45:83-9.

BOHANNAN, H.M.; DISNEY, J.A.; GRAVES, R.C.; KLEIN, S.P.; and LEONE, F.H. (1981): Caries prevalence in the national preventive dentistry demonstration program. P-6625, Santa Monica, CA: The Rand Corporation.

BRUSZT, P. (1959): Relationship of caries incidence in deciduous and permanent dentitions. *J Dent Res* 38:416.

CROSSNER, C.G. and HOLM, H.K. (1977): Saliva tests in the prognosis of caries in children. *Acta Odontol Scand* 35(3):135-9.

DOWNER, M.C. (1991): Description and explanation of the distribution of caries in the population of Europe. In: *Risk Markers for Oral Diseases*. Vol. I. Dental Caries, N.W. Johnson, ed., Cambridge: Cambridge University Press, pp. 100-131.

EPIDEMIOLOGY AND ORAL DISEASE PREVENTION PROGRAM (1989): National Institute of Dental Research, U.S. Department of Health and Human Services, Public Health Service, National Institute of Health, NIH Publication No. 89-2243, Washington.

FOCH, C.B. (1981): A cost analysis plan for the national preventive dentistry demonstration program. N-1670-RWJ. Santa Monica, CA: The Rand Corporation.

GLASS, R.L., ed. (1982): The first international conference on declining prevalence of dental caries. *J Dent Res* 61(Spec Issue):1301-83.

GORDIS, L. (1988): *Epidemiology and Health Risk Assessment*, New York: Oxford. University Press.

HOLM, A.K. (1978): Dental health in a group of Swedish 8-year-olds followed since the age of 3. *Comm Dent Oral Epidemiol* 6:71-7.

JEFFERY, R.W. (1989): Risk Behaviors and Health - Contrasting Individual and Population Perspectives, *Amer Psychologist* 44:1194-1202.

JORDAN, H.V.; LARAWAY, R.; SNIRCH, R.; and MARMEL, M. (1987): A simplified diagnostic system for cultural detection and enumeration of *Streptococcus mutans*. *J Dent Res* 66(1):57-61.

KLEIN, S.P. and BOHANNAN, H.M. (1979): The first year of field activities in the national preventive dentistry demonstration program. R-2356/1 and R-2356/2-RWJ. Santa Monica, CA: The Rand Corporation.

KLEIN, H.; BIMSTEIN, E.; and CHOSACK, A. (1985): Caries prevalence of the primary dentition at age seven: an indicator for future caries prevalence in the permanent dentition. *Pediatr Dent* 3(2):184-5.

KLOCK, B. and KRASSE, B. (1979): A comparison between different methods for prediction of caries activity. *Scand J Dent Res* 87:129-39.

KÖHLER, B. and BRATTHALL, D: (1979). Practical method to facilitate estimation of *Strepotococcus mutans* levels in saliva. *Jour of Clin Microbiol* 9:584-8.

KURAMITSU, H.K. (1987): Recent advances in defining the cariogenicity of mutans streptococci: molecular genetic approaches. *Eur J Epidemiol* 3:257-260.

LECLERCQ, M.H.; BARMES, D.E.; and SARDO INFERRI, J. (1987): Oral Health: global trends and projections. *World Health Stat Quart* 40:116-128.

LITTLETON, N.W. and WHITE, C.L. (1964): Dental findings from a preliminary study of children receiving extended antibiotic therapy, *JADA* 68:520-525.

MILLER, W.D. (1890): *Microorganisms of the Human Mouth*. Philadelphia: S.S. White Dental Mfg. Co.

NATIONAL CARIES PROGRAM, NATIONAL INSTITUTE OF DENTAL RESEARCH. The prevalence of dental caries in United States schoolchildren, 1979-80. The National Dental Caries Prevalence Survey. NIH pub no 82-2245, December 1981.

ROBBINS, L. and HALL, J. (1970): *How to Practice Prospective Medicine*. Indianapolis, Methodist Hospital of Indiana.

RUNDEGREN, J. and ERICSON, T. (1978): Actual caries development compared with expected caries activity. *Comm Dent Oral Epidemiol* 6:97-102.

SCHOENBACH, V.J. (1987): Appraising Health Risk Appraisal, *Amer Jour Pub Health* 77:409-411.

SILNESS, J. and LÖE, H. (1964): Periodontal disease in pregnancy: correlation between oral hygiene and periodontal condition. *Acta Odont Scand* 22:121-135.

STAMM, J.W.; DISNEY, J.A.; GRAVES, R.C.; BOHANNAN, H.M.; and ABERNATHY, J.R. (1988): The University of North Carolina Caries Risk Assessment Study (I: Rationale and Content), *J Pub Health Dent* 48(12):225-232.

STEWART, P.W. and STAMM, J.W. (1991): Classification Tree Prediction Models for Dental Caries Using Clinical, Microbiological and Interview Data, *J Dent Res* 70:1239-1251.

WORLD HEALTH ORGANIZATION (1989). Dental Caries levels at 12 years (mimeograph of data from Global Oral Data Bank). Geneva: WHO.

Saliva Flow and Dental Caries in Aging Adults

RONALD J. BILLINGS

Over the past two decades, it has become increasingly convincing that saliva is indispensable to the integrity of the teeth and mouth tissues (Mandel and Wotman, 1976; Mandel, 1984; Mandel, 1989) and that altered salivary gland function can have adverse consequences on the maintenance of oral health (Baum *et al.*, 1985; Schubert and Izutsu, 1987; Sreebny, 1989). Among middle-age and elderly individuals, the most common manifestations of salivary gland dysfunction are chronic hyposalivation secondary to irradiation for head and neck cancer (Frank *et al.*, 1965; Ben-Aryeh *et al.*, 1975; Dreizen *et al.*, 1976; Brown *et al.*, 1976), diseases such as Sjögren's Syndrome (Scully, 1986; Malmström *et al.*, 1988), and use of certain classes of therapeutic medications (Johnson *et al.*, 1984; Handelman *et al.*, 1986; Sreebny and Schwartz, 1986) [Figure 1]. Among the frequently cited concerns associated with chronic hyposalivation in adults is dental caries (Mandel, 1974; Dreizen and Brown, 1976; Petersen, 1986; Vissink *et al.*, 1988; Baum, 1989).

The goals of this symposium are both important and timely: root surface caries can be a major problem in middle-age and elderly individuals and, concomitantly, there are aging adults who remain highly susceptible to coronal caries (Banting, 1984; Beck, 1984; Banting, 1986; Beck *et al.*, 1988; Hand *et al.*, 1988). Alterations in salivary flow, or composition, or both, in middle-age and elderly adults, may have a role in increased dental caries susceptibility as well as other oral diseases or disorders (Fox *et al.*, 1985).

The occurrence of salivary gland hypofunction and the consequent onset of rampant caries in orofacially irradiated, diseased and institutionalized populations has been well documented (Frank *et al.*, 1965; Bertram, 1967; Dreizen and Brown, 1976). Much less is known about the prevalence of salivary gland hypofunction and its relation to dental caries in the general, non-institutionalized community-dwelling population. For example, the extent and severity of pharmacologically-induced salivary gland hypofunction in the general population have not been reported, even though hundreds of drugs which have the

Figure 1 COMMON CAUSES OF SALIVARY GLAND DYSFUNCTION

Glandular Factors	
Usually Reversible	Usually Irreversible
Obstruction	Radiation*
Inflammation	Degenerative Changes
Infection	Aplasia/Excision
Systemic Factors	
Usually Reversible	Usually Irreversible
Medications*	Autoimmune Exocrinopathies (e.g., Sjogren's Syndrome)*
Psychogenic Disorders (e.g., Depression)	Neurologic Diseases, Disorders
Substance Abuse (e.g., Recreational Drugs, Alcohol, Tobacco)	Various Other Organic Diseases, Disorders

* Major Causes of Salivary Gland Dysfunction in Middle-Age and Elderly Persons

potential to affect salivary gland function have been identified (Bahn, 1972; Sreebny and Schwartz, 1986), and their utilization patterns described (Shapiro *et al.*, 1986; Nelson *et al.*, 1987; Levy *et al.*, 1988).

Salivary Hypofunction in Community-Dwelling Adults

To begin to accumulate a database on this and related questions on the extent and consequences of salivary hypofunction in the general population, a cross-sectional assessment of oral health conditions across a broad age-range of community-dwelling adults was conducted. Seven hundred and ten persons between the ages of 20 and 80+ participated in this study. Although the study sample was not random, every effort was made to select a representative group of community-dwelling persons. Volunteers were drawn from neighborhood health centers, places of business and commerce, universities, and senior citizen centers. Responses to a standardized series of questions on general and oral health, medication use and symptoms of xerostomia were compared with objective measurements of passive and stimulated whole saliva flow. An oral examination of each study participant was performed to determine dentition status and the presence or absence of oral pathology, including coronal and root surface caries, abrasion and erosion. For the purpose of summarizing the data for the present paper, the study sample was arrayed into three age groups (Table 1).

All saliva specimens were collected into pre-weighed plastic tubes. Collection times were recorded and the volume determined gravimetrically. Flow rates

TABLE 1 *Distribution of Sample by Age Group and Gender*

Age Group	*Males*	*Females*	*Combined*
20 - 49	114	265	379
50 - 79 +	98	194	292
80 +	14	25	39
All Ages	226	484	710

were expressed in mL/min. Unstimulated saliva was collected for two minutes. Stimulated saliva was collected for one minute by means of 2% citric acid stimulation, which was swabbed onto the dorsum and lateral borders of the tongue. Extensive preliminary studies determined that a two minute unstimulated and a one minute stimulated saliva collection period yielded approximately the same flow rates as the more lengthy collection periods commonly employed in physiologic studies. In most cases whole saliva flow rates were observed to range from approximately 0 to 1.85 mL/min for unstimulated saliva and from 1 to 3 mL/min for stimulated saliva. Although no defined boundary exists between normal and abnormal flow rates (Dawes, 1987; Ship *et al.*, 1991), values below 0.05 mL/min unstimulated and 0.50 mL/min stimulated would be considered extremely low and values this low occurring together would generally be considered indicative of impaired function. The results of this study, which have been analyzed to date, will be described and the implications of these findings as they may relate to dental caries in the middle-age and elderly community-dwelling population will be discussed.

Health Problems Affecting Saliva Flow

As might be expected, the prevalence of health problems which may affect salivation tended to increase with advancing age (Table 2). The observed decrease in hypertension and diabetes among persons aged 80 and older may reflect a greater mortality from these diseases during earlier periods. Psychogenic disorders resulting from stress, anxiety and menopause may account for the proportionally greater occurrence of this condition among young and middle-age persons.

Medications Affecting Saliva Flow

Many medications have the potential to affect salivary gland function, and to exacerbate oral dryness. As shown in Table 3, there are some fourteen classes of drugs generally ascribed as having this property. The regular use of analgesics, antiarrhythmics, antihypertensives, and diuretics was observed to increase

TABLE 2 *Prevalence (Percent) of Common Chronic Diseases/Disorders with the Potential to Affect Salivary Function by Age Group*

Disease/Disorder	*Age Group*			
	20 - 49	*50 - 79*	*80 +*	*All Ages*
Cardiovascular	2.9	21.9	38.4	12.7
Hypertension	7.1	39.3	33.3	21.8
Arthritis	2.6	22.9	30.7	12.5
Gastrointestinal	9.2	17.4	15.3	13.0
Psychogenic	11.3	13.6	2.5	11.8
Diabetes	2.1	13.0	5.1	6.8
Neurovascular	1.5	4.4	5.1	3.0
Neuromuscular	2.6	3.7	2.5	3.1
Cancer	0.5	4.4	5.1	2.4

TABLE 3 *Hyposalivation-Inducing Drug Categories*

+ Analgesics	+ Antiparkinsons
+ Anorectics	+ Antipsychotics
+ Antiarrhythmics	+ Antispasmodics
+ Anticonvulsants	+ Diuretics
+ Antidepressants	+ Hypnotics
+ Antihistamines	+ Muscle Relaxants
+ Antihypertensives	+ Sedatives

TABLE 4 *Prevalence (Percent) of Daily Use of Medications with the Potential to Affect Salivary Function by Age Group*

Medication Category	*Age Group*			
	20 - 49	*50 - 79*	*80 +*	*All Ages*
Analgesics	4.0	18.8	12.8	10.6
Antiarrhythmics	0.8	18.8	12.8	10.6
Antidepressants	4.5	4.1	5.1	4.4
Antihistamines	2.6	2.1	2.6	2.4
Antihypertensives	3.2	26.4	15.4	13.4
Antispasmodics	0.8	5.5	7.7	3.1
Diuretics	1.8	9.6	12.8	5.6
Hypnotics/Sedatives	1.8	3.4	0	2.4
Muscle Relaxants	1.6	1.7	0	1.5

substantially with age, while the use of antidepressants and antihistamines remained constant (Table 4). Similar proportions of middle-age and elderly used at least one or more hyposalivation-inducing medications on a regular basis (Table 5) and the proportional use differed sharply between the younger and older age groups. The middle-age and elderly groups also consumed about 1.7

TABLE 5 *Prevalence (Percent) of Population Reporting the Regular Use of at Least One Hyposalivation-Inducing Medication*

Age Group	*Males*	*Females*	*Combined*
20 - 49	14.0	14.0	14.0
50 - 79	54.1	49.0	50.7
80 +	42.8	48.0	46.2
All Ages	33.2	29.8	30.9

different types of medication per person. Levy *et al.* (1988) reported similar figures for elderly community-dwelling Iowans. In general, saliva flow decreased as the number of medications with potential hyposalivatory side-effects increased (Table 6). Other investigators have reported similar observations (Thorselius *et al.*, 1988 and Handelman *et al.*, 1989).

Among persons ingesting one or more hyposalivation-inducing medications per day, the majority in each age category had saliva flow rates within generally accepted normal limits, while greater proportions of middle-age and elderly individuals had both a diminished unstimulated and stimulated flow rate than did younger persons (Table 7). Among individuals who reported consuming no medications with hyposalivation-inducing side-effects, a greater proportion had saliva flow rates within normal limits (Table 8) than did medicated persons

TABLE 6 *Saliva Flow Rate by Number of Medications Used*

Number of Drugs Used Daily	*N*	*Unstimulated*	*Stimulated*
0	491	0.22 (0.20)*	2.08 (1.26)
1	116	0.19 (0.20)	1.79 (1.32)
2	62	0.15 (0.12)	1.56 (1.14)
3	32	0.15 (0.17)	1.32 (0.92)
4	6	0.13 (0.15)	1.50 (1.52)
> 4	3	0.12 (0.09)	1.26 (0.50)

* Mean ± S.D.

TABLE 7 *Percent Distribution of Persons with Diminished Saliva Flow by Medication Status and Age Group (One or More Medications Used at Least Once Daily)*

Age Group	*Normal*		*Unstimulated Only < (0.05 mL/min)*		*Stimulated Only < (0.50 mL/min)*		*Both*	
	%	*N*	*%*	*N*	*%*	*N*	*%*	*N*
20 - 49	68.0	36	24.5	13	3.8	2	3.8	2
50 - 79	65.0	96	20.3	30	4.7	7	10.1	15
80 +	55.6	10	11.1	2	22.2	4	11.1	2
All Ages	64.8	142	20.5	45	5.9	13	8.7	19

TABLE 8 *Percent Distribution of Persons with Diminished Saliva Flow by Medication Status and Age Group (No Medication)*

Age Group	*Normal*		*Unstimulated Only < (0.05 mL/min)*		*Stimulated Only < (0.50 mL/min)*		*Both*	
	%	*N*	*%*	*N*	*%*	*N*	*%*	*N*
20 - 49	85.0	277	11.3	37	1.2	4	2.5	8
50 - 79	73.6	106	13.9	20	2.8	4	9.7	14
80 +	66.7	14	9.5	2	4.8	1	19.0	4
All Ages	80.9	397	12.0	59	1.8	9	5.3	26

(Table 7). A somewhat higher than expected proportion of non-medicated individuals had both flows low compared to medicated individuals, and this may have been due to the cross-sectional nature of the study, small cell size (particularly in the elderly), or possibly to undiagnosed or pharmacologically untreated health problems.

Dental Caries and Saliva Flow

As suggested by Baum (1986), reduced salivary function, in otherwise healthy individuals, may or may not have an effect on oral health status. In the present study, the relationship between saliva flow rates and root caries was investigated. As may have been expected, the prevalence of root caries increased with age in both males and females (Table 9). Additionally, the prevalence of root caries tended to be higher among individuals with reduced saliva flow rates (Table 10). However, when the likelihood of presenting with root caries was modeled as a function of both age and saliva flow rate using logistic regression analysis, saliva flow rate did not have a significant effect on the likelihood of presenting with root caries above and beyond that due to age (and those attendant variables confounded with age, e.g., health and medication status). Thus, if attention is restricted to generally healthy individuals of roughly a common

TABLE 9 *Prevalence (Percent) of Root Caries Among Dentate Subjects by Age Group and Gender*

Age Group	*Males*	*Females*	*Combined*
20 - 49	4.4	3.4	3.7
50 - 79	38.5	34.8	36.1
80 +	100.0	58.3	77.3
All Ages	22.4	16.4	18.3
N = 634			

TABLE 10 *Prevalence (Percent) of Root Caries by Saliva Flow Rate*

Saliva Flow Rate (mL/min)				
Unstimulated	*Stimulated*	*N*	*Root Caries*	*No Root Caries*
≥ .2	1.5	433	13.4	86.6
< .2	1.5	119	22.7	77.3
< .1	1.0	50	36.0	64.0
< .05	0.5	31	32.3	67.7
< .01	0.1	1	100.0	0

age, there is no evidence that any significant relationship between saliva flow rate and likelihood of presenting with root caries would be evident among such individuals.

Other recent studies of both coronal and root caries have also reported no significant relationship between the presence of caries and diminished saliva flow (Bergman and Ericson, 1986; Ravald *et al.*, 1986; Söderholm and Birkhed, 1988; Fure and Zickert, 1990; Klock *et al.*, 1990). Thus, one is inevitably drawn to the conclusion that, except in cases of extreme or catastrophic hyposalivation resulting from diseases or disorders (or treatment thereof) which cause complete or near-complete cessation of saliva flow for sustained periods of time, saliva flow alone does not serve well to explain caries experience.

Saliva in the Broader Context of Caries Risk Assessment

That most studies on healthy adults have generally not found a strong relationship between altered salivary function and dental caries should hardly come as a surprise. Several recent publications have either reviewed or identified numerous risk factors associated with caries susceptibility (Kitamura *et al.*, 1986; Beck *et al.*, 1988; Hunter, 1988; Graves *et al.*, 1990; Hunt, 1990; Kingman, 1990; Krasse, 1990). As pointed out by Hunt (1990), because of the multifactorial nature of dental caries, individual risk factors studied separately from the overall pool of risk factors tend to be poor predictors of caries onset.

There are three general classes of risk factors: biological, behavioral and intrinsic (Figure 2). Contained within these three general classes, the number of potential risk factors implicated in caries susceptibility is extensive and each one of these can be further subdivided nearly ad infinitum as amply described by Stamm (this symposium), Hunter (1988), Graves *et al.* (1990), Hunt (1990), Kingman (1990), and Krasse (1990). Interactions among the various protective and pathogenic factors are complex, and sophisticated multivariate methods of analysis will be required to establish caries risk profiles useful to public health workers, researchers, and clinicians. For example, the impact of topically applied fluorides on reducing the risk of rampant caries secondary to radiation-induced hyposalivation is profound (Wescott *et al.*, 1975; Dreizen *et al.*, 1977;

Figure 2 CARIES RISK ASSESSMENT

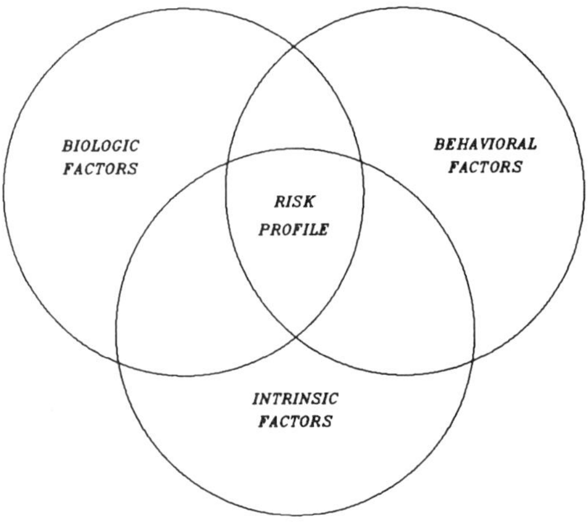

I. Biological Risk Factors
   + Morphology and molecular composition of coronal and root surfaces
   + Availability, oral concentration and distribution of fluoride
   + Plaque microbiology
   + Composition and secretion rate of saliva
   + Heredity

II. Behavioral Risk Factors
   + Personal oral hygiene
   + Dietary Practices
   + Socio-cultural beliefs, attitudes
   + Psychological status
   + Patterns of Dental Care Utilization

III. Intrinsic Risk Factors
   + Sociodemographic
   + Environmental
   + General Health
   + Dexterity
   + Oral Health, including status of dental restorations

Katz, 1982; Meyerowitz *et al.*, 1991). As reported previously, a major reason for this is the prolonged retention time of fluoride in the mouth when the diluting and clearing properties of saliva are absent (Billings *et al.*, 1988). Thus, while the near complete absence of saliva can be isolated as a dominant risk factor in the development of rampant caries in xerostomic individuals, the equation can be balanced and hence the risk profile altered by the protective benefits of fluoride and this rather neatly exemplifies the types of problems encountered in establishing risk profiles, especially for individuals. The role of less than catastrophic cases of hyposalivation in the development of caries risk profiles remains to be elucidated.

Ongoing and Future Studies

Work on the relationship between salivary factors and caries experience is continuing, with three major studies being conducted by researchers in Rochester. First, the methodology of the aforementioned cross-sectional adult survey has been incorporated into a large-scale longitudinal epidemiologic study of middle-age and elderly adults (age 55 and over). A serious limitation of cross-sectional studies attempting to assess the relationship of saliva flow to dental caries is the unknown temporal relationship between flow rates at the time of the study and flow rates during the period of caries development. The longitudinal nature of the current study will permit investigators to observe changes in salivary gland function which may be related to dental caries susceptibility. In a second study, on caries risk assessment in children, the possible role of salivary factors in assessing the risk of future caries onset is being investigated. Finally, a Cariology Center study is attempting to identify salivary factors responsible for pH regulation in plaque among fully-dentate caries-free adults over 55 years of age. This latter study may contribute to understanding the relationship of host resistance to dental caries and may provide a genetic basis which, in combination with local factors such as fluoride levels and microbial profiles, would aid in the identification of individuals at high risk for dental caries prior to the onset of disease.

Mandel and Wotman (1976) have ascribed four theoretical mechanisms by which saliva can affect dental caries: 1) mechanical cleansing of debris and bacteria from tooth surfaces, 2) enhancement of remineralization and inhibition of demineralization, 3) buffering and neutralization of plaque acids, and 4) antibacterial activity against oral microflora. The explicit influence of saliva on the risk of developing caries, whether primary, secondary, or recurrent, remains to be determined. The concentration of many salivary constituents is affected by significant perturbations in flow (Mandel, 1980; Brown *et al.*, 1976; Dreizen *et al.*, 1976); yet, little information is available on how more subtle quantitative and qualitative shifts affect an individuals overall caries risk profile.

In conclusion, more knowledge about the kinds of issues described by Dawes concerning flow, and composition as described by Levine, Oppenheim and Tabak (this symposium) will need to be acquired before salivary factors can be optimally useful in caries risk assessment. As pointed out by Sweeney (1979) and again by Baum *et al.* (1985), mechanisms involved in salivary gland disturbances are still incompletely understood. Further investigations in this area are sorely needed. As also noted by Baum (1981) and reviewed by Beck and Hunt (1985), many methodologic issues related to the study of salivary function must be addressed and overcome. Frequently, clinical studies are so poorly designed and reported as to make meaningful interpretation of the data difficult or impossible. Standardized protocols for the collection and measurement of saliva flow need to be agreed upon and implemented. Known factors, such as the regular use of hyposalivation-inducing medications which have the potential to affect salivary function, must be considered in studies attempting to determine the relationship of salivary function to oral health and, in particular, dental caries. Both the intra- and inter-subject variation in response to medications with hyposalivation-inducing properties is profound. Data not yet completely analyzed from our earlier cross-sectional study on middle-age and elderly adults suggest that, on average, the community-dwelling elderly are much more tolerant of a dry mouth than younger community-dwelling individuals and are less likely to seek professional attention or relief. Coupled with the generally poorer oral hygiene and dietary practices of many elderly persons, the risk of dental caries would be expected to be higher than in younger-adult age groups. Epidemiologic studies on the complex dose-response relationship of hyposalivation-inducing medications to salivary function are needed and could ultimately provide much useful information to both scientists and clinicians.

These are but a few of the many questions remaining to be addressed. A number of additional recommendations for future research on the relationship of saliva to dental caries can be extrapolated from three recent publications: the collaborative NIDR, NIA, VA Research Agenda on Oral Health in the Elderly (1986), the proceeding from the North Carolina Risk Assessment Conference in Dentistry (1990), and the NIDR Long-Range Research Plan for the Nineties (1991).

REFERENCES

BAHN, S.L. (1972): Drug-Related Dental Destruction, *Oral Surg* 49-54.

BANTING, D.W. (1984): Dental Caries in the Elderly, *Gerodontology* 3:55-61.

BANTING, D.W. (1986): Epidemiology of Root Caries, *Gerodontology* 5:5-11.

BAUM, B.J. (1981): Evaluation of Stimulated Parotid Saliva Flow Rate in Different Age Groups, *J Dent Res* 60:1292-1296.

BAUM, B.J. (1986): Salivary Gland Function During Aging, *Gerodontics* 2:61-64.

BAUM, B.J. (1989): Salivary Gland Fluid Secretion During Aging, *JAGS* 37:453-458.

BAUM, B.J.; BODNER, L.; FOX, P.C.; IZUTSU, K.T.; PIZZO, P.A.; and WRIGHT, W.E. (1985): Therapy-Induced Dysfunction of Salivary Glands: Implications for Oral Health, *Spec Care Dentist* 274-277.

BECK, J.D. (1984): The Epidemiology of Dental Diseases in the Elderly, *Gerodontology* 3:5-15.

BECK, J.D. and HUNT, R.J. (1985): Oral Health Status in the United States: Problems of Special Patients, *J Dent Educ* 49:407-425.

BECK, J.D.; KOHOUT, F.; and HUNT, R.J. (1988): Identification of High Caries Risk Adults: Attitudes, Social Factors and Diseases, *Int Dent J* 38:231-238.

BEN-ARYEH, H.; GUTMAN, D.; SZARGEL, R.; and LAUFER, D. (1975): Effects of Irradiation on Saliva in Cancer Patients, *Int J Oral Surg* 4:205-210.

BERGMAN B. and ERICSON G. (1986): Cross-Sectional Study of Patients Treated with Removable Partial Dentures with Special Reference to the Caries Situation, *Scand J Dent Res* 94:436-442.

BERTRAM, U. (1967): Xerostomia: Clinical Aspects, Pathology and Pathogenesis, *Acta Odontol Scand* 49(Supp.):31-124.

BILLINGS, R.J.; MEYEROWITZ, C.; FEATHERSTONE, J.D.B.; ESPELAND, M.A.; FU, J.; COOPER, L.F.; and PROSKIN, H.M. (1988): Retention of Topical Fluoride in the Mouths of Xerostomic Subjects, *Caries Res* 33:306-310.

BROWN, L.R.; DREIZEN, S.; RIDER, L.J.; and JOHNSTON, D.A. (1976): The Effect of Radiation-Induced Xerostomia on Saliva and Serum Lysozyme and Immunoglobulin Levels, *Oral Surg* 41:83-92.

DAWES, C. (1987): Physiological Factors Affecting Salivary Flow Rate, Oral Sugar Clearance, and the Sensation of Dry Mouth in Man, *J Dent Res* 66:648-653.

DREIZEN, S. and BROWN, L.R. (1976): Xerostomia and Dental Caries, In: *Microbial Aspects of Dental Caries*, Vol. 1, H.M. Stiles, W.J. Loesche, T.C. O'Brien, Eds., Washington, D.C.: Information Retrieval Inc., 263-273.

DREIZEN, S.; BROWN, L.R.; HANDLER, S.; and LEVY, B.M. (1976): Radiation-Induced Xerostomia in Cancer Patients: Effect on Salivary and Serum Electrolytes, *Cancer* 38:273-278.

DREIZEN, S.; BROWN, L.R.; DALY, T.E.; and DRANE, J.B. (1977): Prevention of Xerostomia-Related Dental Caries in Irradiated Cancer Patients, *J Dent Res* 56:99-104.

FOX, P.C.; VAN DER VEN, P.F.; SONIES, B.C.; WEIFFENBACH, J.M.; and BAUM, B. J. (1985): Xerostomia: Evaluation of a Symptom with Increasing Significance, *JADA* 110:519-525.

FRANK, R.M.; HERDLEY, J.; and PHILIPPE, E. (1965): Acquired Dental Defects and Salivary Gland Lesions After Irradiation for Carcinoma, *JADA* 70:868-883.

FURE, S. and ZICKERT, I. (1990): Root Surface Caries and Associated Factors, *Scand J Dent Res* 98: 391-400.

GRAVES, R. C.; DISNEY, J.; STAMM, J. W.; ABERNATHY, J. R.; and BOHANNAN, H. M. (1990): Physical and Environmental Risk Factors in Dental Caries, In: *Risk Assessment in Dentistry*, J.D. Bader, Ed., Chapel Hill: University of North Carolina Dental Ecology.

HAND, J.S.; HUNT, R.J.; and BECK, J.D. (1988): Coronal and Root Caries in Older Iowans: 36-Month Incidence, *Gerodontics* 4:136-139.

HANDELMAN, S.L.; BARIC, J.M.; ESPELAND, M.A.; and BERGLUND, K.L. (1986): Prevalence of Drugs Causing Hyposalivation in an Institutionalized Geriatric Population, *Oral Surg Oral Med Oral Pathol* 62:26-31.

HANDELMAN, S.L.; BARIC, J.M.; SAUNDERS, R.H.; and ESPELAND, M.A. (1989): Hyposalivatory Drug Use, Whole Stimulated Salivary Flow, and Mouth Dryness in Older, Long-Term Care Residents, *Spec Care Dentist* 12-18.

HUNT, R. J. (1990): Behavioral and Sociodemographic Risk Factors for Caries, In: *Risk Assessment in Dentistry*, J.D. Bader, Ed., Chapel Hill: University of North Carolina *Dental Ecology.*

HUNTER, P.B. (1988): Risk Factors in Dental Caries, *Int Dent J* 38:211-217.

JOHNSON, G.; BARENTHIN, I.; and WESTPHAL, P. (1984): Mouthdryness Among Patients in Longterm Hospitals, *Gerodontology* 3:197-203.

KATZ, S. (1982): The Use of Fluoride and Chlorhexidine for the Prevention of Radiation Caries, *JADA* 104:164-170.

KINGMAN, A. (1990): Statistical Issues in Risk Models for Caries, In: *Risk Assessment in Dentistry*, J.D. Bader, Ed., Chapel Hill: University of North Carolina Dental Ecology.

KITAMURA, M.; KIYAK, H.A.; and MULLIGAN, K. (1986): Predictors of Root Caries in the Elderly, *Community Dent Oral Epidemiol* 14:34-38.

KLOCK B.; SVANBERG M.; and PETERSSON L.G. (1990): Dental Caries, Mutans Streptococci, Lactobacilli, and Saliva Secretion Rate in Adults, *Community Dent Oral Epidemiol* 18: 249-252

KRASSE, B (1990): Microbiological and Salivary Risk Factors, In: *Risk Assessment in Dentistry*, J.D. Bader, Ed., Chapel Hill: University of North Carolina Dental Ecology, 51-61.

LEVY, S.M.; BAKER, K.A.; SEMLA, T.P.; and KOHOUT, F.J. (1988): Use of Medications with Dental Significance by a Non-Institutionalized Elderly Population, *Gerodontics* 4:119-125.

MALMSTRÖM, M.J.; SEGERBERT-KONTTINEN, M.; TUOMINEN, T.S.; HIETANEN, J.H.; WOLF, J.E.; SANE, J.I.; and KONTTINEN, Y.T. (1988): Xerostomia Due to Sjögren's Syndrome, *Scand J Rheumatology* 17:77-86.

MANDEL, I.D. (1974): Relation of Saliva and Plaque to Caries, *J Dent Res* 53:246-266.

MANDEL, I.D. (1980): Sialochemistry in Disease and Clinical Situations Affecting Salivary Glands, *CRC Crit Rev Clin Lab Sci* 12:321-366.

MANDEL, I.D. (1984): Oral Defenses and Disease: Salivary Gland Function, *Gerodontology*, 3:47-54.

MANDEL, I.D. (1989): The Role of Saliva in Maintaining Oral Homeostasis, *JADA* 119:298-304.

MANDEL, I.D. and WOTMAN, S. (1976): The Salivary Secretions in Health and Disease, *Oral Sci Rev* 8:25-47.

MEYEROWITZ, C.; FEATHERSTONE, J.D.B.; BILLINGS, R.J.; EISENBERG, A.D.; FU, J.; SHARIATI, M.; and ZERO, D.T. (1991): Use of an Intra-Oral Model to Evaluate 0.05% Sodium Fluoride Mouthrinse in Radiation-Induced Hyposalivation, *J Dent Res* 70:894-898.

NELSON, J.F.; BARNES, G.P.; TOLLEFSBOL, R.G.; and PARKER, W.A. (1987): Prevalence and Significance of Prescription Medication Usage Among Gerodontic Patients, *Gerodontology* 6:17-22.

PETERSEN, J.K. (1986): Xerostomia, *Scand J Rheumatology* 61:185-189.

RAVALD, N.; HAMP S-E; and BIRKHED D. (1986): Long-Term Evaluation of Root Surface Caries in Periodontally Treated Patients, *J Clin Periodontol* 13:758-767.

SCHUBERT, M.M. and IZUTSU, K.T. (1987): Iatrogenic Causes of Salivary Gland Dysfunction, *J Dent Res* 66:680-688.

SCULLY, C. (1986): Sjögren's Syndrome: Clinical and Laboratory Features, Immunopathogenesis, and Management, *Oral Surg Oral Med Oral Pathol* 62:510-523.

SHAPIRO, S.; AVERY, K.T.; and CARPENTER, R.D. (1986): Drug Utilization by a Non-Institutionalized Ambulatory Elderly Population, *Gerodontics* 2:99-103.

SHIP, J.A.; FOX, P.C.; and BAUM, B.S. (1991): How Much Saliva is Enough? Normal Function Defined, *JADA* 122:63-69.

SÖDERHOLM, G. and BIRKHED, D. (1988): Caries Predicting Factors in Adult Patients Participating in a Dental Health Program, *Community Dent Oral Epidemiol* 16:374-377.

SWEENEY, E.A. (1979): Salivary Flow and Composition in Relation to Dental Caries - Methods and Problems in Studying this Relationship in Humans and Animals, Proceedings *Saliva and Dental Caries*, I. Kleinberg, S.A. Ellison, and I.D. Mandel, Eds., Sp. Supp. Microbiology Abstracts, pp. 183-190.

SREEBNY, L.M. (1989): Recognition and Treatment of Salivary Induced Conditions, *Int Dent J* 39:197-204.

SREEBNY, L.M. and SCHWARTZ, S.S. (1986): A Reference Guide to Drugs and Dry Mouth, *Gerodontology* 5:75-99.

THORSELIUS, I.; EMILSON, C.G.; and OSTERBERG, T. (1988): Salivary Conditions and Drug Consumption in Older Age Groups of Elderly Swedish Individuals, *Gerodontics* 4:66-70.

U.S. DEPARTMENT OF HEALTH AND HUMAN SERVICES, National Institute of Dental Research. NIDR Long-Range Research Plan for the Nineties. Bethesda, Md.: NIH, 1990. (NIH Publ. No. 90-1188).

UNIVERSITY OF NORTH CAROLINA - CHAPEL HILL, Department of Dental Ecology. Risk Assessment in Dentistry. Proceedings of a Conference at the University of North Carolina, Chapel Hill, held June 2-3, 1989. Chapel Hill: University of North Carolina Dental Ecology, 1990.

VETERANS ADMINISTRATION, Department of Medicine and Surgery. A Research Agenda on Oral Health in the Elderly. Washington, D.C.: Veterans Administration, 1986.

VISSINK, A.; PANDERS, A.K.; 'S-GRAVENMADE, E.J.; and VERMEY, A. (1988): The Causes and Consequences of Hyposalivation, *Ear, Nose and Throat J* 67:166-176.

WESCOTT, W.B.; STARCKE, E.N.; and SHANNON, I.L. (1975): Chemical Protection Against Postirradiation Dental Caries, *Oral Surg* 40:709-719.

Caries in Renal Dialysis Patients

CYRIL MEYEROWITZ

Much attention has been focused on the generation of acid in plaque, as a major etiological factor in dental caries. Less attention has been given to the formation of alkali, although it is frequently observed that plaque not exposed to sugar for more than 24 hours has a pH value as much as one unit higher than the surrounding saliva (Kleinberg and Jenkins, 1964). This section will cover the literature relating to caries experience in renal dialysis subjects. It will describe a clinical study on caries-related parameters in this population who have chronically elevated urea levels in serum and saliva.

Elevated urea levels are a consistent feature of chronic renal failure, a progressive loss of renal function. In this condition there is retention of the constituents normally excreted in the urine, for example urea, creatinine, uric acid and phosphorus among other substances. The most common causes of chronic renal failure are chronic glomerulonephritis, interstitial nephritis and diabetic glomerulosclerosis. (Kurtz and Johnson, 1984; Burton and Walls, 1987). Chronic renal failure in the United States is generally treated by life-long maintenance dialysis or renal transplantation. It affects approximately 10,000 to 15,000 new patients every year in the United States.

A number of investigators have described the oral features of patients with chronic renal failure who are undergoing dialysis. Prominent among these is low caries prevalence. Kirkpatrick and Morton (1971) examined nineteen patients on dialysis whose mean age was 35.8 years. They reported that these patients had a reduced mean number of decayed teeth, when compared with a control group, comprising routine plastic surgery cases (mean number of decayed teeth = 2.0 in the dialysis group vs. 2.6 in the control group). A low caries prevalence in 100 adult patients with chronic renal failure was reported by Mercer *et al.* (1973) and Renson and Mercer (1973). However, there was no control group for comparison, and no actual data on caries prevalence was provided in these abstracts. The dental condition of 52 children with chronic renal failure was compared to that of 52 children with normal renal function (Jaffee *et al.*, 1986). Caries prevalence was significantly less in the chronic renal failure group, DMFS = 2.71

(SD = 3.78) vs. 5.84 (SD = 4.53) than in the control group. These studies extend the case reports in the literature which described similar findings (Chow and Peterson, 1979; Woodhead *et al.*, 1982). It is clear that information comparing the prevalence of dental caries in adult patients with chronic renal failure to that of a matched control groups is very sparse.

The reported low caries prevalence in chronic renal failure subjects is surprising in view of their recommended dietary intake. These patients maintain an adequate caloric intake by increasing their carbohydrate consumption, often in the form of cakes, cookies and candy, which are recommended *ad libitum,* while limiting their intake of protein to reduce nitrogenous waste (Heard *et al.*, 1978; Chow and Peterson, 1979; Renson, 1986). In addition, a reduction in stimulated saliva flow rates has been reported in chronic renal failure patients (Epstein *et al.*, 1980). This reduction in saliva flow coupled with the increased consumption of fermentable carbohydrates could be expected to lead to an enhanced risk for caries development, however available evidence indicates that this does not occur (Kirkpatrick and Morton, 1971; Mercer *et al.*, 1973; Jaffee *et al.*, 1986).

The low caries prevalence observed has been attributed to the high salivary urea levels found in these subjects (Peterson *et al.*, 1985; Jaffee *et al.*, 1986). As Kleinberg and others have shown, the exposure of dental plaque to urea results in a rapid rise in pH due to the breakdown of urea to ammonia (Kleinberg, 1967; Singer and Kleinberg, 1983). The generation of ammonia, primarily from urea with contributions from arginine and proline peptides, may be an important factor in the pathogenesis of dental caries. (Kleinberg *et al.*, 1982; Peterson *et al.*, 1985; Curtis and Kemp, 1984). The effect of high salivary urea levels on plaque pH has been investigated in a clinical study of children with chronic renal failure (Peterson *et al.*, 1985). These investigators demonstrated that chronic renal failure subjects had significantly more alkaline baseline plaque pH values than controls; and, although the fall in number of pH units after exposure to carbohydrates did not differ, minimum pH in chronic renal failure subjects did not fall below values considered to be cariogenic levels (pH 5.5). It is unclear whether the differences in response can be attributed solely to enhanced buffering capacity, or a difference in the amount and type of acids produced, or major changes in plaque flora. Details available currently in studies on children is equivocal (MacFadyen *et al.*, 1984, 1985).

In addition to reductions in stimulated flow rates previously mentioned, the presence of high urea concentrations in whole and individual gland, stimulated and unstimulated salivary secretions from chronic renal failure subjects has been described (Shannon *et al.*, 1977; Epstein *et al.*, 1980; Shasha *et al.*, 1983). The ratio of parotid salivary urea levels to serum urea levels is approximately 0.66 with a near-perfect correlation (r = 0.97) (Shannon *et al.*, 1977).

Data presented by Peterson *et al.* (1985) suggests that the concentration of fluoride in ductal saliva may be increased in chronic renal failure subjects, although these authors do not comment on this finding or its implications. Persons with chronic renal failure excrete fluoride less efficiently than do patients with normal renal function (Spiers, 1981). The influence of this phenomenon on salivary fluoride and plaque levels has received scant attention.

We know that the composition of saliva can influence the ecology of the microflora and the biochemical activity of plaque. It has been suggested that the high salivary urea levels and resultant alkaline plaque influences plaque microflora and the metabolic activity (Kirkpatrick and Morton, 1971; Chow and Peterson, 1979; Peterson *et al.*, 1985). In this context it is of interest to observe that *S. sanguis* (Carlsson and Griffith, 1974; Cowman *et al.*, 1979) can use ammonia as a sole source of nitrogen.

The influence of rinsing with a urea-based solution for mineralizing early caries enamel lesions was studied by Pearce *et al.* (1983) and Gallagher *et al.* (1984). They observed that the members of the genera actinomyces, bifadabacterium, staphylococcus and streptococcus could breakdown urea. They reported no lasting effect on the flora following several days of rinsing with the urea-containing preparation. It was suggested that the urea did not remain in the mouth for a sufficient length of time to exert an ecological effect because it was rapidly metabolized. Elevated levels of calcium, phosphorus and fluoride in plaque were reported following this rinsing procedure. The influence of chronically elevated levels of salivary urea on the microbial composition of plaque has not been explored. The availability of a special population who have chronically elevated levels of salivary urea offers a unique opportunity to study the ecological pressure exerted by urea, a substance with major cariostatic potential.

In a clinical study conducted in Rochester, NY, it was hypothesized that prolonged elevations of salivary urea, as found in chronic renal failure subjects, affects the caries process and alters the oral environment. This chapter reports on the preliminary results of this study as related to the following specific aims:

1. Measuring salivary flow rates in patients with chronic renal failure and determining the concentration of urea, calcium, phosphorus and fluoride in the salivary secretions;
2. Determining the concentration of urea, ammonia, calcium phosphate and fluoride in the dental plaque of chronic renal failure subjects;
3. Determining the populations of *Streptococcus sanguis*, *Streptococcus mutans*, lactobacilli, enterobacteria, and urease-producing organisms in plaque and saliva from chronic renal failure subjects.

Urea, ammonia, calcium phosphate and fluoride in plaque and saliva were selected for study because of their influence on the onset and progress of caries. The organisms studied were selected either because of their association with the etiology of dental caries, or because of the expectation of seeing some of the ecological pressure being exerted by the chronically elevated levels of salivary urea.

Study Design

Subjects between the ages of 25 to 70 years were included in the study. The rationale for this is described below.

The hypothesis that the high urea levels found in chronic renal failure patients leads to a reduction in dental caries suggests that the longer the duration of renal failure the greater the impact on caries experience. Older subjects with a longer history of elevated urea levels, therefore, would be more likely to demonstrate a greater reduction in caries than would be observed in a younger population (except, of course, children of high caries attack years who are not represented in the population available). Based on our records we estimated that for subjects between the ages of 25 to 70 years the mean length of time from the onset of elevated serum urea levels to dialysis plus the time on dialysis is approximately 9 years. The onset of high urea levels is defined as two sequential serum urea levels which are greater than 40 mg % (normal values are 5-15 mg %). Subjects on dialysis are maintained with serum urea levels which are 3 to 5 times that found in the normal population.

Diabetic subjects were excluded from the study because diabetes affects salivary function (Harrison and Bowen, 1987), has extensive multisystem involvement, and greatly reduces life expectancy in these subjects (Hutchinson *et al.*, 1982). Similarly, subjects with diseases such as lupus erythematosis and amyloidosis, which have multi-system involvement, were excluded to allow for more accurate control group matching.

Subjects who had a course of antibiotics within the most recent two-month period were excluded due to the effect of antibiotics on plaque microflora.

The study design was cross sectional with paired matched controls. Each subject in the study population was matched with a control. Matching was done for: a) age (5 year spans); b) gender; c) race; d) minimum of 10 teeth and number of teeth plus or minus 25%; e) utilization of dental care (the frequency and nature of dental visit over the past years were determined, lifelong residency in a fluoridated community and use of fluoride products); f) number of antihypertensive medications.

Although important in the etiology of caries, we did not match for diet because of the great difficulty associated with taking accurate and meaningful diet histories and because it has been well documented by others and in our population that renal failure subjects consume large quantities of fermentable carbohydrates which would predispose to an increased caries attack. Any reductions in caries prevalence seen in the renal failure subjects will tend to be much more conservative had the groups been matched for dietary intake.

Clinical Examinations

All study subjects had plaque and saliva sampling done during the 30 minutes immediately preceding dialysis. All saliva collections were done over ice more than two hours after the last meal and standardized for the morning between 9:00 - 11:30 AM. The sequence of the examination was: 1) unstimulated whole saliva sample, 2) plaque sampling, 3) stimulated parotid sample.

Plaque Sampling

Three plaque samples were done in the following fashion:

a. Sample 1 was taken from the maxillary teeth close to the parotid duct. This sample was quick frozen in dry ice and transported to the lab for determination of ammonia and urea composition.
b. Sample 2 was taken similarly from a position close to the parotid duct and stored on ice for microbiological determination.
c. Sample 3 was a pooled plaque sample of greater than 2 mg and was used for calcium phosphate and fluoride determination.

Saliva Sampling

a. Whole Saliva Collection - The method described by Bertram (1967) was utilized. A 5 minute sample was taken and divided into three aliquots. Aliquot 1 and 2 were quick frozen in dry ice for ammonia and urea determination. Aliquot 3 was chilled and used for the microbiology, calcium, phosphate, and fluoride determinations.
b. Parotid Saliva Sample - Using modified Lashley cups (Curby, 1953) a stimulated sample using 2% citric acid applied to the lateral border of the tongue every 30 seconds was collected. The initial 2 minute sample was discarded and the following five minutes collected over ice and divided into three aliquots for ammonia, urea, calcium, phosphate, and fluoride determinations as done for the whole unstimulated saliva sample.

Laboratory Analysis

The concentration of urea, ammonia, calcium, phosphate and fluoride in plaque and salivary secretions was done in the laboratory using standardized techniques:

a. Fluoride was determined using the Taves diffusion technique and a fluoride reference electrode.

b. Urea concentration was determined using a colometric technique described by Crocker (1967) using a sigma-diagnostics blood, urea, nitrogen procedure #535.
c. Ammonia was done using an ammonia specific electrode Orion model 9512.
d. Calcium concentrations were determined by atomic absorption spectrophotometry.
e. Phosphate determination was done using an ammonium molybdate technique described by Hess and Durr 1975.

Microbiology

a. *Streptococcus mutans* - the population of these organisms was determined using the glucose - sucrose - potassium tellurite - bacitracin agar medium described by Tanzer *et al.*, 1984. Serotypes were identified using highly specific antisera used previously (Thompson *et al.*, 1980).
b. Total cultivable flora (TCF) - blood agar was inoculated and incubated anaerobically in gas packs.
c. *Streptococcus sanguis* populations were estimated on the high sucrose differential medium described by deStoppelaar *et al.*, 1969.
d. Lactobacillus populations were determined using Ragosa SL Agar.
e. Urea-producing organisms were estimated using a modification of Christensen (1946) (urea agar base).
f. Actinomyces populations were estimated on the selected medium described by Ellen and Balcorzak (1975).

Results

The results from 31 subjects on renal dialysis and 24 control subjects will be reported on this preliminary study. The gender distribution for the dialysis group was 19 males and 12 females, and 14 males and 10 females for the control group.

The mean age for the dialysis subjects was 48.7 years and 47.8 years for the controls. The mean years on dialysis for the experimental subjects was 6.2 years. The mean number of hyposalivatory drugs was 0.33 for the dialysis group and 0.21 for the control group.

Saliva Flow Rates

The table below depicts the salivary flow rates for unstimulated whole saliva flow and stimulated parotid flow. Renal dialysis subjects had significantly lower flow rates for unstimulated whole saliva and stimulated parotid flow than control subjects.

	Dialysis Mean (SD)	*Control Mean (SD)*	*P Value*
Unstimulated whole saliva flow mL/min	0.45 (0.34) n = 27	0.75 (0.53) n = 24	0.02
*Stimulated parotid flow mL/min	0.27 (0.18) n = 21	0.75 (0.56) n = 24	0.0005
*2% citric acid stimulation			

Saliva and Plaque Urea

The following table depicts the salivary and plaque urea concentrations in unstimulated whole saliva, stimulated parotid saliva, and plaque. Significantly higher concentrations of urea were found in unstimulated whole saliva and stimulated parotid saliva from dialysis subjects when compared with control subjects. The plaque urea concentration in renal dialysis subjects was significantly elevated. The concentration of urea in the plaque of control subjects was below the limits of detection.

	Dialysis Mean (SD)	*Control Mean (SD)*	*P Value*
Unstimulated whole saliva Urea mg/dl	46.70 (18.70) n = 25	3.72 (3.70) n = 24	> 0.00001
Stimulated parotid saliva Urea mg/dl	73.60 (26.40) n = 18	6.73 (5.00) n = 23	> 0.00001
Plaque Urea μg/mg	6.75 (16.80) n = 25	Not detected n = 22	

Saliva and Plaque Ammonia

The next table shows the saliva and plaque ammonia concentration in unstimulated whole saliva, stimulated parotid saliva, and plaque of renal dialysis and control subjects. Significantly higher concentrations of ammonia were found in the salivary secretions and plaque of the renal dialysis subjects as compared with the control subjects:

	Dialysis Mean (SD)	*Control Mean (SD)*	*P Value*
Unstimulated whole saliva NH_3 mg/dl	28.2 (22.40) n = 22	8.05 (12.70) n = 23	0.0005
Stimulated parotid saliva NH_3 mg/dl	5.93 (12.10) n = 19	3.11 (3.34) n = 22	0.02
Plaque NH_3 μg/mg	27.50 (4.04) n = 19	1.81 (1.93) n = 23	

Fluoride Analysis

The fluoride concentration in whole unstimulated saliva, parotid stimulated saliva, and plaque of renal dialysis subjects was significantly higher than that found in the control subjects:

	Dialysis Mean (SD)	*Control Mean (SD)*	*P Value*
Unstimulated whole saliva Fluoride μg/mL	0.17 (0.09) n = 23	0.08 (0.02) n = 22	0.0004
Stimulated parotid saliva μg/mL	0.12 (0.05) n = 16	0.05 (0.03) n = 22	0.000008
Plaque fluoride μg/g	19.60 (13.80) n = 26	12.50 (8.21) n = 23	0.03

Saliva and Plaque Calcium

The following table depicts the concentration of calcium in unstimulated whole saliva, stimulated parotid saliva and plaque of renal dialysis subjects and controls. The concentration of calcium in stimulated parotid saliva was significantly elevated in the renal dialysis subjects as compared with the control subjects:

	Dialysis Mean (SD)	*Control Mean (SD)*	*P Value*
Unstimulated whole saliva Ca mM/L	1.01 (0.29) n = 25	0.85 (0.35) n = 23	0.08
Stimulated parotid saliva Ca mM/L	0.71 (0.29) n = 16	0.53 (0.14) n = 23	0.01
Plaque Ca μg/mg	2.55 (2.42) n = 26	1.62 (2.32) n = 24	0.10

Saliva and Plaque Phosphate

Table 6 depicts the concentration of phosphate in unstimulated whole saliva, stimulated parotid saliva and plaque of renal dialysis subjects and controls. The concentration of phosphate was significantly higher in stimulated parotid saliva and plaque of renal dialysis subjects as compared to control subjects:

	Dialysis Mean (SD)	*Control Mean (SD)*	*P Value*
Unstimulated whole saliva PO_4 mM/L	5.50 (1.92) n = 25	5.03 (3.21) n = 24	0.5
Stimulated parotid saliva PO_4 mM/L	5.31 (2.53) n = 24	3.25 (0.85) n = 24	0.0005
Plaque PO_4 μg/mg	9.51 (7.30) n = 24	2.61 (1.96) n = 24	0.00005

Microbiology Data

The microbiology assessments of plaque and saliva for the renal dialysis (E) and control (C) subjects are shown below. These data are expressed as colony forming units (C.F.U.) × 10^6. In both saliva and plaque, *S. sanguis* counts were elevated in the renal dialysis subjects as compared with the control subjects. Dialysis subjects also had a greater number of urease positive organisms.

		Plaque			*Saliva*		
		Mean	*SD*	*%*	*Mean*	*SD*	*%*
TCF	C	37.5	34.3	100	250	327	100
	E	33.3	28.8	100	100	95	100
Lactobacillus	C	0.47	1.16	1.25	0.27	0.54	0.11
	E	0.99	4.52	2.97	0.25	0.42	0.25
S. sanguis	C	0.0075	0.0257	0.02	0.77	1.67	0.31
	E	0.259	1.06	0.77	1.63	3.54	1.63
A. viscosus	C	3.33	4.12	8.88	6.16	5.90	2.46
	E	1.59	1.89	4.77	2.0	2.2	2.0
S. mutans	C	0.616	1.04	1.64	0.41	0.66	0.16
	E	0.354	1.01	1.06	0.67	1.28	0.67
Urease	C		–			–	
	E		+			+	

Discussion

These preliminary results indicate that subjects with chronic renal failure have an interesting and unusual combination of factors that influence caries activity. Their high consumption of carbohydrates and diminished flow rates, as demonstrated in the study, would be expected to lead to a greater enhanced risk of caries. However, as these preliminary results demonstrate, they have high concentrations of salivary and plaque urea, ammonia, and fluoride, accompanied by increases in calcium and phosphate which would have a caries inhibiting effect. Completion of the study will provide data on coronal and root caries in dialysis subjects as compared with matched controls and on assessment of the ability of plaque from chronic renal failure patients to lower the pH value and sugar and determine the acid end-product. Further assessment of the ecology of the microflora will help to determine the influence of chronic exposure of urea on these organisms.

REFERENCES

BERTRAM, U. (1967): Xerostomia. Clinical Aspects, Pathology and Pathogenesis, *ACTA Odont Scand* 25:1-126.

BURTON, P.R. AND WALLS, J. (1987): Selection-adjusted Comparison of Life-expectancy of Patients on Continuous Ambulatory Peritoneal Dialysis, Haemodialysis, and Renal Transplantation, *Lancet* 1:1115-1119.

CARLSSON, J. and GRIFFITH, C.J. (1974): Fermentation Products and Bacterial Yields in Glucose-limited and Nitrogen-limited Cultures of Streptococci, *Arch Oral Biol* 19:1105-1109.

CHOW, M.H. and PETERSON, D.S. (1979): Dental Management for Children with Chronic Renal Failure Undergoing Hemodialysis Therapy, *Oral Surg Oral Med Oral Pathol* 48:34-38.

CHRISTENSEN, W.B. (1946): Urea Decomposition as a Means of Differentiating Proteus and Paracolon Cultures from Each Other and from Salmonella and Shigella types. *J Bacteriol* 52:461-466.

COWMAN, R.A.; SCHAEFER, S.J.; FITZGERALD, R.J.; ROSNER, D.; SHKLAIR, I.L.; and WALTER, R.G. (1979): Differential Utilization of Proteins in Saliva from Caries-active and Caries-free Subjects as Growth Substrates by Plaque-forming Streptococci, *J Dent Res* 58:2019-2027.

CROCKER, C.L. (1967): Rapid Determination of Urea Nitrogen in Serum of Plasma Without Deproteinization, *Amer J Med Techn* 33:361-365.

CURBY, W.A. (1953): Device for Collection of Human Parotid Saliva, *J Lab Clin Med* 41:493-496.

CURTIS, M.A. and KEMP, C.W. (1984): Nitrogen Metabolism in Dental Plaque. In: *Cariology 1983*, Cariology Today International Congress in Honor of Professor Dr. Hans R. Mehlemann, B. Guggenheim, Ed., Basel: Karger, pp. 212-222.

DE STOPPELAAR, J.D.; VAN HOUTE, J.; and DIRKS, O.B. (1969): The Relationship between Extracellular Polysaccharide-producing Streptococci and Smooth Surface-Caries in 13-Year-Old Children, *Caries Res* 3:190-199.

ELLEN, R.P. and BALCERZAK-RACZKOWSKI, I.B. (1975): Differential Medium for Detecting Dental Plaque Bacteria Resembling *Actinomyces viscosus* and *Actinomyces naeslundii*, *J Clin Microbiol* 2:305-310.

EPSTEIN, S.R.; MANDEL, I.; and SCOPP, I.W. (1980): Salivary Composition and Calculus Formation in Patients Undergoing Hemodialysis, *J Periodontol* 51: 336-338.

GALLAGHER, I.H.C.; PEARCE E.I.F.; and HANCOCK, E.M. (1984): The Ureolytic Microflora of Immature Dental Plaque Before and After Rinsing with a Urea-based Mineralizing Solution, *J Dent Res* 63:1037-1039.

HARRISON, R. and BOWEN, W.H. (1987): Flow Rate and Organic Constituents of Whole Saliva in Insulin-dependent Diabetic Children and Adolescents, *Pediatr Dent* 9:287-291.

HEARD, JR., E.; STAPLES, A.F.; and CZERWINSKI, A.W. (1978): The Dental Patient with Renal Disease: Precautions and Guidelines, *JADA* 96:792-796.

HESS, H.H. and DURR, J.E. (1975): Assay of Inorganic and Organic Phosphorus in the 0.1-5 Nanomole Range, *Anal Biochem* 63:607-613.

HUTCHINSON, T.A.; THOMAS, D.C.; and MACGIBBON, B. (1982): Predicting Survival in Adults with End-stage Renal Disease: An Age Equivalence Index, *Ann Intern Med* 96:417-423.

JAFFEE, E.C.; ROBERTS, G.J.; CHANTLER, C.; and CARTER, J.E. (1986): Dental Findings in Chronic Renal Failure, *Br Dent J* 160:18-20.

KIRKPATRICK, T.J. and MORTON, J.B. (1971): Factors Influencing the Dental Management of Renal Transplant and Dialysis Patients, *Br J Oral Surg* 9:57-64.

KLEINBERG, I. (1967): Effect of Urea Concentration on Human Plaque pH Levels *in situ*, *Arch Oral Biol* 12:1457-1484.

KLEINBERG, I. and JENKINS, G.N. (1964): The pH of Dental Plaques in the Different Areas of the Mouth Before and After Meals and Their Relationship to the pH and Rate of Flow of Resting Saliva, *Arch Oral Biol* 9:493-516.

KLEINBERG, I.; JENKINS, G.N.; CHATTERJEE, R.; and WIJEYEWEERA, L. (1982): The Antimony pH Electrode and Its Role in the Assessment and Interpretation of Dental Plaque pH, *J Dent Res* 61:1139-1147.

KURTZ, S.B. and JOHNSON, W.J. (1984): A Four-year Comparison of Continuous Ambulatory Peritoneal Dialysis and Home Hemodialysis: A Preliminary Report, *Mayo Clin Proc* 59:659-662.

MACFADYEN, E.E.; WEETMAN, D.A.; DUNN, M.F.; MURPHY, A.V.; BEATTIE, T.J.; and GEDDES, D.A.M. (1985): Dental Parameters of Children with Impaired Renal Function: Saliva and Plaque Constituents for Acid Base Balance, *Caries Res* 19:190-191, Abst. No. 110.

MACFADYEN, E.E.; WEETMAN, D.A.; MURPHY, A.V.; DUNN, M.F.; and GEDDES, D.A.M. (1984): Dental Status of Children Attending a Renal Unit, *J Dent Res* 63:507, Abst. No. 158.

MERCER, C.E. and RENSON, C.E. (1973): Routine Dental Treatment of Hemodialysis and Renal Transplant Patients, *J Dent Res* 52:965-966, Abst. No. 135.

PEARCE, E.I.F.; SCHAMSCHULA, R.G.; and COOPER, M.H. (1983): Increases in-Fluoride, Calcium, and Phosphate in Dental Plaque Resulting from the Use of a Mineralizing Mouthrinse Containing Urea and Monofluoraphosphate, *J Dent Res* 62:818-820.

PETERSON, S.; WOODHEAD, J.; and CRALL, J. (1985): Caries Resistance in Childrcn with Chronic Rcnal Failurc: Plaquc pH, Salivary pH, and Salivary Composition, *Pediatr Res* 19:796-799.

RENSON, C.E. (1986): letter to the editor, *Br Dent J* 160:187-188.

RENSON, C.E. and MERCER, C.E. (1973): Dental Needs of a Group of Hemodialysis and Renal Transplant Patients, *J Dent Res* 52:966, Abst. No. 136.

SHANNON, I.L.; FELLER, R.P.; EKNOYAN, G.; and SUDDICK, R.P. (1977): Human Parotid Saliva Urea in Renal Failure and During Dialysis, *Arch Oral Biol* 22:83-86.

SHASHA, S.M.; HANNA, B.A.; ANGEL, A.; and GUTMAN, D. (1983): Salivary Content in Hemodialysed Patients, *J Oral Med* 38:67-70.

SINGER, D.L. and KLEINBERG, I. (1983): Quantitative Assessment of Urea, Glucose and Ammonia Changes in Human Dental Plaque and Saliva Following Rinsing with Urea and Glucose, *Arch Oral Biol* 28:923-929.

SPIERS, R.L. (1981): Fluorides: Systemic Balance and Cariostatic Mechanisms. In: *Dental Caries: Aetiology, Pathology, and Prevention*, L.M. Silverstone, N.W. Johnson, J.M. Hardie, and R.A.D. Williams, Eds., London: Macmillan Press, Ltd., pp. 228-248.

TANZER, J.M.; BÖRJESSON, A.-C.; LASKOWSKI, L.; KURASZ, A.B.; and TESTA, M. (1984): Glucose-sucrose-potassium Tellurite-bacitracin Agar, an Alternative to Mitis Salivarius-bacitracin Agar for Enumeration of *Streptococcus mutans, J Clin Microbiol* 20:653-659.

THOMSON, L.A.; LITTLE, W.A.; BOWEN, W.H.; SIERRA, L.I.; AGUIRRER, M.; and GILLEPSIE, G. (1980): Prevalence of *Streptococcus mutans* Serotypes, *Actinomyces*, and Other Bacteria in the Plaque of Children, *J Dent Res* 59:1581-1589.

WOODHEAD, J.C.; NOWAK, A.J.; CRALL, J.J.; and ROBILLARD, J.E. (1982): Dental Abnormalities in Children with Chronic Renal Failure, *Pediatr Dent* 4:281-285.

Determinants of Virulence in Dental Plaque

J. van Houte

The problem of dental caries, a bacterial infectious disease, is a complex ecological one. Not surprisingly, diligent study over the years has identified a great variety of host- and environmental factors of potential influence on this disease. Rather than engaging in a broad discussion of these factors which has been done very ably by others (Mandel, 1979; Marsh, 1989), I will focus here on only a few of them. In this regard I will stay within close range of the dogma of dental caries etiology. Also, only coronal caries will be dealt with since determinants of root caries will be discussed by Dr. Ellen.

As depicted in a classic diagram by Keyes and Jordan (1963), the triad of factors indispensable for caries activity consists of the microbiota (dental plaque), the diet (carbohydrates) and the host and (susceptible) teeth; caries development requires the simultaneous presence of all three factors. This factorial triad identifies the bacterial flora of dental plaque as its most obvious determinant of virulence (cariogenicity). Here we encounter immediately a controversial issue in most quarters, namely the importance of the "mutans" streptococci as caries-etiologic agents. In my view the present state of knowledge permits only speculation about the true impact of these organisms on caries development in the human population.

The view of "mutans" streptococci as the most potent, the major, or perhaps the sole caries-etiologic agents is based on a now massive amount of information that has accumulated during the last 25 years. Most of our present knowledge pertains to *S. mutans* and *S. sobrinus* and much information has come from populations in which *S. mutans* greatly outnumbers *S. sobrinus* or other "mutans" streptococci; also, species have been differentiated in only a few studies although some important inter-species differences exist. We will use therefore, generally, the term "mutans" streptococci (MS) for the present discussion.

This study was supported by USPHS Research Grants DE-07009 and DE-07493 from the National Institute of Dental Research, National Institute of Health, Bethesda, MD 20892.

Evidence for the MS as caries-etiologic agents can be placed in three categories: (1) physiological cell traits, (2) cariogenic potential in experimental animals, and (3) association of oral cell numbers with caries. The positive correlation between the plaque levels of MS and coronal caries development is well established; plaque in caries-free subjects contains often only low, or sometimes undetectable, levels of MS whereas in caries-positive subjects the MS are often more widespread in plaque (more "infected sites") and in higher proportions (of the total flora); they are also often more numerous in caries-associated plaque or in caries lesions than in plaque associated with the clinically-sound enamel surface (Hamada and Slade, 1980; van Houte, 1980; Loesche, 1986). This emergence of the MS in plaque,i.e., the proliferation of cells attached to the tooth surface to significant proportions, appears to require dietary carbohydrate; access to host-derived energy sources appears to be limited for these organisms and in animals or humans their prolonged maintainance in other than small numbers requires dietary carbohydrate (de Stoppelaar *et al.*, 1970; Cornick and Bowen, 1972). It is an important fact that because caries development and the emergence of the MS require both dietary carbohydrate, they are unavoidably linked. Animal studies have also established the high cariogenic potential of the MS which is of a multi-surface nature when the diet contains sucrose (Tanzer, 1989). For caries development in humans, therefore, MS can be considered as a (very sensitive) indicator (Krasse, 1985) as well as a perpetrator. An extreme example of this is "nursing bottle caries," a form of rampant caries affecting particularly the upper front teeth, which results from a high-frequency exposure to carbohydrate; this disease is associated with plaque with extremely high or sometimes "pure cultures" of MS (van Houte *et al.*, 1982).

Two prominent putative cariogenic determinants of the MS that must be considered in relation to their emergence in plaque are the sucrose-mediated synthesis of extracellular glucans and the tolerance to an acidic plaque pH. The view of sucrose as the "arch criminal" of caries shortly after the re-discovery of "*S. mutans*" in the mid-1960's (Newbrun, 1967) was predicated upon the uniqueness of sucrose as a substrate for extracellular glucan synthesis rather than the prominence of its consumption among the common dietary carbohydrates. In spite of much study, however, I do not think that we have resolved the critical issue of the unique role of sucrose in human caries development as mediated by extracellular glucan; clarification of the mechanisms by which glucan may exert its effect is also needed.

Since the establishment of the link between sucrose-mediated glucan synthesis and plaque formation by MS in rodents (Krasse *et al.*, 1967), studies of the significance of glucan have focused primarily on its effect on the colonization of these organisms on the teeth. Soon thereafter it was recognized also that glucans can form a major component of the structural interbacterial matrix of plaque (Guggenheim, 1970) and it was postulated that insoluble glucan in plaque could constitute a barrier to the outward diffusion of bacterial acids formed in plaque and, hence, could enhance plaque's acidity and cariogenic potential (McNee *et al.*, 1982).

In evaluating the effect of glucan on tooth surface colonization, plaque formation by and plaque proportions of MS should be considered separately. In rodents, voluminous plaque formation on smooth tooth surfaces, necessary for caries induction on these surfaces, is associated specifically with sucrose as a substrate (Tanzer, 1989); the same may be true for smooth tooth surfaces in humans (Carlsson, 1967; Carlsson and Sundstrom, 1968). For human tooth fissures, however, which are most prone to caries, the situation is much less clear. The results from studies of the cariogenicity or the colonization of MS in fissures of glucose- and sucrose-fed rats are equivocal (van Houte and Russo, 1986a). However, effective colonization of these organisms in fissures of glucose-fed rats does clearly occur. Such colonization is not due to mechanical cell entrapment. This is indicated, for example, by the widely-varying colonization ability among strains of non-mutans streptococci in molar fissures of sucrose-fed germ-free rats (Drucker *et al.*, 1984; van Houte and Russo, 1986b). Evidence suggests also that *S. mutans* can initially adhere to and persist on the tooth pellicle, or even reach plaque proportions of 1% or more under conditions that appear not to involve glucan; this may not be the case for *S. sobrinus* which appears, more than *S. mutans*, to be dependent on adhesive interactions involving glucan (Carlsson, 1967; de Stoppelaar *et al.*, 1970; Gibbons *et al.*, 1986; Schilling *et al.*, 1989).

By promoting voluminous plaque formation, glucan synthesis may increase the total numbers of MS per given tooth surface area but this is not accompanied necessarily by an increase of their proportions in the more voluminous plaque mass (Carlson, 1967). The question may be raised as to how cell-associated or cell-free enzymatic synthesis of glucan, short of toxic effects on other bacteria, could lead to the conquest of a major part of the plaque territory by the MS. Such predominance could also, or instead, be associated with one of their other traits, their acid tolerance, i.e. their capacity for survival, growth and adaptation as well as acidogenesis in an acidic milieu (Carlsson, 1989). Frequent consumption of carbohydrates, conducive to caries development as well as the emergence of the MS, may provide these highly acid-tolerant organisms with a selective advantage over most of the other less acid-tolerant microflora when the plaque milieu is frequently acidified (van Houte, 1980; Denepitiya and Kleinberg, 1984; Loesche, 1986; van Houte and Russo, 1986a). According to this concept, the essential condition for the emergence of the MS is not dietary sucrose or carbohydrate availability *per se*, but frequently-recurring acidic episodes in dental plaque that accompany frequent carbohydrate consumption. Direct support for this concept exists (Svanberg, 1980; Bradshaw *et al.*, 1989).

Evidence suggesting that extracellular glucan can affect plaque's cariogenic potential as an acid diffusion-limiting matrix component has been reported

(Hojo *et al.*, 1976; Taubman *et al.*, 1983). However, other studies with human plaque or pure cell masses of *Streptococcus sanguis* or *S. mutans* and diffusants such as sucrose, sorbitol or acetate have not revealed a special diffusion-limiting property of bacterial extracellular glucan (McNee *et al.*, 1982; Dibdin *et al.*, 1983; Tatevossian, 1985). Other recent studies with cell masses of MS with varying cell density and volume of glucan-containing interbacterial matrix space do suggest that glucans in plaque may enhance its acidity and cariogenicity but by a different process (Zero *et al.*, 1986; Dibdin and Shellis, 1988; van Houte *et al.*, 1989). Cell masses of MS with a high glucan content are of low cell density with cells widely apart (van Houte *et al.*, 1989); such glucan-mediated cell spacing can also occur in plaque *in vivo* in rats (van der Hoeven, 1974) as well as in humans (Carlsson and Sundstrom, 1968). In one study with an intra-oral enamel demineralization model (Brudevold *et al.*, 1984) subjects carried a palatal appliance with blocks of bovine enamel which were covered by a cell mass of MS; an increased volume of the glucan-rich matrix space was associated with a prolonged depression of the cell mass pH and increased enamel demineralization after a rinse with glucose solution (Zero *et al.*, 1986). In another, *in vitro,* study, pH profiles of different cell masses were determined with a model which permits vertical penetration of peripherally-applied glucose through the cell mass and pH evaluation at different depths within the cell mass; an increased volume of the glucan-rich matrix was associated with an earlier initiation and an increased rate of pH drop in the cell mass depth; the glucose supply to the cells in the cell masses with negligible glucan and high cell density in particular appeared to be restricted severely for an increase in the glucose concentration enhanced the onset and rate of the pH drop (van Houte *et al.*, 1989). Evaluation in this and another *in vitro* study (Dibdin and Shellis, 1988) of low and high-glucan cell masses with respect to factors such as diffusion, buffering capacity, extracellular fluid volume fraction and porosity suggests that the enhanced glucan-associated pH drop in cell masses is based on two key factors. First, glucan-associated enhanced spacing of cells causes a greater porosity of the cell mass due to the lower organic density of the matrix content relative to that of the cells. Second, the carbohydrate supply to the cells in the cell masses is generally restricted and allows acidogenesis only at a rate below maximum velocity. However, an increase of the matrix volume by glucan allows a higher amount of glucose to pass through. This leads to a higher bacterial acid production rate, a quicker penetration of glucose deeper in the cell mass and an enhanced pH drop in the peripheral as well as deeper cell mass regions. This concept is supported further by recent studies with the intra-oral Brudevold model (Fu *et al.*, 1990; 1991).

Collectively, the above considerations suggest at least three different ways in which sucrose-mediated glucan synthesis may promote caries development. Voluminous plaque induction as well as a glucan-enriched plaque matrix may particularly play a role on smooth tooth surfaces; the effect in fissures may be much less or only on the location of caries development. Further study of the *in vivo* significance of both aspects as well as the mechanisms involved appears desirable. It should be noted that other plaque bacteria besides the MS can produce glucan or other extracellular polymers (Birkhed *et al.*, 1979; van Houte, 1983). In principle, effects of the plaque matrix can be mediated by a variety of host-derived and bacterial products. The issue of a specific effect of glucan on the plaque proportions of MS appears also to require further study.

Any theory of dental caries etiology must reckon with the classic finding of Stephan (1944) concerning the pH response of dental plaque to brief sugar exposure. Stephan showed that this response *in vivo* has a typical profile consisting of a rapid decrease of the pH from the initial "resting" level to a minimum and a slower return of the pH to the initial level. He demonstrated also that the pH range in which this profile is located becomes increasingly lower with increasing caries activity. Over the years it has become clear that host factors such as saliva can have a major effect on the plaque pH profile in humans (Jenkins, 1979). However, different plaque pH responses during a short "Stephan" test may not be due only to a varying local effect of saliva. For example, the plaque pH profile in rodents can be manipulated readily by the mere oral implantation of different acidogenic plaque-forming test organisms (Charlton *et al.*, 1971). Similarly, the *in vitro* pH response of human plaque from different sources to sugar shows wide variation of the pH drop rate and pH minimum reached; under the conditions employed this response reflects essentially the capacity of the microbiota for acidogenesis and acid tolerance and the buffering capacity of the plaque (Igarashi *et al.*, 1987; van Houte *et al.*, 1991a).

The evidence now available suggests instead that the pH response and cariogenicity of human plaque is determined fundamentally by its microbial composition and that not all plaques possess a sufficient pH-lowering capacity for caries induction (van Houte, 1980; Loesche, 1986). Consequently, a shift in plaque flora composition is prerequisite for a change in plaque's pH-lowering capacity. As a framework for further study of core issues, it may be postulated further that the acid tolerance of the bacterial flora functions in this respect as a crucial determinant. Thus, the acid production rate at acidic plaque pH values is a direct function of bacterial acid tolerance; the lowest pH that can be reached in plaque is therefore a function of those acidogenic organisms with the highest acid tolerance. From a mechanistic standpoint the caries process may be formulated as a dietary carbohydrate-modified bacterial infectious disease. More frequent carbohydrate consumption causes a chain reaction involving a more frequent plaque acidification, and in turn a shift towards higher proportions of more acid-tolerant organisms; the latter, in turn, cause an increase of plaque's acid production capacity at acidic pH values and thus a lowering of the potential pH minimum; this, in turn, increases the probability of a net loss of tooth mineral over time. This process may progressively increase, level off, or reverse itself depending on the level of carbohydrate consumption (van Houte, 1980).

At present, the only plaque organisms that appear to fit well in the above scenario are the MS and the acidogenic, highly acid-tolerant lactobacilli which exhibit, likewise, a dependency on dietary carbohydrate for their oral colonization as well as a positive correlation with caries activity (van Houte, 1980). The demise of the lactobacilli as major caries-etiologic agents in the 1950's reflects essentially their generally low prevalence and concentration in caries-associated plaque. Identification of the cariogenic plaque bacteria presents great difficulties for various reasons. A foremost one is that plaque bacteria form a high-low hierarchy regarding many putative cariogenic traits including acidogenesis, acid tolerance, extra- and intracellular polymer synthesis, and so on (Tanzer, 1989); MS may only possess top hierarchical status with respect to these traits. Also, other factors besides plaque can affect caries activity, whereas plaques with a varying flora and acidogenic potential can induce caries at different rates (the factor time).

Nevertheless, mounting evidence indicates that besides the MS other plaque organisms may play a role in caries development. There is now more than anecdotal evidence that human caries activity can be associated with plaque in which MS are either undetectable or present in small proportions (de Stoppelaar *et al.*, 1969; Boyar *et al.*, 1989; Marsh *et al.*, 1989; MacPherson *et al.*, 1990). Also, a variety of plaque bacteria, notably many strains of the so numerous non-mutans streptococci, exhibit considerable cariogenic potential in experimental animals (Willcox *et al.*, 1990).

In past studies of this heterogeneous group of predominant non-mutans streptococci, divided often conveniently in *S. sanguis* and *S. mitis* or "other streptococci," no positive correlation with caries was observed for any of the "species" or group (Loesche, 1986). This finding was co-responsible for the view that among the streptococcal flora only the MS merit serious consideration as caries-etiologic agents. It should be noted that all these correlation studies were based on colonial morphology of the organisms on growth agar plates as a means of their identification rather than on their more caries-relevant acidogenic properties. Recently, final pH in sugar broth was used as a selection criterion instead. In this manner, a segment of the non-mutans streptococci in human plaque, capable of acidogenesis at a low pH, could be readily identified (van Houte *et al.*, 1991b; van Houte, unpublished). Strains in this segment yield a final pH in Phenol Red Dextrose Broth between 4.05 and 4.4 with about one-half of the strains yielding a pH below 4.2; by comparison strains of S. mutans yield a final pH between 3.95 and 4.10. Strains in this segment (final pH below 4.4) are very numerous in plaque and outnumber the MS, even in the case of caries-associated plaque, by a wide margin until the levels of the MS reach about 5% or higher. The plaque levels of these non-mutans streptococci are lower in plaque from caries-free than in plaque from caries-positive subjects and their levels in plaque exhibit also a positive correlation with its pH-lowering potential *in vitro*. These correlations do not exist for the total of the non-mutans streptococci (final pH range between 4.05 and above 5.0). Consequently, increased pH-lowering ability of plaque and caries-conducive conditions are correlated with a shift among the non-mutans streptococci towards strains with a low final pH. These findings strengthen further the earlier-noted link between the acid tolerance of the plaque flora and plaque's pH-lowering and cariogenic potential. In view of the difficulties with the taxonomy of oral streptococci, the identity of the strains with a low final pH is presently unclear.

Non-mutans streptococci with a low final pH can be considered as a second-echelon category of potentially-cariogenic plaque organisms. The issue of the caries-etiologic role of MS has two distinct aspects. The first is their contribution normally during caries development. The second is the effect of their elimination from plaque on caries development with all other conditions remaining the same. Based on their acidogenic properties and demonstrated cariogenic potential, it seems not unreasonable to suppose that the second-echelon non-mutans streptococci could contribute substantially to caries development particularly when the MS have not attained great numerical predominance in plaque. If the MS were eliminated from plaque, the non-mutans streptococci could be similarly responsible for caries development, albeit at a lower rate perhaps, particularly, if their further emergence in plaque would be facilitated by the absence of the MS.

A cardinal feature of dental caries is that it is highly localized. Preferentially-affected dentition sites include deep fissures, pits, grooves, and areas in-between the teeth. These have been considered traditionally as locations where, more than in others, effective plaque build-up and prolonged exposure to dietary carbohydrate can occur. The localization of caries can also be readily observed on smooth tooth surfaces; in areas near the gingival margin an area may be carious whereas the area right next to it on the same surface is sound; moreover, the carious and sound areas may be both covered with plaque (Duchin and van Houte, 1978). If caries is highly localized and correlated specifically with elevated MS levels, the earlier discussed link between caries activity, emergence of MS and dietary carbohydrate exposure would suggest also a higher exposure of carious than of sound tooth surface areas to carbohydrate. It appears, however, that recognition of this possibility, although obvious for the whole dentition of caries-free and caries-active subjects, has been much less obvious for carious and sound areas in the same dentition. In fact, as mentioned earlier, similarity between carious and sound tooth surface areas with respect to plaque organisms such as *S. sanguis* or *S. mitis* has been interpreted generally as indicating their lack of involvement in caries development; this interpretation implies that all other (local) conditions affecting both types of areas are considered to be similar. If this were the case, this would disconnect the conditions for carbohydrate exposure and the emergence of MS; this may be true for caries development in absence of significant MS levels.

The possibility that, instead, the locally-prevailing environment of carious and sound tooth surface areas is significantly different is a highly plausible one. Each tooth surface area can then be viewed as a unique entity with respect to the determinants of caries. This concept finds support in the past and recent literature on the role of saliva in caries etiology. Thus, the potential major effect of saliva on the bacterial composition, pH profile and cariogenic potential of plaque has been long recognized (Jenkins, 1979; McNamara *et al.*, 1979; Kleinberg *et al.*, 1982). An example of this is the lower anterior dentition area. When compared to other dentition areas it is characterized by: (1) a relatively high salivary exposure of, particularly, the lingual tooth surfaces due to the proximity of the orifices of the submandibular/ sublingual glands, (2) a relatively low pH-lowering potential of plaque (Kleinberg and Jenkins, 1964; Kleinberg *et al.*, 1982), (3) relatively low levels of MS and non-mutans streptococci capable of acidogenesis at low pH (Keene *et al.*, 1981, 1990; Lindquist and Emilson, 1990, van Houte *et al.*, 1991b) and, (4) a relatively low level of caries activity (Backer-Dirks, 1961; Carlos and Gittelsohn, 1965).

Studies with markers such as fluoride ion, KCl, glucose and sucrose suggest further that salivary clearance varies markedly within the mouth e.g., tongue versus vestibulum or anterior versus posterior part as well as in different local sites within the dentition (Kellaway, 1960; Goulet *et al.*, 1985; Briste and Lagerlof, 1987; Weatherell *et al.*, 1988; Dawes and Weatherell, 1990; Disabato-Mordarski *et al.*, 1991). Local differences in salivary flow rate, translated into a varying velocity by which the salivary film which covers the plaque periphery is replaced (Dawes, 1989; Dawes *et al.*, 1989), may manifest themselves in local differences with respect to the exposure of plaque to carbohydrate (Sundstrom, 1979) and to salivary buffers and salivary substrates for base production (Wijeyeweera and Kleinberg, 1989), as well as the clearance from plaque of different products such as acids. These differences may be related to factors such as the location of the salivary ducts, the salivary secretion rate, the anatomy of the mouth, the movement of the oral musculature, shape and size of spaces (fissures, interdental), and so on. Studies of the site- and subject-specificity of salivary clearance and its relation to the triad of factors indispensible for caries development may help to formulate more precisely what is meant by the description of fissures, for example, as "retentive," "stagnant," or "sheltered from oral cleansing forces." Finally, in the case of the lower anterior dentition area, it is tempting to include the effect of saliva in the earlier-described framework of caries as a dietary-modified bacterial infectious disease in a commanding role as a modifyer of plaque's exposure to dietary carbohydrate, plaque's bacterial composition and its pH-lowering and cariogenic potential; and, to extend this concept to caries development or the absence thereof in other parts of the dentition as well.

REFERENCES

BACKER DIRKS, O. (1961): Longitudinal Dental Caries Study in Children 9-15 Years of Age, *Arch Oral Biol* 6:94-108.

BIRKHED, D.; ROSELL, K.G.; and BOWDEN, G.H. (1979): Structure of Extracellular Polysaccharides Synthesized from Sucrose by *Neisseria* Isolated from Human Dental Plaque, *Arch Oral Biol* 24:63-66.

BOYAR, R.M.; THYLSTRUP, A.; HOLMEN, L.; and BOWDEN, G.H. (1989): The Microflora Associated with the Development of Initial Enamel Decalcification Below Orthodontic Bands *in vivo* in Children Living in a Fluoridated-water Area, *J Dent Res* 68:1734-1738.

BRADSHAW, D.J.; McKEE, A.S.; and MARSH, P.D. (1989): Effects of Carbohydrate Pulses and pH on Population Shifts Within Oral Microbial Communities *in vitro*, *J Dent Res* 68:1298-1302.

BRISTE, A. and LAGERLOF, F. (1987): The Diluting Effect of Saliva on the Sucrose Concentration in Different Parts of the Human Mouth After a Mouth-Rinse with Sucrose, *Arch Oral Biol* 32:755-756.

BRUDEVOLD, F.; ATTARZADEH, F.; TEHRANI, A.; VAN HOUTE, J.; and RUSSO, J. (1984): Development of a New Intraoral Demineralization Test, *Caries Res* 18:421-429.

CARLOS, J.P. and GITTELSOHN, A.M. (1965): Longitudinal Studies of the Natural History of Caries, *Arch Oral Biol* 10:739-751.

CARLSSON, J. (1967): Presence of Various Types of Non-haemolytic Streptococci in Dental Plaque and in Other Sites of the Oral Cavity in Man, *Odont Rev* 18:55-74.

CARLSSON, J. and SUNDSTROM, B. (1968): Variations in Composition of Early Dental Plaque Following Ingestion of Sucrose and Glucose, *Odont Rev* 19:161-169.

CARLSSON, J. (1989): Microbial Aspects of Frequent Intake of Products with High Sugar Concentrations, *Scand J Dent Res* 97:110-114.

CHARLTON, G.; FITZGERALD, D.B.; and KEYES, P.H. (1971): Hydrogen Ion Activity in Dental Plaques of Hamsters During Metabolism of Sucrose, Glucose and Fructose, *Arch Oral Biol* 16:655-661.

CORNICK, D.E.R. and BOWEN, W.H. (1972): The Effect of Sorbitol on the Microbiology of the Dental Plaque in Monkeys (Macaca Irus), *Arch Oral Biol* 17:1637-1648.

DAWES, C. (1989): An Analysis of Factors Influencing Diffusion from Dental Plaque into a Moving Film of Saliva and the Implications for Caries, *J Dent Res* 11:1483-1488.

DAWES, C.; WATANABE, S.; BIGLOW-LECOMTE, P.; and DIBDIN, G.H. (1989): Estimation of the Velocity of the Salivary Film at Some Different Locations in the Mouth, *J Dent Res* 68:1479-1482.

DAWES, C. and WEATHERELL, J.A. (1990): Kinetics of Fluoride in the Oral Fluids, *J Dent Res* 69(Spec Iss):638-644.

DENEPITIYA, L. and KLEINBERG, I. (1984): A Comparison of the Acid-base and Aciduric Properties of Various Serotypes of the Bacterium Streptococcus mutans Associated with Dental Plaque, *Arch Oral Biol* 29:385-393.

De STOPPELAAR, J.D.; VAN HOUTE, J.; and BACKER DIRKS, O. (1969): The Relationship Between Extracellular Polysaccharide-Producing Streptococci and Smooth Surface Caries in 13-Year-Old Children, *Caries Res* 3:190-199.

De STOPPELAAR, J.D.; VAN HOUTE, J.; and BACKER DIRKS, O. (1970): The Effect of Carbohydrate Restriction on the Presence of *Streptococcus mutans*, *Streptococcus sanguis* and Iodophilic Polysaccharide-Producing Bacteria in Human Dental Plaque, *Caries Res* 4:114-123.

DIBDIN, G.H.; WILSON, C.M.; and SHELLIS, R.P. (1983): Effect of Packing Density and Polysaccharide to Protein Ratio of Plaque Samples Cultured *in vitro* Upon Their Permeability, *Caries Res* 17:52-58.

DIBDIN, G.H. and SHELLIS, R.P. (1988): Physical and Biochemical Studies of *Streptococcus mutans* Sediments Suggest New Factors Linking the Cariogenicity of Plaque with Its Extracellular Polysaccharide Content, *J Dent Res* 67:890-895.

DISABATO-MORDARSKI, T.;WOLFF, M.; and KLEINBERG, I. (1991): Saliva Changes in Embrasures in Different Regions of the Human Dentition During the Swallowing Cycle. *J Dent Res* (Spec.Iss) 70:406, Abst 1122.

DUCHIN, S. and VAN HOUTE, J. (1978): Relationship of *Streptococcus mutans* and Lactobacilli to Incipient Smooth Surface Dental Caries in Man, *Arch Oral Biol* 23:779-798.

DRUCKER, D.B.; SHAKESPEARE, A.P.; and GREEN, R.M. (1984): *In vivo* Dental Plaque-Forming Ability and Relative Cariogenicity of the Bacteria *Streptococcus mitis* and *Streptococcus sanguis* I and II in Mono-Infected Gnotobiotic Rats, *Arch Oral Biol* 29:1023-1031.

FU, J.; ZERO, D.T.; DASS, A.; ANNE, K.M.; and CAVARETTA, G.M. (1990): Effect of Plaque Thickness on Acid Production, *J Dent Res* 69:318 Abst. 1677.

FU, J.; ZERO, D.T.; ANNE, K.M.; and DASS. A. (1991): Effect of Plaque Thickness on Glucose Retention and Acid Production, *J Dent Res* 70:493, Abst. 1815.

GIBBONS, R.J.; COHEN, L. and HAY, D.I. (1986): Strains of *Streptococcus mutans* and *Streptococcus sobrinus* Attach to Different Pellicle Receptors, *Infect Immun* 52:555-561.

GOULET, D.; BRUDEVOLD, F.; TEHRANI, A.; and ATTARZADEH, F. (1985): Sugar Clearance from Saliva and Intra-oral Spaces, *J Dent Res* 64:411-415.

GUGGENHEIM, B. (1970): Extracellular Polysaccharides and Microbial Plaque, *Intern Dent J* 20:657-678.

HAMADA, S. and SLADE, H.D. (1980): Biology, Immunology and Cariogenicity of *Streptococcus mutans*, *Microbiol Rev* 44:331-384.

HOJO, S.; HIGUCHI, M.; and ARAYA, S. (1976): Glucan Inhibition of Diffusion in Plaque. *J Dent Res* 55:169.

IGARASHI, K.; HAMADA, Y.; NISHIMAKI, H.; SAKURAI, S.; and KAMIYAMA, K. (1987): The acidogenic Potential of Plaque from Sound Enamel, White Spot Lesions, and Cavities in Children, *Pediat Dentristry* 9:212-215.

JENKINS, G.N. (1979): Salivary Effects on Plaque pH. In: *Saliva and Dental Caries*, I. Kleinberg,S.A. Ellison, I.D. Mandel, Eds., New York, Information Retrieval, Inc., pp. 307-322.

KEENE, H.J.; HORTON, I.M.; and HANDLER, S.F. (1981): *Streptococcus mutans* Approximal Plaque Index as a New Epidemiologic Tool for Defining the Parameters of *Streptococcus mutans* Infection in Human Populations, *Arch Oral Biol* 26:345-355.

KEENE, H.J.; FOLSOM, K.S.; BASEL, D.A.; and PUENTE, E.S. (1990): Primary Reservoirs of *Streptococcus mutans* and Their Relationship to Caries Experience in Adults with Good Oral Hygiene, *Oral Microbiol Immunol* 5:19-23.

KELLAWAY, R.W. (1960): The Clearance of Liquid Glucose Solutions from Anterior Interproximal Spaces, *Aust Dent J* 5:140-148.

KEYES, P.H. and JORDAN, H.V. (1963): Factors Influencing the Initiation, Transmission, and Inhibition of Dental Caries. In: *Mechanisms of Hard Tissue Destruction*, R.S. Harris, Ed., New York; Academic Press, pp. 261-283.

KLEINBERG, I. and JENKINS, G.N. (1964): The pH of Dental Plaques in the Different Areas of the Mouth Before and After Meals and Their Relationship to the pH and Rate of Flow of Resting Saliva, *Arch Oral Biol* 9:493-516.

KLEINBERG, I., JENKINS, G.N.; CHATTERJEE, R. and WIJEYEWEERA, L. (1982): The Antimony pH Electrode and Its Role in the Assessment and Interpretation of Dental Plaque pH, *J Dent Res* 61:1139-1147.

KRASSE, B.; EDWARDSSON, S.; SVENSSON, I.; and TRELL, L. (1967): Implantation of Caries-Inducing Streptococci in the Human Oral Cavity, *Arch Oral Biol* 12:231-236.

KRASSE, B. (1985): *Caries Risk. A Practical Guide for Assessment and Control*, Chicago, Quintessence Publishing Co., Inc.

LINDQUIST, B. and EMILSON, C.G. (1990): Distribution and Prevalence of Mutans Streptococci in the Human Dentition, *J Dent Res* 69:1160-1166.

LOESCHE, W.J. (1986): Role of *Streptococcus mutans* in Human Dental Decay, *Microbiol Revs* 50:353-380.

MACPHERSON, L.M.D.; MACFARLENE, T.W.; and STEPHEN, K.W. (1990): An Intra-oral Appliance Study of the Plaque Microflora Associated with Early Enamel Demineralization, *J Dent Res* 69:1712-1716.

MANDEL, I.D. (1979): In Defense of the Oral Cavity. In: *Saliva and Dental Caries*, I. Kleinberg, S.A. Ellison, I.D. Mandel, Eds., New York, Information Retrieval, Inc., pp. 473-491.

MARSH, P.D. (1989): Host Defenses and Microbial Homeostasis: Role of Microbial Interactions, *J Dent Res* 68(Spec Iss):1567-1575.

MARSH, P.D.; FEATHERSTONE, A; MCKEE, A.S.; HALLSWORTH, A.S.; ROBINSON, C.; WEATHERELL, J.A.; NEWMAN, H.N.; and PITTER, A.F.V. (1989): A Microbiological Study of Early Caries of Approximal Surfaces in Schoolchildren, *J Dent Res* 68:1151-1154.

MCNAMARA, T.F.; FRIEDMAN, B.K.; and ROTH, P. (1979): Salivary Access as an Ecological Determinant. In: *Saliva and Dental Caries*, I. Kleinberg, S.A. Ellison, I.D. Mandel, Eds., New York, Information Retrieval, Inc., pp. 211-225.

MCNEE, S.G.; GEDDES, D.A.M.; WEETMAN, D.A.; SWEENEY, D.; and BEELEY, J.A. (1982): Effect of Extracellular Polysaccharides on Diffusion of NaF and ^{14}C-sucrose in Human Dental Plaque and in Sediments of the Bacterium *Streptococcus sanguis* 804 (NCTC 10904), *Arch Oral Biol* 27:981-986.

NEWBRUN, E. (1967): Sucrose, the Arch Criminal of Dental Caries, *Odont Revy* 18:373-386.

SCHILLING, K.M.; BLITZER, M.H.; and BOWEN, W.H. (1989): Adherence of *Streptococcus mutans* to Glucans Formed in situ in Salivary Pellicle, *J Dent Res* 68:1678-1680.

STEPHAN, R.M. (1944): Intra-oral Hydrogen-ion Concentrations Associated with Dental Caries Activity, *J Dent Res* 23:257-266.

SUNDSTROM, F. (1979): Influence of Saliva on the Availability of Carbohydrate Substrate. In: *Saliva and Dental Caries*, I. Kleinberg, S.A. Ellison, I.D. Mandel, Eds., New York, Information Retrieval, Inc., pp. 323-331.

SVANBERG, M. (1980): *Streptococcus mutans* in Plaque After Mouth-rinsing with Buffers of Varying pH Value, *Scand J Dent Res* 88:76-78.

TANZER, J.M. (1989): On Changing the Cariogenic Chemistry of Coronal Plaque, *J Dent Res* 68:1576-1587.

TATEVOSSIAN, A. (1985): The Effects of Heat Inactivation, Tortuosity, Extracellular Polyglucan and Ion-Exchange Sites on the Diffusion of 14[C]-Sucrose in Human Dental Plaque Residue *in vitro*, *Arch Oral Biol* 30:365-371.

TAUBMAN, M.A.; SMITH, D.J.; EBERSOLE, J.L.; and HILLMAN, J.D. (1983): Protective Aspects of Immune Response to *Glucosyltransferase, in Relation to Dental Caries. In: Glucosyltransferases, Glucans, Sucrose, and Dental Caries*. R.J. Doyle and J.E. Ciardi, Eds., Sp. Supp., Chemical Senses, pp. 249-258.

VAN DER HOEVEN, J.S.; MIKX, F.H.M.; PLASSCHAERT, A.J.M.; KONIG, K.G.; and MALTHA, J.C. (1974): The Interaction of *Actinomyces viscosus* with Oral Streptococci in Plaque of Gnotobiotic Rats. Ecological Significance of Antibacterial Activity in Plaque. Ph.D. Thesis, University of Nymegen, The Netherlands, pp. 1-18.

VAN HOUTE, J. (1980): Bacterial Specificity in the Etiology of Dental Caries, *Intern Dent J* 30:305-326.

VAN HOUTE, J.; GIBBS, G.; and BUTERA, C. (1982): Oral Flora of Children with "Nursing Bottle Caries," *J Dent Res* 61:382-385.

VAN HOUTE, J. (1983): Bacterial Adherence in the Mouth, *Revs of Infect Dis* 5:659-669.

VAN HOUTE, J. and RUSSO, J. (1986a): Factors Influencing the Cariogenicity of *Streptococcus mutans*. In: *Molecular Microbiology and Immunobiology of Streptococcus mutans*. S. Hamada, S. M. Michalek, H. Kiyono, L. Menaker and J.R. McGee, Eds., Amsterdam, Elsevier Science Publishers, pp.157-169.

VAN HOUTE, J. and RUSSO, J. (1986b): Variable Colonization by Oral Streptococci in Molar Fissures of Monoinfected Gnotobiotic Rats, *Infect Immun* 52:620-622.

VAN HOUTE, J.; RUSSO, J.; and PROSTAK, K.S. (1989): Increased pH-lowering Ability of *Streptococcus mutans* Cell Masses Associated with Extracellular Glucan-rich Matrix Material and the Mechanisms Involved, *J Dent Res* 68:451-459.

VAN HOUTE, J.; SANSONE, C.; GHOREISHI, J.; KENT, R.L.; and SOPARKAR, P. (1991a): Evaluation of the *in vitro* pH-lowering Potential and Microbial Composition of Human Dental Plaque From Sound and Carious Coronal Tooth Surfaces, *J Dent Res* 70:544, Abst. 2227.

VAN HOUTE, J.; SANSONE, C. and KENT, R.L. (1991b): Correlation Between *in vitro* pH-lowering potential of Human Plaque and Proportions of Mutans Streptococci and Highly-Acid Tolerant Non-mutans Streptococci, *J Dent Res* 70:544, Abst. 2226.

WEATHERELL, J.A.; DUGGAL, M.S.; ROBINSON, C.; and CURZON, M.E.J. (1988): Site-specific Differences in Human Dental Plaque pH After Sucrose Rinsing, *Arch Oral Biol* 33:871-873.

WIJEYEWEERA, R.L. and KLEINBERG, I. (1989): Arginolytic and Ureolytic Activities of Pure Cultures of Human Oral Bacteria and Their Effects on the pH Response of Salivary Sediment and Dental Plaque *in vitro*, *Arch Oral Biol* 34:43-53.

WILLCOX, M.D.P.; DRUCKER, D.B. and GREEN, R.M. (1990): *In vivo* Dental Plaque-Forming Ability and Cariogenicity of the Bacterium Streptococcus bovis in Gnotobiotic Rats, *Arch Oral Biol* 35:163-166.

ZERO, D.T.; VAN HOUTE, J.; and RUSSO, J. (1986): The Intra-oral Effect on Enamel Demineralization of Extracellular Matrix Material Synthesized from Sucrose by *Streptococcus mutans*, *J Dent Res* 65:918-923.

Alternatives to Conventional Clinical Caries Trials

DAVID W. BANTING

What is a Clinical Trial?

Clinical trials date back to the eighteenth century when James Lind evaluated six treatments (a quart of cider/ day, 25 drops of elixir of vitriol three times/ day on an empty stomach, two spoonfuls of vinegar three times/ day, one-half pint of seawater/ day, an electuary of garlic, mustard, balsam of Peru and myrrh and two oranges and one lemon/ day) among twelve seamen with scurvy (Bull, 1959). After six days, the two seamen using the oranges and lemon were suddenly and visibly better such that one returned to active duty and the other was assigned to nurse the others. Despite these dramatic and conclusive results, almost 50 years elapsed before the British Navy supplied lemon juice to its ships! The concept of randomization was not introduced until 1926 when Fisher first used this technique in agricultural research but the first randomized clinical trial was conducted by the Medical Research Council on streptomycin for the treatment of pulmonary tuberculosis in 1948 (Pocock, 1983).

Clinical trials possess the following fundamental characteristics:

(a) a clinical trial is a planned experiment where the investigator manipulates or controls the important aspects of the study design;
(b) subjects are followed over time from a well-defined baseline point. Therefore, a clinical trial is prospective although all study subjects are rarely followed from a common calendar date;
(c) an active intervention is applied to some subjects in a uniform fashion. This is the 'test' group;
(d) another group of subjects receives no active intervention, a placebo (a placebo would now only be employed if there was no currently accepted standard treatment), or the currently accepted standard of intervention (treatment). This is the 'control' group.;

(e) clinical trials are conducted on human beings; and
(f) ideally, clinical trials include randomization of subjects into 'treatment' and 'control' groups. Randomization is a technique which controls for bias associated with known, unknown and unmeasured variables (as opposed to bias associated with known variables such as age and sex and specific differences which can be controlled by other methods such as stratification). Randomization is not a perfect tool in eliminating sources of bias but, in the long term, is generally effective.

How Do Clinical Trials Differ From Other Types of Studies?

Clinical trials are by no means the only type of study that allows an investigator to examine the relationship and determine the degree of association between two or more variables. Clinical trials represent one of three major study types. All three types of studies select a sample from a larger target population and, therefore, the type of study reveals the method of sampling (Fleiss, 1986).

If a sample of n subjects is selected and then the presence or absence of an event A and the presence or absence of a factor B are determined for each subject, this study design exemplifies a crossectional survey. In these types of studies, both the event in question and the suspected factor are determined at the same time. An example would be a study of the association of dental caries with the condition of the periodontium as determined by a single clinical examination. These types of studies are relatively straightforward and are usually completed within a short period of time. The major limitation of crossectional surveys is their inability to determine any temporal relationship between the factor and the event.

Another type of study selects a predetermined number (n) of subjects who possess characteristic A and a predetermined number (m) of subjects without characteristic A. If characteristic A is a risk factor and the subjects are followed forward in time, the study is known as a prospective cohort or follow-up study. If characteristic A is the response variable and the study subjects are traced back in time to determine how many possessed the risk factor, the study is classified as a retrospective case-control study. In general, prospective and retrospective studies are more informative than a crossectional study of equal sample size.

The third type of study is the comparative clinical trial. Clinical trials are particularly well-suited for intervention and etiological studies because exposure can be controlled experimentally, particularly with respect to temporal sequencing (i.e. the exposure precedes the event). Futhermore, the effect of factors not controlled within the clinical trial can be minimized through the random assignment process. This done, the effect observed can confidently be attributed to the factor under study. Thus, unlike the other types of studies, it is possible to state with a high degree of certainty whether treatment influences outcome. This is why both the Federal Drug Administration and the American Dental Association require data from clinical trials in order to approve products and devices for use by the general public.

However, clinical trials are extremely labor intensive and, therefore, are very expensive in terms of dollars, time and human resources. Usually the decision to conduct a clinical trial is a judgement call based on many factors, not the least of which is the 'misery' index of the disorder. That is, the disorder has a high enough incidence to affect a substantial proportion of the general population so that an attack upon it will obviously promote the public good. Or, if infrequent, the disorder has a devastating outcome. Clinical trials are also undertaken when either existing interventions are unknown or, if known, are not efficacious, possess undesirable side effects, are expensive or all of the above.

None of these conditions relate to dental caries or anticarious agents, at least at this time.

Furthermore dental caries investigators are now faced with one or more of the following perplexing problems:

(a) dental caries, in both children and adults, is found in a much smaller segment of the population. 79% of 9, 10 and 11 year old children have an annual decayed and filled surface caries increment of zero and, therefore, 21% of the children account for all of the disease incidence (DePaola, 1990). Similarily, between 22% and 35 % of adults have evidence of active or restored root caries (Stamm *et al.*, 1990).

(b) dental caries most often occurs in only one or two sites per subject annually. 75% of children with a positive caries increment have just one or two carious sites (DePoala, 1990).

(c) depending on the presence or absence of certain etiologic factors such as a specific type of microorganism, not all sites in a subject are equally at risk of dental caries (Tanzer, 1990).

(d) the response of multiple sites within subjects to a risk factor or a treatment although correlated, is not identical.

(e) exposure to a risk factor or a treatment is usually considered to be subject-specific (i.e. a professional fluoride gel treatment represents an exposure for all of the teeth in a mouth) but a pit and fissure sealant is site-specific). And,

(f) co-variables can be both subject-specific and site-specific (i.e. age and sex are common to all teeth but the environment around any tooth may vary widely).

What are the Alternatives?

1. Some Old Tricks

Some efficiency in clinical trials can be gained by using only subjects who have a high likelihood of experiencing the event. This concept is not new and has been used extensively in the past. Subjects representing high risk, special populations (the chronically ill, diabetics, primitive populations, radiated subjects) have much higher dental caries prevalence rates and the occurrence rate of an event is maximized if these groups are studied. But, the results cannot readily be extrapolated to the general population. Although it may be demonstrated that a particular intervention is effective in a high-risk population under highly controlled experimental conditions, less reliable information is available regarding how efficacious that treatment would be in the general population under unsupervised conditions.

Fortunately, extensive research in risk assessment is now providing investigators with the tools to select subjects from the general population who are at the greatest risk of dental caries. Sophisticated statistical modelling of suspected risk factors and the development and refinement of clinical diagnostic tests are most helpful in selecting high-risk subjects from among the general population. For example, investigators at North Carolina have demonstrated that a logistic regression model using clinical, microbial and sociological independent variable can correctly classify 78% of children most at risk of dental caries (Disney *et al.*, 1991).

When the event is rare, the frequency can be increased by selecting other, more frequently observed endpoints. For instance, initial decalcification (white spot lesions) could be used to define dental caries rather than the more traditional cavitation. Redefining dental caries as white spot lesions increases the number of events (at least for crown caries) but it carries with it several significant disadvantages. Firstly, it assumes that white spot lesions are caries or that white spot lesions inevitably progress to dental caries given favorable conditions. Secondly, it raises questions regarding the definition and measurement of white spot lesions particularly when the white spot lesion is considered part of a dynamic relationship between demineralization and remineralization (Graves, 1990; Katz, 1990) . Unreliable measurement of the response variable increases the sample size necessary to detect a specified treatment difference (Fleiss, 1986).

There are many examples of dental research where the subject has been used as his/her own control. Clinical trials of pit and fissure sealants and dental floss are just two of them. In these studies, contralateral teeth or quadrants are used as the sampling unit. This type of design relies on the clinical observation that caries occurs in a bilaterally symmetrical fashion in both teeth and, perhaps more importantly, surfaces. However, Lewis *et al.* (1980) demonstrated that surprisingly large deviations from bilaterality occur with incidence data. About one-half of the surface pairs did not become carious in the same year of observation. However, bilaterality increases as the length of the interval between the baseline and subsequent examinations increases and Lewis recommends an observation period of at least four years in order to rule out lack of simultaneous decay as an explanation of observed differences between test and control contralateral surfaces.

Another commonly employed design (which also uses the subject as his/her own control) is the crossover design. Crossover studies have been more popular in periodontal studies than caries trials because some periodontal diseases are reversible (i.e. have no permanent adverse effects) and, therefore, there is no "carry-over" of treatment effect from one treatment interval to the next.

Both of these designs have the delightful feature of requiring no more than one half the number of subjects required by the conventional parallel group clinical trial to observe the same magnitude of treatment effect. Therefore, they are more efficient and less expensive.

However, there are very few interventions where the effect is completely reversible. In fact, the objective should be to develop interventions that are permanent. Futhermore, the very low incidence of dental caries today (even in high risk groups) prolongs the time needed to observe an effect and this can have an adverse effect on subject retention. And, it seems, we can no longer assume that caries will occur bilaterally within a reasonable observation period (two or three years). Therefore, the subject as his/her own control and crossover designs, for all their efficiency, are now less well-suited to the study of dental caries and these designs will have limited usefulness in future caries research.

2. A New Approach

A third, but essentially untried, alternative is to use the site (i.e. the tooth or the tooth surface) as the sampling unit. Caries researchers who undertake clinical trials should explore the advantages that can be gleaned from the fact that a dentate subject usually possesses more than one tooth (the average number of teeth in U.S. adults is 23.6) and each tooth has four or five surfaces. Periodontists have realized the time and sample size advantages of studying sites rather than subjects particularly when there may be as many as 192 sites to be measured per subject in periodontal trials.

If the site is to be used as the unit of observation some important adjustments must be made. Mainland (1963) correctly points out that individual teeth in any mouth are not independent and that treating them as replicate measurements amounts to counting the same thing over again and can produce misleading results. Imrey (1986), Fleiss (1987) and others correctly argue that teeth within the same mouth cannot be expected to respond independently because host factors, such as immune response, diet and nutrition, saliva flow, composition and distribution, the indigenous microflora, oral hygiene practices, concomitant disease and other factors influence all teeth. The issue in question, as far as these and other statisticians are concerned, is that conventional statistical methods assume that the observations are independent and, therefore, cannot be applied to the analysis of individual teeth (or surfaces) within a mouth.

Although teeth (or surfaces) within a mouth are unquestionably affected by host factors which are more similar within a mouth than between mouths, there is also considerable variation in the local environment surrounding a tooth surface, a tooth or a group of teeth which would render that tooth (or surface) more or less susceptible to disease or more or less responsive to treatment. The fact that all teeth in a mouth are not equally at risk of dental caries appears to depend on the characteristics, conditions and dynamics of: the number and type of microorganisms colonizing the tooth (surface), the salivary flow rate and type of saliva, plaque fluid composition, pH and the calcium concentration, pellicle composition and stage of development,tooth type and surface characteristics and probably many other factors.

If the site is to be used as the sampling unit, we must expand our thinking in two important areas:

(a) the research question being asked, and
(b) our concept of exposure.

Imrey (1986), in discussing the appropriate unit of observation, suggests that it is often more relevant to frame research questions in terms of sites than in terms of subjects. For example, it may be of interest to know whether the number or proportion of carious sites is reduced more by one treatment than another, or varies according to some subject-specific environmental or genetic trait. In other words, the hypothesis states that the caries rate is the same in both exposure groups in contrast to the traditional hypothesis which states that the proportion of subjects with at least one carious lesion is the same. In the conventional clinical trial, sites within subjects are summarized and we are interested in people exhibiting or not exhibiting the response; whereas when the site is the unit of observation, we are interested in sites which exhibit or do not exhibit the response regardless of which subject they are in.

Exposure has traditionally been considered to be subject-specific. If a subject was assigned to the treatment group, all teeth (surfaces) were exposed to the treatment and, if a subject was assigned to the control group, no teeth (surfaces) were exposed to the treatment. Similarly, risk (i.e. the presence of a prognostic factor such as mutans Streptococci) is usually defined as the presence of the microorganism in the saliva. However, not all teeth (surfaces) in a subject would be colonized by that microorganism and, therefore, not all subjects are equally at risk assuming that subjects with more teeth (surfaces) colonized

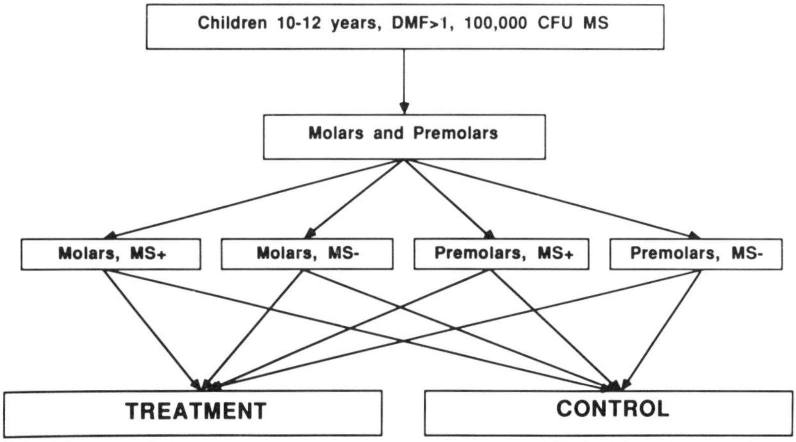

Figure 1 Design of a site-specific clinical trial to test a varnish

by a microorganism considered to be the etiologic agent must be at greater risk. Unfortunately, our present level of technological sophistication does not allow us to determine whether there is a gradient of risk associated with increased numbers of sites exhibiting the prognostic factor (i.e. something akin to a dose-response effect).

Another issue in site-specific observation relates to whether a treatment or factor can be applied to only some teeth (surfaces) and not others within the same mouth. The answer is probably ''yes'' but new and innovative methods of delivery of treatments must be developed to ensure that the effect remains local such that no other teeth (surfaces) would be inadvertently exposed to the treatment through saliva contamination or other means of transmission. There is considerable room here for research and development.

An example might be helpful at this point (Figure 1). Suppose we wished to test the efficacy of a varnish containing histanin for reducing pit and fissure caries in children using a site-specific approach. Our hypothesis would state that there is no difference in the proportion (or number) of treated and control sites with pit and fissure caries. The investigators would be prudent to select a sample population which is at higher risk of dental caries yet otherwise representative of the target population. Based on risk assessment studies, the investigators might select children of a specific age-group or age-range who have evidence of previous dental caries and who demonstrate a level of at least 100,000 colony forming units (CFU) of mutans Streptococci (MS) by means of a saliva test. Therefore, age, previous caries experience and the presence of the risk factor would constitute the minimal inclusion criteria.

Once selected, these children would be subjected to a baseline clinical examination to determine (a) which teeth were available for study and (b) the presence/absence of mutans Streptococci in the occlusal pits and fissures of the available teeth using some suitable test. In fact, defining the presence of the prognostic variable as two consecutive positive test results might be considered because of the high false positive rate for microbiological sampling. The presence or absence of mutans Streptococci would then be used as a stratification variable at this point in the design of the study and as a co-variable in the analysis phase.

The molar and premolar teeth in the subjects would then be randomized to treatment and control groups, the treatment would be applied to the treatment group teeth and a placebo would be applied to the control teeth. The occurrence of the event (dental caries) would then be recorded at several points in time - usually over a two-year period. Univariate analysis is quite straightforward except that the statistical test employed must be adjusted to take into account that several teeth are clustered within the same subject and, therefore, cannot be considered to be independent in their reaction to the treatment (Laster, 1985; Blomqvist, 1985; Imrey, 1986; Fleiss *et al.*, 1987; Donner and Banting, 1988, 1989).

Selecting the tooth as the unit of observation and employing a slightly different concept of exposure does not interfere with other design considerations of the clinical trial such as:

(1) the end point to be used as the outcome variable;
(2) the method of measurement of the risk factors and covariables;
(3) employing a variable observation period (e.g. time to the event) instead of the more conventional fixed observation period (e.g. 12 months, 24 months);
(4) the type, frequency and quantity of treatment;
(5) performing an interim analysis; and
(6) using both univariate and multivariate statistical tests in the analysis;

Perhaps the most difficult aspect of using the site as the unit of observation is thinking in terms of sites rather than subjects in framing the question. Let's consider another example (Figure 2). Suppose we wish to determine the effect of root polishing on the incidence of root caries hypothesizing that roots left untreated are at greater risk than those which are highly polished. This time, we would select a sample of dentate subjects with gingival recession, evidence of previous dental caries experience and the presence of the etiological risk factor. From the baseline examination teeth with no visible root caries, at least 3mm of recession and the presence of the risk factor on the facial surface would be identified. These teeth would then be randomly assigned to treatment and control

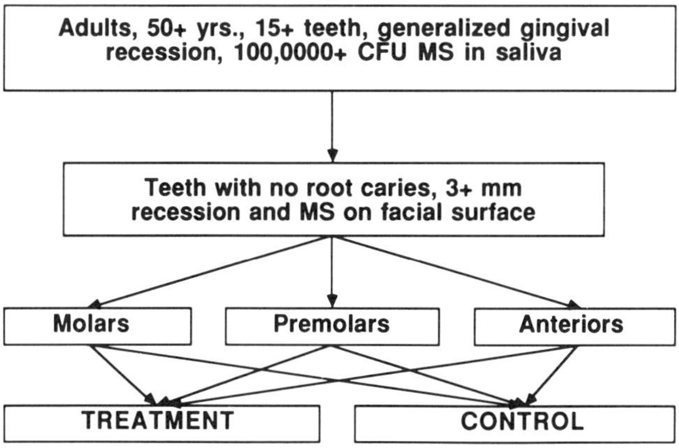

Figure 2 Design of a site-specific clinical trial on root caries

groups. We may first wish to stratify the teeth by tooth and surface type in an attempt to balance the groups thereby controlling for potentially confounding factors. These same teeth would be reexamined for root caries after an appro priate observation period (one and two years) and then comparisons made between treated and control teeth. In this study, root polishing is considered to be the exposure. Exposure, therefore, is tooth-specific. We must refrain from the temptation of posing the traditional research hypothesis which states that the caries experience in subjects with and without root polishing is the same. The more appropriate hypothesis states that the root caries rate for polished and non-polished teeth is the same.

This alternative clinical trial design compares treated and control sites; but in different subjects realizing, of course, that responses for teeth within the same subject are not independent. The basic difference relative to the conventional clinical trial design is that comparisons are site-specific as opposed to subject-specific. However, there are many other differences between subject-specific and site-specific clinical trial designs which have not been presented in this paper due to space limitations (Table 1).

The approach outlined here is just in its earliest (conceptual) stage of development and has not been extensively tested in the field. Nevertheless, clinical trials using the site as the unit of observation provide an intriguing alternative to the conventional (parallel group) clinical trial and other design modifications such as the split-mouth and cross-over techniques. However, significant progress and sophistication of this design must await advances in other areas such as diagnostic criteria, the ability to apply and limit the effect of treatments to single or multiple sites within the same mouth without contaminating other sites and the development of multivariate statistical methodology which

Table 1
A COMPARISON OF SOME CHARACTERISTICS OF CONVENTIONAL AND SITE-SPECIFIC CLINICAL TRIALS

CHARACTERISTIC	*CONVENTIONAL*	*SITE-SPECIFIC*
Response	sum or average across all subjects	relates to sites only
Exposure	equal for all sites in test group subjects	limited to test sites within subjects
Covariables	treated as subject-specific	both subject and site-specific
Question	relates to subjects	relates to sites
Sample size	usually large, particularly if incidence is low	more sites but fewer subjects required
Analysis	traditional, non-parametric and parametric methods	requires adjustment to traditional methods to allow for multiple sites in the same subject
Assumptions	exposure and susceptibility are constant for all sites and subjects	the similarity between any two sites within the same subject is constant
Case Definition	may vary depending on the number of sites affected/subject	relates to sites only
Limitations	size, cost, feasibility	analysis, interpretation, contamination of treatment effect

will allow for the simultaneous consideration of both subject-specific and site-specific variables.

REFERENCES

BLOMQVIST, N. (1985): On the Choice of Computational Unit in Statistical Analysis, *J Clin Periodontol*, 12:873-876.

BULL, J.P. (1959): The Historical Development of Clinical Therapeutic Trials, *J Chronic Dis.* 10:218-248.

DEPAOLA, P.F. (1990): Measurement Issues in the Epidemiology of Dental Caries, In: *Risk Assessment in Dentistry*, J. D. Bader, Ed., Chapel Hill: University of North Carolina Dental Ecology, pp. 19-26.

DISNEY, J.A.; GRAVES, R.; STAMM, J.W.; and BOHANNAN, H.M. (1991): UNC Caries Risk Assessment Study Prediction Models, IADR *Prog & Abst* 70: No. 745.

DONNER, A. and BANTING, D.W. (1988): Analysis of Site-Specific Data in Dental Studies, *J Dent Res* 67:1392-1395.

DONNER, A. and BANTING, D.W. (1989): Adjustment of Frequently Used Chi-square Procedures for the Effect of Site -to-site Dependencies in the Analysis of Dental Data, *J Dent Res* 68:1350-1354.

FLEISS, J.L. (1981): *Statistical Methods for Rates and Proportions*, Second Edition, New York: John Wiley & Sons, pp.19-26.

FLEISS, J.L. (1986): *The Design and Analysis of Clinical Experiments*, New York: John Wiley & Sons, p. 5.

FLEISS, J.L.; PARK, M.H.; and CHILTON, N.W. (1987): Within-mouth Correlations and Reliabilities for Probing Depth and Attachment Level, *J Periodontol* 58:460-463.

GRAVES, R.C. (1990): Physical and Environmental Risk Factors in Dental Caries, In: *Risk Assessment in Dentistry*, J.D. Bader, Ed., Chapel Hill: University of North Carolina Dental Ecology, pp. 37-47.

IMERY, P.B. (1986): Considerations in the Statistical Analysis of Clinical Trials in Periodontics, *J Clin Perio* 13:517-528.

KATZ, R.V. (1990): Reactor Paper: Measurement Issues in the Epidemiology of Dental Caries, In: *Risk Assessment in Dentistry*, J.D. Bader, Ed., Chapel Hill: University of North Carolina Dental Ecology, pp. 27-28.

LASTER, L.L. (1985): The Effect of Subsampling Sites Within Patients, *J Periodontol Res* 20:91-96.

LEWIS, D.W.; SHAUGHNESSY, S.; and HOWLEY, T.P. (1980): *Bilaterality of Dental Caries on Premolar and Second Molar Teeth—A Four Year Study*, Toronto, Department of Community Dentistry, Dental Health Services and Epidemiology Research Unit.

POCOCK, S.J. (1983): *Clinical Trials: A Practical Approach*, Chichester: John Wiley & Sons, p.17.

STAMM, J.W,; BANTING, D.W.; and IMREY, P.B. (1990): Adult Root Caries Survey of Two Similar Communities with Contrasting Natural Water Fluoride Levels, *JADA* 120:143-149.

TANZER, J.M. (1990): Why is Prediction of Risk for Caries by Microbiological Monitoring Problematic? In: *Risk Assessment in Dentistry*, J.D. Bader, Ed., Chapel Hill: University of North Carolina Dental Ecology, pp. 62-66.

MICROBIOLOGY/PLAQUE

Adhesion and Cohesion of Plaque Microflora: A Function of Microbial Fimbriae and Fibrils?

ARNOLD S. BLEIWEIS* AND PETRA C.F. OYSTON

Different sites in the oral cavity are colonized by distinct populations of bacteria. All exposed surfaces of the mouth, including teeth, periodontal tissues and tongue, have specific organisms associated with them. Selectivity of a species for a particular niche may in part be influenced by specificity of adhesion to particular substrata, especially in the case of the early colonizers of the oral cavity. Subsequent bacteria may be able to adhere not only to the surfaces of the mouth, but also to other bacteria which are already adhering to the surfaces.

Bacteria entering the mouth and the surfaces of the oral cavity are coated by salivary proteins which adsorb to form pellicles. These proteins must be considered when studying microbial adhesion in the mouth. In addition, saliva contains secretory IgA antibodies which bind to bacteria thus preventing adhesion. However, a number of oral bacteria produce IgA1 proteases capable of cleaving secretory IgA1 molecules at the hinge region to generate Fab and Fc fragments (Kilian and Reinholdt, 1986; Mulks, 1985; Plaut, 1983). Fab fragments have been detected in plaque (Ahl and Reinholdt, 1991) and whereas IgA antibodies inhibit adhesion of bacteria, Fab fragments have little or no effect (Kilian *et al.*, 1988; Mulks, 1985; Reinholdt and Kilian, 1987). Therefore, IgA proteases may play a great role *in vivo* in the adhesion of oral bacteria.

Several models are available for studying *in vitro* adhesion of oral microbes. Adhesion to the tooth surface has been studied using enamel (Ørstavik *et al.*, 1974) and hydroxyapatite beads (Clark *et al.*, 1978) which can be coated with a pellicle of salivary proteins similar to that found on teeth (Eggen and Rolla, 1982). The adhesion of bacteria to epithelial surfaces has been studied using the buccal epithelial cell model developed by Gibbons and van Houte (1971).

* To whom correspondence should be addressed
Work described in this paper is supported by NIH grant R37-DE-08007 to A.S.B.

The adhesion of oral bacteria has received much attention. If the attachment of these bacteria is understood, it may be possible to control plaque formation and thus reduce the risk of caries and periodontal disease.

Streptococcus salivarius

S. salivarius is an early colonizer of the oral cavity and is isolated in large numbers from the tongue dorsum and buccal epithelium. Two serotypes, Lancefield group K+ and K-, are present in almost equal proportions in the mouth.

K+ strains possess three classes of adhesin (Weerkamp and McBride, 1980, Weerkamp and Jacobs, 1982). The first group mediates in host-related adherence and aggregation reactions, haemagglutination and adhesion to buccal epithelial cells, and is known as the host attachment factor (HAF) or Antigen C. The second adhesin mediates in coaggregation with *Veillonella*, and is therefore known as the Veillonella-binding protein (VBP) or Antigen B, while the final group mediates coaggregation with *Fusobacterium nucleatum*. In contrast, K- strains do not haemagglutinate, agglutinate with saliva and have a reduced affinity for buccal epithelial cells (Weerkamp and McBride, 1980).

While K- strains are fimbrate, K+ strains possess fibrils (Handley *et al.*, 1984). The fibrillar strains are structurally complex. *S. salivarius* HB was shown to possess protease-sensitive short fibrils of 91, 72 and 63 nm in length, and long protease-resistant fibrils of 178 nm (Weerkamp *et al.*, 1986). Immunoelectron microscopy revealed Antigen B and Antigen C to be located in the fibrillar layer of *S. salivarius* HB, on separate classes of fibril, 91 nm and 72 nm in length respectively (Weerkamp *et al.*, 1986). The functions of the other fibril classes are not known.

Little is known about the nature of the receptors for VBP or HAF. Coaggregation with veillonellae is not affected by simple sugars or saliva, but is partially inhibited by galactose analogues (Weerkamp and McBride, 1980).

K+ strains can therefore attach directly in the oral cavity by HAF or can attach to adherent *Veillonella* already present in plaque. Interspecies coaggregation to produce structured microbial ecosystems may have developed as specific pairs of organisms can benefit from close physical association. For example, extracellular lactate inhibits glycolysis in a strain of *S. salivarius*, and removal of the lactate by *Veillonella parvula* stimulated glycolysis significantly (Hamilton and Ng, 1983). Therefore, close association would benefit both coaggregating partners.

S. salivarius demonstrates that bacteria may simultaneously display more than one adhesin, each with specific binding properties. The cell surface adhesins mediate attachment to receptors which can be located on the host surface, allowing adhesion, or on another bacterium, allowing coaggregation. This gives the organism an increased opportunity of being incorporated into a niche in the oral cavity.

Actinomyces species

Actinomyces viscosus and *Actinomyces naeslundii* are early colonizers of clean tooth surfaces and are among the principle species isolated from supragingival plaque. These organisms possess two types of fimbriae involved in adhesion to oral surfaces and coaggregation with other bacterial species (Cisar *et al.*, 1981, 1983; Cisar, 1982; Revis *et al.*, 1982).

Type 1 fimbriae mediate adhesion to saliva-coated hydroxyapatite (SCHA), and therefore probably to teeth *in vivo*. Proline-rich proteins (PRP) present in human parotid saliva and part of the pellicle on teeth may serve as receptors for adhesins of Type 1 fimbriate actinomyces (Gibbons and Hay, 1988; Gibbons *et al.*, 1988). Only adsorbed PRPs act as receptors for *A. viscosus*. When present in soluble form, they do not interact with the fimbriae. Possibly, PRPs undergo conformational changes when they adsorb to expose hidden regions to which the fimbriae can bind. Gibbons (1989) referred to these receptors as "cryptitopes."

Type 2 fimbriae bind to mammalian cells by interacting with galactose termini of cell surface glycoproteins and glycolipids (Cisar *et al.*, 1981; Costello *et al.*, 1979). Type 2 fimbriae can haemagglutinate, but it is neuraminidase-dependent, the neuraminidase exposing galactose residues to which fimbriae can bind (Costello et al., 1979). These fimbriae can interact with salivary glycoproteins adsorbed to latex beads to aggregate them, and this process is inhibited by lactose (Gabriel *et al.*, 1985). Type 2 fimbriae also mediate coaggregation with *S. sanguis, S. mitis* and *S. morbillorum* in a lactose-inhibitable manner (Kolenbrander *et al.*, 1983; Kolenbrander and Williams, 1981, 1983).

When mutants defective in the ability to express either or both fimbrial types were compared for their ability to colonize the oral cavities of volunteers (Clark, 1985), the wild type was recovered in higher numbers than any of the mutants. Type 1 fimbriate mutants were better able to colonize teeth than mutants only expressing Type 2 fimbriae. Mutants lacking fimbriae were virtually undetected. Therefore, Type 1 fimbriae were more efficient at binding bacteria to the tooth surface than Type 2 fimbriae, but Type 2 fimbriae still mediated adhesion. This may have been due to Type 2 fimbriae binding to other bacteria already present on teeth and coaggregation resulting in the incorporation of the bacteria into plaque.

The different binding properties of the fimbriae may explain the distribution of the *Actinomyces* in the mouth. Using monospecific antibodies to Type 1 or Type 2 fimbriae, Cisar et al (1985) found the majority of the actinomyces on epithelial surfaces such as the tongue to have only Type 2 fimbriae, but some were present which possessed both types. In contrast, Type 2 fimbriate organisms were rare in plaque, the majority labelling with both Type 1 and Type 2 antibodies. The Type 2 fimbriae therefore allow binding to epithelial cells and streptococci in plaque on teeth, while Type 1 fimbriae are responsible for adhesion to the tooth surface.

Streptococcus mutans

S. mutans has been strongly implicated as a causative organism of dental caries (Hamada and Slade, 1980). Dietary sucrose is essential for accumulation of mutans streptococci on teeth and initiation of carious lesions on smooth enamel surfaces. *S. mutans* synthesizes large amounts of glucans from sucrose and possesses a glucan-binding lectin (GBL) and glucosyltransferases (GTF) capable of binding to glucans. The interaction of cell-bound GBL and GTF with insoluble glucans in plaque could promote cohesion between streptococci and allow accumulation on teeth (Gibbons and van Houte, 1975). However, initial adhesion to teeth may not involve glucans and a model was proposed by Staat *et al.* (1980) where protein-mediated attachment to pellicle components would be followed by glucan-dependent accumulation of *S. mutans* in plaque.

Streptococcal surface proteins involved in interactions with salivary glycoproteins have been identified. Serotype c organisms express a protein of approximately 185 kDa designated antigen I/II (Russell *et al.*, 1980; Zanders and Lehner, 1981), antigen B (Russell, 1979, 1980), IF (Hughes *et al.*, 1980), MSL-1 (Demuth *et al.*, 1990a), PAc (Okahashi *et al.*, 1989a, 1989b) and P1 (Forester *et al.*, 1983) which mediates attachment to agglutinin-coated hydroxyapatite (ACHA) (Lee *et al.*, 1989; Koga *et al.*, 1990). Analogous proteins have been described for *S. sobrinus* serotypes d and g strains (Spa A or PAg), *S. mutans* serotype f strains (SR) and *S. sanguis* strains (SSP-5) (Abiko *et al.*, 1989; Holt *et al.*, 1982; Okahashi *et al.*, 1986; Ackermans *et al.*, 1985; Demuth *et al.*, 1988).

P1 is associated with fibrils on the *S. mutans* surface (Ayakawa *et al.*, 1987). The P1-like proteins are believed to function as adhesins *in vivo* enabling *S. mutans* to bind to the salivary pellicle on teeth and to other plaque bacteria (Douglas and Russell, 1984; Gibbons, 1984; Lee *et al.*, 1989; McBride *et al.*, 1984). The binding of agglutinin is calcium-dependent and can be inhibited by the presence of lactose and fucose (Demuth *et al.*, 1990).

The *spaP* gene encoding P1 has been cloned from strain NG5 into *E. coli* (Lee *et al.*, 1988). A similar gene *pac* encoding the 190 kDa PAc protein was also cloned from strain MT8148 (Okahashi *et al.*, 1989a). Comparison of the two sequences reveals a high degree of homology (Kelly *et al.*, 1989; Okahashi *et al.*, 1989b). The cloned *spaP* and *pac* genes possess their own promoters and a Shine-Delgarno sequence precedes the open reading frame (Lee *et al.*, 1988; Okahashi *et al.*, 1989b). P1 and PAc proteins share a number of features when predicted amino acid sequences are compared: an N-terminal signal peptide; an alanine-rich or A region in the amino terminal third of the molecule; a proline-rich or P region in the central portion of the molecule; a C terminal proline-rich region believed to span the cell wall and a potential transmembrane domain of hydrophobic amino acids followed by a charged cytoplasmic tail.

Secondary structure prediction indicates that the A region is likely to be alpha-helical (Okahashi *et al.*, 1989b). A similar structure has been proposed for the M protein of group A streptococci (Phillips *et al.*, 1981). The antiphagocytic effect of M protein may be due to the alpha-helical structure (Phillips *et al.*, 1981) and it is possible that the A region of *S. mutans* P1 protein may have a similar property.

When the *spaP* gene was examined from various serotype c strains in a restriction fragment length polymorphism (RFLP) study, the gene was found to be highly conserved except for a central variable (V) region (Brady *et al.*, 1991). RFLP analysis revealed two types of V-region. Isolates were either *pac*-like or *spaP*-like. The significance of the V region is not yet known and the occurrence of the two types was independent of geographic origin.

The *spaP* gene encoding the P1 protein was disrupted by insertional inactivation and transformed into the serotype c strain NG8 to produce a mutant designated 834 (Lee *et al.*, 1989). Strain 834 no longer produced P1 and did not possess fibrils which had been observed on NG8 (Lee *et al.*, 1989) and was no longer able to bind to ACHA (Bleiweis *et al.*, 1990).

Some *S. mutans* strains express P1, but do not retain it on the cell surface (Ayakawa *et al.*, 1987). Strain GS5 produces a truncated protein of 155 kDa which is released into the supernatant. Nonretention is not due to loss of the DNA sequence coding the membrane anchor and wall-spanning regions (Brady *et al.*, 1991). Strains NG5 and Ingbritt 162 are also nonretainers, but they release the full 185 kDa protein. The reason why P1 is not anchored in the surface of many common streptococcal strains is not known.

Due to the importance of this organism in tooth decay, much interest has been focused on the development of a vaccine against *S. mutans*. Lehner *et al.* (1981) found antigen I/II (P1) to be an effective caries vaccine in monkeys, and passive immunization with monoclonal antibodies against this antigen also protected against caries in both monkeys (Lehner *et al.*, 1985) and humans (Ma and Lehner, 1990). There was concern expressed about the suitability of a vaccine based on the P1-like proteins as antibodies produced against *S. mutans* whole cells were reported to cross-react with heart tissue (van de Rijn *et al.*, 1976; Ferretti *et al.*, 1980; Hughes *et al.*, 1980; Russell, 1980; Forester *et al.*, 1983). However, subsequent evidence now suggests that surface components other than P1 may be responsible (reviewed by Russell and Wu, 1990). For example, Ayakawa *et al.*, (1987) and Smith *et al.* (1984) failed to detect heart cross-reactivity using monoclonal antibodies to P1. Also, isogenic mutants with defective *spaP* genes were still able to cross-react with heart tissue, the cross-reactivity possibly being attributable to 45 or 62 kDa membrane proteins (Bleiweis *et al.*, 1990). In addition, *S. rattus* serotype b does not possess a surface protein resembling P1 but can still elicit heart cross-reactive antibodies (van de Rijn *et al.*, 1976).

Streptococcus sanguis

S. sanguis is one of the first bacterial species to colonize the tooth surface and is one of the predominant bacteria in human coronal plaque and gingival crevices (Gibbons and van Houte, 1975). *S. sanguis* strains must therefore have a high affinity for the salivary pellicle on teeth. Pellicles contain a small number of high affinity neuraminidase-sensitive receptors and a larger number of lower affinity neuraminidase-insensitive receptors for *S. sanguis* (Gibbons *et al.*, 1983). When the adhesion of *S. sanguis* strain 12 and a non-aggregating variant 12na were examined, both strains were able to adhere to SCHA. Strain 12na would not bind to the neuraminidase-sensitive receptor, but instead bound to a receptor which was inactivated by preincubation at pH5 (Morris and McBride, 1984).

When examined by negative staining, the majority of *S. sanguis* strains possess peritrichous fibrils, a few possess tufts of fibrils and very occasional strains carry fimbriae (Handley *et al.*, 1985). The peritrichously fibrillar strains are able to coaggregate with *A. viscosus* and *A. naeslundii* and are better able to adhere to SCHA than tufted strains (Wyatt *et al.*, 1987). The most highly adherent strain, CR834, possesses fimbriae in addition to peritrichous fibrils. Fimbriae have also been observed on strain FW213 (Fives-Taylor and Thompson, 1985). Chemical mutagenesis of this strain was used to produce mutants with an impaired ability to adhere to SCHA. In general, loss of adherence coincided with loss of fimbriae, although two of the seventeen mutants still expressed fimbriae. These may have been defective in adhesion. Although adhesion had been impaired, several mutants were still able to aggregate in the presence of saliva and to coaggregate with actinomyces indicating that adhesion and aggregation are distinct phenomena and adherence may be associated with fimbriae while aggregation is not. Antisera to the fimbriae were able to inhibit the adhesion of FW213 to SCHA (Fachon-Kalweit *et al.*, 1985).

Ganeshkumar *et al.* (1988) cloned an adhesin of *S. sanguis* strain 12 which mediates attachment to SCHA via the pH-sensitive receptor. A 36 kDa protein designated *S. sanguis* adhesin B (Ssa B) was used to raise polyclonal antibodies in rabbits which were able to block adhesion of *S. sanguis* 12na to SCHA. However, adhesion of strain 12 was only weakly inhibited, confirming the two-site binding model proposed by Morris and McBride (1984). Immunogold labelling of *S. sanguis* with polyclonal IgG to Ssa B resulted in labelling of the tips of the densely packed short fibrils carried by the organism (Ganeshkumar *et al.*, 1988). The long fibrils carry the adhesin which recognizes the neuraminidase-sensitive receptor, as shown by adhesion-inhibition experiments using antibodies raised to the long fibrils (Morris *et al.*, 1987).

An adhesin of *S. sanguis* strain M5 (SSP-5) was cloned by Demuth *et al.* (1988) and transformed into *Enterococcus faecalis* conferring both agglutinin binding and salivary agglutination abilities onto the transformant (Demuth et al, 1989). The 205 kDa protein is antigenically related to *SpaA* from *S. sobrinus*,

P1 of *S. mutans* serotype c and SR of *S. mutans* serotype f (Demuth *et al.*, 1988; Ogier *et al.*, 1990). SSP-5 binds agglutinin in a calcium-dependent fashion and is inhibited by neuraminidase treatment of the salivary agglutinin and by simple sugars containing sialic acid, showing that SSP-5 is the adhesin which recognizes the neuraminidase-sensitive receptor and that sialic acid is the primary ligand involved (Demuth *et al.*, 1990a). The nucleotide and deduced amino acid sequences of SSP-5 are highly homologous to the P1 protein of *S. mutans* discussed above. However, the proteins are not identical and their specificity differs. *S. sanguis* requires much higher levels of agglutinin for aggregation than *S. mutans* (Malamud *et al.*, 1983). Binding of SSP-5 to agglutinin is sensitive to pretreatment of agglutinin with neuraminidase, while binding by *S. mutans* is unaffected, and SSP-5 binds sialic acid while the *S. mutans* adhesin binds fucose and lactose (Levine *et al.*, 1978, 1987; Demuth *et al.*, 1990a, 1990b).

Surface Proteins as Virulence Factors

The descriptions of the morphologically distinctive surface proteins on oral pathogens presented above would predict that they play an important role in colonization and human caries-formation. Certainly, these proteins appear to bind to salivary proteins or to other oral microorganisms. Recent studies of the M protein fibrillar antigen of *Streptococcus pyogenes*, however, has thrown doubt on the role of that prominent structure in virulence. Caparon *et al.* (1991) recently demonstrated that M+ and M- isogenic pairs of *S. pyogenes* strains show no difference in adherence to human epithelial cells or to fibronectin receptors. Courtney and Hasty (1991), using this same isogenic pair of *S. pyogenes* strains, found that each strain aggregated in human saliva and each adsorbed the salivary agglutinin also responsible for *S. sanguis* aggregation and adherence. Thus, it can be concluded that the role of the prominent M protein of *S. pyogenes* in adherence *in vivo* is still not clear.

But what is the role of antigen P1 of *S. mutans* in oral colonization *in vivo*? In collaboration with Dr. W.H. Bowen, University of Rochester, we compared the abilities of *S. mutans* NG8 and its isogenic sister strain 834 to colonize and cause caries in rats fed a cariogenic (56% sucrose) diet. Previous studies had shown that rat saliva contains an agglutinin similar in specificity and chemical properties to the human mucin (Brack and Reynolds, 1987) and that colonization of the rat oral cavity was in part related to the ability of a streptococcal strain to react with this protein (Brack and Reynolds, 1988). One agglutination-negative strain, GS5, which cannot anchor P1 to its cell surface, however, nevertheless colonized rats as well as those strains retaining this surface fibril. Our own studies revealed that both NG8 and 834 could bind to artificial dextran pellicles on hydroxyapatite beads, but the P1- mutant was unable to bind to parotid saliva-coated beads. *In vivo,* however, these strains colonized rats, either intact or desalivated, to similar extents. Likewise, caries scores revealed no differences in the virulence of this isogenic pair (Bowen *et al.*, 1991).

From these data, we conclude that the ability to colonize is a complex, multifactorial process. The elimination of a single "virulence factor" does not necessarily render the microbe unable to infect. Yet, these surface proteins undoubtedly have been retained to perform key functions which await our discovery.

REFERENCES

ABIKO, Y.; HAYAKAWA, M.; AOKI, H.; SAITO, S.; and TAKIGUCHI, H. (1989): Cloning of the gene for cell-surface protein antigen A from *Streptococcus sobrinus* (serotype d), *Arch Oral Biol* 34:571-575.

ACKERMANS, F.; KLEIN, J.P.; OGIER, J.A.; BAZIN, H.; CORMONT, F.; and FRANK, R.M. (1985): Purification and characterization of a saliva-interacting cell wall protein from *Streptococcus mutans* serotype f by using monoclonal antibody immunoaffinity chromatography, *Biochem J* 228:211-217.

AHL, T. and REINHOLDT, J. (1991): Detection of immunoglobulin A1 protease-induced Fabα fragments on dental plaque bacteria, *Infect Immun* 59:563-569.

AYAKAWA, G.Y.; BOUSHELL, L.W.; CROWLEY, P.J.; ERDOS, G.W.; McARTHUR, W.P.; and BLEIWEIS, A.S. (1987): Isolation and characterization of monoclonal antibodies specific for antigen P1, a major surface protein of mutans streptococci, *Infect Immun* 55:2759-2767.

BLEIWEIS, A.S.; LEE, S.F.; BRADY, L.J.; PROGULSKE-FOX, A.; and CROWLEY, P.J. (1990): Cloning and inactivation of the gene responsible for a major surface antigen of *Streptococcus mutans*. *Arch Oral Biol* 35 (Suppl):15-23.

BOWEN, W.H.; SCHILLING, K.; GIERTSEN, E.; PEARSON, S.; LEE, S.F.; BLEIWEIS, A.; and BEEMAN, D. (1991): Role of a cell surface-associated protein in adherence and dental caries, *Infect Immun* 59:4606-4609.

BRACK, C.M. and REYNOLDS, E.C. (1987): Characterization of a rat salivary sialoglycoprotein complex which agglutinates *Streptococcus mutans*, *Infect Immun* 55:1264-1273.

BRACK, C.M. and REYNOLDS, E.C. (1988): Colonization of rat molar teeth by mutans streptococci with different salivary agglutination characteristics, *Arch Oral Biol* 33:695-699.

BRADY, L.J.; CROWLEY, P.J.; MA, J.K-C.; KELLY, C.; LEE, S.F.; LEHNER, T.; and BLEIWEIS, A.S. (1991): Restriction fragment length polymorphisms and sequence variation within the *spaP* gene of *Streptococcus mutans* serotype c isolates, *Infect Immun* 59:1803-1810.

CAPARON, M.G.; STEPHENS, D.S.; OLSEN, A.; and SCOTT, J.R. (1991): Role of M protein in adherence of Group A streptococci, *Infect Immun* 59:1811-1817.

COURTNEY, H.S. and HASTY, D.L. (1991): Aggregation of Group A streptococci by human saliva and effect of saliva on streptococcal adherence to host cells, *Infect Immun* 59:1661-1666.

CISAR, J.O.; BARSUMIAN, E.L.; CURL, S.H.; VATTER, A.E.; SANDBERG, A.L.; and SIRAGANIAN, R.P. (1981): Detection and localization of a lectin on *Actinomyces viscosus* T14 by monoclonal antibodies, *J Immunol* 127:1318-1322.

CISAR, J.O.; CURL, S.H.; KOLENBRANDER, P.E.; and VATTER, A.E. (1983): Specific absence of type 2 fimbriae on a coaggregation-defective mutant of *Actinomyces viscosus* T14V, *Infect Immun* 40:759-765.

CISAR, J.O.; BRENNAN, M.J.; and SANDBERG, A.L. (1985): Lectin-specific interaction of *Actinomyces* fimbriae with oral streptococci. In: Molecular Basis of Oral Microbial Adhesion, S.E. Mergenhagen and B. Rosan, Eds., Washington D.C.: *ASM*, pp. 159-163.

CLARK, W.B. (1985): Actinomyces fimbriae and adherence to hydroxyapatite. In: *Molecular Basis of Oral Microbial Adhesion*, S.E. Mergenhagen and B. Rosan, Eds., Washington D.C.: ASM, pp. 103-108.

CLARK, W.B.; BAMMANN, L.L.; and GIBBONS, R.J. (1978): Comparative estimates of bacterial affinities and adsorption sites on hydroxyapatite surfaces, *Infect Immun* 19:846-853.

COSTELLO, A.H.; CISAR, J.O.; KOLENBRANDER, P.E.; and GABRIEL, O. (1979): Neuraminidase-dependent haemagglutination of human erythrocytes by human strains of *Actinomyces viscosus* and *Actinomyces naeslundii*, *Infect Immun* 26:563-572.

DEMUTH, D.R.; DAVIS, C.A.; CORNER, A.M.; LAMONT, R.J.; LEBOY, P.S., and MALAMUD, D. (1988): Cloning and expression of a *Streptococcus sanguis* surface antigen that interacts with human salivary agglutinin, *Infect Immun* 56:2484-2490.

DEMUTH, D.R.; BERTHOLD, P.; LEBOY, P.S.; GOLUB, E.E.; DAVIS, C.A.; and MALAMUD, D. (1989): Saliva-mediated aggregation of *Enterococcus faecalis* transformed with a *Streptococcus sanguis* gene encoding the SSP-5 surface antigen, *Infect Immun* 57:1470-1475.

DEMUTH, D.R.; GOLUB, E.E.; and MALAMUD, D. (1990a): Streptococcal-host interactions: structural and functional analysis of a *Streptococcus sanguis* receptor for a human salivary glycoprotein, *J Biol Chem* 265:7120-7126.

DEMUTH, D.R.; LAMMEY, M.S.; HUCK, M.; LALLY, E.T.; and MALAMUD, D. (1990b): Comparison of *Streptococcus mutans* and *Streptococcus sanguis* receptors for human salivary agglutinin, *Microbial Pathogen* 9:199-211.

DOUGLAS, C.W.I. and RUSSELL, R.R.B. (1984): Effect of specific antisera upon *Streptococcus mutans* adherence to saliva-coated hydroxyapatite, *FEMS Microbiol Lett* 25:211-214.

EGGEN, K.E. and ROLLA, G. (1982): Interaction between human saliva and various hydroxyapatite surfaces, *Nordisk Ontodontologisk Forening* (Abs) - Annual Meeting 114.

FACHON-KALWEIT, S.; ELDER, B.L.; and FIVES-TAYLOR, P. (1985): Antibodies that bind to fimbriae block adhesion of *Streptococcus sanguis* to saliva-coated hydroxyapatite, *Infect Immun* 48:617-624.

FERRETTI, J.J.; SHEA, C.; and HUMPHREY, M.W. (1980): Cross-reactivity of *Streptococcus mutans* antigens and human heart tissue, *Infect Immun* 30:69-73.

FIVES-TAYLOR, P. and THOMPSON, D.W. (1985): Surface properties of *Streptococcus sanguis* FW213 mutants non-adherent to saliva-coated hydroxyapatite, *Infect Immun* 47:752-759.

FORESTER, H.; HUNTER, N.; and KNOX, K.W. (1983): Characteristics of a high molecular weight extracellular protein of *Streptococcus mutans*, *J Gen Microbiol* 129:2779-2788.

GABRIEL, O.; HEEB, M.J.; and HINRICHS, M. (1985): Interaction of the surface adhesins of the oral *Actinomyces* spp. with mammalian cells. In: *Molecular Basis of Oral Microbial Adhesion*, S.E. Mergenhagen and B. Rosan, Eds., Washington D.C.: ASM, pp. 45-52.

GANESHKUMAR, N.; SONG, M.; and MCBRIDE, B.C. (1988): Cloning of a *Streptococcus sanguis* adhesin which mediates binding to saliva-coated hydroxyapatite, *Infect Immun* 56:1150-1157.

GIBBONS, R.J. (1984): Adherent interactions which may affect microbial ecology in the mouth, *J Dent Res* 63:378-385.

GIBBONS, R.J. (1989): Bacterial adhesion to oral tissues: a model for infectious diseases, *J Dent Res* 68:750-760.

GIBBONS, R.J. and VAN HOUTE, J. (1971): Selective bacterial adherence to oral epithelial surfaces and its role as an ecological determinant, *Infect Immun* 3:567-573.

GIBBONS, R.J.; ETHERDEN, I.; and MORENO, E.C. (1983): Association of neuraminidase-sensitive receptors and putative hydrophobic interactions with high affinity binding sites for *Streptococcus sanguis* C5 in salivary pellicles, *Infect Immun* 42:1006-1012.

GIBBONS, R.J. and HAY, D.I. (1988): Human salivary acidic proline-rich proteins and statherin promote the attachment of *Actinomyces viscosus* LY7 to apatitic surfaces, *Infect Immun* 56:439-445.

GIBBONS, R.J.; HAY, D.I.; CISAR, J.O.; and CLARK, W.B. (1988): Adsorbed salivary proline-rich protein 1 and statherin: receptors for type 1 fimbriae of *Actinomyces viscosus* T14V-J1 on apatitic surfaces, *Infect Immun* 56:2990-2993.

HAMADA, S. and SLADE, H.D. (1980): Biology, immunology and cariogenicity of *Streptococcus mutans*, *Microbiol Rev* 44:331-384.

HAMILTON, I.R. and NG, S.K.C. (1983): Stimulation of glycolysis through lactate consumption in a resting cell mixture of *Streptococcus salivarius* and *Veillonella parvula*, *FEMS Microbial Lett* 20:61-65.

HANDLEY, P.S.; CARTER, P.L.; and FIELDING, J. (1984): *Streptococcus salivarius* strains carry either fibrils or fimbriae on the cell surface, *J Bacteriol* 157:64-72.

HANDLEY, P.S.; CARTER, P.L.; WYATT, J.E.; and HESKETH, L.M. (1985): Surface structures (peritrichous fibrils and tufts of fibrils) found on *Streptococcus sanguis* strains may be related to their ability to coaggregate with other oral genera, *Infect Immun* 47:217-227.

HOLT, R.G.; ABIKO, Y.; SAITO, S.; SMORAWINSKA, J.; HANSEN, J.B.; and CURTISS, R. III (1982): *Streptococcus mutans* genes that code for extracellular proteins in *Escherichia coli* K12, *Infect Immun* 38:147-156.

HUGHES, M.; MacHARDY, S.M.; SHEPPARD, A.J.; and WOODS, N.C. (1980): Evidence for an immunological relationship between *Streptococcus mutans* and human cardiac tissue, *Infect Immun* 27:576-588.

KELLY, C.; EVANS, P.; BERGMEIER, L.; LEE, S.F.; PROGULSKE-FOX, A.; HARRIS, A.C.; AITKEN, A.; BLEIWEIS, A.S.; and LEHNER, T. (1989): Sequence analysis of the cloned streptococcal antigen I/II, *FEBS Lett* 258:127-132.

KILIAN, M. and REINHOLDT, J. (1986): Interference with IgA defense mechanisms by extracellular bacterial enzymes. In: *Medical Microbiology* Volume 5, C. Easmon and J. Jeljaszewics, Eds., London: Academic Press, pp. 173-208.

KILIAN, M.; MESTECKY, J.; and RUSSELL, M.W. (1988): Defense mechanisms involving Fc-dependent functions of immunoglobulins A and their subversion by bacterial immunoglobulin A proteases, *Microbiol Rev* 52:296-303.

KOGA, T.; OKAHASI, N.; TAKAHASHI, I.; KANAMOTO, T.; ASAKAWA, H; and IWAKI, M. (1990): Surface hydrophobicity, adherence, and aggregation of cell surface protein antigen mutants of *Streptococcus mutans* serotype c, *Infect Immun* 58:289-296.

KOLENBRANDER, P.E. and WILLIAMS, B.L. (1981): Lactose-reversible coaggregation between oral actinomyces and *Streptococcus sanguis*, *Infect Immun* 33:95-102.

KOLENBRANDER, P.E. and WILLIAMS, B.L. (1983): Prevalance of viridans streptococci exhibiting lactose-inhibitable coaggregation with oral actinomyces, *Infect Immun* 41:449-459.

KOLENBRANDER, P.E.; INOUYE, Y.; and HOLDEMAN, L.V. (1983): New *Actinomyces* and *Streptococcus* coaggregation groups among human oral isolates from the same site, *Infect Immun* 41:501-506.

LEE, S.F.; PROGULSKE-FOX, A.; and BLEIWEIS, A.S. (1988): Molecular cloning and expression of a *Streptococcus mutans* major surface protein antigen, P1 (I/II), in *Escherichia coli, Infect Immun* 56:2114-2119.

LEE, S.F.; PROGULSKE-FOX, A.; ERDOS, G.W.; PIACENTINI, D.A.; AYAKAWA, G.Y.; CROWLEY, P.J.; and BLEIWEIS, A.S. (1989): Construction and characterization of isogenic mutants of *Streptococcus mutans* deficient in major surface protein antigen P1 (I/II), *Infect Immun* 57:3306-3313.

LEHNER, T.; RUSSELL, M.W.; CALDWELL, J.; and SMITH, R. (1981): Immunization with purified protein antigens from *Streptococcus mutans* aginst dental caries in rhesus monkeys, *Infect Immun* 34:407-415.

LEHNER, T.; CALDWELL, J.; and SMITH, R. (1985): Local passive immunization by monoclonal antibodies against streptococcal antigen I/II in the prevention of dental caries, *Infect Immun* 50:796-799.

LEVINE, M.J.; HERZBERG, M.C.; LEVINE, M.S.; ELLISON, S.A.; STINSON, M.W.; LI, C.; and VAN DYKE, T. (1978): Specificity of salivary-bacterial interactions: role of terminal sialic acid residues in the interaction of salivary glycoprotein with *Streptococcus sanguis* and *Streptococcus mutans*, *Infect Immun* 19:107-115.

LEVINE, M.; REDDY, M.; TABAK, L.; LOOMIS, R.; BERGEY, E.; JONES, P.; COHEN, R.; STINSON, M.; and AL-HASHIMI, I. (1987): Structural aspects of salivary glycoproteins, *J Dent Res* 66:423-441.

MA, J.K-C. and LEHNER, T. (1990): Prevention of colonization of *Streptococcus mutans* by topical application of monoclonal antibodies in human subjects, *Arch Oral Biol* 35 (Suppl):115-122.

MALAMUD, D.; GOLDMAN, R.; and TAICHMAN, N.S. (1983): Modulation of bacterial aggregation by PMN and platelet extracts, *Inflammation* 7:133-144.

McBRIDE, B.C.; SONG, M.; KRASSE, B.; and OLSSON, J. (1984): Biochemical and immunological differences between hydrophobic and hydrophilic strains of *Streptococcus mutans*, *Infect Immun* 44:68-75.

MORRIS, E.J. and McBRIDE, B.C. (1984): Adhesion of *Streptococcus sanguis* to saliva-coated hydroxyapatite: evidence for two binding sites, *Infect Immun* 43:656-663.

MORRIS, E.J.; GANESHKUMAR, N.; SONG, M.; and McBRIDE, B.C. (1987): Identification and preliminary characterization of a *Streptococcus sanguis* fibrillar glycoprotein, *J Bacteriol* 169:164-171.

MULKS, M.H. (1985): Microbial IgA proteases. In: *Bacterial enzymes and virulence*, I.A. Holder, Ed., Boca Raton, FL, CRC Press, pp.81-104.

OGIER, J.A.; WACHSMAN, D.; SCHÖLLER, M.; LEPOIVRE, Y.; and KLEIN, J.P. (1990): Molecular characterization of the gene *sr* of the saliva interacting protein from *Streptococcus mutans* OMZ 175, *Arch Oral Biol* 35 (Suppl):25-31.

OKAHASHI, N.; KOGA, T.; and HAMADA, S. (1986): Purification and immunochemical properties of a protein antigen from serotype g *Streptococcus mutans*, *Microbiol Immunol* 30:34-47.

OKAHASHI, M.; SASAKAWA, C.; YOSHIKAWA, M.; HAMADA, S.; and KOGA, T. (1989a): Cloning of a surface protein antigen gene from serotype c *Streptococcus mutans*, *Mol Microbiol* 3:221-228.

OKAHASHI, N.; SASAKAWA, C.; YOSHIKAWA, M.; HAMADA, S.; and KOGA, T. (1989b): Molecular characterization of a surface protein antigen gene from serotype c *Streptococcus mutans*, implicated in dental caries, *Mol Microbiol* 3:673-678.

ØRSTAVIK, D.; KRAUS, F.; and HENSHAW, L. (1974) *In vitro* attachment of streptococci to the tooth surface, *Infect Immun* 9:794-800.

PHILLIPS, G.; FLICKER, P.; COHEN, C.; MANJULA, B.; and FISCHETTI, V.A. (1981): Streptococcal M protein: α-helical coiled-coil structure and arrangement on the cell surface, *Proc Natl Acad Sci USA* 78:4689-4693.

PLAUT, A.G. (1983): The IgA1 proteases of pathogenic bacteria, *Ann Rev Microbiol* 37:603-622.

REINHOLDT, J. and KILIAN, M. (1987): Interference of IgA protease with the effect of secretory IgA in adherence of oral streptococci to saliva-coated hydroxyapatite, *J Dent Res* 66:492-497.

REVIS, G.J.; VATTER, A.E.; CROWLE, A.J.; and CISAR, J.O. (1982): Antibodies against the Ag2 fimbriae of *Actinomyces viscosus* T14V inhibit lactose-sensitive bacterial adherence, *Infect Immun* 36:1217-1222.

RUSSELL, M.W; BERGMEIER, E.D.; ZANDERS, E.D.; and LEHNER, T. (1980): Protein antigens of *Streptococcus mutans*: purification and properties of a double antigen and its protease-resistant component, *Infect Immun* 28:486-493.

RUSSELL, M.W. and WU, H. (1990): *Streptococcus mutans* and the problem of heart cross-reactivity, *Crit Revs in Oral Biol Med* 1:191-205.

RUSSELL, R.R.B. (1979): Wall-associated antigens of *Streptococcus mutans*, *J Gen Microbiol* 114:109-115.

RUSSELL, R.R.B. (1980): Distribution of cross-reactive antigens A and B in *Streptococcus mutans* and other oral streptococci, *J Gen Microbiol* 118:383-388.

SMITH, R.; LEHNER, T.; and BEVERLEY, P.C.L. (1984): Characterization of monoclonal antibodies to *Streptococcus mutans* antigenic determinants I/II, I, II and III and their serotype specificities, *Infect Immun* 46:168-175.

STAAT, R.H.; LANGLEY, S.D.; and DOYLE, R.J. (1980): *Streptococcus mutans* adherence: presumptive evidence for protein-mediated attachment followed by glucan-dependent cellular accumulation, *Infect Immun* 27:675-681.

VAN DE RIJN, I.; BLEIWEIS, A.S.; and ZABRISKIE, J.B. (1976): Antigens in *Streptococcus mutans* cross-reactive with human heart muscle, *J Dent Res* 55C:59-64.

WEERKAMP, A.H. and McBRIDE, B.C. (1980): Characterization of the adherence properties of *Streptococcus salivarius, Infect Immun* 29:459-468.

WEERKAMP, A.H. and JACOBS, T. (1982): Cell wall-associated protein antigens of *Streptococcus salivarius*: purification, properties and function in adherence, *Infect Immun* 38:233-242.

WEERKAMP, A.H.; HANDLEY, P.S.; BAARS, A.; and SLOT, J. (1986): Negative staining and immunoelectron microscopy of adhesion-deficient mutants of *Streptococcus salivarius* reveal that the adhesive protein antigens are separate classes of cell surface fibril, *J Bacteriol* 165:746-755.

WYATT, J.E.; HESKETH, L.M.; and HANDLEY, P.S. (1987): Lack of correlation between fibrils, hydrophobicity and adhesion for strains of *Streptococcus sanguis* biotypes I and II, *Microbios* 50:7-15.

ZANDERS, E.D. and LEHNER, T. (1981): Separation and characterization of a protein antigen from cells of *Streptococcus mutans*, *J Gen Microbiol* 122:217-225.

Molecular Biology of *Streptococcus mutans* Virulence

HOWARD K. KURAMITSU,
MARIA SMORAWINSKA, AND
YOSHIHISA YAMASHITA

The central role of *Streptococcus mutans* in the development of human dental caries is now well established (Loesche, 1986). A variety of biochemical approaches have identified several properties of the organisms which appear to contribute to their cariogenic potential: (a) aciduricity at pH levels observed in cariogenic plaque; (b) strong acidogenicity; (c) ability to synthesize water-insoluble glucan polymers in the presence of dietary sucrose; (d) attachment to the tooth pellicle. However, for the most part, these properties have been inferred to be important in caries formation and direct experimental proof for such a role *in vivo* is still lacking.

Verification of the role of a potential virulence factor in disease production can best be obtained by constructing specific mutants of the pathogen followed by testing of each mutant in a suitable animal model system. Defined bacterial mutants can be constructed by initially isolating the gene for a putative virulence factor, insertionally inactivating the gene, and replacement of the wild-type copy of the gene with its defective counterpart following gene transfer. Utilizing this approach a number of defined mutants of *S. mutans* have been constructed (Curtiss, 1985; Macrina *et al.*, 1990) and some have been examined in rodent model systems (Barletta *et al.*, 1988; Schroeder *et al.*, 1989). However, many of the potential virulence factors of *S. mutans* have not yet been examined in a comparable rigorous manner (Table 1).

We wish to express our thanks to numerous investigators who shared unpublished data with us. Work carried out in this laboratory was supported in part by National Institutes of Health grants DE03258 and DE09039.

TABLE 1 *S. mutans genes implicated in cariogenicity*

Gene	*Proposed role*	*Specific mutants*	*Animal model*
ldh	Acidogenicity	No	No
ATPase	Aciduricity	No	No
PAc	Colonization	Yes	In progress
gtfB	Colonization	Yes	In progress
gtfC	Colonization	Yes	In progress
gtfD	Colonization	Yes	Yes
ftf	Reserve nutrient	Yes	Yes
gbp	Colonization	Yes	No
glg	Reserve nutrient	Yes	In progress
fruA	Reserve nutrient	Yes	In progress

Evaluation of Specific Mutants of S. mutans in Animal Model Systems

Although it is reasonable to assume that lactic acid production by *S. mutans* is an important cariogenic factor, mutants defective in only lactic acid production have yet be constructed for testing in animal models. The mutants which are available (Hillman, 1978) have been isolated following chemical mutagenesis and it is possible that these mutants might possess other undetected alterations which could be relevant to cariogenesis. However, the recent isolation of the lactic dehydrogenase (*ldh*) gene from strain JH1000 (Hillman *et al.*, 1990) now makes it possible to construct specific LDH$^-$ mutants for further testing.

Biochemical analysis (Bender *et al.*, 1986) has also suggested that the H^+-translocating ATPases of *S. mutans* play an important role in the aciduricity of these organisms. More recently, fragments of the gene coding for the beta-subunit of this complex have been isolated (Faustoferri and Quivey, 1990). Therefore, it should be possible to construct mutants of *S. mutans* which are defective in this activity for direct testing of this hypothesis *in vitro* and in the rodent model system.

Besides fermentation of dietary sugars, *S. mutans* strains may also produce lactic acid following degradation of reserve polysaccharides (Loesche, 1986). Therefore, fructans synthesized by the *ftf* gene product, FTF (fructosyltransferase), of *S. mutans* as well as intracellular glycogen could be potential virulence factors for these organisms. However, mutants defective in FTF activity have been demonstrated to produce caries at the same rate as the parental organism in the rat model (Schroeder *et.al.*, 1989; Kuramitsu and Bowen, unpub. results). In contrast, preliminary results (Harris and Curtiss, unpub. results) suggest that mutants defective in glycogen synthesis (*glg* mutants) are defective in cariogenesis. In addition, mutants which are defective in the fructanase gene, *fru*A, are currently under evaluation in the rat caries model (Burne, person. commun.).

Colonization of tooth surfaces by mutans streptococci is presumably dependent upon both sucrose-dependent and independent mechanisms (Loesche, 1986). The latter phenomena appears to be mediated by proteins (adhesins) associated with the cell surface of *S. mutans* (Gibbons *et al.*, 1986). Several of the genes coding for potential adhesins (designated P1, B, antigen I/II, or PAc) have recently been isolated and sequenced (Lee *et al.*, 1988; Okahashi *et al.*, 1989; Demuth *et al.*, 1990). In addition, a mutant defective in one of the putative adhesins has been recently constructed from its corresponding gene and is currently being testing in the rat caries system (Bleiweis, see this volume).

A significant amount of data has accumulated implicating glucosyltransferases (GTFs) as virulence factors for the mutans streptococci (Loesche, 1986). Based on Southern blot analysis of a variety of human isolates of *S. mutans* (Chia *et al.*, 1991; Y. Sato, person. commun.), it has been suggested that the majority of these strains express three distinct *gtf* genes (Fig. 1). Previous results have demonstrated that two of the genes, *gtf*B and *gtf*C, are required for sucrose dependent attachment to smooth surfaces *in vitro* (Aoki *et.al.*, 1986; Hanada and Kuramitsu, 1988) while the third gene, *gtf*D, is dispensible (Hanada and Kuramitsu, 1989). However, caution should be exercised in extrapolating *in vitro* colonization results to the oral cavity since at least one *S. mutans* strain, UA101, does not colonize smooth surfaces *in vitro* in the presence of sucrose (Yamashita and Kuramitsu, unpub. results) while inducing significant levels of caries in rats (Barletta *et al.*, 1988). Interestingly, strain UA101 expresses only a single GTF-I enzyme from a gene which appears to have been derived from homologous recombination between the *gtf*B and C genes.

In order to assess the relative contribution of each of the three *S. mutans gtf* gene products in cariogenesis in the rat model, each insertionally inactivated gene has been transferred into either strains UA130 or UA101 following transformation to create mutants defective in each gene. These mutants have been implanted into rats (in collaboration with W. Bowen, Univ. of Rochester) and preliminary results indicate that, like the *in vitro* system, mutants defective in the *gtf*D gene coding for the primer-dependent GTF-S produce as much caries as the parental organism while *gtf*B and C mutants induce significantly less caries in rats fed a high sucrose-containing diet.

The demonstration of a glucan-binding protein (GBP) in culture fluids of *S. mutans* (Russell, 1979) has suggested the possibility that this protein may play a role in sucrose-dependent colonization of tooth surfaces. The recent isolation and sequencing of the *gbp* gene coding for this protein (Banas *et al.*, 1990) clearly indicates that the GBP is a specific gene product and not a peptide fragment generated from proteolysis of a GTF (Wong *et al.*, 1990). Mutants of

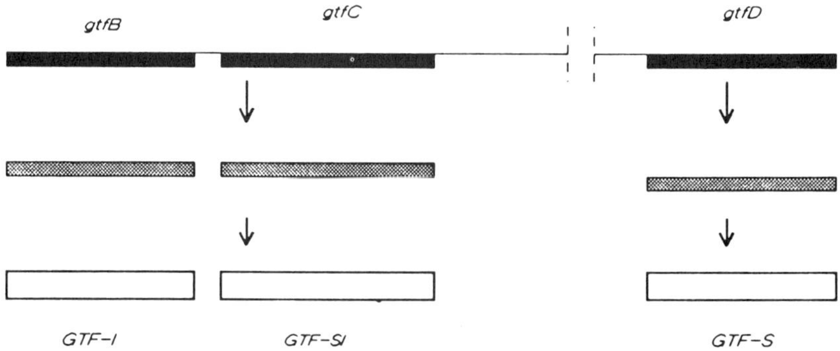

Fig. 1. Organization of the *gtf* genes contained on the chromosome of most strains of *S. mutans.* [black box], genes; [XXXX], mRNA; [open box], proteins.

S. mutans defective in the *gbp* have been constructed and appear to colonize smooth surfaces *in vitro* as well as the parental organism (J. Ferretti, person. commun.). However, such mutants have yet to be tested in animal model systems. Therefore, the role of the GBP in colonization *in vivo* remains to be established.

Potential Utilization of Molecular Biological Approaches in Caries Prevention

Differentiating the cariogenic potential of S. mutans isolates—Although a preliminary report suggested that there are differences in the cariogenic potential of naturally occuring strains of *S. mutans* (Kohler and Krasse, 1988), it is not clear whether or not such differences can be correlated with the caries experience of individuals harboring such strains. One factor preventing such a determination has been the difficulty in differentiating between different strains of *S. mutans*. However, the recent development of RFLP (restriction fragment length polymorphism) techniques for *S. mutans* (Caufield and Walker, 1989) has now made it possible to readily distinguish between different strains of these organisms. Therefore, it now should be possible to examine distinct strains of these organisms in an animal model to determine if the resulting caries is a reflection of the caries experience of individuals carrying these strains. In addition, a comparison of the different strains might reveal additional virulence factors which have gone undetected up to now.

Identification of caries susceptible children—Despite the impressive decline in the incidence of dental caries in most modern societies, a significant number

TABLE 2 *Specificity of S. mutans DNA probes*

	Hybridization[a]					
Probe	*S. mutans*	*S. sob.*[b]	*S. sal.*	*S. gord.*	*A. vis.*	*P.ging.*
gtfB	+	−	−	−	−	−
gtfD	+	−	−	−	−	−
ftf	+	−	−	−	−	−

[a]Southern blot hybridization with the *S. mutans GS5 probes were carried out under relatively high stringency conditions.*

[b]*S. sob, Streptococcus sobrinus; S. sal., Streptococcus salivarius; S. gord., Streptococcus gordonii; A. vis, Actinomyces viscosus; P. ging., Porphyromonas gingivalis.*

of children still remain at high risk of developing dental caries (Krasse, 1985). Although there are multiple factors which influence the development of this disease, preliminary findings have suggested that monitoring the levels of *S. mutans* in saliva can provide one means of identifying individuals at high risk of developing caries (Krasse, 1985). However, quantitation of these organisms in salivary samples cannot be carried out conveniently in a dentist's office. Nevertheless, the recent development of DNA probes to detect infectious agents suggests that this technology can be applied to rapidly quantitate *S. mutans* levels in salivary samples. In our laboratory we have constructed several DNA probes which can differentiate *S. mutans* from other organisms commonly isolated from the human oral cavity (Smorawinska and Kuramitsu, manu. submitted; Table 2). With the current rapid development of probe technology it is likely that these or equivalent (ie., ribosomal RNA) probes could be developed for quantitating *S. mutans* in saliva in dental practise.

Novel anticaries strategies—Since some of the individuals who experience high caries rates are not effectively protected by current anticaries strategies (oral hygiene, fluoridation, etc.), alternative anticaries procedures may prove useful to effectively treat these individuals. Several new approaches based on the utilization of molecular biological approaches are currently under investigation. Reduction in the levels of *S. mutans* in the oral cavity could be produced by vaccination, by adminstration of inhibitors of *S. mutans* growth (bacteriocins), or by neutralizing virulence factors (mutanase). Genes coding for *S. mutans* cell surface proteins could be incorporated into attenuated *Salmonella* strains for utilization as an anticaries vaccine (Curtiss *et al.*, 1988). Alternatively, genes coding for anti-*S. mutans* bacteriocins or inhibitors of plaque formation (mutanases) could be engineered into noncariogenic plaque bacteria (*Streptococcus sanguis*) in order to inhibit the colonization of teeth by *S. mutans*. Likewise, replacement therapy strategies based on genetically engineered organisms may be utilized to reduce or neutralize cariogenic *S. mutans* in the oral cavity (see R. Quivey's paper). Although none of these new approaches has yet to be tested in animal model systems, each of these has the potential of providing additional strategies to further reduce the incidence of dental caries.

REFERENCES

AOKI, H.; SHIROZA, T.; HAYAKAWA, M.; SATO, S.; and KURAMITSU, H.K. (1986): Cloning of a *Streptococcus mutans* glucosyltransferas gene coding for insoluble glucan synthesis. *Infect Immun* 53:587-594.

BANAS, J.A.; RUSSELL, R.R.B.; and FERRETTI, J.J. (1990): Sequence analysis of the gene for the glucan-binding protein of *Streptococcus mutans* Ingbritt. *Infect Immun* 58:667-673.

BARLETTA, R.; MICHALEK, S.M.; and CURTISS III, R. (1988): Analysis of the virulence of *Streptococcus mutans* serotype c *gtf*A mutants in the rat model system. *Infect Immun* 56:322-330.

BENDER, G.R.; SUTTON, S.V.W.; and MARQUIS, R.E. (1986): Acid tolerance, proton permeabilities, and membrane ATPases of oral streptococci. *Infect Immun* 53:331-338.

CAUFIELD, P.W. and WALKER, T.M. (1989): Genetic diversity within *Streptococcus mutans* evident from chromosomal DNA restriction fragment polymorphisms. *J Clin Microbiol* 27:274-276.

CHIA, J.-S.; HSU, T.-Y.; TENG, L.-J.; CHEN, J.-Y.; HAHN, L.-J.; and YANG, C.-S.. (1991): Glucosyltransferase gene polymorphism among *Streptococcus mutans* strains. *Infect Immun* 59:1656-1660.

CURTISS, R. III. (1985): Genetic analysis of *Streptococcus mutans* virulence. *Curr Top Microbiol Immun* 118:253-277.

CURTISS, R. III; GOLDSCHMIDT, R.M.; FLETCHALL, N.B.; and KELLY, S.M. (1988): Avirulent *Salmonella typhimurium* delta *cya* delta *crp* oral strains expressing a streptococcal colonization and virulence antigen. *Vaccine* 6:155-160.

DEMUTH, D.R.; LAMMEY, M.S.; HUCK, M.; LALLY, E.T.; and MALAMUD, D. (1990): Comparison of *Streptococcus mutans* and *Streptococcus sanguis* receptors for human salivary agglutinin. *Microbiol Path* 9:199-211.

FAUSTOFERRI, R.C. and QUIVEY, R.G. (1990): Cloning and DNA sequence determination of streptococcal ATPases. *J Dent Res* 69 (Spec. Issue):376.

GIBBONS, R.J.; COHEN, L.; and HAY, D.I.(1986): Strains of *Streptococcus mutans* and *Streptococcus sobrinus* attach to different pellicle receptors. *Infect Immun* 52:555-561.

HANADA, N. and KURAMITSU, H.K. (1988): Isolation and characterization of the *Streptococcus mutans gtf*C gene, coding for synthesis of both soluble and insoluble glucans. *Infect Immun* 56:1999-2005.

HANADA, N. and KURAMITSU, H.K. (1989): Isolation and characterization of the *Streptococcus mutans gtf*D gene, coding for primer-dependent soluble glucan synthesis. *Infect Immun* 57:2079-2085.

HILLMAN, J.D. (1978): Lactate dehydrogenase mutants of *Streptococcus mutans*: isolation and preliminary characterization. *Infect Immun* 21:206-212.

HILLMAN, J.D.; DUNCAN, M.J.; and STASHENKO, K.P. (1990): Cloning and expression of the gene encoding the fructose-1,6-diphosphate-dependent L-(+)-lactate dehydrogenase of *Streptococcus mutans*. *Infect Immun* 58:1290-1295.

KOHLER, B. and KRASSE, B. (1988): Human strains of mutans streptococci show different cariogenicity. *J Dent Res* 67 (Spec. Issue):343.

KRASSE, B. (1985): *Caries Risk*. Quintessence Books, Chicago, Il.

LEE, S.F.; PROGULSKE-FOX,A.; and BLEIWEIS, A.S. (1988): Molecular cloning and expression of a *Streptococcus mutans* major surface protein antigen, P1 (I/II), in *Escherichia coli*. *Infect Immun* 56:2114-2119.

LOESCHE, W.J. (1986): Role of *Streptococcus mutans* in human dental decay. *Microbiol Revs* 50:353-380.

MACRINA, F.L.; DERTZBAUGH, M.T.; HALULA, M.C.; KRAH III, E.R.; and JONES, K.R. (1990): Genetic approaches to the study of oral microflora: a review. *CRC Crit. Rev. Oral Biology and Med* 1:207-227.

OKAHASHI, N.; SASAKAWA, C.; YOSHIKAWA, M.; HAMADA, S.; and KOGA, T. (1989): Cloning of a surface protein antigen gene from serotype c *Streptococcus mutans*. *Mol Microbiol* 3:221-228.

RUSSELL, R.R.B. (1979): Glucan-binding proteins of *Streptococcus mutans* serotype c. *J Gen Microbiol* 112:197-201.

SCHROEDER, V.A.; MICHALEK, S.M.; and MACRINA, F.L. (1989): Biochemical characterization and evaluation of virulence of a fructosyltransferase-deficient mutant of *Streptococcus mutans* V403. *Infect Immun* 57:3560-3569.

WONG, C.; HEFTA, S.A.; PAXTON, R.J.; SHIVELY, J.E.; and MOOSER, G. (1990): Size and subdomain architecture of the glucan-binding domain of sucrose: 3-α-D-glucosyltransferase from *Streptococcus sobrinus*. *Infect Immun* 58:2165-2170.

Arginine Deiminase and Alkali Generation in Plaque

R.E. MARQUIS, R.A. BURNE, D.T. PARSONS AND A.E. CASIANO-COLÓN

Everyone in the cariology field is familiar with Stephan curves which show the rapid drop in plaque pH value following a sugar challenge and the more gradual rise in pH after glycolytic acid production subsides. The subsequent pH rise can be attributed to a number of processes. Diffusion of acid products from plaque into saliva, even though it may be restricted by stagnant layers, clearly is important and may involve protonated acids, unprotonated acids and protons. The buffering influence of plaque, and at a distance of saliva, serves to moderate glycolytic pH drops but also moderates subsequent pH increases. Bacteria are the predominant buffer agents in plaque, and acid-base titration curves for plaque are very similar to those for bacterial cells. Plaque fluid also contains buffers (Margolis, 1990), but of course, the buffering capacity of the fluid is much less per unit volume than that of the bacterial mass. Fig. 1 presents data for buffer capacities (μmol H^+/pH unit/g cell dry weight) for cells of *Streptococcus mutans* GS-5 in the pH range from 4.0 to 9.5. Generally, there are only relatively small differences in buffering profiles among various bacterial types, including extreme acidophiles or alkaliphiles. In the acid range, there is a peak of buffering at a pH value of about 6.0. However, the cells are buffering over the entire range, and even at a pH value of 5.0, at which buffering is minimal in the acid range, the capacity is still some 178 μmol H^+/pH unit/g dry weight. Most of the buffering in this range is probably due to carboxyl groups of bacterial polymers, which have average pK_a values of about 4.5, but with the range of values expected for polymer networks exhibiting large electrostatic effects. In the alkaline range, buffering is low between pH values of about 7.0 and 8.0, but then rises at higher pH because of titration of amino groups in biopolymers. The

The work of the authors was supported by U. S. Public Health Service grants DE07003 and DE06127 from the National Institute of Dental Research.

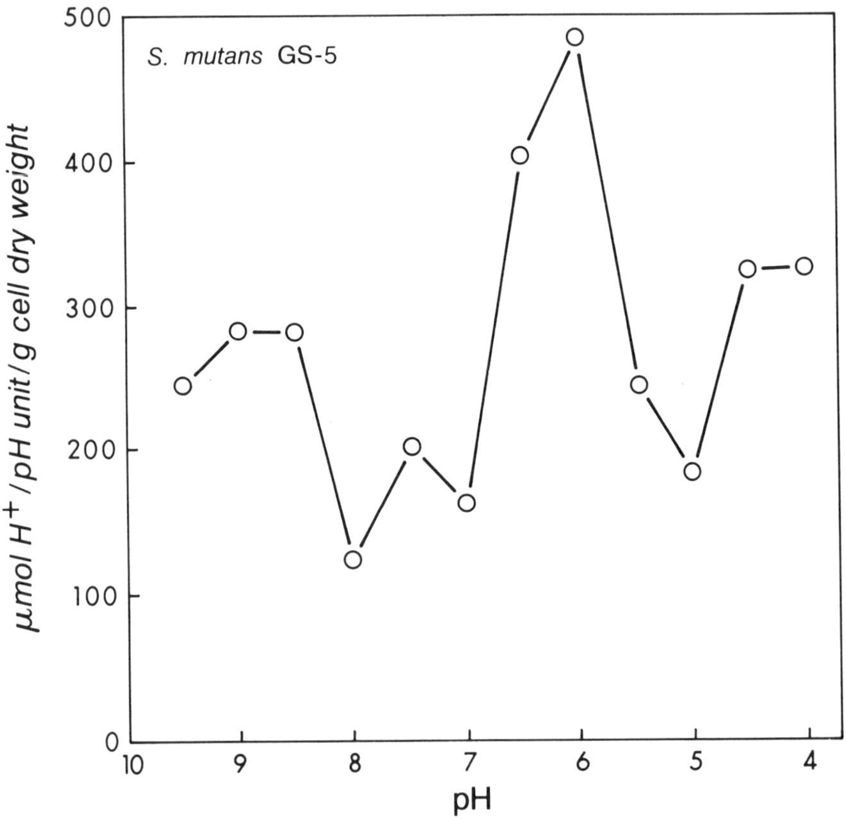

Figure 1 Buffering capacities of permeabilized cells of *S. mutans* GS-5. Cells were permeabilized with 10% butanol before being used for acid-base titrations.

data shown in Fig. 1 are similar to those obtained, for example, by Krulwich *et al.* (1985) for *Escherichia coli* and *Bacillus* organisms. The data, then, can be expected to reflect the overall buffering behavior of plaque bacteria and not just *S. mutans*. Bicarbonate is not a common buffer for bacteria, but of course, is for saliva. Organic phosphates buffer only at low pH values not generally encountered in plaque. If there is dissolution of apatites during acidification, this process also will contribute to pH rise. However, as the pH of plaque increases, the tendency is for mineralization, which would then moderate pH rise.

The other major factor in pH rise in plaque is base-generating metabolism of the flora. This metabolism is considered by many to be of major importance in the overall cariogenicity of plaque. For example, Wijeyeweera and Kleinberg (1989) have proposed " . . . that a deficiency in base formation, especially that from arginine, may be as great or a greater risk for the development of dental caries as excessive formation of acid from fermentable carbohydrate.'' The major base in plaque is ammonia, and levels detected in plaque fluid range from about 1 to 43 mmol/L (Dawes, 1984; Edgar and Higham, 1990). This variation in level is to be expected in relation to variations in bacterial metabolism, host factors and in loss of ammonia from plaque. Plaque may also contain basic, amino compounds such as ornithine and polyamines. The identified sources for plaque ammonia include ureolysis, Stickland fermentation reactions and the major focus of this paper, the arginine deiminase system (ADS).

The importance of urea hydrolysis in ammonia production in plaque remains somewhat unresolved. Urea hydrolysis clearly occurs in saliva, where *Streptococcus salivarius* is a major player (Sissons *et al.*, 1990). However, it has been more of a problem to identify the major ureolytic bacteria in plaque. Salako and Kleinberg (1989) have implicated *Haemophilus parainfluenzae*, *Actinomyces naeslundii*, *Actinomyces viscosus* and coagulase-negative staphylococci with indication that *H. parainfluenzae* is the major contributor to ureolytic activity.

Curtis *et al.* (1983) detected 5-aminovaleric acid in plaque, initially from monkeys, and concluded that plaque bacteria could carry out Stickland fermentations with coupled oxidation-reductions of amino acids. Reduction of proline or ornithine would yield 5-aminovalerate but also NH_3 and CO_2. The organisms most implicated in this activity were peptostreptococci, although other organisms could be involved.

Many bacteria are able to respond to acid or alkaline conditions with increased activities of amino-acid decarboxylases or deamidases, as shown many years ago by Gale and Epps (1942) for *Escherichia coli* and *Micrococcus luteus*. Similar responses have not been well characterized for oral bacteria except for the ADS, which can be induced at remarkably low pH values and has remarkable acid tolerance (Marquis *et al.*, 1987). In the mouth the supply of arginine for the system can be from the diet or from the degradation of salivary proteins or proteins from crevicular fluid. Many plaque bacteria can grow on saliva agar and so must be able to derive their nutrients from degradation of salivary peptides and glycoproteins (De Jong and Van der Hoeven, 1986)). Even an organism such as *S. mutans*, which requires supplementation with carbohydrate to grow on saliva agar, still has proteolytic activity. In fact, many oral streptococci can free carbohydrates from mucins to supply fuel for growth or other functions (Van der Hoeven *et al.*, 1990). Results of a recent study by Homer *et al.* (1990) indicate that proteins such as casein and bovine serum albumin are degraded by the common oral streptococci, and Rogers and Reynolds (1990) have shown that nearly all of the amino acid residues of alpha$_{s1}$-casein with the exception of tyrosine, can be utilized by *Streptococcus sanguis* P_4A_7. Earlier, Rogers *et al.* (1988) had shown that this same organism can degrade small arginine-containing peptides to release arginine, which was then degraded via the ADS. The organisms of subgingival plaque associated with periodontal disease are noted for being highly proteolytic, and organisms such as *Treponema denticola* also have the

ADS for catabolism of arginine or arginine-containing peptides released by proteolysis (Blakemore and Canale-Parola, 1976).

Physiology and Genetics of the ADS

Our major orientation in studying the ADS is for developing implantable, base-producing bacterial strains for use in moderating the cariogenicity of plaque. These strains could be either hyperproducing *S. sanguis* or *S. mutans* to which genes for the ADS have been transferred to render them ADS-positive. Because of the peculiarities of the ADS and the need to make implantable strains competitive with the natural population, we have had to undertake detailed characterization of the system, mainly in *S. sanguis* NCTC 10904, but also in *S. rattus* FA-1 and *T. denticola*.

As indicated, arginine catabolism is considered to be a major source of ammonia in plaque, and the ADS is the major system in oral bacteria for arginolysis. The ADS-positive organisms commonly in plaque include: *S. sanguis, S. gordonii, S. rattus, S. milleri, S. mitis* biovar 2, *S. anginosus, A. naeslundii, L. fermentum,* and in some people, enterococci. In general, the less acid-tolerant plaque bacteria have the ADS, and one of its main functions is to protect the organisms against acid damage (Casiano-Colón and Marquis, 1988). These organisms are considered to be desirable in terms of having plaque with low cariogenic potential. One of the basic tenants of ecology is that Nature abhors a vacuum. Therefore, a non-harmful flora is much more desirable than no flora, and the establishment of a flora dominated by organisms such as *S. sanguis* can be considered a major defence against caries. This view can be applied to root caries as well as to coronal caries, especially now that the microbiology of root caries is moving in the direction of considering mutans streptococci as major pathogens. A role for ammonia production in relation to gingivitis or periodontal disease has not been established, although clearly the flora associated with these diseases have the potential to degrade arginine to produce ammonia.

Much of our current information on the biochemistry and physiology of the ADS is summarized in Fig. 2. As shown, arginine can enter the cell via an arginine/ornithine antiporter (Driessen *et al.*, 1987; Driessen and Konings, 1990). This exchange does not require ATP, so the organism does not expend ATP gained from arginolysis for substrate uptake. The antiport is neutral also in relation to acid-base exchange. Organisms such as *S. sanguis* appear to have two arginine transport systems (Ferro *et al.*, 1983) - the antiporter and a constitutive system, presumably used when the ADS is repressed to bring in arginine, which is a required amino acid for the organism.

The first step in degradation is catalyzed by the enzyme arginine deiminase (ADase) in a reaction which is essentially irreversible with K_{eq} = ca. 10^5 (Sta-

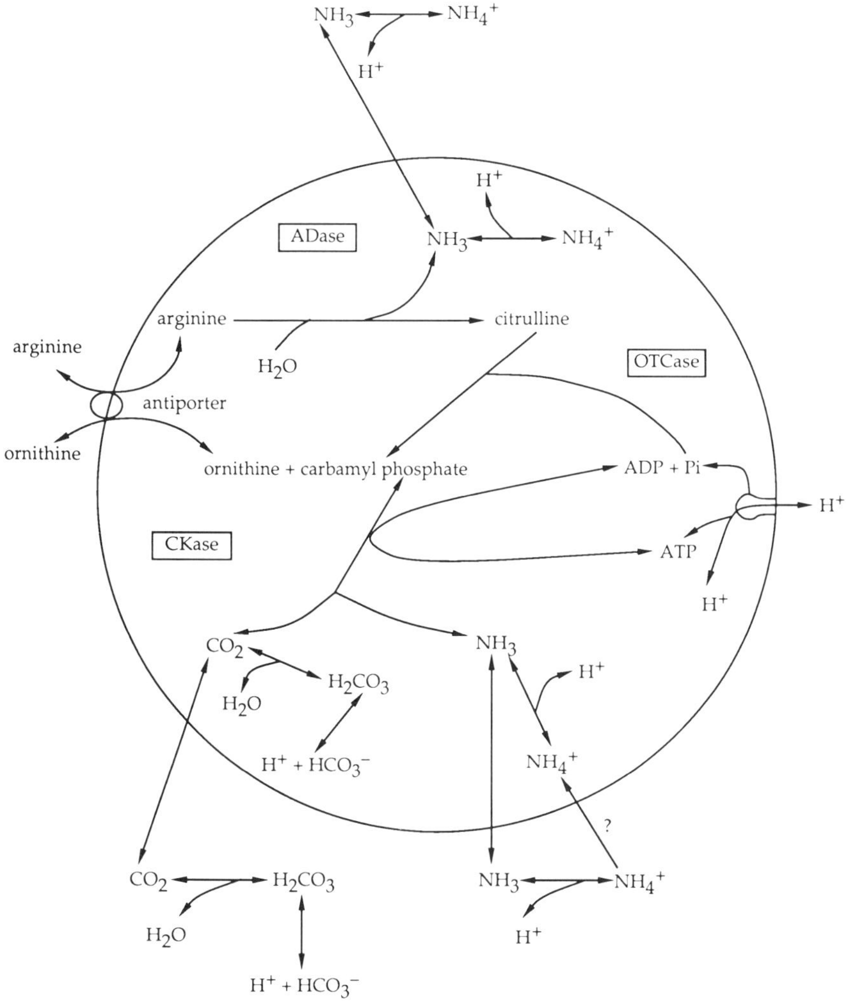

Figure 2 Current views of the biochemistry and physiology of the arginine deiminase system in the lactic-acid bacteria.

lon, 1972). One mol of ammonia per mol of arginine is released. The other product, citrulline is degraded to ornithine and carbamyl phosphate in a reaction catalyzed by catabolic ornithine carbamyl transferase (OTCase). Some organisms can use citrulline as substrate for the ADS, but generally, its transport into the cell is very slow, and citrulline degradation will not support growth. Finally, carbamyl phosphate can be degraded in a reversible reaction catalyzed by catabolic carbamate kinase (CKase) to yield ammonia and CO_2. The reaction is coupled to synthesis of ATP. Carbamyl phosphate can also serve as phosphate donor in formation of glucose-1-phosphate (Keevil *et al.* 1984) for glycogen synthesis.

As mentioned, the major function of the ADS in organisms such as *S. sanguis* appears to be for protection against acid damage rather than supplying ATP for growth, although the organism can grow rather feebly with arginine as sole fuel. The ADS is repressed in the presence of sugars such as glucose because of catabolite repression. Therefore, in the usual sort of laboratory culture the ADS is repressed during the growth phase and derepressed after growth has ceased. The genes for the ADS could be considered *pex* genes, that is, genes normally activated only after exponential growth.

The products of the ADS important for cell acid-base physiology include CO_2, NH_3 and ATP. The cell membrane is permeable to CO_2, which reacts with water to form carbonic acid, with resultant acidification of the cell or its environment. However, in an open system, CO_2 is lost to the atmosphere, and so its acidification potential is lost, especially at acid pH values. The cell membrane is highly permeable also to NH_3 (Kleiner, 1985). However, NH_3 can combine with protons to form NH_4^+ ($pK_a = 9.27$). If this association occurs within the cell, one proton is removed, and the cytoplasmic pH value rises. NH_4^+ can substitute for intracellular K^+ (Buurman *et al.*, 1989), and so is functional. If the association with a proton occurs outside of the cell, the environmental pH value is elevated. In organisms such as *E. coli*, NH_4^+ can re-enter the cell via the high-affinity Kdp system for K^+ (Buurman *et al.*, 1991), and a futile cycle can be initiated. Since NH_3 is a weak base, its distribution between the cell and the environment is determined by ΔpH across the cell membrane. It then serves to discharge ΔpH. However, for an ammonia-producing organism in an acid environment with a relatively alkaline cytoplasm, the dissipation of ΔpH is due to an increase in environmental pH rather than to acidification of the cytoplasm. Moreover, for organisms such as *S. sanguis*, these effects on ΔpH may not be energetically very important because ATP is generated primarily at the substrate level and not by ATP synthase (F_1F_0ATPase).

The other product of the ADS is ATP, and especially in non-growing cells, the ATP can be used for extrusion of protons through the F_1F_0ATPase. The production of 2 molecules of NH_3 would result in the neutralization of 2 protons. The production of 1 ATP could result in extrusion of 1 to 3 protons depending on the ATP/H^+ coupling ratio, which still has not been fully resolved. Thus, for each molecule of arginine catabolized, the cell can neutralize two protons and extrude 1 to 3 protons.

The genes of the ADS of *S. sanguis* NCTC10904 have been cloned (Burne *et al.*, 1989), initially on a 13 kpb fragment in phage lambda, and gene order was then determined by use of subclones in plasmid pMK4. The genes for the three enzymes of the system were found to be contiguous and were designated *arc*A (ADase), *arc*B (OTCase) and *arc*C (CKase). It appeared that *arc*AB and *arc*C were divergently transcribed from two promoters. Thus, although the genes are contiguous and the system can be coordinately derepressed, the *arc*C gene appears to have its own promoter, possibly to allow for independent synthesis of carbamyl phosphate for biosynthetic processes. The gene for the antiporter has not been mapped, but it was determined that the gene(s) for the cobalt-activated aminopeptidase produced by the organism (Casiano-Colón and Marquis, 1990) is not associated with the ADS cluster.

The *arc*A gene was subsequently transferred to *S. mutans* UA130 (Burne *et al.*, 1989, 1990) initially by means of genetic transformation with the vector pVA856. The gene was expressed well in the mutans organism, but the genetic construction was unstable. A genetically more stable construction was obtained by introducing the *arc*A gene into the mutans chromosome at the *gtf*A locus. However, in the chromosome, the gene was very poorly expressed. Thus, it appears that ADS genes can be introduced into *S. mutans* but that ways need to be devised to circumvent regulatory restriction by the new host. The current focus is on ADS genes of *S. rattus*, which are less subject to catabolite repression (Burne *et al.*, 1991). Yet another possibility is to use genes from *T. denticola*, in which the ADS serves primarily for ATP synthesis and so is expressed even in the presence of glucose (Caldwell *et al.*, 1990).

REFERENCES

BLAKEMORE, R. P. and CANALE-PAROLA, E. (1976): Arginine Catabolism by *Treponema denticola*, *J Bacteriol* 128:616-622.

BURNE, R. A.; PARSONS, D. T.; and MARQUIS, R. E. (1989): Cloning and Expression in *Escherichia coli* of the Genes of the Arginine Deiminase System of *Streptococcus sanguis* NCTC 10904, *Infect Immun* 57:3540-3548.

BURNE, R. A.; PARSONS D. T.; and MARQUIS, R. E. (1991): Environmental Variables Affecting Arginine Deiminase Expression in Oral Streptococci. In: *Streptococcal Genetics*, G. Dunny, P.P. Cleary, L.L. McKay Ed., Washington, D. C.: American Society for Microbiology, 276-280.

BUURMAN, E. T.; PENNOCK, J.; TEMPEST, D. W.; JOOST TEIXEIRA de MATTOS, M.; and NEIJSSEL, O. M. (1989): Replacement of Potassium Ions by Ammonium Ions in Different Micro-organisms Grown in Potassium-limited Chemostat Culture, *Arch Microbiol* 152:58-63.

BUURMAN, E. T.; JOOST TEIXEIRA de MATTOS, M.; and NEIJSSEL, O.M. (1991): Futile Cycling of Ammonia Ions via the High Affinity Potassium Uptake System (Kdp) of *Escherichia coli*, *Arch Microbiol* 155:391-395.

CALDWELL, C. E.; BURNE, R. A.; and MARQUIS, R. E. (1990): Partial Characterization of the Arginine Deiminase System of *Treponema denticola*, *J Dent Res* 69:184 (Abst. 602).

CASIANO-COLÓN, A. and MARQUIS, R. E. (1988): Role of the Arginine Deiminase System in Protecting Oral Bacteria and an Enzymatic Basis for Acid Tolerance, *Appl Environ Microbiol* 54:1318-1324.

CASIANO-COLÓN, A. E. and MARQUIS, R. E. (1990): Cobalt-activated Aminopeptidase from *Streptococcus sanguis* NCTC 10904, *Curr Microbiol* 21:317-323.

CURTIS, M. A.; KEMP, C. W.; ROBRISH, S. A.; and BOWEN, W. H. (1983): Stickland Reactions in Dental Plaque, *Infect Immun* 42:431-433.

DAWES, C. (1984): Inorganic Constituents of Saliva in Relation to Caries. In: *Cariology Today*, B. Guggenheim, Ed., Basel: Karger, pp. 70-74.

DE JONG, M. H. and VAN DER HOEVEN, J. S. (1987): The Growth of Oral Bacteria in Saliva, *J Dent Res* 66:498-505.

DRIESSEN, A. J. M.; POOLMAN, B.; KIEWIET, R.; and KONINGS, W. N. (1987): Arginine Transport in *Streptococcus lactis* is Catalyzed by a Cationic Exchanger, *Proc Natl Acad Sci* USA 84:6093-6097.

DRIESSEN, A. J. M. and KONINGS, W. (1990): Energetic Problems of Bacterial Fermentations: Extrusion of Metabolic End Products. In: *Bacterial Energetics*, T. A. Krulwich, Ed., San Diego: Academic Press, Inc., pp. 449-478.

EDGAR, W. M. and HIGHAM, S. M. (1990): Plaque Fluid as a Bacterial Milieu, *J Dent Res* 69:1332-1336.

FERRO, K. J.; BENDER, G. R.; and MARQUIS, R. E. (1983): Coordinately Repressible Arginine Deiminase System in *Streptococcus sanguis*, *Curr Microbiol* 9:145-149.

GALE, E. F. and EPPS, H. M. R. (1942): The Effect of the pH of the Medium during Growth on the Enzymatic Activities of Bacteria (*Escherichia coli* and *Micrococcus lysodeikticus*) and the Biological Significance of the Changes Produced, *Biochem J* 36:600-618.

HOMER, K. A.; WHILEY, R. A.; and BEIGHTON, D. (1990): Proteolytic Activity of Oral Streptococci, *FEMS Microbiol Lett* 67:257-260.

KEEVIL, C. W.; MARSH, P. D.; and ELLWOOD, D.C. (1984): Regulation of Glucose Metabolism in Oral Streptococci Through Independent Pathways of Glucose 6-phosphate and Glucose 1-phosphate Formation, *J Bacteriol* 157:560-567.

KLEINER, D. (1985): Bacterial Ammonium Transport, *FEMS Microbiol Rev* 32:87-100.

KRULWICH, T. A.; AGUS, R.; SCHNEIER, M.; and GUFFANTI, A. A. (1985): Buffering Capacity of Bacilli That Grow at Different pH Ranges, *J Bacteriol* 162:768-772.

MARGOLIS, H. C. (1990): An Assessment of Recent Advances in the Study of the Chemistry and Biochemistry of Dental Plaque Fluid, *J Dent Res* 69:1337-1342.

MARQUIS, R. E.; BENDER, G. R.; MURRAY, D. R.; and WONG, A. (1987): Arginine Deiminase System and Bacterial Adaptation to Acid Environments, *Appl Environ Microbiol* 53:198-200.

ROGERS, A. H.; ZILM, P. S.; GULLY, N. J.; and PFENNING, A.L. (1988): Response of a *Streptococcus sanguis* Strain to Arginine-containing Peptides, *Infect Immun* 56:687-692.

ROGERS, A. H. and REYNOLDS, E. C. (1990): The Utilization of Casein and Amino Acids by *Streptococcus sanguis* P_4A_7 in Continuous Culture, *J Gen Microbiol* 136:2545-2550.

SALAKO, N. O. and KLEINBERG, I. (1989): Incidence of Selected Ureolytic Bacteria in Human Dental Plaque from Sites with Differing Salivary Access, *Arch Oral Biol* 34:787-791.

SISSONS, C. H.; PERINPANAYAGAM, H. E. R.; HANCOCK, E. M.; and CUTRESS, T. W. (1990): pH Regulation of Urease Levels in *Streptococcus salivarius*, *J Dent Res* 69:1131-1137.

STALON, V. (1972): Regulation of the Catabolic Ornithine Carbamoyltransferase of *Pseudomonas fluorescens* A Study of the Allosteric Interactions, *Eur J Biochem* 29:36-46.

VAN DER HOEVEN, J. S.; VAN DEN KIEBOOM; and CAMP, P. J. M. (1990): Utilization of Mucin by Oral *Streptococcus* species, Antonie van Leeuwenhoek 57:165-172.

WIJEYEWEERA, R. L. and KLEINBERG, I. (1989): Acid-base pH Curves *In Vitro* with Mixtures of Pure Cultures of Human Oral Microorganisms, *Arch Oral Biol* 34:55-64.

Ecological Determinants of Dental Root Surface Caries

RICHARD P. ELLEN

Ecology: the discipline of biology which encompasses the relationship between organisms and their environment. Ecological determinants of dental root surface caries can be investigated and discussed on many levels, and whether or not root caries is a unique biological entity probably depends on the ecological scale being considered. On the microbiological scale, the local events within the microcosm of the root surface - gingival interface determine the outcome, health or caries, for an individual site. To be unique, the pathogenesis of caries at this site would have to differ significantly from that on coronal surfaces; this issue is certainly open to debate. On the macrobiological scale, the physiological, social, and behavioral events surrounding root caries active individuals must be considered, and it is on this ecological plane that some determinants of root caries activity might differ considerably. The purpose of this critical review is to examine both the micro- and macro-environmental influences which set root caries apart from coronal caries, so that research resources can be targeted toward testing new and specific hypotheses, rather than merely replicating the wealth of preceding coronal caries research for roots.

Root caries is caries on roots, a statement difficult to deny. Yet a whole generation of research has been invested in trying to disprove this hypothesis on the pathogenesis side. Although there have been several attempts to determine a unique microbial etiology for dental root caries, there has been very little evidence generated that distinguishes the pathogenesis of caries apical to the cemento-enamel junction from that coronal to it. Just like their predecessors, clinical microbiologists have now conducted both cross-sectional and longitudinal studies of the microbiota on carious and noncarious roots in humans and, with few exceptions, they have found no major, fundamental differences, even though the root surface microbiota is not as well defined and perhaps more variable. (for review, see Bowden, 1990).

Although the higher organic content of cementum than enamel has led some to hypothetically assign proteolysis a role in root caries, a growing body of evidence is accumulating to confirm that net demineralization of root surfaces is the significant event in root caries pathogenesis. While it is possible that a wider variety of bacteria might contribute sufficient acid for demineralization of cementum than of enamel, as these mineralized tissues differ in their critical pH, microradiography and histopathology of both natural and experimentally induced root lesions has yielded little to distinguish them from coronal lesions (Frank *et al.*, 1989; Nyvad *et al.*, 1989). Therefore, the microbiota contributing significantly to root caries would be expected to contain acidogenic and aciduric species which would emerge in an environment conducive to demineralization. Indeed, morphologically, the microorganisms detected deep within the invasive front of root lesions and situated among intact collagen fibrils are predominantly Gram-positive, just like in the dentin of coronal lesions (Frank *et al.*, 1989).

The idea that root caries might be unique microbiologically can be traced to an era when it was considered appropriate to generalize results from rodent experimental caries models to humans. The observation that periodontal disease and associated root caries were transmissible but distinct infections from coronal caries in hamsters and germfree rats was a profound finding (Jordan, 1971). It prompted the survey of the human oral microbiota for bacteria resembling the newly described *Odontomyces* (now *Actinomyces*) *viscosus* of hamsters. Rather quickly thereafter, human isolates, including those from root caries lesions in human teeth, were shown to induce similar lesions in rodents (Jordan and Hammond, 1972; Jordan *et al.*, 1972). Even though streptococci, including *Streptococcus mutans*, were frequently isolated, the predominance of filamentous bacteria in carious root debris from extracted human teeth and the filamentous nature of the plaques overlying human root lesions (Jordan and Hammond, 1972; Sumney and Jordan, 1974) fostered the concept that root lesions were microbiologically distinct from coronal lesions, which were so often associated with elevated levels of streptococci, especially mutans streptococci, near the surface and Gram-positive rods, especially lactobacilli, deep within the dentin. Indeed, a pleomorphic rod, genus *Arthrobacter*, which had never previously been described in the oral microbiota, was found at the advancing front in the dentin of root lesions . . . with no lactobacilli in sight (Sumney and Jordan, 1974). Together, these findings suggested that the environment of root surfaces somehow allowed a more periodontally and perhaps proteolytically oriented microbiota to emerge, rather different from that found more coronally on enamel surfaces. Yet all these studies were nonquantitative, based on the identification of predominant colony types in established lesions of extracted teeth rather than the enumeration of the predominant isolates themselves. Thus, in the mid-seventies, the research environment had evolved to be ready to accept *A. viscosus* (and other filamentous bacteria) as the primary root caries pathogen(s). Almost predictably, the first quantitative survey of the predominant microbiota of plaque overlying root lesions supported this hypothesis by finding 100% of these lesions colonized by *A. viscosus*, with a mean percent hovering 40% (Syed *et al.*,

1975). *Streptococcus mutans* was not found in all lesions, a finding which was emphasized thereafter, but few noticed that when it was present, it constituted a very high percentage of the microbiota. Although quantitative, the study of Syed and coworkers (1975), like all the preceding studies, had no controls, no healthy roots with which to compare.

We now know *A. viscosus* to be a rather ubiquitous species. Cariogenic or not, its wide distribution on both carious and noncarious surfaces has defied attempts to incriminate it in human root caries etiology by numerical association alone. Presumably in clinical microbiology research the strongest evidence for etiological significance of a species would be its greater association with diseased than healthy states, especially if such an association were to be established longitudinally over the period of disease onset. During the past 15 years, there have been several controlled cross-sectional comparisons of carious and sound roots as well as a few longitudinal studies documenting caries initiation on initially sound roots. Virtually all of these studies have suggested a stronger association of mutans streptococci with carious than sound roots but not necessarily all carious roots (Bowden *et al.*, 1990; Brown *et al.*, 1986; Emilson *et al.*, 1988; Fure *et al.*, 1987; Keltjens *et al.*, 1987, 1988; van Houte *et al.*, 1990). The longitudinal surveys have associated either the detection frequency or proportional distribution of mutans streptococci in plaques or their recovery per mL saliva with root caries susceptibility of subjects and sites (Ellen *et al.*, 1985a; MacEntee *et al.*, 1990; Ravald *et al.*, 1981, 1986). One treatment study monitored the reduction in mutans streptococci concomitant with the arrest of root caries activity (Billings *et al.* 1985). Another aciduric genus, *Lactobacillus*, has also been associated with root cariogenic situations in longitudinal studies, although the association has not been as strong as that for mutans streptococci (Ellen *et al.*, 1985a; Ravald *et al.*, 1986).

What became of *A. viscosus* in the controlled investigations? Virtually none of the comparative studies was able to demonstrate a numerical association betweeen human root caries and *A. viscosus* detection frequency and/or proportions in plaque. In our longitudinal study of hospitalized older adults, there was no difference in the mean proportions of any of the monitored species and root caries initiation, either on a site or subject basis (Ellen *et al.* 1985b). Although further analysis of detection frequencies revealed a clear association of elevated root caries risk for mutans streptococci alone or in combination with lactobacilli (Ellen *et al.*, 1985a), the data for *A. viscosus* was not published for comparison. Figures 1-3 and tables 1 and 2 illustrate different ways to try to relate *A. viscosus* to root caries onset in the population studied by us.

Analyzing detection frequencies for surfaces becoming carious or remaining caries-free yielded no differences for *A. viscosus* but found a closer association with noncarious than carious root surfaces for *Actinomyces naeslundii*, a taxonomically close relative which also had been shown previously to induce root lesions in rodents (Fig.1). Analyzing the data by concentrating on samples

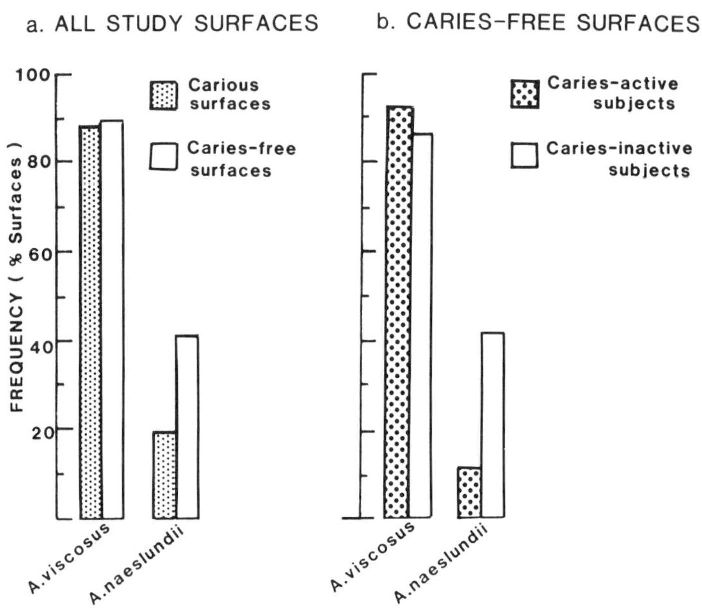

Figure 1 Isolation frequency of *A. viscosus* and *A. naeslundii* on previously caries-free roots diagnosed as carious and those remaining caries-free during a longitudinal study. Bars represent the mean for seven sampling sessions spaced 4 months apart. 1a: Stippled bars represent carious surfaces, those on which an unfilled carious lesion was detected at the clinical examination following the microbial sampling session. Open bars represent surfaces which were caries-free. 1b: Isolation frequency for only the roots which remained caries-free. Stippled bars represent caries-free surfaces in caries-active subjects. Open bars represent caries-free roots in caries-inactive subjects. Data derived from 16 caries-active and 29 caries-inactive subjects (Ellen *et al.*, 1985).

which were outliers, those with ''superhigh'' proportional counts one or two standard deviations above the mean, also yielded no association, beyond random expectation, with root surfaces or subjects experiencing new root lesions (Table 1). Categorizing the proportional counts into ranges and trying to relate the frequency distribution of the categories to the onset of caries also yielded equivocal findings (Table 2). Even tracing the fluctuations in *A. viscosus* proportions on individual roots, for sampling sessions leading up to the clinical detection of caries, found an approximately equal number of samples which had rising and falling proportions (Figs. 2 and 3). There is simply no way that the data from our longitudinal study of hospitalized adults with high root caries activity or the data from several subsequent cross-sectional studies could be interpreted to support *A. viscosus* as an indicator species for root caries in

TABLE 1 *Distribution of Samples With High A. Viscosus Count Data* Relative to the Mean at Each Sampling Session: Association With Caries Activity*

Session	% Microbiota Mean (± st. dev.)	No. Surfaces > 1 St. Dev. Above Mean Caries-acive subjects (N = 59)	Caries-inactive subjects (N = 91)	Ratio expected (59/91 = 0.65)
1	8.1±12.7	4	13	0.31
2	7.7±16.2	7	10	0.70
3	6.8±15.0	5	8	0.63
4	6.3±13.0	6	13	0.46
5	3.9±10.5	2	6	0.33
6	7.3±14.4	4	8	0.50
7	7.0±14.4	2	8	0.25
	Total	30**	66	0.45

* Samples with *A. viscosus proprtions > 1 standard deviation above the mean were considered to have high counts*
** 13 of these 30 were carious surfaces

humans. Yet is it cariogenic in humans? Or, as recently discussed by Bowden (1990), are heterogeneous species or cariogenic biotypes hidden within our current definition of what is currently named "*A. viscosus*"?

Although rearrangements in classification will undoubtedly cast doubt on previous clinical microbiology studies which used identification schemes which may now be outdated, there is emerging data to suggest either that there are metabolically different *A. viscosus* biotypes colonizing carious and noncarious roots or that carious roots select for metabolic adaptations of the *A. viscosus* strains established on them. *Actinomyces viscosus* growing in colonies on a variety of dietary carbohydrates is known to depress colony pH considerably, a demonstration of its acidogenicity within dense communities; yet there are differences

TABLE 2 *Distribution of Microbial Count Data For Surfaces Becoming Carious*

	Number of surfaces with % flora 0	< 1%	1-10%	> 10%
Just prior to caries diagnosis				
A. viscosus	3	7	8	8
A. naeslundii	21	4	0	1
All times prior to caries diagnosis				
A. viscosus	9	26	23	15
A. naeslundii	60	11	1	1

* includes all observations of all roots which became carious (n = 26, of 150 surfaces) up to and including the session just prior to clinical caries detection

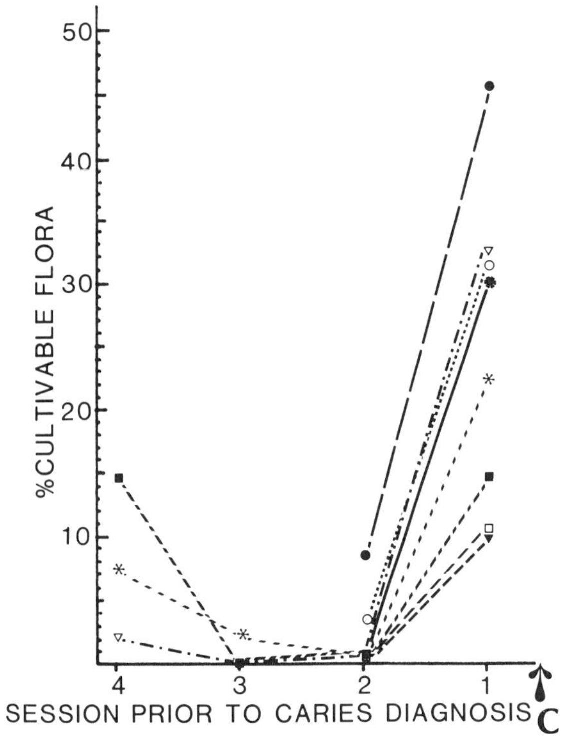

Figure 2 Temporal fluctuations in the percentage of *A. viscosus* in the cultivable microbiota of the eight surfaces which became carious during a longitudinal study and which had increasing *A. viscosus* proportions in the sampling session leading up to caries detection (C). Data derived from Ellen *et al.*, 1985.

among *A. viscosus* strains in their ability to produce acid in colonies from lactose and starch (Ellen and Onose, 1978). Over the past several years, Komiyama *et al.* (1986, 1988) have demonstrated a difference in sugar metabolism for *A. viscosus* strains freshly isolated from carious and noncarious roots of humans. The strains from carious roots are more acidogenic and aciduric. Over a wide pH range, they both synthesize and degrade more intracellular glycogen and produce more acid over a longer period following depletion of exogenous carbohydrate. These observations do not prove that some strains or biotypes of *A. viscosus* are more cariogenic than others. They suggest a few hypotheses which bear on the ecology of root lesions and why *A. viscosus* might really be cariogenic in that environment, even though numerical count data defy such a conclusion.

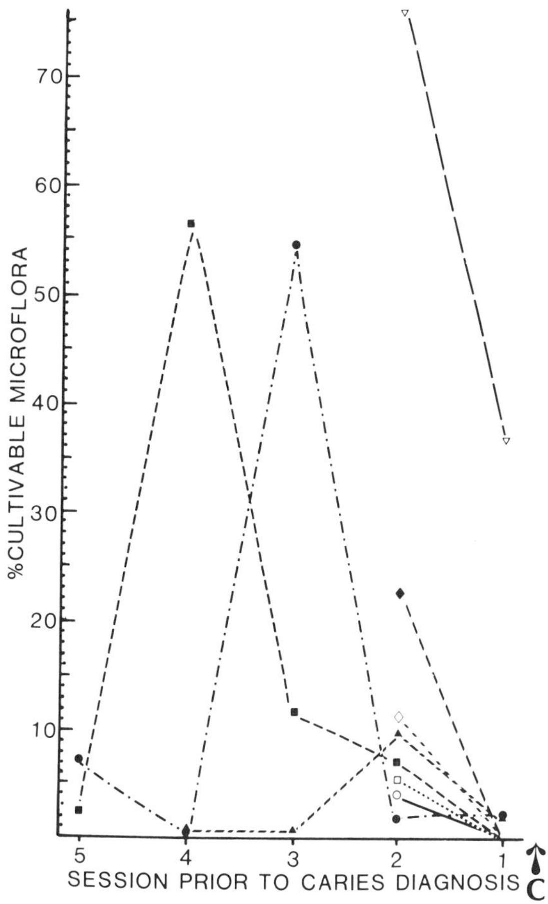

Figure 3 Temporal fluctuations in percent *A. viscosus* for the eight carious surfaces which had decreasing *A. viscosus* proportions leading up to caries detection (C). Data derived from Ellen *et al.*, 1985.

Figure 4 is a flow diagram which illustrates a few possibilities raised by Komiyama's data. Regardless whether *A. viscosus* strains are naturally "cariogenic" or "noncariogenic", properties which can only be substantiated by proving whether or not they cause caries, populations of *A. viscosus* on roots would be subjected to selection pressures of the local environment. In low root caries risk individuals (see below), the accumulation of *A. viscosus* among other bacteria on roots might be inconsequential, for the ecosystem neither favors nor selects for strains which have cariogenic properties (aciduric, glycogen

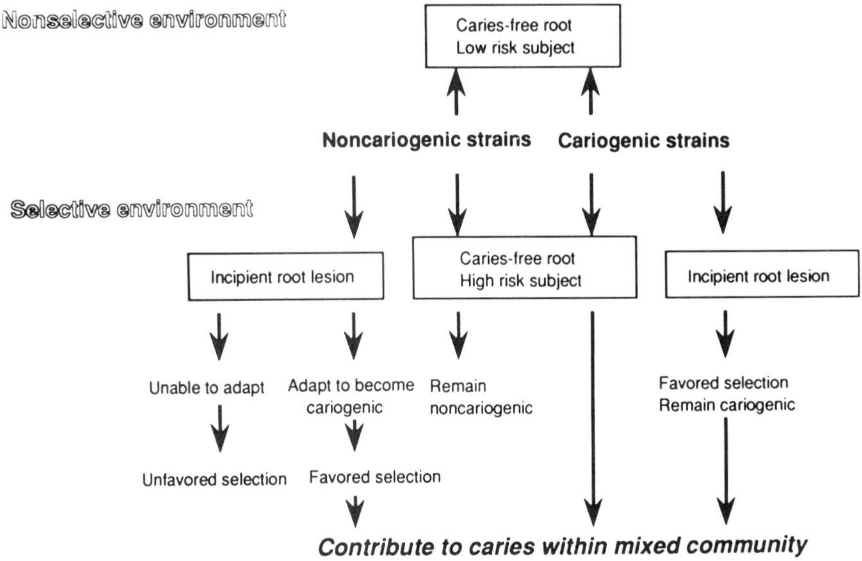

Figure 4 Flow diagram of how the environment of an incipient root lesion or the environment of caries-free roots within a high caries risk host might impose selection pressures to influence the emergence of cariogenic strains or to induce the up-regulation of cariogenic traits in strains of a potentially acidogenic species, like *A. viscosus*. The diagram is hypothetical but based on observations of Komiyama *et al.* (1986, 1988) that *A.viscosus* strains isolated from root caries lesions are more aciduric, glycogen synthetic, and acidogenic than strains isolated from caries-free roots. The root surface environment of low risk hosts would probably present a nonselective environment in terms of favoring the emergence of species or strains with cariogenic properties.

synthetic, and glycolytic), nor does it support the initiation of carious lesions. On roots of high caries risk individuals, where hygiene is poor, dietary carbohydrate intake is frequent, buffering is weak, and other acidogenic bacteria are on the scene, *A. viscosus* strains with cariogenic properties would be favored. This may derive from the selected elimination of "noncariogenic" biotypes or the induced adaptation of *A. viscosus* to up-regulate aciduric and glycolytic properties. Such a scenario implies that ecological determinants for root caries on the microbiological scale virtually mimic those established for coronal caries and that "cariogenicity" (among populations within a mixed community or even of individual bacteria in the community) might be inducible by an environment created by the host. Indeed, recent demonstrations that desalivation of rodents leads to the emergence and interhost transmission of more virulent (cariogenic) streptococci supports the concept of selective pressures imposed by reduction in salivary flow and buffering effect (Madison *et al.*, 1990, 1991). Previous observations of microbial community shifts in postirradiation xerosto-

TABLE 3 *Composite Profile of a High Root Caries Risk Individual*

Biological	
	Older age
	Mutans streptococci and lactobacilli on exposed roots
	Elevated mutans/lactobacilli counts per ml. saliva
	Low salivary buffering capcity
	Prolonged sugar clearance time
Medical	
	Many exposed root surfaces
	Unmet periodontal treatment needs
	Previous root and coronal caries experience
	Taking xerostomic medications
Behavioral	
	Frequent fermentable carbonhydrate intake
	Infrequent dental care
	Insufficent personal dental hygiene
	Use of tobacco
Social	
	Lifelong in low fluoride area

mia patients and pH-induced selective microbial emergence in mixed chemostat cultures also support such a concept. Therefore, determinants of the health status of root surfaces are probably driven most strongly by the macrobiological environment: What determines who is at risk for root caries?

Risk models for root surface caries are beginning to emerge from both cross-sectional and longitudinal analytical epidemiology studies (for review, see Beck, 1990). There is not enough information tying together these disparate studies, which target different types of populations, have different sampling frames, and use different variables and methods of measurement. However, a composite profile of a "typical" root caries risk individual can be listed if variables of common interest are considered.

Table 3 lists four categories of variables defining a host's environment and which have been associated as potential indicators of root caries risk: biological, medical, behavioral, and social. The biological variables place on a subject scale those factors discussed as significant on the microbiological site scale. Individuals more heavily infected with aciduric and acidogenic bacteria and whose saliva is weak at buffering acids are more likely to be at higher risk. The medical variables include conditions of health and disease which might predispose an individual to elevated root caries activity or create the physically selective environment. Supragingival exposure, perhaps recent exposure, of root surfaces is a prerequisite for root caries, and the most common scenario is exposure due to the attachment loss and recession associated with periodontal disease or its treatment (Banting *et al.*, 1985; Beck, 1990; Emilson *et al.*, 1988; Keltjens *et al.*, 1988; Ravald *et al.*, 1984, 1986; Vehkalahti, 1987). Recent animal experiments have confirmed the cariogenicity of *A. viscosus*, alone or in combination with *Streptococcus sobrinus*, on roots exposed by gingivectomy (Firestone *et al.*, 1989). To the microbiota, being thrust into a supragingival environment must present an enormous challenge to adapt. Reduction of salivary flow carries an elevated risk, and the frequent consumption of multiple, potentially xerostomic medications by older adults would contribute to such risk (Kitamura *et al.*, 1986). Prolonged sugar clearance time (Ravald *et al.*, 1986), by salivary or other causes, would also indicate elevated risk. Debilitating medical conditions leading to dependence on caregivers for daily hygiene services might also be considered a medical risk indicator (Banting *et al.*, 1985; Beck *et al.*, 1988). Medical conditions requiring prolonged hospitalization should not be underestimated for their compounding the effects of other risk variables. For example, Hase *et al.* (1987) reported a much prolonged sugar clearance time for elderly hospitalized adults than nonhospitalized, age matched subjects.

The behavioral variables contributing to risk seem to be "negative" dental behaviors of frequent dietary carbohydrate intake, substandard oral hygiene practices, smoking, and infrequent professional care (Beck, 1990; Beck *et al.* 1988; Locker *et al.*, 1989; Ravald *et al.* 1986; Vehkalahti and Paunio, 1988). The latter three may also be indirectly associated by contributing to periodontal disease progression. Smoking probably also causes a dry mouth feeling, which might be alleviated by frequent use of sugared candies or lozenges. A social factor documented in a few studies is lifelong residence in less than optimally fluoridated areas (Hunt *et al.*, 1989; Stamm *et al.*, 1990). Indeed, living in a highly fluoridated area seems to offer additonal protection from root caries (Burt *et al.*, 1986).

The significance of this risk cluster is more than hypothetical. In a single longitudinal study in which subjects treated for periodontitis were followed for 12 years, Ravald (1992) has reported that those at highest risk for developing root caries had a combination of several variables at levels above a threshold discriminating high risk from low risk. Among 27 of the original 35 subjects who started the study, those with more than 5 new lesions accounted for most of the instances (75%) when above threshold values were found. Those variables most often found above the threshold were salivary counts of mutans streptococci and lactobacilli, dietary habit index, and plaque score. Variables with the highest positive predictive values were salivary secretion rate, plaque score, % exposed surfaces with new lesions, and dietary habit index. All of Ravald's significant variables can be linked in some way to an environment which would be selective for aciduric microorganisms.

Returning to the word "ecology", it is important to consider the relationship of persons most highly at risk for root caries to their environment. What is it about older individuals, other than their more frequently exposed root surfaces, which places them at elevated risk? For many, the risks are low, for they display few of the indicators summarized above. However, in any population of individuals, there is a small cohort especially susceptible to dental diseases, which is evident in longitudinal root caries studies (Banting *et al.*, 1985; Hand *et al.*, 1988; Ravald *et al.*, 1984, 1986). Those at risk for root caries might be victims of their environment and their era. Today's older adults grew up in an era when dentistry focused on extraction or repair instead of prevention. The "inevitability" of becoming "long in the tooth" and developing associated problems are probably more acceptable to today's than tomorrow's older adults. They also became more habituated to smoking habits and to the taste of "real" rather than sugarless snacks. For example, Vehkalahti and Paunio (1988) have documented sweetened coffee drinking as a behavior often associated with older adults with root caries in Finland. No one has yet thought of studying the habits and attitudes of older dentists or comparing their knowledge of root caries prevention and management with that of recent graduates. What if older adults were more likely to gravitate toward the peer comfort of older dentists or to stay with a now aged family dentist with little appreciation for root caries? Would such an "environment" be conducive to elevated root caries risk? For those debilitated or dependent on caretakers in collective living centers or hospitals, the environmental pressures toward elevated caries activity can be profound. For example, the caries attack rate for the hospitalized population studied by Banting, Fillery, and me (1985) was much higher than that reported in independent community dwellers elsewhere. These are the ecological determinants, if there are any, which might distinguish root caries as a distinct entity from coronal caries.

The Future, A Changing Global Ecology

Although future generations will retain more natural teeth to older age, there are environmental changes at work to limit the risk of a rise in the root caries incidence. The contributions of both previous periodontal disease and coronal caries activity should be expected to decline. More individuals have grown up lifelong in artificially fluoridated areas or using fluoride supplements, rinses, and dentifrices. The current generation reaching middle age has grown up taking antibiotics for a variety of medical and dental indications. The proportion of the population smoking is declining. The use of noncariogenic sugar substitutes has become an institution. What was once a movement toward dependence on institutional homes for the elderly might become a movement toward living independently, with more community services for the homebound. There is certainly an elevated expectation of a right to optimum health and health care in our society. Therefore, developed countries might be developing the appropriate environments to select for greater numbers of individuals of low caries risk. Such individuals will likely offer fewer opportunities within the microenvironment of the gingiva - root surface interface for the selection of a cariogenic microbiota or for bacteria to express their cariogenicity.

Unfortunately, as in other issues in today's global ecology, noxious by-products are often exported across political boundaries. The growing populations in the third world are probably not prepared to manage a growing caries problem . . . nor might caries seem an important priority. Perhaps the established prevalence of periodontal diseases in developing countries will combine with caries-conducive environmental factors exported by the global market economies of the industrialized countries (e.g. sugar and tobacco) and be compounded by the dental care attitudes which were once faced by our current older generation. The fallout of such a situation would maintain ecological pressures for high levels of root caries risk in economically poor countries. Therefore, if new approaches to limit the environmental determinants of root caries are to be considered, a more global attitude should prevail, one which is logical and ecological.

REFERENCES

BANTING, D.W.; ELLEN, R.P.; and FILLERY, E.D. (1985): A Longitudinal Study of Root Caries: Baseline and Incidence Data, *J Dent Res* 64:1141-1144.

BECK, J. (1990): The Epidemiology of Root Surface Caries, *J Dent Res* 69:1216-1221.

BECK, J.D.; KOHOUT, F.; and HUNT, R.J. (1988): Identification of High Caries Risk Adults: Attitudes, Social Factors and Diseases, *Int Dent J* 38:231-238.

BILLINGS, R.J.; BROWN, L.R.; and KASTER A.G. (1985): Contemporary Treatment Strategies for Root Surface Dental Caries, *Gerodontics* 1:20-27.

BOWDEN, G.H.W. (1990): Microbiology of Root Surface Caries in Humans, *J Dent Res* 69:1205-1210.

BOWDEN, G.H.W.; EKSTRAND, J.; McNAUGHTON, B.; and CHALLACOMBE, S.J. (1990): The Association of Selected Bacteria with the Lesions of Root Surface Caries, *Oral Microbiol Immunol* 5:346-351.

BROWN, L.R.; BILLINGS, R.J.; and KASTER, A.G. (1986): Quantitative Comparisons of Potentially Cariogenic Microorganisms Cultured from Noncarious and Carious Root and Coronal Tooth Surfaces, *Infect Immun* 51:765-770.

BURT, B.A.; ISMAIL, A.I.; and EKLUND, S.A. (1986): Root Caries in an Optimally Fluoridated and a High Fluoridated Community, *J Dent Res* 65:1154-1158.

ELLEN, R.P.; BANTING, D.W.; and FILLERY, E.D. (1985a): *Streptococcus mutans* and *Lactobacillus* Detection in the Assessment of Dental Root Surface Caries Risk, *J Dent Res* 64:1245-1249.

ELLEN, R.P.; BANTING, D.W.; and FILLERY, E.D. (1985b): Longitudinal Microbiological Investigation of a Hospitalized Population of Older Adults with a High Root Caries Risk, *J Dent Res* 64:1377-1381.

ELLEN, R.P. and ONOSE, H. (1978): pH Measurements of *Actinomyces viscosus* Colonies Grown in Media Containing Dietary Carbohydrates, *Arch Oral Biol* 23:105-109.

EMILSON, C.-G.; KLOCK, B.; and SANFORD, C.B. (1988): Microbial Flora Associated with Presence of Root Surface Caries in Periodontally Treated Patients, *Scand J Dent Res* 96:40-49.

FIRESTONE, A.R.; GRAVES, C.N.; and FEAGIN, F.F. (1989): Caries on Root Surfaces Exposed Following Gingivectomy in Conventional Rats Infected with *Streptococcus sobrinus* and *Actinomyces viscosus*, *J Periodontol* 60:624-627.

FRANK, R.M.; STEUER, P.; and HEMMERLE, J. (1989): Ultrastructural Study on Human Root Caries, *Caries Res* 23:209-217.

FURE, S.; ROMANIED, M.; EMILSON, C.-G.; and KRASSE, B. (1987): Proportions of Streptococcus mutans, Lactobacilli, and Actinomyces spp.in Root Surface Plaque, *Scand J Dent Res* 95:119-123.

HASE, J.C.; BIRKHED, D.; GRENNERT, M.-L.; and STEEN, B. (1987): Salivary Glucose Clearance and Related Factors in Elderly People, *Gerodontics* 3:146-150.

HAND, J.S.; HUNT, R.J.; and BECK, J.D. (1988): Coronal and Root Caries in Older Iowans: 36-Month Incidence, *Gerodontics* 4:136-139.

HUNT, R.J.; ELDREDGE, J.B.; and BECK, J.D. (1989): Effect of Residence in a Fluoridated Community on the Incidence of Coronal and Root Caries in a Older Adult Population, *J Publ Health Dent* 49:138-141.

JORDAN, H.V. (1971): Rodent Model Systems in Periodontal Disease Research, *J Dent Res* 50:236-242.

JORDAN, H.V. and HAMMOND, B.F. (1972): Filamentous Bacteria Isolated from Human Root Surface Caries, *Arch Oral Biol* 17:1333-1342.

JORDAN, H.V.; KEYES, P.H.; and BELLACK, S. (1972): Periodontal Lesions in Hamsters and Gnotobiotic Rats Infected with *Actinomyces* of Human Origin, *J Periodontal Res* 7:21-28.

KELTJENS, H.M.A.M; SCHAEKEN, M.J.M.; VAN DER HOEVEN, J.S.; and HENDRIKS, J.C.M. (1987): Microflora of Plaque from Sound and Carious Root Surfaces, *Caries Res* 21:193-199.

KELTJENS, H.M.A.M; SCHAEKEN, M.J.M.; VAN DER HOEVEN, J.S.; and HENDRIKS, J.C.M. (1988): Epidemiology of Root Surface Caries in Patients Treated for Periodontal Diseases, *Community Dent Oral Epidemiol* 16:171-174.

KITAMURA, M.; KIYAK, H.A.; and MULLIGAN, K. (1986): Predictors of Root Caries in the Elderly, *Community Dent Oral Epidemiol* 14:34-38.

KOMIYAMA, K.; KHANDELWAL, R.L.; and DUNCAN, D.E. (1986): Glycogen Synthetic Abilities of *Actinomyces viscosus* and *Actinomyces naeslundii* Freshly Isolated from Dental Plaque Over Root Surface Caries Lesions and Non-Caries Sites, *J Dent Res* 65:899-902.

KOMIYAMA, K.; KHANDELWAL, R.L.; and HEINRICH, S.E. (1988): Glycogen Synthetic and Degradative Activities by *Actinomyces viscosus* and *Acintomyces naeslundii* of Root Surface Caries and Noncaries Sites, *Caries Res* 22:217-225.

LOCKER, D.; SLADE, G.D.; and LEAKE, J.L. (1989): Prevalence of and Factors Associated with Root Decay in Older Adults in Canada, *J Dent Res* 68:768-772.

MADISON, K.M.; BOWEN, W.H.; PEARSON, S.K.; and FALANY, J.L. (1990): Caries Incidence in Intact Rats Infected with *Streptococcus sobrinus* via Transmission from Desalivated Cagemates, *J Dent Res* 69:1154-1159.

MADISON, K.M.; BOWEN, W.H.; PEARSON, S.K.; and FALANY, J.L. (1991): Enhancing the Virulence of Streptococcus sobrinus in Rats, *J Dent Res* 70:38-43.

MACENTEE, M.I.; WYATT, C.C.L., and MCBRIDE, B.C. (1990): Longitudinal Study of Caries and Cariogenic Bacteria in an Elderly Disabled Population, *Community Dent Oral Epidemiol* 18:149-152.

NYVAD, B.; TEN CATE, J.M. and FEJERSKOV, O. (1989): Microradiography of Experimental Root Surface Caries in Man, *Caries Res* 23:218-224.

RAVALD, N.: Root Caries Risk and Caries Control in Periodontal Patients. pp. 121-136 in: *Periodontal Care for Older Adults*, R.P. Ellen, Ed. Toronto: Canadian Scholars' Press, 1992.

RAVALD, N. and HAMP, S.-E. (1981): Prediction of Root Surface Caries in Patients Treated for Advanced Periodontal Disease, *J Clin Periodontol* 8:400-414.

RAVALD, N.; HAMP, S.-E.; and BIRKHED, D. (1986): Long-term Evaluation of Root Surface Caries in Periodontally Treated Patients, *J Clin Periodontol* 13:758-767.

STAMM, J.W.; BANTING, D.W.; and IMREY, P. (1990): Adult Root Caries Survey of Two Similar Communities with Contrasting Natural Water Fluoride Levels, *JADA* 120:143-149.

SUMNEY D.L. and JORDAN, H.V. (1974): Characterization of Bacteria Isolated from Human Root Surface Carious Lesions, *J Dent Res* 53:343-351.

SYED, S.A.; LOESCHE, W.J.; PAPE, H.L. Jr.; and GRENIER, E. (1975): Predominant Cultivable Flora Isolated from Human Root Surface Caries Plaque, *Infect Immun* 11:727-731.

VAN HOUTE, J.; JORDAN, H.V.; LARAWAY, R.; KENT, R.; SOPARKAR, P.M.; and DEPAOLA, P.F. (1990): Association of the Microbial Flora of Dental Plaque and Saliva with Human Root-Surface Caries, *J Dent Res* 69:1463-1468.

VEHKALAHTI, M. (1987): Occurence of Root Caries and Factors Related to It, *Proc Finnish Dent Soc* 83:Suppl IV.

VEHKALAHTI, M. and PAUNIO, I.K. (1988): Occurence of Root Caries in Relation to Dental Health Behavior, *J Dent Res* 6:911-914.

Adaptations in Dental Plaque

D. T. Zero

In simplistic terms dental caries can be considered as a victory of demineralization over remineralization at a localized tooth site. The determinants of the course of the battle are a complex series of events many of which have been described at this conference. The focus of this paper will be on adaptation by plaque microorganisms to changes in the oral environment which influence the cariogenic potential of dental plaque.

Adaptation is a phenomenon which is found in almost all life forms and largely determines the ability of a species to survive in a particular environment. To persist on the tooth surface, plaque microorganisms must adapt to a wide range of environmental conditions many of which are unique to a particular site. The local ecology and metabolic activity of bacteria adjacent to the tooth surface are of primary importance to dental caries. The fermentation of dietary carbohydrates by plaque bacteria results in the production of organic acids, mainly lactic acid, which lowers the pH value of dental plaque and provides the driving force for demineralization of the tooth. The objective of this paper is to attempt to establish that dental caries, for the most part, is a consequence of successful adaptation by oral bacteria to an acid environment.

The pioneering work of Stephan (1944) clearly demonstrated the relationship between the caries activity and the pH-lowering ability of dental plaque. Plaque from individuals with a high caries activity had a lower resting pH and a larger and more prolonged pH depression after sugar challenge than plaque from individuals with low caries experience. Most noticeable from the Stephan (pH/time) curves is that there is a downward shift of the entire curve for the high caries active groups. Therefore, it can be inferred that the plaque bacteria in a caries active individual have adapted to a low pH environment.

This investigation was supported in part by USPHS Research Grant DE-07793 From the National Institute of Dental Research, National Institutes of Health, Bethesda, MD 20892

My appreciation is extended to Mrs. Jean Fu and Mrs. Kathleen Anne for all their hard work in conducting the research, and to Dr. Odette Aguirre Zero for helpful suggestions in preparation of the manuscript.

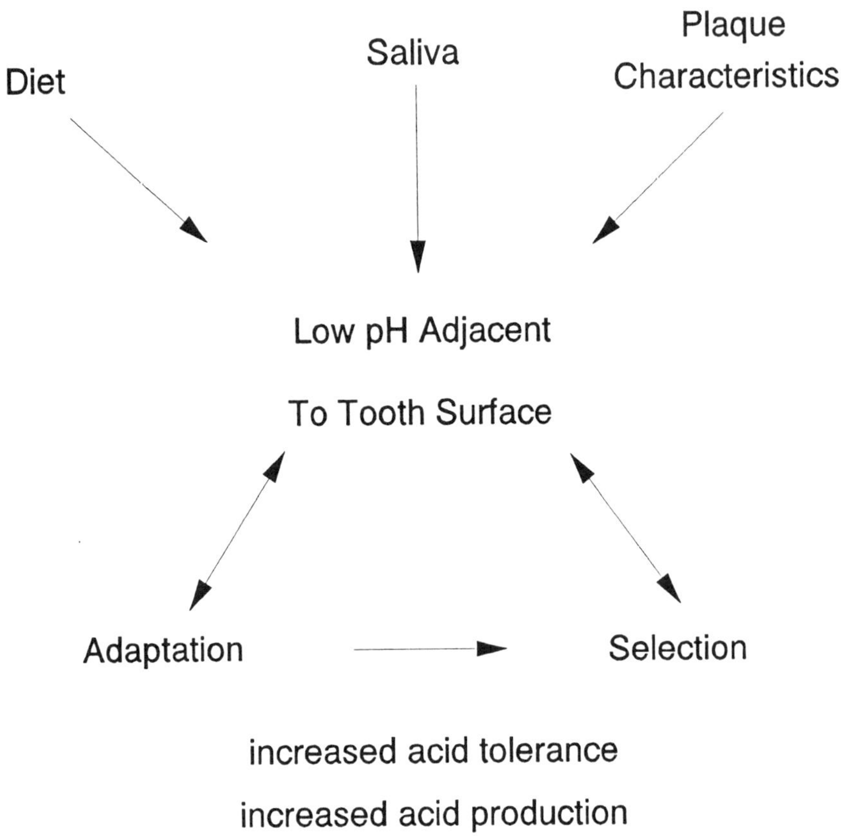

Figure 1 Diagram of the factors involved in the development of a cariogenic plaque.

I will initially review the role of the diet, saliva, and plaque characteristics in the development of a low pH environment adjacent to the tooth surface, which will also provide some insight into the nature of the adaptive response by plaque microorganisms (see Fig. 1). Adaptation by oral bacteria to fluoride exposure will not be discussed in detail. This topic has recently been reviewed (Bowden, 1990; Hamilton, 1990a). Furthermore, recent evidence suggests that fluoride adaptation may not occur *in vivo* (van Loveren *et al.*, 1990).

Diet

The relationship between frequent ingestion of sugar-containing foods and dental caries is well established (Bowen and Birkhed, 1986). Diet has a direct influence on the metabolic activity of plaque microorganisms and thus on plaque pH values. A number of studies have demonstrated that in the presence of diets high in fermentable carbohydrates there is an increase in the relative numbers of *S. mutans* and lactobacilli, and a depression of *S. sanguis* in plaque (Bibby, 1976, van Houte, 1980). It was postulated that the low pH generated by the high carbohydrate diet gave a selective advantage to the more aciduric microorganisms. This contention has been supported by laboratory studies using batch culture by Harper and Loesche (1984) and continuous culture by Bowden and Hamilton (1987, 1989). An important study by Bradshaw *et al.* (1989), using mixed community continuous cultures pulsed with glucose, eloquently demonstrated that low pH generated from carbohydrate metabolism, and not the availability of carbohydrate, was responsible for observed shifts to a aciduric and acidogenic microbial community.

The use of sugar substitutes is a widely accepted approach for caries prevention which can also influence plaque ecology. Most research in this area has focused on the effects of two sugar alcohols: sorbitol which is considered hypo-acidogenic, and xylitol which is considered non-acidogenic and may interfere with glucose metabolism (Waler *et al.*, 1984). These sugar substitutes can exert a major effect on plaque ecology by reducing the frequency of between-meal plaque pH depressions, thus creating a shift away from a predominantly acid environment (Loesche, 1985). There is some evidence that frequent exposure to sorbitol may actually increase the levels of mutans streptococci (MS) in plaque since MS can ferment it while most plaque microorganisms cannot (Soderling *et al.*, 1989; Kalfas *et al.*, 1990). Interestingly, sorbitol adaptation has not been associated with increased caries activity (Birkhed *et al.*, 1990), suggesting that the metabolic state of plaque may be more important than its composition. Adaptation to frequent ingestion of xylitol has not been observed.

Studies of tube-fed humans by Littleton *et al.* (1967) and tube fed monkeys by Bowen (1974) have shown that plaque formed over prolonged periods of time in the absence of dietary carbohydrate loses its pH lowering potential. These studies found reduced numbers of streptococci and lactobacilli with tube feeding; however, the inability to form significant levels of acid must be mainly explained by an alteration in the metabolic properties of plaque bacteria. It is also possible that enhanced buffering of plaque prevented the fall in pH values following exposure to sugar.

Short-term clinical studies in which the diet was modified have shown that a high-sucrose diet enhanced the acidogenic potential of dental plaque compared to a low sucrose diet. Scheie *et al.* (1984) reported that 3 weeks of dietary supplementation with high levels of sucrose increased the pH lowering capacity of plaque compared to a diet which restricted sucrose ingestion. Furthermore, the prevalence of *S. mutans* was not affected by this short-term diet modification. Sgan-Cohen *et al.* (1988) in a similar study, found that a 48 h high sugar diet significantly enhanced the pH lowering potential of plaque compared with a low

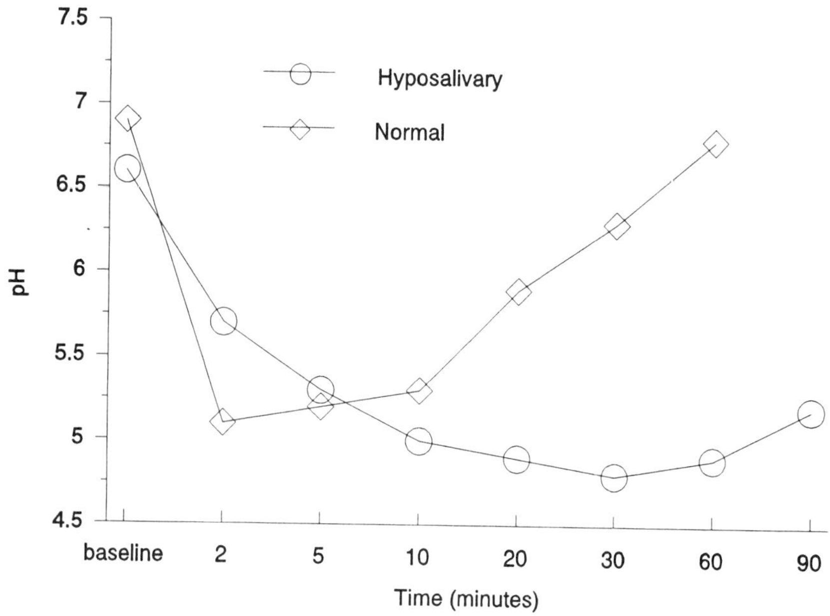

Figure 2 Plaque pH response after 10% sucrose rinse of subjects with normal salivary flow rates compared with subjects with greatly reduced salivary flow rates (n = 5).

sugar diet. These rapid shifts in the acidogenic potential of plaque cannot be solely explained by changes in plaque composition.

Saliva

Saliva has long been considered as an important modifying factor in caries development, mainly due to its role in oral clearance of carbohydrate containing foods and beverages, and its ability to neutralize plaque acids. New evidence presented at this conference (see Dawes: ''Ebb and Flow of the Salivary Tide'') on salivary film thickness and site-specific difference in salivary flow speed has advanced our understanding of how saliva modifies plaque pH values and influences the caries process. The importance of saliva is most dramatically seen in individuals with radiation-induced hyposalivation who experience rapidly progressing dental caries in the absence of fluoride therapy (Brown *et al.*, 1975).

The results from a study comparing radiation-induced hyposalivatory individuals with individuals with normal salivary flow are shown in Fig. 2 (Meyerowitz and Zero, 1988). The graph clearly shows a prolonged pH depression in the hyposalivatory subjects after challenge with 10% sucrose. Also noteworthy was the slower rate of pH fall in the hyposalivatory subjects.

Studies of the general population have not found a strong correlation between salivary flow rate and caries activity (Mandel, 1974). It has become clear that changes in caries activity will become apparent only in extreme cases of salivary dysfunction. Saliva has many beneficial properties which help to maintain the pH of plaque in the neutral range (Mandel, 1987). However, the most direct and important effect of saliva on plaque pH is mediated by the clearance of dietary carbohydrates. Using a drug-induced hyposalivation model, Hase and Birkhed (1988) reported that there is a critical salivary flow rate (0.14 mL/min for unstimulated and 0.62 mL/min for stimulated whole saliva) below which sugar clearance is greatly compromised. These investigators also found an association between low salivary flow rate and prolonged plaque pH depression after sugar challenge.

Clinical studies have shown an increase in aciduric bacteria (*S. mutans* and lactobacilli) associated with greatly reduced salivary flow rates in radiation-induced xerostomic individuals (Brown *et al.*, 1975; Dreizen *et al.*, 1977) and with prolonged salivary sugar clearance in hospitalized elderly (Hase *et al.*, 1987). A recent study by Madison *et al.* (1990) has shown an increase in total streptococcal and lactobacillus populations in surgically desalivated rats. These investigators have also demonstrated the expression of increased virulence in strains of *S. sobrinus* passaged through surgically desalivated rats (Madison *et al.*, 1991).

Plaque Characteristics

Dental plaque varies greatly in composition and thickness and thus must be considered as a heterogenous microbial ecosystem in which the diffusion of solutes results in the segregation of plaque into discrete micro-environments. Gradients in the concentration of nutrients, oxygen levels, cations, metabolic acid and base end products, oxidation reduction potential, and pH affect the growth and metabolism of microorganisms found in a particular plaque strata (Marsh and Keevil, 1986).

Acid production by plaque bacteria due to fermentation of dietary carbohydrates has a direct relationship to the expression of dental caries and is a major determinant of plaque ecology. While the optimum pH for glycolytic activity has been generally reported to be close to neutral (Marsh and Keevil, 1986; Hamilton, 1986; de Soet *et al.*, 1989), the products of glycolysis rapidly lower plaque pH creating a sub-optimal condition for bacterial metabolism. The ability of plaque bacteria to sustain glycolytic activity in an increasingly acid environment is a prerequisite for caries-associated virulence. Several studies have shown that plaque bacteria differ in their acidogenic and aciduric properties (Harper and Loesche, 1983; Denepitiya and Kleinberg, 1984; de Soet *et al.*, 1989) and thus the composition of plaque has a major influence on the rate of acid production and plaque pH.

The thickness of plaque is established by: the adhesive nature of the bacteria and their extracellular products; anatomical factors (pits and fissures, interproximal embrasure form); oral hygiene practices; iatrogenic factors, such as, placement of orthodontic bands, restorations and appliances; and the state of physical activity of the host (tongue and cheek movements). The thickness of plaque is an important and often overlooked factor in the establishment of a low pH adjacent to the tooth surface. When plaque is collected in clinical bacteriologic studies little regard is given to the fact that discrete micro-environments exist at different depths of plaque.

The thickness, diffusion characteristics and metabolic activity of plaque largely determines how much carbohydrate substrate reaches the innermost plaque layer adjacent to the tooth. This environment changes frequently and rapidly, mainly because of fluctuation in carbohydrate availability due to dietary habits of the host. Dawes and Dibdin (1986) used a mathematical model to simulate the interrelationships among sucrose concentration in saliva, plaque thickness and pH changes at the enamel surface. This model predicts that salivary sugar concentration is the main determinant of the optimum plaque thickness that will allow the achievement of the minimum possible pH at the enamel surface. Based on this model they predict that very thin and very thick plaque films produce less acid challenge to the tooth.

Work by our group has also addressed the issue of plaque thickness and sugar diffusion using an intraoral caries model (Zero *et al.*, 1992). The model consists of a palatal appliance which holds eight bovine enamel blocks each covered by a test plaque prepared by harvesting cultures of *S. mutans*. Plaque thickness is established by the dimensions of a plastic holder which is 5 mm wide. Access to the test plaque by saliva and substrate is via a 0.5 mm recess on both sides of the plastic holder.

Fig. 3 depicts the results of a study comparing two different types of test plaque which illustrates the importance of plaque thickness and diffusion properties. A non-glucan plaque was prepared from Todd Hewitt broth and a glucan-containing plaque was prepared from the same broth supplemented with 2.0% sucrose. The change in surface microhardness of bovine enamel was used as an indirect measure of the extent of enamel demineralization occurring at enamel sites corresponding to plaque of different thickness (0.5 mm, 1.5 mm and 2.5 mm). For the non-glucan plaque, which is mainly *S. mutans* cell packed together, demineralization was detected only at the 0.5 mm plaque thickness site, while the glucan plaque resulted in demineralization at a thicker plaque layer (2.5 mm). The maximum demineralization occurred at a plaque thickness of 0.5 mm after a 10% glucose rinse which is identical to that predicted by the Dawes and Dibdin model referred to earlier. Our most recent work using HPLC analysis of test plaque samples collected from superficial and deeper plaque layers, has shown that the presence of glucan in plaque resulted in an increased rate of glucose diffusion and thus acid production at deeper plaque layers (Fu *et al.*, 1991).

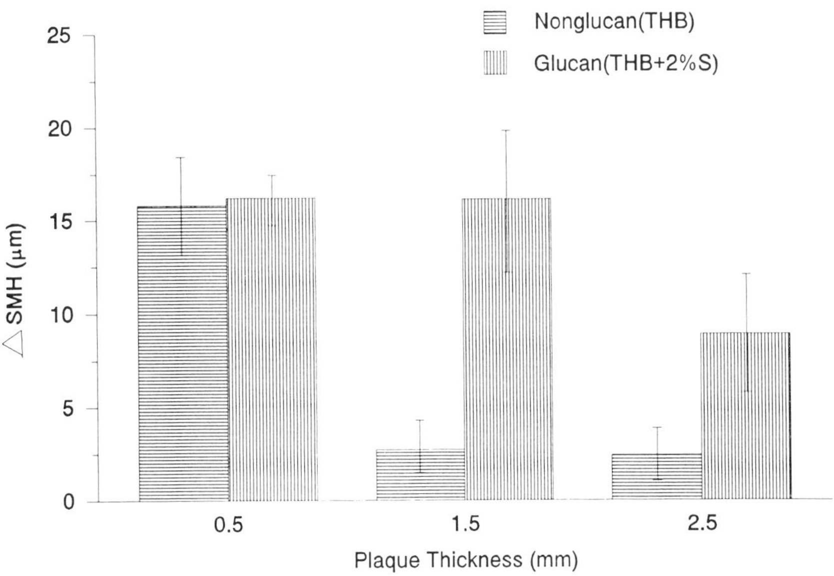

Figure 3 Comparison of a non-glucan *S. mutans* test plaque consisting of packed cells with a glucan-containing *S. mutans* test plaque consisting of cells interspersed with glucan using the intraoral enamel demineralization test. The extent of demineralization (change in surface microhardness) was measured at three sites on enamel blocks corresponding to effective plaque thicknesses of 0.5 mm, 1.5 mm and 2.5 mm. The 45 min tests were initiated with a 10% glucose rinse.

The above findings provide direct experimental evidence on the effect of plaque thickness on enamel demineralization. Furthermore, they confirm and expand on previous reports which attribute the enhanced demineralizing potential of glucan-containing plaque (Zero *et al.*, 1986a) to greater glucose penetration into plaque (Dibdin and Shellis, 1988; van Houte *et al.*, 1989).

In summary, diet, salivary flow rate and buffering capacity, and plaque composition, thickness and diffusion properties are the major factors in establishing a low pH environment adjacent to the tooth surface sufficient to cause demineralization and exert strong environmental pressure on plaque microorganisms (see Fig. 1).

Adaptation to Low pH Conditions

A change to a plaque with increased cariogenic potential may be ascribed to: genetic alteration of plaque bacteria to a more virulent form (acquisition of new genes, mutation, decryptifying existing genes); change in plaque composition to more acidogenic and aciduric microorganisms; or a generalized physiologic adaptation of plaque microorganisms in response to environmental pressure. A genetic mutation would require many generations to be expressed in plaque and there is no experimental evidence supporting this contention. Changes in plaque composition in response to environmental changes are well documented (see above). However, domination by select microorganisms of known aciduric properties, such as MS and lactobacilli, has been observed only in extreme situations and in many cases these organisms are not associated with caries activity (Boyar *et al.*, 1989, Marsh *et al.*, 1989). As discussed above, the shift to a plaque with increased acidogenic potential can occur very rapidly (Sgan-Cohen *et al.*, 1988). The extent of the response suggests that more than a few select microorganisms are involved and that adaptation may involve a larger percentage of the plaque microflora. Also, the speed of the response to an environmental change suggests that a physiologic adaptation is involved.

Hamilton (1986) reported that *S. mutans* 2452, after growth in continuous culture for 5 days at pH 7.0, could adapt to a gradual natural fall in culture pH to 4.8 brought about by the formation of acid end-products. This strain could not tolerate an artificially imposed rapid pH fall to 4.8. In contrast, in a clinical study, repeated mouth rinses with a phosphoric buffer solution (pH 3.9) over a 14 day period were found to significantly increase the percentage of *S. mutans* found in dental plaque (Svanberg, 1980). Together, these studies suggest that microorganisms growing in the mouth are better able to adapt to pH extremes than microorganisms growing in continuous culture.

Studies of the virulence properties of MS using the intraoral model described earlier have lead us to also investigate the adaptive response of MS to growth under low pH conditions. We have studied the glycolytic activity of two strains of MS, *S. mutans* IB-1600 and *S. sobrinus* 6715-13 grown in batch culture under different pH conditions (Zero *et al.*, 1990, 1991). The environmental pH during growth was lowered by reducing the buffering capacity of the basal TTY medium (Hamada and Torii, 1978). The modified medium contained 1/8 of the concentration of buffering salts found in the basal medium. The glycolytic activity of washed cell suspensions of the test strains was measured at constant pH levels of 7 and 5 using a pH stat. Both 18 h stationary phase cultures and log phase cultures were studied. As shown in the Table, growth in low pH conditions enhanced the glycolytic activity of the *S. mutans* test strains, confirming the results from a previous study where continuous cultures were used (Hamilton and Ellwood, 1978). More recent studies in our laboratory have shown that acid-adapted *S. mutans* cells rapidly de-adapt when grown under neutral pH conditions (Zero *et al.*, 1991; Satou *et al.*, 1992). Thus, the increased glycolytic activity appears to be part of a physiologic adaptation to growth at low pH.

Surprisingly, the glycolytic activity of the *S. sobrinus* test strain was not influenced by the growth pH condition, but did exhibit enhanced glycolytic activity when grown in a medium containing sucrose compared to growth in medium containing glucose (Table). A possible explanation is that this particular

TABLE *Glycolytic Activity of S. mutans IB-1600 and S. sobrinus 6715-13 Under Different Batch Culture Conditions*

	S. mutans IB-1600			*S. sobrinus 6715-13*		
		pH Stat Condition			*pH Stat Condition*	
Growth Condition	*tpH***	*pH = 7.0*	*pH = 5.0*	*tpH*	*pH = 7.0*	*pH = 5.0*
Stationary Phase Cells						
TTY basal medium	6.6	0.23*	0.15*	6.6	0.14*	0.13*
+ 0.2% glucose		(0.02)	(0.02)		(0.01)	(0.03)
TTY modified medium***	4.8	0.41	0.29	4.7	0.14	0.07
+ 0.2% glucose		(0.07)	(0.04)		(0.10)	(0.07)
TTY basal medium	6.6	0.24	0.10	6.7	0.90	0.36
+ 0.2% sucrose		(0.04)	(0.08)		(0.40)	(0.10)
TTY modified medium	4.9	0.65	0.43	4.9	0.72	0.31
+ 0.2% sucrose		(0.21)	(0.12)		(0.07)	(0.07)
Log Phase Cells						
TTY basal medium	7.0	0.37	0.16	7.3	0.58	0.13
+ 0.2% glucose		(0.04)	(0.04)		(0.06)	(0.03)
TTY modified medium	5.6	0.80	0.60	6.1	0.58	0.44
+ 0.2% glucose		(0.03)	(0.03)		(0.03)	(0.01)

*Mean(SD), glycolytic rate (μmol acid/mg protein/min), n = 3
**Terminal culture pH
***1/8 the concentration of buffering salts found in basal medium

strain of *S. sobrinus* does not have the ability to tolerate growth at low pH unless growth is accompanied by the synthesis of glucan which may afford the cells protection against an acid environment. Further experimentation is need to establish whether these findings are unique to the specific strains of *S. mutans* and *S. sobrinus* studied, or whether they can be generalized to the MS subgroups of *S. mutans* and *S. sobrinus*.

We also noted that *S. mutans* cells grown under low pH conditions had glycolytic activity from an endogenous carbohydrate source (IPS) in the absence of an exogenous carbohydrate challenge (Zero *et al.*, 1990). Interestingly, the *S. sobrinus* test strain did not exhibit synthesis of IPS when grown at low pH values. The importance of endogenous substrate in relationship to acid adaptation is uncertain. However, as will be discussed later, it is necessary to have an energy source to drive the proton-translocating membrane ATPase (H^+/ATPase) to regulate intracellular pH. Intracellular polysaccharides may provide energy at a time when exogenous substrate is lacking and the external pH remains low.

Possible Mechanisms for Acid Adaptation

Adaptation to acidic pH conditions may be mediated by a number of changes in cell physiology. The regulation of cytoplasmic pH is essential for cell function. Bacteria have developed a number of strategies to maintain intracellular pH in the optimal range, which include low intrinsic proton (H^+) permeability of the cell membrane, active transport of H^+, production of bases, and the relatively high buffering capacity of the cytoplasm (Booth, 1985).

There is limited evidence of an adaptive change (decrease) in the proton permeability of cell membranes of strains of *S. mutans* in response to growth in an acidic environment (Hamilton and Buckley, 1991). Stronger support exists for adaptation to acidic conditions by proton transport mechanisms. The H^+/ATPase has been correlated with the acid tolerance of strains of *S. mutans* and lactobacilli (Bender *et al.*, 1986; Bender and Marquis, 1987). More recent reports have found increased H^+/ATPase activity associated with decreased pH of the growth condition in chemostat studies (Hamilton and Buckley, 1991; Belli and Marquis, 1991).

Closely coupled with increased H^+/ATPase activity is an increased energy demand required to drive proton extrusion (Harold and Altendorf, 1974). It has been proposed that the rate-limiting step in carbohydrate metabolism is sugar transport and not the glycolytic pathway (Keevil *et al.*, 1986). The phosphoenolpyruvate-dependent sugar phosphotransferase system (PTS) has been well characterized and is thought to be the major route of sugar transport by *S. mutans* (Vadeboncoeur *et al.*, 1991). The PTS appears to be a high-affinity energy-conserving system which is most active under conditions of sugar limitation (Lodge and Jacobson, 1988). However, the PTS is repressed by growth at low pH. Hamilton and Ellwood (1978) observed that *S. mutans* cells grown in continuous culture had a 3-fold higher rate of acid production and nearly a 10-fold lower glucose-PTS activity when grown at pH 5.5, when compared with cells grown at pH 6.5. In a subsequent study (Ellwood *et al.*, 1979), the same investigators reported that PTS activity alone was not capable of supporting growth of *S. mutans* under conditions of excess glucose in continuous culture experiments. Based on these findings, they proposed that *S. mutans* has a secondary uptake system other than the PTS for transport of glucose into the cell.

Hamilton and St. Martin (1982) have proposed a mechanism for the secondary transport system where the transport of glucose occurs by a proton symport mechanism in response to a proton motive force (PMF) created by the extrusion of protons via the membrane-bound H^+/ATPase. It has also been suggested that lactate-coupled proton flow is another possible mechanism for proton transport, supporting the development of a PMF (Keevil *et al.*, 1986).

The importance of a PMF-driven secondary sugar transport system has recently been questioned. Daspher and Reynolds (1990) reported that a PMF-linked glucose transporter was not found in *S. mutans* Ingbritt and that non-PTS glucose transport could be explained by simple diffusion not involving a membrane carrier. Furthermore, it was suggested that glucose transport may not be rate-limiting for glycolysis. Continuous culture studies with *S. mutans* Ingbritt and *S. sobrinus* ATCC 27352 failed to maintain significant pH gradients when growing at low pH (pH 5.0) (Hamilton, 1990b). This finding suggests that other forms of adaptation to acidic conditions may be operational. Hamilton and Buckley (1991) reported limited evidence of increased acid tolerance of glycolytic enzymes of *S. mutans* Ingbritt when grown at low pH in continuous culture.

The synthesis of IPS may be another important acid adaptation mechanism. Carlson (1986) suggested that the capacity for storing IPS may have an advantage for bacteria existing in an environment characterized by an acidic pH and intermittent nutrient supply. Studies have associated the ability of oral bacteria to synthesize IPS with increased acidogenicity (van Houte et al., 1969) and increased caries activity (Gibbons and Socransky, 1962; Zero *et al.*, 1986b). As discussed above, *S. mutans* IB-1600 was found to have increased acid production from endogenous carbohydrate when grown at a low pH, while the *S. sobrinus* 6715-13 did not exhibit significant endogenous activity. The capacity to store IPS when grown in an acidic pH condition appears to be associated with acidogenic potential and may be part of an adaptive response to an acidic environment. Storage of IPS could be envisaged as a fail-safe system to ensure that an energy source is available to drive the H^+/ATPase proton translocation at a time when exogenous carbohydrate has been depleted and the environmental pH remains low. This scenario is likely to occur at deeper layers of plaque. Plaque bacteria found in deeper plaque adjacent to the tooth surface contain large amounts of IPS, and exhibit cell wall thickening which may also be considered an adaptive response to an unfavorable environment (van Houte and Saxton, 1971).

It has also been proposed that the production of insoluble extracellular polysaccharide (EPS) is an adaptation to high levels of dietary sucrose (Donoghue and Newman, 1976). It was proposed that anions incorporated in the EPS restrict the access of extracellular acid to the bacterial cells. As discussed above, *S. sobrinus* may benefit from this form of adaptation. Soluble EPS may also serve as a reserve energy source.

Another possible mechanism to regulate pH is the neutralization of acid via base production. Marquis *et al.* (1987) have reported evidence of base production by the arginine deiminase system in a variety of oral streptococci which was associated with their acid tolerance. Wijeyeweera and Kleinberg (1989) have related the acidogenic properties of plaque to differences in the proportions of arginolytic and non-arginolytic plaque bacteria. Although base formation may contribute to the maintenance of intracellular pH homeostasis and extracellular environmental pH, it must be considered of secondary importance, due to the predominant role that fermentation of dietary carbohydrate plays in oral ecology and dental caries. Furthermore, the influence of base formation may be self-limiting in that higher numbers of arginolytic bacteria will result in increased competiton for a limited amount of substrate (salivary arginine).

In summary, plaque bacteria with greater acid tolerance may result from a number of adaptive mechanisms operating in response to an acid environment. One of the important consequences of adaptation to low pH is increased energy demands, which requires increased glycolytic activity and thus, acid production. It is still unclear whether this response is mediated by enhanced sugar uptake or an alteration of glycolytic enzyme activity. Increased acid production in response to low pH sets off a cascade in which the pH of plaque gets lower and lower over time, ultimately leading to caries formation. The initial phase of the development of a plaque with cariogenic potential is most likely to be driven by organisms other than *S. mutans* and lactobacilli, since these microorganisms tend to be in relatively low numbers. Eventually plaque bacteria with the best mechanism(s) for acid adaptation or constitutive aciduricity are given a survival advantage over other bacteria. *S. mutans* may be considered as the prototype of plaque bacteria in regard to adaptation to low pH environment, although it is likely that other plaque bacteria also respond in similar manner but not to the same degree. Lactobacilli may be examples of microorganisms which are intrinsically acid tolerant and which only reach significant numbers in plaque when there is an extreme selective advantage due to a predominantly acidic environment. It is plausible that both adaptation and selection play important roles in the development of a cariogenic plaque. However, acid adaptation resulting in a more acidogenic plaque may be the driving force which leads to selection (see Fig. 1).

Conclusions:

1. We know that specific laboratory strains of *S. mutans* show an ability to adapt to low pH conditions when grown in batch culture and continuous culture. This appears to be related in part to increased proton-translocating ATPase activity although other adaptive mechanisms are likely to be involved. We don't know whether these adaptive mechanisms are operational in the mouth in a plaque ecosystem. We don't know how universal they are in different strains and species found in plaque. Therefore, studies using fresh isolates are required.
2. We know that specific laboratory strains of *S. mutans* have increased glycolytic activity when grown at low pH due to increased energy requirements. There is still a major question as to the mechanism(s) involved and how adaptation to low pH is regulated. Intracellular polysaccharide synthesis and utilization may be part of the adaptation strategy by aciduric bacteria, and may also be linked to the regulation of glycolytic activity.
3. We know something about the physiologic range of response to various well controlled conditions by a few bacterial strains based on continuous culture studies. We know very little about what physiologic responses occur when cells are packed closely together in a heterogenous community such as dental plaque with rapidly changing ecology. This suggests the need for further development of *in situ* and *in vitro* plaque models.
4. Based on clinical bacteriologic studies we know that mutans streptococci can be associated with dental caries. However, the expression of increased acid tolerance and glycolytic activity, which are major virulence factors, appear to vary between strains and are greatly influenced by culturing technique, especially the pH of the growth condition. Therefore, to move our understanding of the microbiology of dental caries forward, we need to combine the classification and counting of bacteria with studies of their physiologic properties mainly in regard to acid tolerance and acidogenicity.

REFERENCES

BELLI, W.A. and MARQUIS, R.E. (1991): Adaptation of *Streptococcus mutans* and *Enterococcus hirae* to Acid Stress in Continuous Culture, *Appl Environ Microbol* 57:1134-1138.

BENDER, G.R. and MARQUIS, R.E. (1987): Membrane ATPases and Acid Tolerance of *Actinomyces viscosus* and *Lactobacillus casei*, *Appl Environ Microbiol* 53:2124-2128.

BENDER, G.R.; SUTTON, S.V.W.; and MARQUIS, R.E. (1986): Acid Tolerance, Proton Permeabilities, and Membrane ATPases of Oral Streptococci, *Infect Immun* 53:331-338.

BIBBY, B.G. (1976): Influence of Diet on the Bacterial Composition of Plaques. In: Proceedings, *Microbial Aspects of Dental Caries*, H.M. Stiles, W.J. Loesche, and T.C. O'Brien, Eds., Sp. Supp. *Microbiology Abstracts*, Washington, D.C.: Information Retrieval Inc. pp. 477-489.

BIRKHED, C.; SVENSATER, G.; and EDWARDSSON, S. (1990): Cariological Studies of Individuals with Long-Term Sorbitol Consumption, *Caries Res* 24:220-223.

BOOTH, I.R. (1985): Regulation of Cytoplasmic pH in Bacteria, *Microbiol Rev* 49:359-378.

BOWDEN, G.H.W. (1990): Effects of Fluoride on the Microbial Ecology of Dental Plaque, *J Dent Res* 69 (Spec Iss):653-659.

BOWDEN, G.H.W. and HAMILTON, I.R. (1987): Environmental pH as a Factor in the Competition Between Strains of the Oral Streptococci *Streptococcus mutans*, *S. sanguis*, and *S. mitior* Growing in Continuous Culture, *Can J Microbiol* 33:824-827.

BOWDEN, G.H.W. and HAMILTON, I.R. (1989): Competition Between *Streptococcus mutans* and *Lactobacillus casei* in Mixed Continuous Culture, *Oral Microbiol Immunol* 4:57-64.

BOWEN, W.H. (1974): Effect of Restricting Oral Intake to Invert Sugar or Casein on the Microbiology of Plaque in Macaca Fascicularis (Irus), *Arch Oral Biol* 19:231-239.

BOWEN, W.H. and BIRKHED, D. (1986): Dental Caries: Dietary and Microbiology Factors. In: *Systematized Prevention of Oral Disease; Theory and Practice*, L. Granath and W.D. McHugh, Eds., Boca Raton: CRC, pp. 19-41.

BOYAR, R.M.; THYLSTRUP, A.; HOLMEN, L.; and BOWDEN, G.H.(1989): The Microflora Associated with the Development of Initial Enamel Decalcification Below Orthodontic Bands *in vivo* in Children Living in a Fluoridated-Water Area, *J Dent Res* 68:1734-1738.

BRADSHAW, D.J.; MCKEE, A.S.; and MARSH, P.D. (1989): Effects of Carbohydrate Pulses and pH on Population Shifts Within Oral Microbial Communities *in vitro*, *J Dent Res* 68:1298-1302.

BROWN, L.R.; DREIZEN, S.; HANDLER S.; and JOHNSTON, D.A. (1975): Effect of Radiation-induced Xerostomia on Human Oral Microflora, *J Dent Res* 54:740-750.

CARLSSON, J. (1986): Biochemical Aspects on the Ecology of *Streptococcus mutans*. In: *Molecular Microbiology and Immunobiology of Streptococcus mutans*, S. Hamada, S.M. Michalek, H. Kiyono, L. Menaker and J.R. McGee, Eds., Elsevier Science Publishers BV (Biomedical Division), pp. 93-103.

DASHPER, S.G. and REYNOLDS, E.C. (1990): Characterization of Transmembrane Movement of Glucose and Glucose Analogs in *Streptococcus mutans* Ingbritt, *J Bacteriol* 172:556-563.

DAWES, C. and DIBDIN, G.H. (1986): A Theoretical Analysis of the Effects of Plaque Thickness and Initial Salivary Sucrose Concentration on Diffusion of Sucrose into Dental Plaque and its Conversion to Acid During Salivary Clearance, *J Dent Res* 65:89-94.

DE SOET, J.J.; TOORS, F.A.; and DE GRAAFF, J. (1989): Acidogenesis by Oral Streptococci at Different pH Values, *Caries Res* 23:14-17.

DENEPITIYA, L. and KLEINBERG, I. (1984): A Comparison of the Acid-Base and Aciduric Properties of Various Serotypes of the Bacterium *Streptococcus mutans* Associated with Dental Plaque, *Arch Oral Biol* 29:385-393.

DIBDIN, G.H. and SHELLIS, R.P. (1988): Physical and Biochemical Studies of *Streptococcus mutans* Sediments Suggest New Factors linking the Cariogenicity of Plaque with its Extracellular Polysaccharide Content, *J Dent Res* 67:890-895.

DONOGHUE, H.D. and NEWMAN, H.N. (1976): Effect of Glucose and Sucrose on Survival in Batch Culture of *Streptococcus mutans* C67-1 and a Noncariogenic Mutant, C67-25, *Infect Immun* 13:16-21.

DREIZEN, S.; BROWN, L.; DALY, T.; and DRANE, J. (1977): Prevention of Xerostomia-related Dental Caries in Irradiated Cancer Patients, *J Dent Res* 56:99-106.

ELLWOOD, D.C.; PHIPS, P.J.; and HAMILTON, I.R. (1979): Effect of Growth Rate and Glucose Concentration on the Activity of the Phosphoenolpyruvate Phosphotransferase System in *Streptococcus mutans* Ingbritt Grown in Continuous Culture, *Infect Immun* 23:224-231.

FU, J.; ZERO, D.T.; ANNE, K.M.; and DASS, A. (1991): Effect of Plaque Thickness on Glucose Retention and Acid Production, *J Dent Res* 70:493, Abst. 1815.

GIBBONS, R.J. and SOCRANSKY, S.S. (1962): Intracellular Polysaccharide Storage by Organisms in Dental Plaques, Its Relation to Dental Caries and Microbial Ecology of the Oral Cavity, *Arch Oral Biol* 7:73-80.

HAMADA, S. and TORII, M. (1978): Effect of Sucrose in Culture Media on the Location of Glucosyltransferase of *Streptococcus mutans* and Cell Adherence to Glass Surfaces, *Infect Immun* 20:592-599.

HAMILTON, I.R. (1986): Growth, Metabolism and Acid Production by *Streptococcus mutans*. In: *Molecular Microbiology and Immunobiology of Streptococcus mutans*, S. Hamada, S.M. Michalek, H. Kiyono, L. Menaker and J.R. McGee Eds., Elsevier Science Publishers BV (Biomedical Division), pp. 145-155.

HAMILTON, I.R. (1990a): Biochemical Effects of Fluoride on Oral Bacteria, J Dent Res 69 (Spec Iss):660-667.

HAMILTON, I.R. (1990b): Maintenance of Proton Motive Force by *Streptococcus mutans* and *Streptococcus sobrinus* During Growth in Continuous Culture, *Oral Microbiol Immunol* 5:280-287.

HAMILTON, I.R. and BUCKLEY, N.D. (1991): Adaptation by *Streptococcus mutans* to Acid Tolerance, *Oral Microbiol Immunol* 6:65-71.

HAMILTON, I.R. and ELLWOOD, D.C. (1978): Effects of Fluoride on Carbohydrate Metabolism by Washed Cells of *Streptococcus mutans* Grown at Various pH Values in a Chemostat, *Infect Immun* 19:434-442.

HAMILTON, I.R. and ST. MARTIN, E.J. (1982): Evidence for the Involvement of Proton Motive Force in the Transport of Glucose by a Mutant of *Streptococcus mutans* Strain DR 0001 Defective in Glucose-Phosphoenolpyruvate Phosphotransferase Activity, *Infect Immun* 36:567-575.

HAROLD, F.M. and ALTENDORF, K. (1974): Cation Transport in Bacteria: K^+, Na^+ and H^+, *Current Topics Membrans Transp* 5:2-50.

HARPER, D.S. and LOESCHE, W.J. (1983): Effect of pH Upon Sucrose and Glucose Catabolism by the Various Genogroups of *Streptococcus mutans*, *J Dent Res* 62:516-531.

HARPER, D.S. and LOESCHE, W.J. (1984): Growth and Acid Tolerance of Human Dental Plaque Bacteria, *Arch Oral Biol* 29:843-848.

HASE, J.C.; BIRKHED, D.; GRENNERT, M-L.; and STEEN, B. (1987): Salivary Glucose Clearance and Related Factors in Elderly People, *Gerodontics* 3:146-150.

HASE, J.C. and BIRKHED, D. (1988): Salivary Glucose Clearance, Dry Mouth and pH Changes in Dental Plaque in Man, *Arch Oral Biol* 33:875-880.

KALFAS, S.; SVENSATER, G.; BIRKHED, D.; and EDWARDSSON, S. (1990): Sorbitol Adaptation of Dental Plaque in People with Low and Normal Salivary-secretion Rates, *J Dent Res* 69:442-446.

KEEVIL, C.W.; MCDERMIN, A.S.; MARSH, P.D.; and ELLWOOD, D.C. (1986): Protonmotive Force Driven 6-Deoxyglucose Uptake by the Oral Pathogen *Streptococcus mutans* Ingbritt, *Arch Microbiol* 146:118-124.

LITTLETON, N.W.; MCCABE, R.M.; and CARTER, C.B. (1967): Studies of Oral Health in Persons Nourished by Stomach Tube-II, *Arch Oral Biol* 12:601.

LODGE, J. and JACOBSON, G.R. (1988): Starvation-Induced Stimulation of Sugar Uptake in *Streptococcus mutans* is Due to an Effect on the Activities of Preexisting Proteins of the Phosphotransferase System, *Infect Immun* 56:2594-2600.

LOESCHE, W.J. (1985): The Rationale for Caries Prevention Through the Use of Sugar Substitutes, *Int Dent J* 35:1-8.

MADISON, K.M.; BOWEN, W.H.; PEARSON, S.K.; and FALANY, J.L. (1990): Caries Incidence in Intact Rats Infected with *Streptococcus sobrinus* via Transmission from Desalivated Cagemates, *J Dent Res* 69:1154-1159.

MADISON, K.M.; BOWEN, W.H.; PEARSON, S.K.; and FALANY, J.L. (1991): Enhancing the Virulence of *Streptococcus sobrinus* in Rats, *J Dent Res* 70:38-43.

MANDEL, I.D. (1974): Relation of Saliva and Plaque to Caries, *J Dent Res* 53 (Supp No. 2):246-266.

MANDEL, I.D. (1987): The Functions of Saliva, *J Dent Res* 66 (Spec Iss):623-627

MARQUIS, R.E.; BENDER, G.R.; MURRAY, D.R.; and WONG, A. (1987): Arginine Deiminase System and Bacterial Adaptation to Acid Environments, *Appl Environ Microbiol* 53:198-200.

MARSH, P.D.; FEATHERSTONE, A.; MCKEE, A.S.; HALLSWORTH, A.S.; ROBINSON, C.; WEATHERELL, J.A.; NEWMAN, H.N.; and PITTER, A.F.V. (1989): A Microbiological Study of Early Caries of Approximal Surfaces in Schoolchildren, *J Dent Res* 68:1151-1154.

MARSH, P.D. and KEEVIL, C.W. (1986): Environmental Regulation of Glycolysis in Dental Plaque. In: *Factors Relating to Demineralization and Remineralization of the Teeth*, S.A. Leach, Eds., Oxford, England: IRL Press Limited, pp. 51-59.

MEYEROWITZ, C. and ZERO, D.T. (1988): Plaque pH Depression and Recovery in Hyposalivatory Subjects, *J Dent Res* 67:279, Abst. 1331.

SATOU, N.; ZERO, D.T.; SATOU, J.; FU, J.; and SHINTANI, H. (1992): Acidogenicity of Streptococci Grown at Different Chemostat pH Conditions, *J Dent Res* 71:734, Abst.1748.

SCHEIE, A.A.; ARNEBERG, P.; ORSTAVIK, D.; and AFSETH, J. (1984): Microbial Composition, pH-Depressing Capacity and Acidogenicity of 3-Week Smooth Surface Plaque Developed on Sucrose-Regulated Diets in Man, *Caries Res* 18:74-86.

SGAN-COHEN, H.D.; NEWBRUN, E.; HUBER, R.; TENENBAUM, G.; and SELA, M.N. (1988): The Effect of Previous Diet on Plaque pH Response to Different Foods, *J Dent Res* 67:1434-1437.

SODERLING, E.; MAKINEN, K.K.; CHEN, C-Y.; PAPE, JR., H.R.; LOESCHE, W.; and MAKINEN, P-L. (1989): Effect of Sorbitol, Xylitol, and Xylitol/Sorbitol Chewing Gums on Dental Plaque, *Caries Res* 23:378-384.

STEPHAN, R.M. (1944): Intra-Oral Hydrogen-Ion Concentrations Associated with Dental Caries Activity. *J Dent Res* 23:257-266.

SVANBERG, M. (1980): *Streptococcus mutans* in Plaque After Mouth-Rinsing with Buffers of Varying pH Value, *Scand J Dent Res* 88:76-78.

VADEBONCOEUR, C.; ST. MARTIN, S.; BROCHU, D.; and HAMILTON, I.R. (1991): Effect of Growth Rate and pH on Intracellular Levels and Activities of the Components of the Phosphoenolpyruvate: Sugar Phosphotransferase System in *Streptococcus mutans* Ingbritt, *Infect Immun* 59:900-906.

VAN HOUTE, J. (1980): Bacterial Specificity in the Etiology of Dental Caries, *Int Dent J* 30:305-326.

VAN HOUTE, J.; RUSSO, J.; and PROSTAK, K.S. (1989): Increased pH-Lowering Ability of *Streptococcus mutans* Cell Masses Associated with Extracellular Glucan-rich Matrix Material and the Mechanisms Involved, *J Dent Res* 68:451-459.

VAN HOUTE, J. and SAXTON, C.A. (1971): Cell Wall Thickening and Intracellular Polysaccharide in Microorganisms of the Dental Plaque, *Caries Res* 5:30-43.

VAN HOUTE, J.; WINKLER, K.C.; and JANSEN, H.M. (1969): Iodophilic Polysaccharide Synthesis, Acid Production and Growth in Oral Streptococci, *Arch Oral Biol* 14:46-61.

VAN LOVEREN, C.; LAMMENS, A.J.; and TEN CATE, J.M. (1990): Development and Establishment of Fluoride-Resistant Strains of *Streptococcus mutans* in Rats, *Caries Res* 24:337-343.

WALER, S.M.; ROLLA, G.; ASSEV, S.; and CIARDI, J.E. (1984): The Effect of Xylitol on Plaque Metabolism, *Swed Dent J* 8:155-161.

WIJEYEWEERA, R.L. and KLEINBERG, I. (1989): Acid-Base pH Curves *in vitro* with Mixtures of Pure Cultures of Human Oral Microorganisms, *Arch Oral Biol* 34:55-64.

ZERO, D.T.; ANNE, K.M.; CAVARETTA, G.M.; and FU, J. (1990): Effect of Growth at Low pH on Virulence of *S. mutans*, *J Dent Res* 69:318, Abst. 1680.

ZERO D.T.; ANNE, K.M.; and FU, J. (1991): Adaptive Response of *S. mutans* to Growth at Low pH, *J Dent Res* 70:493, Abst. 1814.

ZERO, D.T.; FU, J.; ANNE, K.M.; CASSATA, S.; MCCORMACK, S.M.; and GWINNER, L.M. (1992): An Improved Intra-oral Enamel Demineralization Test Model for the Study of Dental Caries, *J Dent Res*, 71 (Spec Iss): 871-878.

ZERO, D.T.; VAN HOUTE, J.; and RUSSO, J. (1986a): The Intra-oral Effect on Enamel Demineralization of Extracellular Matrix Material Synthesized From Sucrose by *Streptococcus mutans*, *J Dent Res* 65:918-923.

ZERO, D.T.; VAN HOUTE, J.; and RUSSO, J. (1986b): Enamel Demineralization by Acid Produced From Endogenous Substrate in Oral Streptococci, *Arch Oral Biol* 31:229-234.

Oral Ecological Disasters: The Role of Short-Term Extracellular Storage Polysaccharides

R. A. BURNE

Like many tissues in the body, the integrity of oral tissue is dependent on the peaceful coexistence between microbes and their host. Sterility of the tissues is not a prerequisite for health, but rather a dynamic interaction exists between ameliorative processes and deleterious compounds and enzymes, elicited by both the host and its parasites, in which the structural integrity of tissue undergoes some minor flux, but retains characteristic function, composition, and appearance. Health deteriorates and disease ensues following perturbation of the normal ecologic balance between host defenses, environmental conditions, and microbial activities, which in some manner results in damage to host tissue. In the case of oral diseases, such as dental caries or periodontal diseases, the progression from health to disease entails subtle changes in microflora, environment, and supporting tissues, often involving intervals of disease activity interspersed with quiescent periods. The molecular events underlying disease development are complex and multifaceted, requiring the structural and biochemical interactions of host and parasite components. The ecologic succession from a ''healthy flora'' to a ''cariogenic flora'' involves the temporal organization of various events and the spatial distribution of microenvironments within the plaque biofilm which cooperate to foster the emergence of cariogenic communities. And, although these events in plaque are largely dictated by the microbes, the biofilm community is continually subjected to, and must respond to tremendous environmental instability as a result of extrinsic factors, e.g. host diet, physico-mechanical forces, and variable access of nutrients, salivary components, host defense molecules, oxygen tension, and so forth to the biofilm.

Despite a general understanding of the microbial and chemical events leading to the induction of a carious lesion, it is only recently that the molecular aspects of the process have begun to be dissected. Structure/function relationships of salivary proteins, and bacterial adhesins and exoenzymes has progressed through the use of recombinant DNA technology and sensitive biochemical and immunologic methods. Interactions of bacteria with the tooth surface mediated by macromolecules, and the role of bacterial coaggregation in establishment and accumulation of dental plaque are becoming defined (Gibbons, 1984, Schilling *et al.*, 1989, Banas *et al.* 1990, Larrimore *et al.* 1983; Kolenbrander *et al.*, 1985; Koga *et al.* 1990). As many of these interactions are characterized, it remains apparent that the molecular forces driving the maturation process toward the emergence of a cariogenic microflora are poorly understood. Definition of the changes which occur as cariogenic plaque develops have been refractile to dissection by traditional means because of the complexity of the microbial communities (Ellen *et al.* 1985; Brown *et al.* 1986; Keltjens *et al.* 1987; Bowden *et al.* 1990; van Houte *et al.* 1990), the lack of understanding of the phenotypic characteristics of individual niches within the film, and the difficulties in preserving the spatial and functional organization of the biofilm communities (Hamilton, W., 1987; Wimpenny, 1983). Other difficulties further complicate the study of dental plaque ecology, such as the site specificity of the disease. The location of a carious lesion is of prime consideration since access to saliva changes dramatically in relation to site in the mouth (Dawes *et al.* 1989). Moreover, the relative contribution of bacterial virulence traits can vary as a function of the lesion site. For example, data from the rat caries model indicate that the GTF's of *S. mutans* appear to be critical for most smooth-surface caries, but are not required for the induction of interproximal or occlusal caries (Freedman and Tanzer, 1982, Tanzer *et al.*, 1985). The study of plaque communities also necessitates discrimination between active and quiescent lesions, since the composition and characteristics of the plaque communities fluctuate (Ritz, 1965; Bowden *et al.* 1979; Ellen *et al.*, 1985). These and other considerations notwithstanding, it is reasonable to speculate that the interactions leading to the emergence of a cariogenic microflora have similar or overlapping control points which can be targeted with compounds capable of perturbing key developmental events within the biofilm that lead to caries. Identifying these factors lies not only in molecular definition of the critical virulence determinants of plaque bacteria, but also in elucidating the phenotypic characteristics and capabilities of these bacteria, specifically within individual communities in the dental plaque matrix.

Organisms in the mouth are continually subjected to radical changes in environmental pH, sugar concentrations, Eh, oxygen tension, and immune and non-immune defenses. Central to understanding the processes which govern ecologic succession in dental plaque is the realization that the microbial constituents of dental plaque are not phenotypically static, and must respond rapidly and efficiently with altered expression patterns of many genes to the challenges imposed from their surroundings. As a consequence of the unique characteristics of biofilms, as well as the environmental pressures and microbial reflexes within these elaborate communities, organisms tend to be quite distinct phenotypically from laboratory-cultured counterparts (Hamilton, W., 1987; Costerton *et al.* 1987). A variety of experiments have consistently supported that there are important differences in the physiology, metabolic rates, surface composition, exopolysaccharide synthesis machinery, and expression of virulence by sessile (adherent) populations when compared with planktonic (free-growing) organisms (Wimpenny, 1983; Costerton *et al.*, 1987; Hamilton, W., 1987). Indirect evidence supports that this is true for plaque streptococci.

There have been a limited number of experiments performed to determine what influence environmental conditions have on the envelope and enzyme profiles of the oral streptococci, and especially *S. mutans*. The results of these experiments indicate that these bacteria display remarkable plasticity in their surface composition, cellular physiology, and exoenzyme profiles in response to altered growth conditions. Importantly, the expression of those determinants which are thought to be prime contributors to virulence is markedly altered as a function of pH, carbohydrate substrate, and growth domain. For example, insoluble glucosyltransferase activity increases considerably as a total proportion of glucan synthetic activity as the growth rate of the organisms increases (Keevil *et al.*, 1983; Walker *et al.*, 1984) Expression of the major surface adhesin, P1, and of lipoteichoic acids (LTA), secretion of P1 and LTA, and adherence to saliva-coated hydroxylapatite (sHA) are regulated by the growth rate, pH, and carbon sources in continuous culture (Hardy *et al.*, 1981; Jacques *et al.*, 1981; Rosan *et al.* 1982; Keevil *et al.*, 1983; Knox and Wicken, 1985). Other virulence attributes of *S. mutans*, such as the activities of the F_1F_0 proton-translocating ATPase (Belli and Marquis, 1991) and the glucose phosphotransferase system (Hamilton, I., 1987; Hamilton and Buckley, 1991) are modulated by growth pH and carbohydrate source. Perhaps more significant than the steady state characteristics of *S. mutans* are the transition state responses of the organism, which occur when nutrient-limited streptococci are suddenly pulsed with excess nutrients. These sudden additions of nutrient presumably mimic what occurs in plaque during meals and snacks, and at least *in vitro,* some transitions elicit phenotypic responses by *S. mutans* which are uncharacteristic of steady state cells. Often, the biosynthetic capabilities for a particular determinant during transition, and specifically shift-up conditions, far exceed the capacity of the organism to produce the determinant under steady state conditions (Walker *et al.* 1982). In addition to regulation by nutrient availability and other environmental factors, immobilization of *S. mutans* at a solid surface, as occurs in plaque biofilm via interactions with host macromolecules at the tooth surface or through binding to other bacteria, also influences the phenotypic properties of the organism. *In vitro,* adherence of *S. mutans* to sHA has been shown to alter the levels of transcriptional fusions to the *ftf* gene (Hudson and Curtiss, 1990). So, there is solid evidence that oral streptococci are quite adaptable to fluxes in the environment which mimic conditions the bacteria would encounter in the human mouth. These characteristics have likely evolved as a result of ecologic pressures generated *in vivo* which will have selected for organisms with the ability to persistently colonize at the tooth surface.

At this juncture, a distinction should be made between rapid, temporary alterations in expression of specific determinants and slower, less transient, adaptation responses of *S. mutans*. The ability of *S. mutans* to respond to environmental alterations, such as intermittent pulses of carbohydrate, with altered synthesis of catabolic pathways in most cases probably would involve rapid, readily-reversible transcriptional or translational modulation governed by discrete regulatory components. On the other hand, adaptation of the cells to growth at low pH likely involves the control of multiple regulons and probably a restructuring of lipid components. These adaptive alterations appear to require a number of generations to become established, as does reversal to the unadapted phenotype (Hamilton and Buckley, 1991; Belli and Marquis, 1991). And although these two types of adaptation can be differentiated, the regulatory pathways controlling the rapid alterations in the levels of specific gene products and the adaptation of cells to persistent environmental conditions probably overlap and are strongly interdependent. For example, once adaptation to acid environments has occured, the response profiles of the exopolysaccharide metabolism machinery or expression of adhesins may be quite different than those at neutral pH values. This type of condition-specific control of gene expression would have ramifications in the maturation and conditioning of the plaque matrix, as well as in the pathogenesis of the infection. The precise functions of modulation of specific genes in the ecology of dental plaque are not understood, but hypotheses can be put forth, based on the patterns of regulation seen *in vitro,* which would help to predict *in vivo* strategies for gene regulation and their teleologic significance. For instance, the up-regulation of insoluble glucan synthetic activity with increases in growth rate (Walker *et al.* 1984) may mimic an *in vivo* response by *S. mutans* to sucrose and nutrient additions which would result in the synthesis of a more adherent polysaccharide. Such a response may be desirable since it could facilitate the firm establishment of the organisms and aid in recruitment of other organisms which could bind to the GTF/glucan/saliva matrix.

Factors Contributing to Emergence of *S. mutans*

It is becoming increasingly clear that the prime ecological determinant for organisms in establishing a niche in cariogenic plaque is aciduriance (Bender *et al.* 1986, Bowden and Hamilton, 1987, McDermid *et al.*, 1986). Further, although survival at low pH is a critical determinant, the ability to actively metabolize in acidic conditions probably contributes to the emergence of a species as a member of the cariogenic microflora, as well as to the ability of a species to contribute to caries formation. Organisms which can grow at low pH values have the opportunity to outcompete species in which metabolism was arrested by acidification. Also, continued metabolism at low pH would perpetuate the acidic environment with the consequences of selecting for aciduric bacteria and of effecting further demineralization of the tooth enamel. Despite the importance of aciduricity, it is also clear that the pathogenic potential of *S. mutans* is of a multifactorial nature (Kuramitsu, 1987). A variety of factors work either independently, or in concert to allow *S. mutans* to initiate caries (Hamada and Slade, 1980; Loesche, 1986). Key components in adherence (P1, GTF's) (Schilling *et al.*, 1989; Koga *et al.*, 1990), accumulation (GTF's, GBP) (Banas *et al.*, 1990) and acidurance (ATPase) (Bender *et al.*, 1986) all contribute in some manner to the pathogenic potential of the organism. Another contributor to the ability of *S. mutans* to dominate and to mold a cariogenic environment would be the ability to effectively scavenge sugars and other nutrients at low concentrations (for summary see Chassy, 1983). And, perhaps a major contributor to *S. mutans* pathogenesis, which has been largely overlooked as a key factor in plaque ecology, is the synthesis and degradation of, for lack of a better term, short-term, extracellular, storage polysaccharides (SESP); which in this case are defined as glucans rich in $\alpha(1,6)$ linkages, and $\beta(2,6)$- and ($\beta(2,1)$-linked fructan polymers.

Exopolysaccharide Degradation as an Ecologic Asset

The ability to synthesize and degrade exopolysaccharides in dental plaque may foster the emergence of *S. mutans* in cariogenic flora through multiple mechanisms. The most obvious asset to the bacteria is that the conversion of sucrose to high-molecular-weight polysaccharides prevents the diffusion of fermentable carbohydrate from the plaque matrix. The ability of the bacteria in plaque to access this polysaccharide effectively allows for the use of larger amounts of exogenous carbohydrate. Furthermore, the ability to degrade and metabolize SESP may further enhance the selective pressure for these microbes at low pH. Catabolism of exogenously-derived polysaccharide should drive the community to a more aciduric population since the net effect of the accumulation and subsequent breakdown of plaque SESP would result in creation of a more acidic local environment. The production of larger quantities of acids, over a longer period of time not only is detrimental to the tooth surface, but increases the duration that less aciduric species must try to survive. Longer periods of exposure to acids would result in more organisms being displaced from the community. And although organisms such as *S. sanguis* and *Actinomyces viscosus* have SESP-degrading enzymes, they lack the unique combination of virulence attributes of *S. mutans*. Essentially, then, SESP degradation is yet another mechanism by which *S. mutans* can dominate under conditions which foster enamel demineralization.

Dextranase

S. mutans produces an extracellular dextranase (Dex) of high molecular mass which cleaves α(1,6)-linked glucan polymers to produce oligosaccharides (Guggenheim and Burkhardt, 1974; Barrett *et al.*, 1986). Dex has been demonstrated to contribute to the cariogenic potential of *S. mutans* and *S. sobrinus* (Freedman and Tanzer, 1982; Tanzer *et al.*, 1985; Curtiss *et al.*, 1987; Barrett *et al.*, 1986). Although there is no direct evidence, Dex has been proposed to function in concert with the GTF's as a modifier of extracellular glucans (Guggenheim, 1970). The action of Dex presumably increases the proportion of α(1,3) linkages in plaque glucans, thus helping to create a less water-soluble, more adherent matrix. In doing so, Dex releases oligosaccharides of glucose into the plaque matrix. These small, α(1,6)-linked molecules can then be transported inside the cell where they can be degraded by the *dexB* gene product (Burne *et al.*, 1986), a dextran glucosidase (Russell and Ferretti, 1990). Whether the primary role of Dex is in polymer modification and matrix conditioning or in SESP acquisition is a secondary consideration since Dex will liberate metabolizable sugar in either case. The net effect of the process is that glucose is incorporated into α(1,6) polymers through the action of glucosyltransferases, temporarily shunting carbohydrate into a non-diffusing form which acts as plaque SESP. This is consistent with *in vivo* observations demonstrating the accumulation and subsequent disappearance of dextrans in dental plaques (Gold *et al.*, 1974). However, the precise mechanism of action of Dex and the temporal spacing of the synthesis and degradation of dextrans remain uncharacterized. Support for Dex as an important ecologic determinant can be found in experiments performed by Freedman and Tanzer (1985). Demonstrating that Dex$^-$ *S. mutans* had decreased cariogenic potential in specific pathogen free rats, but that these mutants were as cariogenic as wild-type *S. mutans* in gnotobiotic rats, these authors have postulated that the dextranase of *S. mutans* may facilitate the displacement of organisms which are able to adhere to dextran polymers. Not excluding this proposal, the data can also support the contention that the Dex$^-$ phenotype enhances the competitive abilities of *S. mutans* in a fashion described above. These experiments are of further significance in the sense that they demonstrate the importance of the interactions of bacteria with other bacteria in plaque and clearly show how these interactions can have an influence on the disease process.

Fructanase

The synthesis and breakdown of plaque fructans has received far less attention than glucan metabolism. Yet, following an intake of dietary sucrose, fructans rapidly accumulate in plaque; constituting a large proportion of total plaque polysaccharide (Gold *et al.*, 1974). The fructan biosynthetic capacity of isolated dental plaque is comparable to that for glucans (Higuchi *et al.*, 1970; Gold *et al.* 1974). Also, Rølla *et al.* (1983) have found that the fructan synthesis capabilities of enamel pellicles and whole saliva frequently exceed those of glucan synthesis. The role of fructans as an important plaque SESP is supported by the kinetics of fructan synthesis and degradation. *In vivo* studies in humans have demonstrated that fructans are abundant in dental plaque shortly after a dietary sucrose intake, and their level declines usually within 30-60 minutes after exogenous carbohydrate is exhausted. The presence of fructan hydrolase activity in plaque samples from human volunteers (Manly and Richardson, 1968) and isolated plaque streptococci (DaCosta and Gibbons, 1968; van Houte and Jansen, 1968) presumably accounts for the disappearance of these polymers. So, in fact, fructans are a prominent reservoir of fermentable hexose in dental plaque which are accessible to plaque bacteria through enzymatic hydrolysis.

The majority of fructans in plaque appear to be produced by streptococci and *Actinomyces* species. *S. salivarius* and *A. viscosus* produce copious amounts of a levan-type [predominantly β(2,6)-linked] polysaccharide (Warner and Miller, 1978; Ehrlich *et al.*, 1975; Marshall and Weigle, 1980, Simms *et al.*, 1990), while other plaque streptococci, such as *S. mutans*, *S. sanguis*, and *S. mitior* produce large amounts of an inulin-type [(β(2,1)-linked] fructan (Shimamura *et al.*, 1987; Ebisu *et al.*, 1975). *S. mutans* produces a fructosyltransferase, capable of synthesizing a polymer which is predominantly composed of β(2,1)-linked fructose, with a modest amount of branching by β(2,6)-linkages (Shimamura *et al.*, 1987). This organism also produces an exo β-D-fructofuranosidase, or fructanase (Fru), which can degrade the fructans produced by many oral bacteria (Burne *et al.*, 1987). The gene encoding for this enzyme was isolated and the cloned gene product and the enzyme from *S. mutans* culture supernate was purified (Burne *et al.*, 1987). The characteristics of the fructanase are listed in the Table. Notably, the preferential substrates for the enzyme are β(2,6)-linked fructans, such as those produced by *S salivarius* and *A. viscosus*. The enzyme can function as an invertase, and interestingly, has a pH optimum for sucrose hydrolysis which is lower than that for fructans, which may have implications in sucrose and fructan metabolism in plaque. The molecular basis for this is not clear, but may reflect different sites for substrate binding and catalysis. Based on our data and that of others, we have proposed that this enzyme could represent the extracellular invertase of *S. mutans* (Chassy *et al.*, 1974). Direct evidence proving or disproving should be forthcoming. Genetic regulation of fructanase is complex. It appears to be inducible by substrates and repressible by glucose (Jacques *et al.*, 1985). It also is produced in significant quantities at low growth rates (Jacques *et al.*, 1985). In *S. salivarius*, induction of synthesis after the addition of sucrose is slower than that of FTF (Towsend-Lawson and Bleiweiss, 1991). The repression and delay in expression of fructanase seen *in vitro* is

TABLE *Characteristics of the S. mutans GS-5 fructanase*

Enzyme classification	Exo β-D-fructofuranosidase
Molecular Mass	Approx. 140,000
Cellular location	Extracellular
Substrates (Relative activity)	Levan (100%) Inulin (34%) Sucrose (21%) Raffinose (12%)
pH optima (Substrate)	5.5 (Fructans) 5.0 (Sucrose)
Product from fructans	Fructose
Genetic regulation	Inducible Repressible by glucose Growth rate/pH dependent expression

consistent with *in vivo* observations which indicate that FTF may act on sucrose first, allowing sufficient reserves of polysaccharide to accumulate. Following exhaustion of exogenous carbohydrates, induction and derepression of fructanase synthesis allows for the catabolism of exogenously accumulated fructans.

The fructanase enzyme (Fru) may be a prime determinant in driving ecologic succession. The metabolism of the large amounts of fructan in plaque after sucrose challenge would further acidify plaque and prolong the exposure of the tooth to organic acids. In doing so, the enzyme contributes to the selection of aciduric species, which can metabolize at the lower pH values. The potential for Fru acting as the extracellular invertase of *S. mutans* may amplify the importance of Fru in ecology and sugar metabolism. If Fru is the *S. mutans* extracellular invertase, then it would play a dual role in sucrose metabolism and cariogenicity of *S. mutans*. Recently, we have constructed a Fru-defective *S. mutans* by inactivation of the chromosomal homologue of *fruA* with an insertionally inactivated recombinant gene, and have introduced these mutants into rats fed a high sucrose diet. The results indicate that these strains are not impaired in their cariogenic potential, although additional experiments to test the role of Fru in initiation of caries in interval-fed rats are planned. Should future experimentation support that Fru is an essential virulence determinant for *S. mutans*, targeting of fructanase by specific inhibitors may provide a mechanism to disrupt ecologic succession in plaque.

Conclusions

The oral cavity offers a collection of unique microenvironments for testing and comparing pathogenic strategies of microbes and the role of the differential expression of these determinants in perpetuating colonization, facilitating ecologic emergence, and initiating oral diseases. Current methodologies, hampered by a lack of sufficient sensitivity and specificity, have not permitted the "monitoring" of phenotypic characteristics and specific gene activities of microorganisms in the human mouth. However, existing methodologies combining chemostat culture and the sensitivity of molecular biological techniques will allow the investigator to not only characterize the phenotypic plasticity of organisms in response to altered environmental conditions, but also to begin to understand the molecular strategies for regulating expression of virulence determinants of oral bacteria. Further, recently developed polymerase chain reaction-based techniques (Mullis *et al.*, 1986; Saiki *et al.*, 1988) and approaches involving gene fusions should facilitate the quantification of minute levels of transcriptional activity; such that in the future, it should be possible to actually measure the level of activity of a given gene in response to altering environmental conditions in the human oral cavity. Such techniques would contribute greatly to an understanding of the molecular events underlying disease progression, but also have tremendous implications for diagnostic applications. Further, this knowledge should help substantially toward the development of novel, specific, effective treatment and prophylactic regimens. The vast majority of our current caries treatment and prevention strategies involve attempts to physically remove dental plaque, to modulate remineralization and bacterial acid production and tolerance with fluorides, or to simply seal the tooth by application of synthetic polymers. These methods have been largely effective in the majority of individuals, yet a very significant proportion of the population remains susceptible to caries. Importantly, much more specific and effective means of caries control may present themselves as an understanding of the processes governing the ecologic succession in dental plaque from a "pre-carious" lesion to overt dental caries is realized. Complementary treatments, such as fluoride regimens coupled with specific inhibitors of ecologic succession to a cariogenic microflora are likely to be a very effective means of controlling caries and other oral ecological disasters.

REFERENCES

BANAS, J. A.; RUSSELL R. R. B.; and FERRETTI, J. J. (1990): Sequence Analysis of the Gene for the Glucan-binding Protein of *Streptococcus mutans* Ingbritt, *Infect Immun* 58:667-673.

BARRETT, J. F.; BARRETT, T. A.; and CURTISS, R. III (1986): Biochemistry and Genetics of Dextranase from *Streptococcus mutans*, In: *Proceedings: Molecular, Microbiology, and Immunobiology of Streptococcus mutans*, Amsterdam, The Netherlands, Elsevier Science Publishing, pp. 205-215.

BELLI, W. A. and MARQUIS, R. E. (1991): Adaptation of *Streptococcus mutans* and *Enterococcus hirae* to Acid Stress in Continuous Culture, *Appl Environ Microbiol* 57:1134-1138.

BENDER, G. R.; SUTTON, S. V. W.; and MARQUIS, R. E. (1986): Acid Tolerance, Proton Permeabilities, and Membranes ATPase of Oral Streptococci, *Infect Immun* 53:331-338.

BIRKHED, D.; ROSELL, K. -G.; and GRANATH, K. (1979): Structure of Extracellular Water Soluble Polysaccharides Synthesized from Sucrose by Oral Strains of *Streptococcus mutans*, *Streptococcus salivarius*, *Streptococcus sanguis* and *Actinomyces viscosus*, *Arch Oral Biol* 24:53-61.

BOWDEN, G. H. W. (1990): Microbiology of Root Surface Caries in Humans, *J Dent Res* 69:1205-1210.

BOWDEN, G. H. W.; ELLWOOD, D. C.; and HAMILTON, I. R. (1979): Microbial Ecology of the Oral Cavity, In: *Advances in Microbial Ecology* (Vol.3), M. Alexander, Ed., New York, Plenum Press, pp. 135-217.

BOWDEN, G. H. and HAMILTON, I. R. (1987): Environmental pH as a Factor in the Competition between Strains of the Oral Streptococci *Streptococcus mutans*, *S. sanguis*, and "*S. mitior*" Growing in Continuous Culture, *Can J Microbiol* 33:824-827.

BROWN, L. R.; BILLINGS, R. J.; and KASTER, A. G. (1986): Quantitative Comparisons of Potentially Cariogenic Microorganisms Cultured from Noncarious and Carious Root and Coronal Tooth Surfaces, *Infect Immun* 51:765-770.

BROWN, M. R. W. and WILLIAMS, P. (1985): The Influence of Environment on Envelope Properties Affecting Survival of Bacterial Infections, *Ann Rev Microbiol* 39:527-556.

BURNE, R. A.; RUBINFELD, B.; BOWEN, W. H.; and YASBIN, R. E. (1986): Tight Genetic Linkage of a Glucosyltransferase and Dextranase of *Streptococcus mutans* GS-5, *J Dent Res* 65:1392-1401.

BURNE, R. A.; SCHILLING, K.; BOWEN, W. H.; and R. E. YASBIN. (1987): Cloning and Partial Characterization of a β-D Fructosidase of *Streptococcus mutans* GS-5, In: *Streptococcal Genetics*, J. J. Ferretti and R. Curtiss III Eds., Washington D.C., American Society for Microbiology, pp. 220-224.

BURNE, R. A.; SCHILLING, K.; BOWEN, W. H.; and YASBIN, R. E.(1987): Expression, Purification and Characterization of an Exo-β-D-Fructosidase of *Streptococcus mutans*, *J Bacteriol* 169:4507-4517.

CHASSY, B. M. (1983): Sucrose Metabolism and Glucosyltransferase Activity in Oral Streptococci, In: *Proceedings: Glucosyltransferases, Glucans, Sucrose and Dental Caries (a Special Supplement to Chemical Senses)*, R. J. Doyle and J. E. Ciardi, Eds., Washington, D. C., Information Retrieval, Inc. pp. 3-10.

CHASSY, B.M.; BIELAWSKI, R. M.; BEALL, J. R.; PORTER, E. V.; KRICHEVSKY, M. I.; and DONKERSLOOT, J. A. (1974): Extracellular Invertase in *Streptococcus mutans* and *Streptococcus salivarius*, *Life Sci* 15:1173-1180.

COSTERTON, J. W.; CHENG, K. -J.: GEESEY, G. G.; LADD, T. I.; NICKEL, J. C.; DASGUPTA, M.; and MARRIE, T. J. (1987): Bacterial Biofilms in Nature and Disease, *Ann Rev Microbiol* 41:435-464.

CURTISS, R. III; GOLDSCHMIDT, R.; BARRETT, J.; THOREN-GORDON, M.; SALZBERG, D. J.; MURCHISON, H. H.; and MICHALEK, S. (1987): Genetic Analysis of Surface Proteins Essential for Virulence of *Streptococcus sobrinus*, p 212-216. In: *Streptococcal Genetics*, J. J. Ferretti and R. Curtiss III Eds., Washington D.C., American Society for Microbiology, pp. 212-216.

DACOSTA, T. and GIBBONS, R. J. (1968): Hydrolysis of Levan by Human Plaque Streptococci, *Arch Oral Biol* 13:609-617.

DAWES, C.; WATANABE, S.; BIGLOW-LECOMTE, P.; and DIBDIN, G. H. (1989): Estimation of the Velocity of the Salivary Film at Some Different Locations in the Mouth, *J Dent Res* 68:1479-1482.

EBISU, S.; KEIJIRO, K.; KOTANI, S.; and MISAKA, A. (1975): Structural Differences in the Fructans Elaborated by *Streptococcus mutans* and *Strep. salivarius*, *J Biochem* 78:879-887.

EHRLICH, J.; STIVALA, S. S.; BAHARY, W. S.; GARG, S. K.; LONG, L. W.; and NEWBRUN E. (1975): Levans: Fractionation, Solution Viscosity, and Chemical Analysis of Levans Produced by *Streptococcus salivarius*, *J Dent Res* 54:290-297.

ELLEN, R. P.; BANTING, D. W.; and FILLERY, E. D. (1985): Longitudinal Microbiological Investigation of a Hospitalized Population of Older Adults with a High Root Surface Caries Risk, *J Dent Res* 64:1377-1381.

FREEDMAN, M. L. and TANZER, J. M. (1982): Use of Mutants to Study the Glucan-Associated Pathophysiology of *Streptococcus mutans*, In: *Microbiology-1982*. D. Schlessinger, Ed., Washington, D. C., American Society for Microbiology, pp. 186-190.

GIBBONS, R. J. (1984): Adherent Interactions Which May Affect Microbial Ecology in the Mouth, *J Dent Res* 63:378-385.

GOLD, W.; PRESTON, F. B.; LACHE, M. C.; and BLECHMAN, H. (1974): Production of Levan and Dextran in Plaque *in vivo*, *J Dent Res* 53:442-449.

GUGGENHEIM, B. (1970): Extracellular polysaccharides and microbial plaque, *Int Dent J* 20:657-678.

GUGGENHEIM, B. and BURKHARDT, J. J. (1974): Isolation and Properties of a Dextranase from Streptococcus mutans OMZ176, *Helv Odontol Acta* 18:101-113.

HAMADA, S. and SLADE H. D. (1980): Biology, Immunology, and Cariogenicity of *Streptococcus mutans*. *Microbiol Rev* 44:331-384.

HAMILTON, W. A., (1987): Biofilm: Microbial Interactions and Metabolic Activities, In: *Ecology of Microbial Communities*, Cambridge, England, Society for General Microbiology

HAMILTON, I. R. (1987): Effects of Changing Environments on Sugar Transport and Metabolism by Oral Streptococci, In: *Sugar Transport and Metabolism in Gram-positive Bacteria*, J. Reizer and A. Peterkofsky, Eds. Chichester, England, Ellis Horwood Ltd.

HAMILTON, I. R. and N. D. BUCKLEY (1991): Adaptation by *Streptococcus mutans* to Acid Tolerance, *Oral Microbiol Immunol* 6:65-71.

HIGUCHI, M.; IWANI, Y.; YAMADA, T.; and ARAYA S. (1970): Levan Synthesis and Accumulation by Human Dental Plaque. *Arch Oral Biol* 15:563-567.

HUDSON, M. C. and CURTISS R., III. (1990): Regulation of Expression of *Streptococcus mutans* Genes Important to Virulence, *Infect Immun* 58:464-470.

JACQUES, N. A.; FORESTER, H.; CAMPBELL, L. K.; KNOX, K. W.; and WICKEN, A. J. (1981): Effect of Fructose and Other Carbohydrates on the Surface Properties, Lipoteichoic Acid Production, and Extracellular Proteins of *Streptococcus mutans* Ingbritt Grown in Continuous Culture, *Infect Immun* 31:78-87.

JACQUES, N. J.; MORREY-JONES, J. G.; and WALKER, G. J. (1985): Inducible and Constitutive Production of Fructanase in Batch and Continuous Culture of *Streptococcus mutans*, *J Gen Microbiol* 131:1625-1633.

KEEVIL, C. W.; WEST, A.; MARSH, P. D.; and ELLWOOD D. C. (1983): Batch Versus Continuous Culture Studies of Glucosyltransferase Synthesis in Oral Streptococci, In: *Proceedings: Glucosyltransferases, Glucans, Sucrose and Dental Caries (a Special Supplement to Chemical Senses)*, R. J. Doyle and J. E. Ciardi, Eds., Washington, D. C., Information Retrieval, Inc. pp.189-200.

KELTJENS, H. M. A. M.; SCHAEKEN, M. J. M.; VAN DER HOEVEN, J. S.; and HENDRICKS, J. C. M. (1987): Microflora of Plaque from Sound and Carious Root Surfaces, *Caries Res* 21:193-199.

KNOX, K. W. and WICKEN, A. J. (1985): Environmentally Induced Changes in the Surfaces of Oral Streptococci and Lactobacilli, In: *Molecular Basis of Oral Microbial Adhesion*, S. E. Mergenhagen and B. Eds., Washington, D. C., American Society for Microbiology, pp. 212-219.

KOGA, T.; OKAHASHI, N.; TAKAHASHI, I.; KANAMOTO, T.; ASAKAWA, H.; and IWAKI, M. (1990): Surface Hydrophobicity, Adherence and Aggregation of Cell Surface Protein Antigen Mutants of *Streptococcus mutans* serotype c, *Infect Immun* 58:289-296.

KOLENBRANDER, P. E. and ANDERSEN, R. N. (1985): Use of Coaggregation-defective Mutants to Study the Relationship of Cell-to Cell Interactions and Oral Microbial Ecology, In: *Molecular Basis of Oral Microbial Adhesion*, S. E. Mergenhagen and B. Rosan Eds., Washington, D. C., American Society for Microbiology, pp. 164-171.

KURAMITSU, H. K. (1987): Recent Advances in Defining the Cariogenicity of Mutans Streptococci: Molecular Genetic Approaches, *Eur J Epidem* 3:257-260.

LARRIMORE, S. H.; MURCHISON, H.; SHIOTA, T.; MICHALEK, S. M.; and CURTISS, R., III (1983): *In vitro* and *In vivo* Complementation of *Streptococcus mutans* Mutants Defective in Adherence, *Infect Immun* 42:558-566.

LOESCH, W. J. (1986): Role of *Streptococcus mutans* in Human Dental Decay, *Microbiol Rev* 50:353-380.

MANLY, R. S. and RICHARDSON, D. T. (1968): Metabolism of Levan by Oral Samples, *J Dent Res* 47:1080-1086.

MARSHALL, K. and WEIGEL, H. (1980): Evidence of Multiple Branching in the Levan Elaborated by *Streptococcus salivarius* Strain 51, *Carbohydr Res* 83:321-326.

MCDERMID, A. S.; MCKEE, A. S.; ELLWOOD, D. C.; and MARSH, P. D. (1986): The Effect of Lowering the pH on the Composition and Metabolism of a Community of Nine Oral Bacteria Grown in a Chemostat, *Can J Microbiol* 132:1205-1214.

MULLIS, K.; FALOONA, F.; SCHARF, S.; SAIKI, R.; HORN, G.; and EHRLICH, H. (1986): Specific Enzymatic Amplification of DNA *in vitro*: The Polymerase Chain Reaction, *Cold Spring Harbor Symp Quant Biol* 51:263.

RITZ, H. L. (1967): Microbial Population Shifts in Developing Human Dental Plaque, *Arch Oral Biol* 12:1561-1568.

ROSAN, B.; APPLEBAUM, B.; CAMPBELL, L. K.; KNOX, K. W.; and WICKEN, A. J. (1982): Chemostat Studies of the Effect of Environmental Control on *Streptococcus sanguis* Adherence to hydroxylapatite, *Infect Immun* 35:64-70.

RUSSELL, R. R. B.; SHIROZA, T.; FERRETTI, J. J.; and KURAMITSU, H. K. (1988): Homology of Glucosyltransferase Gene and Protein Sequence from *Streptococcus mutans* and *Streptococcus sobrinus*, *J Dent Res* 67:543-547.

RUSSELL, R. R. B. and FERRETTI, J. J. (1990): Nucleotide Sequence of the Dextran Glucosidase (dexB) Gene of *Streptococcus mutans*, *J Gen Microbiol* 136:803-810

RØLLA, G.; CIARDI, J. E.; EGGEN, K. H.; BOWEN, W. H.; and AFSETH, J. (1983): Free Glucosyl- and Fructosyltransferase in Human Saliva and Adsorption of These Enzymes to Teeth *In Vivo*, In: *Proceedings: Glucosyltransferases, Glucans, Sucrose and Dental Caries (a Special Supplement to Chemical Senses)*. R. J. Doyle and J. E. Ciardi Eds., Washington, D. C., Information Retrieval Inc., pp. 21-29.

SAIKI, R. K.; GELFAND, D. H.; STOFFEL, S.; SCHARF, S. J.; HIGUCHI, R.; HORN, G. T.; MULLIS, K. B.; and EHRLICH, H. A. (1988): Primer-directed Enzymatic Amplification of DNA with a Thermostable DNA Polymerase, *Science* 239:487-491.

SCHILLING, K. M.; BLITZER, M. H.; and BOWEN, W. H. (1989): Adherence of *Streptococcus mutans* to Glucans Formed *in situ* in Salivary Pellicle. *J Dent Res* 68:1678-1680.

SCHROEDER, V. A.; MICHALEK, S. M.; and MACRINA, F. L. (1989): Biochemical Characterization and Evaluation of a Fructosyltransferase-deficient Mutant of *Streptococcus mutans* V403, *Infect Immun* 57:3560-3569.

SHIMAMURA, A.; KENJI, T.; NAGASE, T.; ITO, M.; TSUMORI, H.; and MUKASA, H. (1987): Structural Determination of D-Fructans from *Streptococcus mutans*, Serotype b, c, e, and f Strains, by ^{13}C-N.M.R. Spectroscopy, *Carbhydr Res* 165:150-154.

SIMMS, P. J.; BOYKO, W. J.; and EDWARDS, J. R. (1990): The Structural Analysis of a Levan Produced by *Streptococcus salivarius*. *Carbohydr Res* 208:193-198.

TANZER, J.; M., FREEDMAN, M. L.; and FITZGERALD, R. J. (1985): Virulence of Mutants Defective in Glucosyl Transferase, Dextran-mediated Aggregation, or Dextranase Activity, In: *Molecular Basis of Oral Microbial Adhesion*, S. E. Mergenhagen and B. Rosan Eds., Washington, D. C., American Society for Microbiology, pp. 204-211.

THEILADE, E. (1990): Factors Controlling the Microflora of the Healthy Human Mouth, In: *Human Microbial Ecology*, M. J. Hill and P. D. Marsh, Eds., Boca Raton, Florida, CRC Press Inc.

TOWNSEND-LAWMAN, P. and BLEIWEISS, A. S. (1991): Multilevel Control of Extracellular Sucrose Metabolism in *Streptococcus salivarius* by Sucrose, *J Gen Microbiol* 137:5-13.

VAN HOUTE, J. and JANSEN, H. M. (1968): Levan Degradation by Streptococci Isolated from Human Dental Plaque, *Arch Oral Biol* 13:827-830.

VAN HOUTE, J.; JORDAN, H. V.; LARAWAY, R.; KENT, R.; SOPORKAR, P. M.; and P. F. DEPAOLA. (1990): Association of the Microbial Flora of Dental Plaque and Saliva with Human Root-surface Caries, *J Dent Res* 69:1463-1468.

WALKER, G. J.; BROWN, R. A.; and TAYLOR, C. (1984): Activity of *Streptococcus mutans* α-D-Glucosyltranferases Released Under Various Growth Conditions, *J Dent Res* 63:397-400.

WALKER, G. J.; HARE, M. D.; and MORREY-JONES, J. G. (1982): Effect of Variation in the Growth Conditions on Endo-dextranase Production by *Streptococcus mutans*, *Carbohydr Res* 107:111-122.

WARNER, T. N.; and MILLER, C. H. (1978): Cell-associated Levan of *Actinomyces viscosus*, *Infect Immun* 19:711-719.

WIMPENNY, J. W. T.; LOVITT, R. W.; and COOMBS, J. P. (1983). Laboratory Model Systems for the Investigation of Spatially and Temporally Organised Microbial Ecosystems, In: *Microbes in Their Natural Environments*, J. H. Slater, R. Whittenbury, and J. W. T. Wimpenny, Cambridge England, Cambridge University Press, pp. 423-462.

DIET/NUTRITION/PREVENTION

Effects of Diet and Nutrition on Saliva Composition

DORTHEA A. JOHNSON

The secretions of salivary glands contain fluids, electrolytes and proteins of importance for oral host defense. Saliva is one facet in the caries "triad" and as such, factors which influence saliva production may in turn influence the onset and/or progression of dental caries. Proper and adequate nutrition is an important aspect of salivary gland function. It is suspected that there is a relationship between diet and saliva composition such that a nutritionally mediated compromise of salivary gland function may subsequently alter host resistance. In laboratory animals, studies indicate that several nutritional deficiencies do indeed alter both the quantity and the quality of saliva. Among these are zinc deficiency, vitamin D deficiency, protein-calorie malnutrition, and insufficient caloric intake (see below). Insufficient energy intake and zinc deficiency are categorized as current or potential public health issues in this country (Life Sciences Research Office, DHHS Publication No.(PHS) 89-1255, 1989). And while in the United States and other industrialized countries few individuals exhibit overt nutritional deficiencies, for many nutrients, there are segments of the population "at risk" for a nutritional deficiency. For example, breast fed infants who have minimal exposure to sunlight or individuals suffering from malabsorption diseases may become deficient in Vitamin D (National Research Council, 1989). While individual nutrient deficiencies may affect salivary gland function, other relevant factors include the texture and more than likely "taste" of the diet. There are numerous animal studies which suggest that the texture of the diet and its requirement for mastication have a profound effect on salivary gland function. For the clinician, this aspect of the diet may have a more relevant role in everyday practice.

This review will examine the effects of several nutrient deficiencies on salivary glands with particular emphasis on saliva composition. While there are numerous reports of nutrient deficiencies with associated effects on salivary glands, this review will concentrate on a few studies which have examined the effects on both the gland and saliva. These studies should serve as "models" which illustrate the effects on saliva of nutrient deficiencies. This review will also discuss certain aspects of diet "texture" effects on salivary gland physiology with an emphasis on the influence of diet "texture" on saliva production/composition. A more comprehensive review of diet texture effects can be found elsewhere (Johnson, 1987).

Nutritional Deficiencies

1. Vitamin D. Receptors for vitamin D have been found in both the nuclear and cystolic fractions of the parotid gland (Goodwin *et al.*, 1978; Peterfy and Tenenhouse, 1982). In Vitamin D deficient rats, the volume of parotid fluid secreted in response to either pilocarpine or electrical stimulation of the auriculotemporal nerve is reduced by 50%; the protein and amylase content of saliva is elevated so that overall protein secretion is not altered (Tenenhouse and Afari, 1978; Glijer *et al.*, 1985; Peterfy *et al.*, 1988). Vitamin D deficiency results in both hypocalcemia and hyperparathyroidism, but neither of these cause the noted alterations in saliva (Peterfy *et al.*, 1988). Vitamin D receptors have not been found in the submandibular gland and stimulated secretion of submandibular saliva is unaffected by Vitamin D deficiency (Peterfy and Tenenhouse, 1982; Peterfy *et al.*, 1988)

2. Zinc Deficiency. The submandibular and parotid glands of zinc deficient rats are lower in weight, protein and DNA content (Chaudry and Meyer, 1979; Alvares and Johnson, 1981). The concentrations of the enzymes carbonic anhydrase and alkaline phosphatase are decreased in the submandibular gland, while the activity of several other zinc dependent enzymes remain unaltered (Chaudry and Meyer, 1979; Chaudry *et al.*, 1981). Mixed saliva collected from zinc deficient rats does not show a change in concentration of a zinc-regulated substance, prostaglandin (Bales *et al.*, 1986). In other studies, uniformly stimulated parotid saliva showed a reduction in volume along with an increase in protein concentration (Johnson and Alvares, 1984). Electrophoretic profiles of parotid saliva showed that protein composition was altered. Compared to ad libitum-fed control animals, the acidic proline-rich proteins were reduced by half. However, compared to pair-fed control animals (animals with the same energy intake, see caloric restriction below), amylase, Fraction I and DNase were increased; basic and acidic proline-rich proteins were reduced by more than two-thirds.

3. Caloric Restriction. Rats fed a zinc deficient diet reduce their energy intake because of loss of appetite. To differentiate effects due to the reduction in caloric intake from those due to zinc deficiency, a pair-fed group is included in the experimental design. The daily food intake of these rats is restricted to that consumed by the zinc deficient group. In one study, after four weeks, the daily food intake of these caloric restricted rats was approximately 45% that of ad libitum fed rats (Johnson and Alvares, 1984). The weight of the parotid gland was the same as the zinc deficient rats, but was 26% less than that of ad libitum fed rats. For parotid saliva, the volume collected was less, but the protein concentration was increased by 61%. The protein composition was also changed, but in a manner opposite to that seen in the zinc deficient rats. There was a three fold increase in basic proline-rich proteins while DNase and a protein identified as Fraction I were reduced by a third.

4. Moderate Protein-Energy Deficiency. A severe protein deficiency can be induced in rats by feeding a diet of 0.5% protein. This induces a deficiency state similar to that described in humans as kwashiorkor and the effects of such a deficiency state on rat parotid and submandibular glands have been described (Enwonwu, 1972; Johnson *et al.*, 1977). However, a deficiency of this magnitude is rarely seen in industrialized countries. It is more likely that any protein deficiency seen in industrialized countries would be more moderate in nature and induced by reduced protein and energy intake. In laboratory rats, a moderate protein deficiency can be induced by feeding diets of 5% to 8% protein. Young animals fed such diets appear remarkably healthy, but are much smaller than their littermates fed a protein adequate diet. In young rats, a moderate protein-energy deficiency results in retarded growth of the submandibular gland. The weight of the submandibular gland is less than that of controls and the gland content of protein, DNA and RNA is reduced as well (Menaker and Navia, 1973, 1975). Adult rats fed a low protein diet for three to eight weeks show no effect on the morphology of the submandibular gland (Johansson and Alm, 1989). While the gland weight, and content of DNA are not affected, the gland concentration of protein and the secretory glutamine-rich peptide are reduced (Naini *et al.*, 1989). In young animals, the weight of the parotid gland of rats fed a chemically defined non-pelleted 7% protein diet for three and a half weeks is not different from rats fed a 20% protein diet of similar texture (Johnson *et al.*, 1984). In older animals, the secretory granules of the parotid acinar cells lose their electron dense appearance and become electronlucent (Johansson and Alm, 1989).

There are a few studies with respect to effects of protein energy deficiency on saliva. For whole saliva, the stimulated secretion of fluid and protein is markedly reduced in young rats maintained on protein deficient diets (Menaker and Navia, 1974; Watson and Antal, 1980; Johansson and Ericson, 1987a). Some report that salivary amylase is increased with protein deficiency (Johansson and Ericson, 1987a) while others report reductions (Watson, 1977; Watson and Antal, 1980). With respect to the parotid gland, the volume of parotid saliva collected from young rats fed a 7% protein diet is reduced by 25%, but the concentration and secretion of protein is greater than that of rats fed a 20% protein diet. Parotid saliva protein electrophoretic profiles demonstrate a four-fold increase in basic proline-rich proteins and a 30% to 50% reduction in DNase and proteins identified as FI and FV (Johnson *et al.*, 1984). When protein deficiency is induced in older animals, the rate of secretion is not affected, but the secretion of protein and the concentration of a bacteria-agglutinating glycoprotein are reduced (Johansson and Ericson, 1987b).

5. Dietary Tannins. Tannins are compounds found in various foods (such as tea, red wine, berries, apples, bananas, etc.). They show a marked affinity for proteins high in proline and have the ability to precipitate proteins from solution (Mehansho *et al.*, 1987a). When rats or mice are fed diets high in tannins, the parotid, but not the submandibular, gland shows a marked increase in weight and in the synthesis of basic proline-rich proteins (Mehansho *et al.*, 1983, 1985). When placed on diets of high tannin content, rats initially show a loss in body weight. However, as the parotid glands increase the synthesis of proline-rich proteins, the animals begin to gain weight. It is suggested that the proline-rich proteins interact with the tannins to overcome the negative effects of dietary tannins on protein utilization. In contrast to rats and mice, hamsters fail to thrive when fed a diet high in tannins despite the presence of proline-rich proteins in their saliva. Hamsters fail to respond to dietary tannins by increased synthesis of proline-rich proteins (Mehansho *et al.*, 1987b).

Diet Texture and Taste: Animal Studies

1. Liquid Texture: Gland Effects. In 1964 Hall and Schneyer reported that parotid gland atrophy occurred when adult rats were fed a liquid milk diet. The atrophy was pronounced: a 52% reduction in parotid gland weight within a two week period with most of the decrease occurring within the first four days. At the end of the two week interval, parotid gland acinar cell size was reduced and the gland content of amylase, the major secretory protein, was but 28% that of the chow fed rats. The effect of the liquid diet on submandibular gland weight was much less severe with the reduction averaging 15%. In addition to the decrease in gland weight and the appearance of atrophic acinar cells, the parotid gland contents of DNA and RNA were reduced (25% and 50%, respectively) and the rate of synthesis of secretory proteins was reduced by 70% (Sreebny *et al.*, 1971; Johnson, 1982).

The parotid gland atrophy has been called an atrophy of disuse by Hall and Schneyer (1964). The studies indicate that a liquid diet does not stimulate gland function, particularly protein secretion. The parotid glands of rats fed a solid laboratory chow exhibit a diurnal cycle in gland weight and content of secretory proteins (Sreebny and Johnson, 1969). The acinar cells of the parotid glands of rats fed pelleted diets demonstrate an accumulation of secretory granules during the normal "fasting" daylight hours; during the nocturnal feeding cycle, these stores are released. When rats are fed a liquid diet, the gland content of proteins does not decrease during feeding. In fact, the levels of secretory proteins within the gland remain the same as those of rats from whom food is withheld, indicating that no release occurs with feeding when the diet is liquid (Johnson and

Sreebny, 1971). There is also evidence that protein synthesis which normally increases during the feeding cycle when rats are fed a pelleted diet, decreases when rats are fed the liquid diet (Sreebny *et al.*, 1971). In the absence of protein secretion, there is increased activity of lysosomal enzymes within the acinar cells and an invasion of stroma by macrophages (Johnson and Sreebny, 1977; Hand and Ho, 1981). Many acinar cells show evidence of degeneration. With time, acinar cell morphology returns to normal, although cell size, acinar cell number and protein synthesis are reduced (Sreebny *et al.*, 1971; Hand and Ho, 1981; Johnson, 1982). Cell surface adrenergic and cholinergic receptors are reduced as is the enzyme involved in the synthesis of the parasympathetic neurotransmitter, acetylcholine (Ekstrom, 1973; Schneyer *et al.*, 1987). These gland changes induced by the liquid diet are reversed by returning the rats to the solid laboratory diet (Hall and Schneyer, 1964).

2. Liquid Texture: Saliva Effects. While the effects of a liquid diet on parotid gland are pronounced, secretion of fluid and protein are also affected. In response to a secretory stimulus, either isoproterenol or pilocarpine, the flow of saliva is reduced by 50% for animals fed a liquid diet (Scott *et al.*, 1990). While the concentration of protein in the parotid saliva collected for the first five minutes of secretion does not differ from solid chow fed rats, the protein concentration in saliva collected for 30 minutes is reduced by half (Scott *et al.*, 1990; Johnson, 1982). These changes in protein concentration are accompanied by changes in composition: a near 50% reduction in percent of proteins classified as acidic and basic proline-rich proteins, an 11% decrease in amylase and a 50% increase in DNase and Fraction I (Johnson, 1984). Evidence of changes in composition are supported by recent studies of Zelles *et al.* (1989) who reported an increase in the proportion of amylase mRNA as compared to total mRNA.

3. Bulk Diets: Gland Effects. Wells and Peronace (1967) reported that parotid gland enlargement results if the requirement for food mastication is increased. Mastication can be increased by incorporating non-nutritive cellulose into the diet. Various formulations are used, but the range is usually 30% - 50% cellulose. Some of the diets are pelleted; others are fed in a dry powdered state. With a pelleted diet containing 30% non-nutritive cellulose, rats increase their daily food intake by 45% in order to maintain a constant caloric intake (Johnson and Sreebny, 1982). With the increased food intake, parotid gland weight, content of DNA, RNA, and choline acetyltransferase as well as the rate synthesis of secretory proteins are increased (Johnson and Sreebny, 1973, 1982; Ekstrom, 1974; Hall and Schneyer, 1977). Alpha and beta adrenergic as well as cholinergic cell surface receptors are also increased (Johnson and Cardenas, 1992). The weight of the submandibular gland is not changed by the increase in the bulk content of the diet (Anderson and Smith, 1981).

4. Bulk Diets: Saliva Effects. The protein concentration of stimulated parotid saliva is increased by 50% for animals fed a bulk diet (Johnson and Sreebny, 1982). However, the ratio of individual proteins to total protein does not change and the gel electrophoretic protein profiles are not altered suggesting that the synthesis of all proteins increases in parallel such that the composition remains unaltered (Johnson and Sreebny, 1982).

5. *Neural Regulation of Diet Texture Effects.* Both branches of the autonomic nervous system are involved in the regulation of the effects of "mastication" on parotid gland acinar cell number, size and secretory function. Removal of the parotid gland sympathetic and parasympathetic innervation results in a profound parotid gland atrophy which is the same regardless of whether the rats are fed solid chow or liquid diets (Hall and Schneyer, 1973). For lab chow-fed rats, removal of only the sympathetic innervation results in a 14% decrease in gland weight while the weight loss is 38% following removal of the parasympathetic innervation (Hall and Schneyer, 1973). With parasympathetic, but not sympathetic, denervation acinar cell size is markedly reduced (Schneyer and Hall, 1966). Gland enlargement occurs when rats are switched from a liquid diet to a solid diet or from a solid diet to a bulk diet. However, this enlargement is prevented in the absence of an intact autonomic innervation (Schneyer and Hall, 1975, 1976). The studies suggest that the parasympathetic branch primarily influences the increase in acinar cell number that accompanies the increase in mastication since acinar cell mitotic activity is essentially eliminated in the glands of parasympathetically denervated glands (Schneyer and Hall, 1975, 1976). Thus, the parasympathetic branch appears primarily responsible for acinar cell number and size. With respect to secretion, the parasympathetic branch is more involved in fluid secretion while the sympathetic branch enhances protein secretion (Speirs and Hodgson, 1976; Schneyer, 1974). Other studies suggest that the sympathetic branch may also be of prime importance in the regulation of protein synthesis, particularly the synthesis of acidic and basic proline-rich proteins. The synthesis of this group of proteins is increased by chronic treatment of beta adrenergic agonists (Fernandez-Sorensen and Carlson, 1974; Robinovitch *et al.*, 1977; Muenzer *et al.*, 1979a, 1979b; Johnson, 1984). Conversely, in the absence of an intact sympathetic innervation or when rats are treated with a beta adrenergic antagonists, the synthesis of proline-rich proteins is reduced (Johnson and Cortez, 1988; Proctor *et al.*, 1988; Watson *et al.*, 1990).

A greater understanding of the role of dietary factors on parotid gland fluid and amylase secretion has been obtained from studies in laboratory rabbits. In these studies, cannulas were surgically implanted in the parotid ducts and parotid saliva was collected under a variety of conditions. Using a variety of adrenergic and cholinergic antagonists or selective sympathetic or parasympathetic stimulation, it was established that fluid secretion was primarily a function of the parasympathetic branch while amylase (i.e., protein) secretion was more responsive to sympathetic stimulation (Gjorstrup, 1980a; Asking and Gjorstrup, 1980). In other studies, the effects of "taste" versus "mastication" were evaluated. With the lab pellets, parotid saliva flow rates averaged 0.5 ml/min while the amylase concentration was approximately 180 units/ml (Gjorstrup, 1980b).

With carrots, the flow of saliva was 60% less than with pellets, but the amylase concentration was four fold higher. When the glossopharyngeal nerve (the nerve involved in taste perception) was severed, the secretion of fluid was not affected with chewing either pellets or carrots, but amylase secretion was lowered with chewing carrots (Gjorstrup, 1980a). The authors concluded that chewing led to fluid and amylase secretion via both the parasympathetic and sympathetic branch while ''taste'' resulted in enhanced secretion of amylase via the sympathetic branch. With respect to mastication, other studies demonstrated that the output of saliva was always greatest on the chewing side and that flow was decreased when the pellets were reduced to a mash texture (Anderson *et al.*, 1985). Further studies utilizing strain gauges to measure masticatory force showed that the flow of saliva was directly related to masticatory force (Anderson *et al.*, 1985; Anderson and Hector, 1987; Hector and Tripathi, 1990).

Diet Texture and Taste: Human Studies

1. Neural Regulation of Fluid and Protein Secretion in Humans. If one is to apply the knowledge gained in the animal model system to human beings, it is important to determine if the neural mechanisms regulating fluid and protein secretion are comparable. While the subject of fluid and protein secretion is complex, studies suggest that the primary roles for the sympathetic and parasympathetic branches are similar for human beings and rats/rabbits. Mandel and coworkers (Mandel *et al.*, 1968; Mandel and Katz, 1968) showed that the flow rates of both parotid and submandibular saliva are increased with stimulation by pilocarpine or citric acid, but not with stimulation by isoproterenol. Further, the increase in flow rate with pilocarpine administration, was essentially eliminated by prior administration of atropine. This evidence indicates that fluid secretion is primarily a function of the parasympathetic branch. Gland stimulation via the sympathetic branch was more effective in promoting the secretion of amylase (Mandel *et al.*, 1975). Prior administration of a beta adrenergic antagonist substantially reduced the secretion of amylase in response to isoproterenol indicating that gland stimulation via the beta receptors of the sympathetic branch enhanced the secretion of amylase. Other investigators have confirmed the role of the sympathetic branch in amylase secretion (Speirs *et al.*, 1974). Thus, the neural regulation of protein and fluid secretion in humans seems similar to that established for the rat and rabbit.

2. Texture and Taste Effects on Fluid and Protein Secretion. The role of ''chewing'' and ''taste'' in fluid secretion has been studied in some detail. Schneyer and Levin (1955a, 1955b) established that approximately 26% of the total volume of unstimulated saliva is derived from the parotid gland while the submandibular gland contributes about 69%. With stimulation (1% acetic acid), the contribution of parotid saliva increases to 34% of the total volume. Dawes and Jenkins (1964) established that the ratio of parotid to submandibular saliva varied with the source of stimulation. With substances requiring more vigorous mastication and having little "taste", parotid saliva contributed about 61% of the total volume. With heightened "taste", but little mastication (fruit flavored candy), the contributions of the two glands were nearly equal. In response to a salty stimulus, the volume of parotid saliva was less than that of submandibular saliva. Thus, the parotid gland, as compared to the submandibular gland, responds to food mastication with a greater increase in production of saliva. More recently, Watanabe and Dawes (1988a, 1988b) evaluated whole saliva flow rates for normal consumption of several foods, such as rhubarb pie, boiled rice and carrots. They noted that the volume of saliva produced with rhubarb pie was substantially higher than that for boiled rice or raw carrots and found that "taste" was responsible for about 75% of the whole saliva volume. Separate evaluations of "taste" versus "mastication" on secretion of saliva from the submandibular and the parotid gland were not done in this study. With respect to mastication, studies with parotid saliva suggest that the flow of saliva is directly related to masticatory force and that periodontal mechano-receptors mediate the secretory response since flow rates with masticatory force are considerably reduced when these receptors are anesthetized (Hector and Linden, 1987; Anderson and Hector, 1987).

3. Effects of Decreased Mastication on Saliva. Hall *et al.* (1967) showed that pilocarpine-stimulated flow rates of human parotid saliva were reduced 33% after consuming a diet of liquid metrecal for one week. The concentration of protein and amylase were reduced as well (30% and 29%, respectively). The flow rate of submandibular gland saliva was not affected. The reduction in parotid gland secretion did not occur if the subjects consumed a solid diet of comparable caloric intake. In another series of studies, Johansson *et al.* (1984) collected paraffin stimulated whole saliva from adult women before and at the conclusion of consuming a liquid 300 kcal per day diet for eight days. All women demonstrated a reduction in stimulated flow rates with a mean reduction of 31%. The concentration of amylase and protein in the saliva was not significantly reduced. In a subsequent study, utilizing the same 300 kcal/day liquid diet for one week, half of the subjects were asked to chew 1 gram of paraffin wax for 10 minutes five times a day (Johansson and Ericson, 1986). The "chewing program" did not alter the results. Both groups demonstrated a 25% decrease in stimulated flow rates of whole saliva. Using a diet of higher energy, 900 kcal, Johansson and Ericson (1989) compared the effects of liquid vs solid texture on stimulated and unstimulated secretion rates of whole saliva. Neither was reduced when subjects consumed the solid 900 kcal diet, but significant reductions in both flow rates occurred with the liquid diet. In another study in which the caloric intake was not restricted but the mandible was immobilized for six weeks (following elective orthognathic surgery), stimulated parotid saliva flow rates were reduced by 44% while the protein concentration was reduced by 26% (Menard *et al.*, 1985). As determined by gel scans following protein separation by SDS-PAGE, the content of basic proline-rich proteins was reduced, a response similar to that seen in laboratory rats consuming a liquid diet (Johnson, 1984). Thus, severely restricted mastication leads to changes in fluid and protein secretion analogous to those reported for laboratory rats fed a liquid diet.

4. Effects of Increased Mastication on Saliva. The studies evaluating increased mastication on salivary flow rates are more limited. Some studies have used chewing gum to increase mastication; others have attempted to alter the diet to a firmer texture. With respect to the former, Jenkins and Edgar (1989) reported an increase in unstimulated flow rates for subjects living in Newcastle who chewed four sticks of gum each day for eight weeks. But the findings may be equivocal since the enhanced flow rate did not occur when the same investigators repeated the study in Toronto. In another study, subjects were asked to chew a stick of gum for 10 minutes of each waking hour for a period of two weeks. With this much more vigorous "gum chewing" regimen, every subject (n = 9) showed an increased flow rate for citric acid - stimulated parotid saliva. The protein concentration of parotid saliva was not increased. The flow rates for unstimulated whole saliva were not altered (Hsieh *et al.*, 1990; Dodds *et al.*, 1991).

Studies with diet texture alterations are more difficult to interpret. In one study, participants were counseled by a registered dietitian to implement dietary changes that would necessitate increased mastication during their meals (Dodds and Johnson, 1991). The subjects were asked to follow these suggestions for a limited period of two weeks. Masseter muscle activity was recorded for three days prior to the start of the study and for the last three days of the study. While masseter muscle activity increased 67% during meals in the experimental period, the flow rates for unstimulated whole saliva and citric acid stimulated parotid saliva were not changed. In another study of longer duration and under more controlled conditions, there was a significant increase in the stimulated flow rates of parotid saliva (deMuniz *et al.*, 1983). In this latter study, the diet of 66 children living in a children's home was modified to be "less retentive, less acidogenic, and firmer". In so doing the energy, protein and fat content were increased and the carbohydrate content was reduced. While several dietary parameters were altered, the authors attributed the changes in parotid saliva flow rates to the firmer texture of the diet.

Summary

The studies described above make it abundantly clear that diet and nutrition are important components contributing to salivary gland function. In the animal model (i.e., the laboratory rat), the effects of diet and nutrition on salivary gland physiology has been studied in some depth. As described above, these studies indicate that both the quantity and quality of saliva are affected by diet and nutrition. In the limited studies with human beings, nutrition and dietary effects could only be evaluated on saliva production and composition. However, the findings are remarkably consistent with the observations reported for laboratory animals. Using our knowledge gained in the animal model, it should be possible to conduct specific studies in human beings in an effort to more fully elaborate the "saliva" aspect of the caries "triad". It is hoped that this discussion will provide a basis for investigations of the role of diet and nutrition on salivary composition as it relates to the initiation and progression of dental caries.

REFERENCES

ALVARES, O. and JOHNSON, D. (1981): Effects of Zinc Deficiency on Rat Parotid Gland, *J Oral Pathol* 10:430-435.

ANDERSON, D.J. and HECTOR, M.P. (1987): Periodontal Mechanoreceptors and Parotid Secretion in Animals and Man, *J Dent Res* 66:518-523.

ANDERSON, D.J.; HECTOR, M.P.; and LINDEN, R.W.A. (1985): The Possible Relation Between Mastication and Parotid Secretion in the Rabbit, *J Physiol* 364:19-29.

ANDERSON, L.C. and SMITH, T.L. (1981): Increased Mastication and Submandibular Gland Development in the Rat, *Comp Biochem Physiol* 70A:567-570.

ASKING, B. and GJORSTRUP, P. (1980): Amylase Secretion in Response to Activation of Different Autonomic Receptors in the Rabbit Parotid Gland, *Acta Physiol Scand* 109:407-413.

BALES, C.W.; WANG, M.C.; FREELAND-GRAVES, J.H.; and POBOCIK, R.S. (1986): The Effect of Zinc Deficiency and Food Restriction on Prostaglandin E_2 and Thromboxane B_2 in Saliva and Plasma of Rats, *Prostaglandins* 31:859-868.

CHAUDRY, I.M.; GANDOR, D.W.; and GERSON, S.J. (1981): Reduction of Carbonic Anhydrase Activity in the Submandibular Salivary Glands of Zinc-Deficient Rats, *Arch Oral Biol* 26:399-402.

CHAUDRY, I.M. and MEYER, J. (1979): Response of Submandibular Gland of the Rat to Nutritional Zinc Deficiency, *J Nutr* 109:316-320.

DAWES, C. and JENKINS, G.N. (1964): The Effects of Different Stimuli on the Composition of Saliva in Man, *J Physiol* 170:86-100.

deMUNIZ, B.R.; MARESCA, B.M.; TUMILASCI, O.R.; and PEREC, C.J. (1983): Effects of an Experimental Diet on Parotid Saliva and Dental Plaque pH in Institutionalized Children, *Arch Oral Biol* 28:575-581.

DODDS, M.W.J.; HSIEH, S.C.; and JOHNSON, D.A. (1991): The Effect of Increased Mastication by Daily Gum-Chewing on Salivary Gland Output and Dental Plaque Acidogenicity *J Dent Res* 70:1474-1478.

DODDS, M.W.J. and JOHNSON, D.A. (1991): Increased Mastication by Diet Modification: Effects on Saliva and Plaque, Abstract 11, This Meeting.

EKSTROM, J. (1973): Choline Acetyltransferase and Secretory Responses of the Rat's Salivary Glands After Liquid Diet, *Q J Exptl Physiol* 58:171-179.

EKSTROM, J. (1974): Choline Acetyltransferase Activity in Rat Salivary Glands After Cellulose Rich Diet or Treatment with an Atropine-Like Drug, *Q J Exp Physiol* 59:191-199.

ENWONWU, C.O. (1972): Biochemical and Morphologic Changes in Rat Submandibular Gland in Experimental Protein-Calorie Malnutrition, *Exp Molec Pathol* 16:244-269.

FERNANDEZ-SORENSON, A. and CARLSON, D.M. (1974): Isolation of a ''Proline-Rich'' Protein from Rat Parotid Glands Following Isoproterenol Treatment, *Biochem Biophys Res Commun* 60:240-256.

GJORSTRUP, P. (1980a): Taste and Chewing as Stimuli for the Secretion of Amylase from the Parotid Gland of the Rabbit, *Acta Physiol Scand* 110:295-301.

GJORSTRUP, P. (1980b): Parotid Secretion of Fluid and Amylase in Rabbits During Feeding, *J Physiol* 309:101-116.

GLIJER, B.; PETERFY, C.; and TENENHOUSE, A. (1985): The Effect of Vitamin D Deficiency on Secretion of Saliva by Rat Parotid Gland In Vivo, *J Physiol* 363:323-334.

GOODWIN, D.; NOFF, D.; and EDELSTEIN, S. (1978): The Parotid Gland: A New Target Organ for Vitamin D Action, *Biochim Biophys Acta* 539:249-252.

HALL, H.D.; MERIG,JR., J.J.; and SCHNEYER, C.A. (1967): Metrecal-Induced Changes in Human Saliva, *Proc Soc Exptl Biol Med* 124:532-536.

HALL, H.D. and SCHNEYER, C.A. (1964): Salivary Gland Atrophy in Rat Induced by Liquid Diet, *Proc Soc Exptl Biol Med* 117:789-793.

HALL, H.D. and SCHNEYER, C.A. (1973): Role of Autonomic Pathways in Disuse Atrophy of Rat Parotid, *Proc Soc Exptl Biol Med* 143:19-22.

HALL, H.D. and SCHNEYER, C.A. (1977): Functional Mediation of Compensatory Enlargement of the Parotid Gland, *Cell Tiss Res* 184:249-254.

HAND, A.R. and HO, B. (1981): Liquid-Diet-Induced Alterations of Rat Parotid Acinar Cells Studied by Electron Microscopy and Enzyme Cytochemistry, *Arch Oral Biol* 26:369-380.

HECTOR, M.P. and LINDEN, R.W.A. (1987): The Possible Role of Periodontal Mechanoreceptors in the Control of Parotid Secretion in Man, *Q J Exptl Physiol* 72:285-301.

HECTOR, M.P. and TRIPATHI, P. (1990): The Effect of the Chewing Side on Parotid Amylase Secretion in Conscious Rabbits, *Arch Oral Biol* 35:71-73.

HSIEH, S.C.; DODDS, M.W.J.; and JOHNSON, D.A. (1990): Effect of Increased Mastication on Plaque pH and Parotid Saliva, *J Dent Res* 69:321 (Abst No 1699).

JENKINS, G.N. and EDGAR, W.M. (1989): The Effect of Daily Gum-chewing On Salivary Flow Rates in Man, *J Dent Res* 68:786-790.

JOHANSSON, I. and ALM, P. (1989): Effect of Moderate Protein-Deficiency on Ultrastructure in Parotid and Submandibular Acinar Cells in the Adult Rat, *Scand J Dent Res* 97:505-510.

JOHANSSON, I. and ERICSON, T. (1986): Effect of Chewing on the Secretion of Salivary Components during Fasting, *Caries Res* 20:141-147.

JOHANSSON, I. and ERICSON, T. (1987a): Saliva Composition and Caries Development During Protein Deficiency and receptor Stimulation or Inhibition, *J Oral Pathol* 16:145-149.

JOHANSSON, I. and ERICSON, T. (1987b): Biosynthesis of a Salivary Bacteria-Agglutinating Glycoprotein in the Rat During Protein Deficiency, *Caries Res* 21:7-14.

JOHANSSON, I. and ERICSON, T. (1989): Effects of a 900-kcal Liquid or Solid Diet on Saliva Flow Rate and Composition in Female Subjects, *Caries Res* 23:184-189.

JOHANSSON, I.; ERICSON, T.; and STEEN, L. (1984): Studies on the Effect of Diet on Saliva Secretion and Caries Development: The Effect of Fasting on Saliva Composition of Female Subjects, *J Nutr* 114:2010-2020.

JOHNSON, D.A. (1982): Effect of a Liquid Diet on the Protein Composition of Rat Parotid Saliva, *J Nutr* 112:175-181.

JOHNSON, D.A. (1984): Changes in Rat Parotid Salivary Proteins Associated with Liquid Diet-Induced Gland Atrophy and Isoproterenol-Induced Gland Enlargement, *Arch Oral Biol* 29:215-221.

JOHNSON, D.A. (1987): Regulation of Salivary Glands and Their Secretions by Masticatory, Nutritional, and Hormonal Factors. In: *The Salivary System*, L.M. Sreebny, Ed., Boca Raton, FL: CRC. Press, Inc., pp 135-155.

JOHNSON, D.A. and ALVARES, O.F. (1984): Zinc Deficiency-Induced Changes in Rat Parotid Salivary Proteins, *J Nutr* 114:1955-1964.

JOHNSON, D.A. and CARDENAS, H.L. (1992): Effect of Food Mastication on Rat Parotid Gland Adrenergic and Cholinergic Cell Surface Receptors. Proceedings of a Symposium "Contemporary Developments in Salivary Research," Buffalo, Nov. 1991, *Crit Rev Oral Biol Med* (in press).

JOHNSON, D.A. and CORTEZ, J.E. (1988): Chronic Treatment with Beta Adrenergic Agonists and Antagonists Alters the Composition of Proteins in Rat Parotid Saliva, *J Dent Res* 67:1103-1108.

JOHNSON, D.A.; LOPEZ, H.; and NAVIA, J.M. (1984): Dietary-Induced Changes in Parotid Salivary Proteins and Dental Caries, *J Dent Res* 63:213, Abst. No. 379.

JOHNSON, D.A. and SREEBNY, L.M. (1971): Effect of Food Consistency and Starvation on the Diurnal Cycle of the Rat Parotid Gland, *Arch Oral Biol* 16:177-185.

JOHNSON, D.A. and SREEBNY, L.M. (1973): Effect of Increased Mastication on the Secretory Process of the Rat Parotid Gland, *Arch Oral Biol* 18:1555-1558.

JOHNSON, D.A. and SREEBNY, L.M. (1977): Biochemical Changes in Rat Parotid Gland Lysosomal Enzyme Activities After Isoprenaline or Starvation, *Arch Oral Biol* 22:291-297.

JOHNSON, D.A. and SREEBNY, L.M. (1982): Effect of Increasing the Bulk Content of the Diet on the Rat Parotid Gland and Saliva, *J Dent Res* 61:691-696.

JOHNSON, D.A.; SREEBNY, L.M.; and ENWONWU, C.O. (1977): Effect of Protein-Energy Malnutrition and of a Powdered Diet on the Parotid Gland and Pancreas of Young Rats, *J Nutr* 107:1235-1243.

LIFE SCIENCES RESEARCH OFFICE, FEDERATION OF AMERICAN SOCIETIES FOR EXPERIMENTAL BIOLOGY (1989): *Nutrition Monitoring in the United States—An Update Report on Nutrition Monitoring*. Prepared for the U.S. Department of Health and Human Services, DHHS Publication No. (PHS) 89-1255, Public Health Service, Washington, U.S. Government Printing Office, pp 46.

MANDEL, I.D. and KATZ, R. (1968): The Effect of Pharmacologic Agents on Salivary Secretion and Composition. II. Isoproterenol, Alpha and Beta Adrenergic Blockers, *J Oral Therap Pharmacol* 4:260-269.

MANDEL, I.D.; KATZ, R.; ZENGO, A.; DUTSCHER, A.H.; GREENBERG, R.A.; KATZ, S.; SCHARF, R.; and PINTOFF, A. (1968): The Effect of Pharmacologic Agents on Salivary Secretion and Composition in Man. I. Pilocarpine, Atropine and Anticholinesterases, *J Oral Therap Pharmacol* 4:192-199.

MANDEL, I.; ZENGO, A.; KATZ, R.; and WOTMAN, S. (1975): Effect of Adrenergic Agents on Saliva Composition, *J Dent Res* 54 (Spec Iss B):B27-B33.

MEHANSHO, H.; ANN, D.K.; BUTLER, L.G.; ROGLER, J.; and CARLSON, D.M. (1987b): Induction of Proline-rich Proteins in Hamster Salivary Glands by Isoproterenol Treatment and an Unusual Growth Inhibition by Tannins, *J Biol Chem* 262:12344-12350.

MEHANSHO, H.; BUTLER, L.G.; and CARLSON, D.M. (1987a): Dietary Tannins and Salivary Proline-Rich Proteins: Interactions, Induction, and Defense Mechanisms, *Ann Rev Nutr* 7:423-440.

MEHANSHO, H.; CLEMENTS, S.; SHEARES, B.T.; SMITH, S.; and CARLSON, D.M. (1985): Induction of Proline-rich Glycoprotein Synthesis in Mouse Salivary Glands by Isoproterenol and by Tannins, *J Biol Chem* 260:4418-4423.

MEHANSHO, H.; HAGERMAN, A.; CLEMENTS, S.; BUTLER, L.; ROGLER, J.; and CARLSON, D.M. (1983): Modulation of Proline-rich Protein Biosynthesis in Rat Parotid Glands by Sorghums with High Tannin Levels, *Proc Natl Acad Sci USA* 80:3948-3952.

MENAKER, L. and NAVIA, J.M. (1973): Effect of Undernutrition During the Perinatal Period on Caries Development in the Rat: III. Effects of Undernutrition on Biochemical Parameters in the Developing Submandibular Salivary Gland, *J Dent Res* 52:688-691.

MENAKER, L. and NAVIA, J.M. (1974): Effect of Undernutrition During the Perinatal Period on Caries Development in the Rat: V. Changes in Whole Saliva Volume and Protein Content, *J Dent Res* 53:592-597.

MENAKER, L. and NAVIA, J.M. (1975): Caries Incidence in Well-Fed and Malnourished Rats Treated with Isoproterenol During Development, *Caries Res* 9:83-90.

MENARD, T.; BLOOMQUIST, D.; IZUTSU, K.; JOHNSON, D.; KAUFFMAN, D.; and KELLER, P. (1985): Parotid Salivary Changes Following Orthognathic Surgery, *J Dent Res* 64:326, Abst No 1363.

MUENZER, J.; BILDSTEIN, C.; GLEASON, M.; and CARLSON, D.M. (1979a): Purification of Proline-Rich Proteins From Parotid Glands of Isoproterenol-Treated Rats, *J Biol Chem* 254:5623-5628.

MUENZER, J.; BILDSTEIN, C.; GLEASON, M.; and CARLSON, D.M. (1979b): Properties of Proline-Rich Proteins from Parotid Glands of Isoproterenol-Treated Rats, *J Biol Chem* 254:5629-5634.

NAINI, A.; MORGAN, B.; and MANDEL, I.D. (1989): Effect of Protein Malnutrition on the Composition of Submandibular Glands of Aged Rats, *Arch Oral Biol* 34:985-988.

NATIONAL RESEARCH COUNCIL (U.S.), SUBCOMMITTEE ON THE TENTH EDITION OF THE RDA's (1989) *Recommended Dietary Allowances, 10th Edition, Washington, D.C.: National Academy Press, pp. 23-38, 92-97, 205-211.*

PETERFY, C. and TENENHOUSE, A. (1982): Vitamin D Receptors In Isolated Rat Parotid Acinar Cells, *Biochim Biophys Acta* 721:158-163.

PETERFY, C.; TENENHOUSE, A.; and YU, E. (1988): Vitamin D and Parotid Gland Function in the Rat, *J Physiol* 398:1-13, 1988.

PROCTOR, G.B.; ASKING, B.; and GARRETT, J.R. (1988): Influences of Short-Term Sympathectomy on the Composition of Proteins in Rat Parotid Saliva, *Q J Exptl Physiol* 73:139-142.

ROBINOVITCH, M.R.; KELLER, P.J.; JOHNSON, D.A.; IVERSEN, J.M.; and KAUFFMAN, D.L. (1977): Changes in Rat Parotid Salivary Proteins Induced by Chronic Isoproterenol Administration, *J Dent Res* 56:290-303.

SCHNEYER, C.A. (1974): Role of Sympathetic Pathway in Secretory Activity Induced in Rat Parotid by Feeding, *Proc Soc Exptl Biol Med* 147:314-317.

SCHNEYER, C.A. and HALL, H.D. (1966): Function of Rat Parotid Gland After Sympathectomy and Total Postganglionectomy, *Am J Physiol* 211:943-949.

SCHNEYER, C.A. and HALL, H.D. (1975): Parasympathetic Regulation of Mitosis Induced in Rat Parotid by Dietary Change, *Am J Physiol* 229:1614-1617.

SCHNEYER, C.A. and HALL, H.D. (1976): Neurally Mediated Increase in Mitosis and DNA of Rat Parotid With Increase in Bulk of Diet, *Am J Physiol* 230: 911-915.

SCHNEYER, C.A.; HUMPHREYS-BEHER, M.G.; and HALL, H.D. (1987): Adrenergic and Muscarinic Receptors of Parotid Gland Following Maintenance of Rats on Liquid Diet, *Proc Soc Exptl Biol Med* 184:102-106.

SCHNEYER, L.H. and LEVIN, L.K. (1955a): Rate of Secretion by Individual Salivary Gland Pairs of Man Under Conditions of Reduced Exogenous Stimulation, *J Appl Physiol* 7:508-512.

SCHNEYER, L.H. and LEVIN, L.K. (1955b): Rate of Secretion by Exogenously Stimulation Salivary Gland Pairs of Man, *J Appl Physiol* 7:609-613.

SCOTT, J.; BERRY, M.R.; GUNN, D.L.; and WOODS, K. (1990): The Effects of a Liquid Diet on Initial and Sustained, Stimulated Parotid Salivary Secretion and on Parotid Structure in the Rat, *Arch Oral Biol* 35:509-514.

SPEIRS, R.L.; HERRING, J.; COOPER, W.D.; HARDY, C.C.; and HIND, C.R.K. (1974): The Influence of Sympathetic Activity and Isoprenaline on the Secretion of Amylase from the Human Parotid Gland, *Arch Oral Biol* 19:747-752.

SPEIRS, R.L. and HODGSON, C. (1976): Control of Amylase Secretion in the Rat Parotid Gland During Feeding, *Arch Oral Biol* 21:539-544.

SREEBNY, L.M. and JOHNSON, D.A. (1969): Diurnal Variation in Secretory Components of the Rat Parotid Gland, *Arch Oral Biol* 14:397-405.

SREEBNY, L.M.; JOHNSON, D.A.; and ROBINOVITCH, M.R. (1971): Functional Regulation of Protein Synthesis in the Rat Parotid Gland, *J Biol Chem* 246:3879-3884.

TENENHOUSE, A. and AFARI, G. (1978): Protein Secretion from Parotid Glands of Vitamin D Deficient and Glucocorticoid-Treated Rats, *Biochim Biophys Acta* 538:631-634.

WATANABE, S. and DAWES, C. (1988a): The Effects of Different Foods and Concentrations of Citric Acid on the Flow Rate of Whole Saliva in Man, *Arch Oral Biol* 33:1-5, 1988.

WATANABE, S. and DAWES, C. (1988b): A Comparison of the Effects of Tasting and Chewing Foods on the Flow Rate of Whole Saliva in Man, *Arch Oral Biol* 33:761-764.

WATSON, G.E.; PEARSON, S.K.; FALANY, J.L.; TABAK, L.A.; and BOWEN, W.H. (1990): The Effect of Chronic Propranolol Treatment on Salivary Composition and Caries in the Rat, *Arch Oral Biol* 35:435-441.

WATSON, R.R. (1977): The Effect of in utero Protein Malnutrition and Subsequent Renutrition on Rat Saliva and Some Salivary Enzymes, *Br J Nutr* 38:233-238.

WATSON, R.R. and ANTAL, M. (1980): Effect of Moderate Chronic Protein Deficiency on Rat Salivary Components, *J Nutr* 110:771-777.

WELLS, H. and PERONACE, A.A.V. (1967): Functional Hypertrophy and Atrophy of the Salivary Glands of Rats, *Am J Physiol* 212:247-251.

ZELLES, T.; HUMPHREYS-BEHER, M.G.; and SCHNEYER, C.A. (1989): Effects of Liquid Diet on Amylase Activity and mRNA Levels in Rat Parotid Gland, *Arch Oral Biol* 34:1-7.

Sweeteners and Caries: Some Emerging Issues

JASON M. TANZER

Decay of the roots of teeth is an ancient disease. However, decay of their crowns is relatively modern and, as a worldwide phenomenon, has corresponded chronologically with worldwide distribution and consumption changes for sucrose (Keene, 1981). Tooth decay is an infectious disease powerfully affected by the diet and by the pattern of its consumption by the host. Its dependency on ingestion of fermentable dietary carbohydrate is beyond question. However, caries does not occur in germ-free animals, no matter what their diet (Fitzgerald, 1968; Stiles *et al.*, 1976; Tanzer, 1981; Loesche, 1986; Tanzer, 1986; Tanzer, 1989), thus establishing caries as a fundamentally microbiological phenomenon.

A variety of bacteria present in the human mouth, and specifically on the dentition, have been shown to induce caries in gnotobiotic rats and, to some extent, in other experimental rodent models (Fitzgerald, 1968; Tanzer, 1981). However, to date, the bacterial types known to do so most potently in experimental animals and humans are the so-called mutans group of streptococci (Fitzgerald, 1968; Stiles *et al.*, 1976; Hamada and Slade, 1980; Tanzer, 1981; Loesche, 1986; Tanzer, 1989).

Various mono- and disaccharides found in the human diet support development both of colonization of the dentition and of carious lesions. Sucrose appears to be the most potent of these, as shown by a variety of observations made with both humans and animals in epidemiological, field study, and experimental contexts (Mandel, 1970; Tanzer, 1979; Burt and Ismail, 1986; Tanzer, 1989). While it is apparent that the recent declining prevalence of caries in several western(ized) countries is substantially attributable to increasing fluoride exposure of their populations, it is not clear to what degree the declining caries prevalence in these countries (Glass, 1982; National Institutes of Health, 1987; 1989) and its reported increase in several others (Barmes, 1977; Enwonwu, 1981; Mandel, 1985; Stephen, 1993) may also reflect recent changes of eating patterns or of diet compositions with respect to carbohydrates.

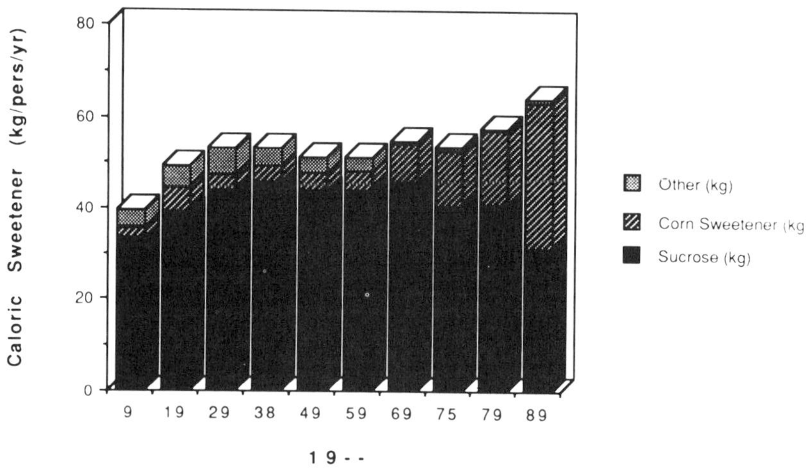

Figure 1. Annual *Per capita* disappearance of major caloric sweeteners in the U.S. at ten-year intervals from 1909-1989. Data from USDA Economic Research Service, 1991.

Since the 1970s, there has been a dramatic decline in the U.S. in the proportion of caloric sweeteners constituted by sucrose and a roughly proportional increase in the amount of high fructose corn sweetener (HFCS), (US Dept. Agriculture, 1991, a, b) (Fig. 1); similar phenomena may be occurring in some western European countries. Conversely, there is suggestion that caries prevalence increase in some societies is associated with worldwide shifts in the commercial production, distribution and consumption of sucrose (Enwonwu, 1981; Gordon and Newbrun, 1986; Licht, 1990).

There are abundant physiological, biochemical, and genetic data on the mutans streptococci, both *in vitro* and in the dental plaques over carious lesions in experimental animals. These allow reasonable characterization of the special interrelationship between virulence expression (cariogenicity) by mutans streptococci, which adhere to and accumulate on the surfaces of teeth, and frequent sucrose consumption (Tanzer *et al.*, 1984; Tanzer, 1989). This work has taken advantage of the ability to study unequivocally mutans-rich, bacteriologically-characterized plaques in animal (and to some extent human) models which develop tooth decay. It allows a pictorial representation of several key elements of these bacteriological phenomena (Fig. 2).

It is a common observation that carious lesions of the teeth are remarkably localized (Fig. 3); the teeth do not decay *en mass.* Similarly, colonization of the teeth by mutans streptococci is also remarkably localized (Ikeda *et al.*, 1973; Gibbons *et al.*, 1974; Duchin and van Houte, 1978). Nonetheless, studies of effects of dietary ingredients on cariogenic plaque have largely failed either to characterize the plaques under study bacteriologically or have chosen to pool

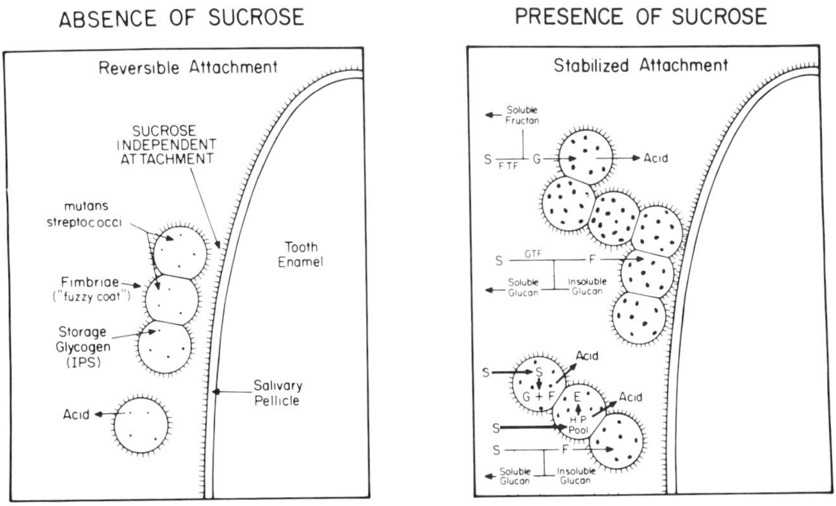

Figure 2. Cartoon representing the association of mutans streptococci with salivary pellicle-coated enamel in the absence (left) and presence (right) of sucrose. While in the absence of sucrose there is reversible adsorption of these bacteria to the tooth surface, there is minimal acid production from exogenous or endogenous substrates and no production of extracellular polysaccharides. By contrast, in the presence of readily fermentable carbohydrate such as constituted by sucrose, glucose or fructose, production of acid occurs from these exogenous substrates, as does the synthesis of intracellular glycogen. However, it is only in the presence of sucrose that the extracellular and cell surface-associated glucosyl- and fructosyl transferases (GTF and FTF, respectively) produce their glucan and fructan products. The insoluble glucan product made *in situ* and remaining associated with the surface of these bacteria are established as responsible for stabilization of their attachment to the tooth surface and are key to virulence expression. These bacteria are capable of growth only in the presence of fermentable carbohydrate. (Reproduced by courtesy of J.M. Tanzer, *J. Dent Res.* 68 (Spec. Iss.): 1576-1587, 1987.)

plaques (both cariogenic ones, gingivitis-related ones, and nonvirulent ones) and to assume that these are cariogenic plaques. Thus, plaques were studied as though the teeth *do* decay *en masse* under *all* plaques. Clearly, this is a grossly flawed assumption. Accordingly, much past and current literature purported to address caries has, in fact, addressed pooled plaque acidogenesis or its inhibition, random tooth surface hardness or its reduction, tooth surface porosity or its reduction, tooth surface demineralization or its remineralization, etc.—but, arguably, not caries (Tanzer, 1991). The relative ease of developing such facile, data-producing models may have misled some into thinking that they were studying the disease, caries, when they were studying a small aspect of the caries process. Only studies of intact animals, human or nonhuman, eating a diet at

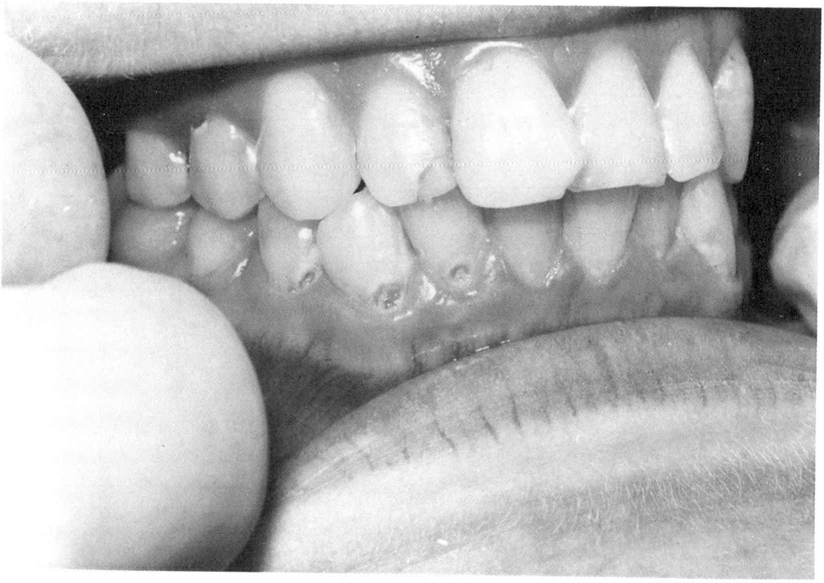

Figure 3. View of dentition of human with carious lesions localized to some buccal and approximal surfaces of teeth. However, there were no occlusal or lingual carious lesions (not shown).

natural frequencies, with teeth colonized by a cariogenic flora, and bathed in an ebbing and flowing salivary sea, protected by host defenses, in a world of transient ecological pressures allows us to comfortably and justifiably speak of studying caries.

There has been great interest, understandably, in market-driven attempts to inhibit the development of or to control dental caries by providing alternative sweeteners to the host. These interests are perhaps a side-effect of commercial attempts to alter the course of diabetes and obesity, surely major health issues affecting well-fed societies (Siebert, 1987). While the consumption of sucrose (or other caloric sweeteners) by such societies has been blamed in both popular press and even in the U.S. Congress for causing or exacerbating these maladies, little evidence supports this view (Bierman *et al.*, 1979). Nonetheless, these anti-obesity and anti-diabetes goals, however shakily founded, have substantially led to commercial interest in the development of a variety of sweeteners for use as substitutes for caloric sweeteners, mainly sucrose and high fructose corn sweetener (HFCS) (Ziesenitz and Siebert, 1987). The use of these food ingredients, presently and prospectively, is limited by their costs, physical and chemical properties, abilities to supply bulk, browning reactions and other phenomena important to food manufacture, sweetness, human tolerance and safety, and, of course, regulatory agency approval. Some of these sweeteners have clearly cariogenic properties, some are non-cariogenic and some may even be anticariogenic. Table 1 lists such caloric and non-caloric sweeteners of greatest interest.

The preponderance of data indicate that glucose and fructose (and, thus, HFCS and invert sugar), and cooked (partially hydrolyzed) corn starch have cariogenic significance, albeit less so than sucrose (Tanzer, 1986; Newbrun, 1990). The sugar alcohols sorbitol (Frostell *et al.*, 1967; Cornick and Bowen, 1972; Glass, 1983) and xylitol (Scheinen and Mäkinen, 1975; Mäkinen, 1989) are essentially non-cariogenic. Emerging data on Lycasin®, a hydrogenated partial hydrolyzate of starch (Rugg-Gunn, 1989), maltitol (Imfeld, 1983), isomaltitol (Imfeld, 1983; Karle and Gehring, 1981), and lactitol (Grenby, 1989), also polyols, suggest their minimal to nil cariogenicity, as do emerging data on Palatinose®(Takazoe, 1989), isomaltulose (Sesaki, *et al.*, 1985), leucrose (Ziesenitz, *et al.*, 1989), and glucosyl sucrose ("coupling sugar") (Ikeda, 1978), bond isomers of sucrose (Table 2). However, because most of these molecules are relatively expensive as bulk sweeteners and are poorly hydrolyzed in and/or absorbed from the small intestine, substitution of them for simple sugars is limited by costs and by adverse effects on the host, especially osmotic diarrhea and flatulence (Siebert, 1987; Ziesenitz and Siebert, 1987), Table 1. Thus, consumption of these sugar substitutes is likely to be essentially limited to use in confections.

Special comments are appropriate about sorbitol, xylitol, and isomaltitol (Palatinit®, Isomalt®) as they are already prominently found in various food products in the USA and abroad. Elegant studies have demonstrated that xylitol is non-cariogenic in humans and animals (Scheinin and Mäkinen, 1975; Mäkinen, 1989). Some workers have even argued that it is anticariogenic, a claim seen by this writer to be weakly supported for humans and not supported by experimental animal data (Bowen and Pearson, 1992). The plaque microflora does not ferment xylitol or use it as a substrate for growth. Some mutans streptococci accumulate xylitol as xylitol-5-phosphate, perhaps using the PEP-dependent PTS system for fructose. However, the xylitol-5-phosphate cannot be channeled along the glycolytic system to yield energy. Rather xylitol phosphorylation is energetically costly to these cells and effectively depletes intracellular energy stores; some have argued that phosphorylated xylitol poisons glycolysis of fermentable substrates (Assev and Rölla, 1984; Trahan *et al.*, 1991). In any case, the non-cariogenicity of xylitol, perhaps based on the inhibition of mutans streptococcal metabolism, and its pleasant taste, foster interest in it from a confectionary standpoint; its costs and laxative effects necessarily limit the dimension and applications of that interest.

Sorbitol is known to be fermented by most mutans streptococci, one of its taxonomic hallmarks. Some have suggested that its consumption is therefore a hazard as a selective pressure for the enrichment of the plaque with mutans streptococci (Loesche, 1984; Birkhed *et al.*, 1987). In fact, evidence of slight

TABLE 1 *Cariogenicity and Gut Absorption of Caloric and Non-Caloric Sweeteners*

Mono-and Disaccharides		*Pentitols and Hexitols*		*Di-, Tri- and Oligo-saccharide Polyols and Bond Isomers*		*Non-caloric, Intense Sweeteners*	
Sweetener	*Caries*	*Sweetener*	*Caries*	*Sweetener*	*Caries*	*Sweetener*	*Caries*
Sucrose	very high	*Xylitol*	nil	*Leucrose*	slight to nil	Na saccharin	slight inhib.
Glucose	high	*Sorbitol*	nil	*Isomaltulose*	slight to nil	Acesulfam K®	-
Fructose	high	*Mannitol*	nil	*Isomaltose*	slight to nil	Aspartame®	nil
HFCS	high			*Nystose*	slight to nil	Sucralose®	nil
Lactose*	slight to mod.			*Isomaltitol*	slight to nil		
Maltose	prob. high			*Maltitol*	slight to nil		
Sorbose	slight			*Lactitol*	slight to nil		
				Hydrogenated starch hydrolysate	slight		
				Glucosyl sucrose	slight		

Italicized sweeteners have limited absorption from gut.
*Variable absorption from gut.

TABLE 2 *Di-, Tri- and Oligo-saccharides, Polyols and Bond Isomers of Interest*

Di-, Tri, and Oligo-saccharide/Polyol/ Bond Isomer	*Components*	*Other Name(s)*
Sucrose	G α (1→2) F	Sugar
Leucrose	G α (1→5) F	
Isomaltulose	G α (1→6) F	Palatinose®
Isomaltose	G α (1→6) G	
Maltitol	G α (1→4) Sorb	Malbitol; Malbit®
Maltose	G α (1→4) G	
Isomaltitol	G α (1→6) Sorb	Palatinit®; Isomalt®
	G α (1→) Man	
Nystose	G α (1→2) F α (1→2) F	"neosugar"

increases of sorbitol-fermenting organisms in the mouths of frequent sorbitol consumers have been reported (Birkhed *et al.*, 1987). However, heavily sorbitol-consuming normal rodents, lower primates, and humans evidence no increase in caries (Frostell *et al.*, 1967; Cornick and Bowen, 1972; Glass, 1983; Birkhed *et al.*, 1987). The metabolic bases of its noncariogenicity appear clear. The mechanisms for transporting sorbitol and dehydrogenating its phosphorylated transport product sorbitol-6-phosphate to the next catabolic intermediate are inducible in the presence of exogenous sorbitol and the simultaneous absence of exogenous sugars, and they are sensitively repressed by exposure to exogenous sugars (Fig. 4 and 5) (Brown and Wittenberger, 1973; Slee and Tanzer, 1983). Further, the catabolic endproducts of sorbitol fermentation include a substantial proportion of non-demineralizing ethanol, and formic acid (Brown and Patterson, 1973), in partial replacement of lactic acid. Therefore, because the host cannot consume sorbitol without the intermittent consumption of various hexoses and sucrose, sorbitol metabolism by at least the mutans streptococci cannot be maintained and thus be cariogenic, a conclusion supported directly by the above clinical and experimental animal data on failure of sorbitol consumption to be cariogenic.

There has been substantial recent interest in the sucrose analog mixture termed isomaltitol (Palatinit®, Isomalt®) (Table 2) because of physical and chemical properties which foster its inclusion in a fairly wide range of food products. Evidence is emerging of its relatively weak or minimal cariogenicity in rodents (Karle and Gehring, 1981) and poor fermentability (Imfeld, 1983). Although similar data could be presented for various other sugar substitutes listed in Table 1, space limitations do not allow review.

Non-caloric or intense sweeteners (Table 1) are, of course, widely used in foods. They constitute 36% of the 3.5 billion dollar food additive market in the U.S. (Bertorelli and Czarnowski-Hill, 1990). Numerous ones have been

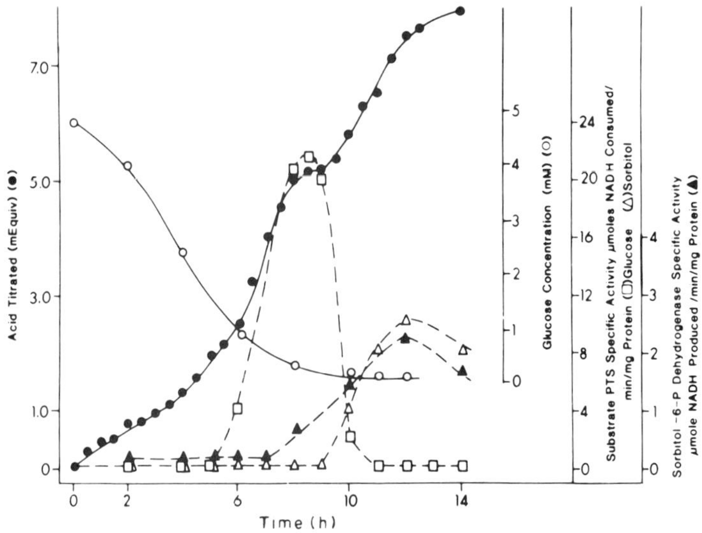

Figure 4. Biphasic ("diauxie") growth and patterns of sequential glucose and sorbitol transport and catabolic enzyme induction/repression when glucose-adapted *S. mutans* is grown in the simultaneous presence of glucose and sorbitol. Note that the sorbitol-specific PTS (the sorbitol transport system) and sorbitol-6-phosphate dehydrogenase (the first enzyme in the sorbitol catabolic pathway) are induced only after glucose has been completely utilized. Acid production is an index of growth for streptococci. (Reproduced by courtesy of A.M. Slee and J.M. Tanzer, *Arch Oral Biol* 28:839-845, 1983.)

developed and continue to be developed. Because of the intensity of their sweetness, they are ideally suited for inclusion in beverages (vehicles in which caloric and less intense sugar substitutes with poor absorption from the gut would provide grossly excessive osmotic challenge and resultant severe diarrhea). Some of these non-caloric sweeteners are used in diverse confections and other foods as a supplement or replacement of relatively unsweet caloric sweeteners. From a cariological viewpoint, there has been greatest interest in Na saccharin, its analog Acesulfam K®, the methylester of aspartylphenylalanine (Aspartame®) and trichlorogalactosucrose (Sucralose®). Only the first three are currently approved for use in the U.S.A. While there are some discrepancies in the literature, it is clear that Na saccharin and Acesulfam K inhibit growth and glycolytic metabolism of mutans streptococci (Slee and Tanzer, 1981; Brown and Best, 1986), not surprising in view of their sulfonamide-like structures, and Sucralose has been reported to inhibit growth and extracellular polysaccharide synthesis by mutans streptococci (Young and Bowen, 1990). Na saccharin but not Aspartame® is caries inhibitory at high concentrations in *ad libitum* fed rats

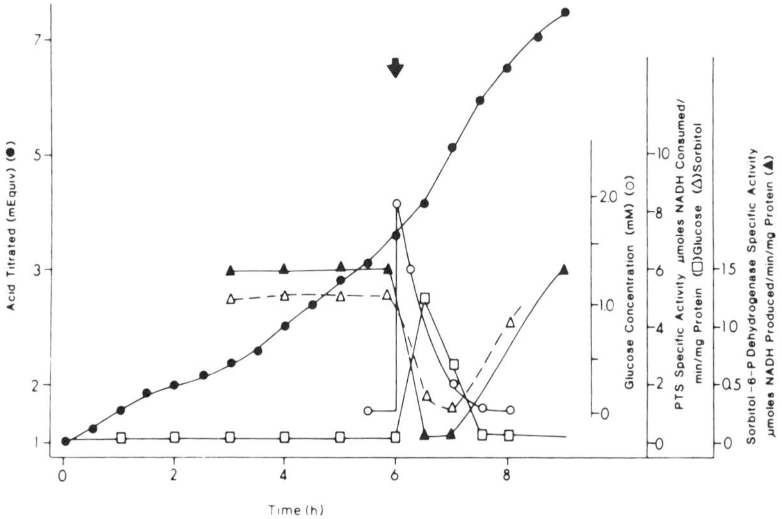

Figure 5. Repression of sorbitol-specific PTS and sorbitol-6-phosphate activity in sorbitol-adapted culture of *S. mutans* by addition of glucose (arrow) to culture medium. (Reproduced by courtesy of A.M. Slee and J.M. Tanzer, *Arch Oral Biol* 28:839-845, 1983.)

which develop high caries scores (Tanzer and Slee, 1983), but it is not detectably anticariogenic in program-fed rats which characteristically develop lower caries scores. Like Sucralose® and Aspartame®, in program-fed rats Na saccharin is noncariogenic (Lout *et al.*, 1988; Bowen *et al.*, 1990a; Bowen *et al.*, 1990b). Some have reported that inclusion of combinations of noncaloric sweeteners in the cariogenic diets of rats mitigates cariogenicity (Ziesenitz *et al.*, 1987). However, the concentrations of these intense sweeteners required to effect this result appear far beyond those found pleasant by humans. Nonetheless, whether repeated human use of low concentration noncaloric sweeteners, having subtle and weak effects on cariogenic plaque metabolism, may ecologically select against cariogens or in some other manner inhibit caries, has not been evaluated.

It is appropriate, lastly, to think about sweeteners in the context of human subjects, mostly adults, who for diverse reasons have compromised salivary secretion. The importance of this is hopefully suggested by Fig. 6. Saliva, like fluoride, as discussed elsewhere in the proceedings of this symposium, tends to pull apart, to dissociate, the three interactive spheres of caries—the tooth, the cariogenic flora and the key substrate for that cariogenic flora embodied by the diet of the host. While "normal" humans and experimental animals clearly develop caries in the presence of intact salivary function, the requirements for its development are stringent and focus most impressively on the colonization of the tooth surface by mutans streptococci, the presentation

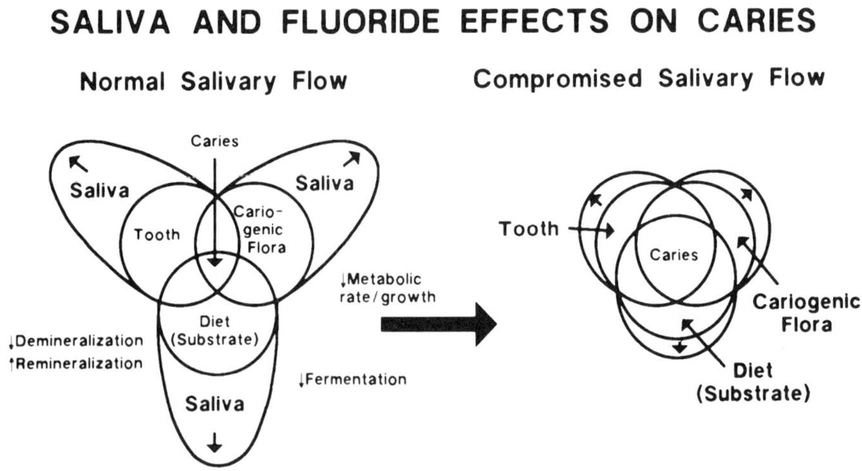

Figure 6. Modification by fluoride and saliva flow of the interaction of susceptible teeth, cariogenic microflora and cariogenic diet (bacterial substrate) required for the induction of caries. Normal salivary secretion, like fluoride, functions to dissociate the three interactive spheres; defective salivary secretion increases interaction of teeth, tooth flora, and diet and promotes caries activity, as suggested by the increased interaction of the spheres in the right figure. (Reproduced by courtesy of J.M. Tanzer, In: J. Bader (ed), *Risk Assessment in Dentistry*, Univ. No. Carolina, 1990. p 62-66.)

to that flora of fermentable carbohydrate, especially sucrose, and the relative lack of tooth surface exposure to fluoride. However, in the absence or deficit of normal salivary function, the saliva-induced dissociation of the interactive spheres of caries is clearly mitigated and the stringency of bacterial, dietary and fluoride requirements for caries induction may well be severely reduced (Tanzer, 1989; 1990; 1991). Indeed, there is a report, admittedly of problematic experimental design and statistical evaluation, which suggests that in salivary flow-deficit status, sorbitol may be cariogenic (Kalfas *et al.*, 1990).

REFERENCES

ASSEV, S. and RÖLLA, G. (1984): Further Studies on the Growth Inhibition of *Streptococcus mutans* OMZ176 by Xylitol, *Acta Path Microbiol Immunol Scand, Sec. B* 94:97-102.

BARMES, D.E. (1977): Epidemiology of Dental Caries, *J Clin Periodontol* 4:80-93.

BERTORELLI, A.M. and CZARNOWSKI-HILL, J.V. (1990): Review of Present and Future Nonnutritive Sweeteners, *Diab Educator* 16:415-422.

BIERMAN, E.L. (1979): Carbohydrates, Sucrose, and Human Disease, *Amer J Clin Nutr* 32 (12 Suppl): 2712-22.

BIRKHED, D.; SVENSÄTER, G.; and EDWARDSSON, S. (1990): Cariological Studies of 14 Individuals with Long-term Sorbitol Consumption, *Caries Res* 24:220-3.

BIRKHED, D.; SVENSÄTER, G; KALFAS, S.; and EDWARDSSON, S. (1987): The Risk of Adaptation of the Oral Microflora to Sorbitol, *Deutsche Zahn Z* 42:S141-S144.

BOWEN, W.H. and PEARSON, S.K. (1992): The Effects of Sucralose, Xylitol and Sorbitol on Remineralization of Caries Lesions in Rats, *J Dent Res* 71:1166-1168.

BOWEN, W.H.; PEARSON, S.K.; and FALANY, J.L. (1990): Influence of Sweetening Agents in Solution on Dental Caries in Desalivated Rats, *Arch Oral Biol* 35:839-844.

BOWEN, W.H.; YOUNG, D.A.; and PEARSON, S.K. (1990b): The Effects of Sucralose on Coronal and Root-surface Caries, *J Dent Res* 69:1485-1487.

BROWN, A.T. and BEST, G.M. (1986): Proposed Mechanism for the Effects of Saccharin on Glucose Metabolism by *Streptococcus mutans*, *Caries Res* 20:406-418.

BROWN, A.T. and PATTERSON, C.E. (1973): Ethanol Production and Alcohol Dehydrogenase Activity in *Streptococcus mutans*, *Arch Oral Biol* 18:127-131.

BROWN, A.T. and WITTENBERGER, C. (1973): Mannitol and Sorbitol Catabolism in *Streptococcus mutans*, *Arch Oral Biol* 18:117-126.

BURT, B.A. and ISMAIL, A.I. (1986): Diet, Nutrition, and Food Cariogenicity, *J Dent Res* 65 (Spec Iss): 1475-1484.

CORNICK, D. and BOWEN, W.H. (1972): The Effect of Sorbitol on the Microbiology of the Dental Plaque of Monkeys (*Macaca irus*), *Arch Oral Biol* 17:1637-1648.

DUCHIN, S. and van HOUTE, J. (1978): Relationship of *Streptococcus mutans* and Lactobacilli in Incipient Smooth Surface Dental Caries in Man, *Arch Oral Biol* 23:779-786.

ENWONWU, C.O. (1981): Review of Oral Disease in Africa and the Influence of Socioeconomic Factors. *Internat Dent J* 31:29-38.

FITZGERALD, R.J. (1968): Dental Caries Research in Gnotobiotic Rats, *Caries Res* 2:139-146.

FROSTELL, G.; KEYES, P.H.; and LARSON, R.H. (1967): Effect of Various Sugars and Sugar Substitutes on Dental Caries in Hamsters, *J Nutrit* 93:65-76.

GIBBONS, R.J.; DePAOLA, P.F.; SPINELL, D.M.; and SKOBE, Z. (1974): Interdental Localization of *Streptococcus mutans* as Related to Dental Caries Experience, *Infect Immun* 9:481-488.

GLASS, R.L. (ed.) (1982): The First International Conference on the Declining Prevalence of Dental Caries, *J Dent Res* 61 (Spec Iss): 1301-1383.

GLASS, R.L. (1983): A Two-Year Clinical Trial of Sorbitol Chewing Gum, *Caries Res* 17:365-368.

GORDON, M. and NEWBRUN, E. (1986): Comparison of Trends in the Prevalence of Caries and Restorations in Young Populations of Several Countries, *Comm Dent Oral Epidemiol* 14:104-109.

GRENBY, T.H. (1989): Research on Lactitol and Dental Health: A Review, Chap. 14. In: *Progress in Sweeteners*, Grenby, T.H., ed. Elsevier Applied Science, London. p 363-379.

HAMADA, S. and SLADE, H.D. (1980): Biology, Immunology, and Cariogenicity of *Streptococcus mutans*, *Microbiol Revs* 44:331-384.

IKEDA, I.; SANDHAM, H.J.; and BRADLEY, E.L., Jr. (1973): Changes in *Streptococcus mutans* and Lactobacilli in Plaque in Relation to the Initiation of Caries in Negro Children, *Arch Oral Biol* 18:555-566.

IKEDA, I.; SHIOTA, T.; McGHEE, J.R.; OTAKE, S.; MICHALEK, S.M.; OCHIAI, K.; HIRASAWA, M.; and SUGIMOTO, K. (1978): Comparison of the Effects of a Coupling Sugar and Sucrose on Certain Metabolic Activities and Caries, *Infect Immun* 19:477-480.

IMFELD, T.N. (1983): Identification of Low Caries Risk Dietary Components, *Monographs in Oral Science* Vol. II. Myers, H.M. (ed.) Karger, Basel.

KALFAS, S; SVENSÄTER, G; BIRKHED, D; and EDWARDSSON, S. (1990): Sorbitol Adaptation of Dental Plaque in People with Low and Normal Salivary-secretion Rates, *J Dent Res* 69:442-446.

KARLE, E.J. and GEHRING, F. (1981): Palatinit und Xylit im Gnotobiotischen Rattenversuch *Deutche Zahn Z.* 36:673-678.

KEENE, H.J. (1981): History of Dental Caries in Human Populations: The First Million Years, In: *Animal Models in Cariology*. Tanzer, J.M. ed. Information Retrieval, Ltd., Washington, D.C. pp 23-40.

LICHT, F.O. (1990): *Sugar and Sweetener Yearbook*. World Sugar Statistics. International Sugar Organization, London and Food and Agriculture Organization, Rome.

LOESCHE, W.J. (1984): The Effect of Sugar Alcohols on Plaque and Saliva Levels of *Streptococcus mutans*, *Swed Dent J* 8:125-135.

LOESCHE, W.J. (1986): Role of *Steptococcus mutans* in Human Dental Decay, *Microbiol Revs* 50:353-380.

LOUT, R.K.; MESSER, L.B.; SOBERAY, A; KAJANDER, K; and RUDNEY, J. (1988): Cariogenicity of Frequent Aspartame and Sorbitol Rinsing in Laboratory Rats, *Caries Res* 22:237-241.

MANDEL, I.D. (1970): Effects of Dietary Modifications on Caries in Humans, *J Dent Res* 49 (Suppl): 1201-1211.

MÄKINEN, K.K. (1989): Latest Dental Studies on Xylitol and Mechanism of Action of Xylitol in Caries Limitation. Chap. 13 In *Progress in Sweeteners*, Grenby, T.H., ed. Elsevier Applied Science, London. pp 331-362.

NATIONAL INSTITUTES OF HEALTH (1987): *Oral Health of United States Adults. The National Survey of Oral Health in U.S. Employed Adults and Seniors: 1985-1986. National Findings*. U.S. Govt. Printing Office, Washington. NIH Pub. No. 87-2868.

NATIONAL INSTITUTES OF HEALTH (1989): *Oral Health of United States Children. The National Survey of Dental Caries in U.S. School Children*, 1986-1987. National and Regional Findings. U.S. Govt. Printing Office, Washington. NIH Pub. No. 89-2247.

NEWBRUN, E. (1990): The Potential Role of Alternative Sweeteners in Caries Prevention, *Israel J Dent Sci* 2:200-213.

RUGG-GUNN, A.J. (1989): Lycasin and the Prevention of Dental Caries. (Chap. 12) In: *Progress in Sweeteners*, Grenby, T.H. ed. Elsevier Applied Science, London. p 311-329.

SASAKI, N.; TOPITSOGLU, V.; TAKAZOE, I.; and FROSTELL, G. (1985): Cariogenicity of Isomaltulose (Palatinose), Sucrose and a Mixture of these Sugars in Rats Infected with *Streptococcus mutans*, *Swedish Dent J* 9:149-155.

SCHEINEN, A. and MÄKINEN, K.K. (1975): Turku Sugar Studies I-XXI. *Acta Odontol Scand* 33 (Suppl 70):1-351.

SIEBERT, G. (ed) (1987): *Zuckersymposium IV Würzburg. 1986. Deutsche Zahnärztliche Z.* 42:S7-S172.

SLEE, A.M. and TANZER, J.M. (1981): The Effect of Sodium Saccharin on the Growth of Cariogenic and Other Selected Plaque-forming Streptococci. In: *Fifth Annual Conference on Foods, Nutrition and Dental Health*, Wayer, E. (ed.), Amer Dent Ass. Chicago pp 25-36.

SLEE, A.M. and TANZER, J.M. (1983): The Repressible Metabolism of Sorbitol (D-glucitol) by Intact Cells of the Oral Plaque-forming Bacterium *Streptococcus mutans*, *Arch Oral Biol* 28:839-845.

STEPHEN, K. (1993): Caries in Young Populations Worldwide. In: *Cariology for the Nineties*, Bowen, W.H. and Tabak, L.A. eds. Rochester: University of Rochester Press. pp. 37-50.

STILES, H.M.; LOESCHE, W.J.; and O'BRIEN, T.C. (eds.) (1976): *Microbial Aspects of Dental Caries*, Information Retrieval, Inc., Washington, pp 878.

TAKAZOE, I. (1989): Palatinose—An Isomeric Alternative to Sucrose. Chap. 6. In: *Progress in Sweeteners*, Grenby, T.H. ed. Elsevier Applied Science, London. pp 143-167.

TANZER, J.M. (1979): Essential Dependence of Smooth Surface Caries on, and Augmentation of Fissure Caries by, Sucrose and *Streptococcus mutans*, *Infect Immun* 25:526-531.

TANZER, J.M. (ed.) (1981): *Animal Models in Cariology*, Information Retrieval, Ltd., Washington, D.C. p 458.

TANZER, J.M. (1986): Testing Food Cariogenicity in Experimental Animals, *J Dent Res* 65 (Spec Iss): 1491-1497.

TANZER, J.M. (1989): On Changing the Cariogenic Chemistry of Coronal Plaque, *J Dent Res* 68 (Spec Iss): 1576-1587.

TANZER, J.M. (1990): Why Is Prediction of Risk for Caries by Microbiological Monitoring Problematic? In: *Risk Assessment in Dentistry*. Bader, J. (ed) Univ. North Carolina, Chapel Hill. pp 62-66.

TANZER, J.M. (1991): Microbiology of Dental Caries. Chap. 22 In: *Contemporary Oral Microbiology and Immunology*, Slots, J. (ed) Mosby-YearBook, St. Louis, pp.377-424.

TANZER, J.M.; FREEDMAN, M.L.; and FITZGERALD, R.J. (1984): Virulence of Mutants Defective in Glucosyl Transferase, Dextran-mediated Aggregation, or Dextranase Activity, In: *Molecular Basis of Oral Microbiol Adhesion*, Mergenhagen, S. and Rosan, B. eds. Amer Soc Microbiol pp 204-211.

TANZER, J.M. and SLEE, A.M. (1983): Saccharin Inhibits Tooth Decay in Experimental Models, *JADA* 106:331-333.

TRAHAN, L.; NERON, S.; and BAREIL, M. (1991): Intracellular Xylitol-phosphate Hydrolysis and Efflux of Xylitol in *Streptococcus sobrinus*, *Oral Microbiol Immunol* 6:41-50.

U.S. DEPT. AGRICULTURE, Economic Research Service, Sweeteners Analysis Section (1991): Sweeteners (Excluding Noncalorics), 1909-1966: Per Capita Consumption.

U.S. DEPT. AGRICULTURE, Economic Research Service, Sweeteners Analysis Section (1991): Caloric and Low Calorie Sweetener, 1967-1990: Per Capita Consumption.

YOUNG, D.A. and BOWEN, W.H. (1990): The Influence of Sucralose on Bacterial Metabolism *J Dent Res* 69:1480-1484.

ZIESENITZ, S.C. and SIEBERT, G. (1987): The Metabolism and Utilization of Polyols and Other Bulk Sweeteners Compared with Sugar. Chap 5. In: *Developments in Sweeteners*, Vol 3. Grenby, T.H. (ed). Elsevier Applied Science, London pp. 109-149.

ZIESENITZ, S.C.; SIEBERT, G.; and IMFELD, T. (1989): Cariological Assessment of Leucrose [D-Glucopyranosyl-(15)-D-Fructopyranose] as a Sugar Substitute, *Caries Res* 23:351-357.

ZIESENITZ, S.C.; SIEBERT, G; and LOTTER, J. (1987): Marked Caries Inhibition in the Sucrose-challenged Rat by a Mixture of Nonnutritive Sweeteners, *Caries Res* 21:141-148.

Genetic Manipulation of the Oral Streptococci

ROBERT G. QUIVEY, JR.; R.C. FAUSTOFERRI; AND P. S. KRIGER

The use of recombinant DNA technology to understand the mechanisms of streptococcal virulence at the molecular level has been vigorously pursued over the last decade. In addition to the use of those techniques to understand the virulence mechanisms of the streptococci, it might be possible to utilize our knowledge to begin thinking about the genetic alteration of the streptococci to directly counter or prevent the initiation of dental disease. In this paper, we will be concerned with the genetic manipulation of the oral streptococci in order to generate highly defined strains for use as replacement bacteria, that is, organisms that will be artificially introduced into the oral cavity for the purpose of preventing or reducing the impact of oral disease. The strategies discussed herein may be useful for the treatment of dental caries but may not be limited to prevention and treatment of disease in the oral cavity.

Historically, interest in replacement therapy can be recalled from the turn of the century, when Eli Metchnikoff extoled the benefits of replacing the intestinal flora with *Lactobacillus bulgaricus*, in order to lengthen lifespan. Though his hypotheses were later disproved, the results from other experiments in the 1960s showed dramatic differences in infant morbidity using a non-virulent strain of *Staphylococcus aureus* to combat hospital nursery infections (Shinefield *et al.*, 1963; Boris *et al.*, 1964; Shinefield *et al.*, 1966; Boris *et al.*, 1968).

More recently, experiments have been undertaken with purpose of eliminating urinary tract and vaginal infections by competitive displacement or bacterial replacement therapy. *In vitro* studies have shown that bacteria indigenous to the urogenital tract were capable of blocking the attachment of pathogenic bacteria to human uroepithelial cells (Bruce *et al.*, 1983; Chan *et al.*, 1984; Chan *et al.*,

The research from our laboratory that has been described herein was supported by NIH/NIDR DE0-RO1-7777, DE0-7003 as part of the Rochester Caries Research Center, and Biomedical Research Support Grant S7RR05403-30.

TABLE *Three strategies for using genetically engineered streptococci to prevent dental caries*

1. Reduction of caries by reducing plaque acids
2. Reduction of caries by increasing plaque pH values
3. Delivery of novel therapeutic agents *in situ*

1985; Reid *et al.*, 1985; Reid *et al.*, 1987). Their studies demonstrated the ability of *Lactobacillus casei* to block the infection of bladder and kidney tissues by uropathogenic bacteria (*E. coli, Pseudomonas aeruginosa,* and *Klebsiella pneumoniae*) in rats. Thus the results of those studies underscored the concept that bacteria can competitively exclude the invasion of host sites by pathogens. Subsequent experiments have shown that bacteria, contained in vaginal washes from healthy monkeys, could be extremely effective in combating *E. coli* infections in infected monkeys; thus, providing additional evidence that naturally occurring bacteria can exclude pathogens (Herthelius *et al.*, 1989).

With this background, it is not surprising that replacement therapy strategies for combatting oral disease were being explored. Earlier work in this endeavor, by numerous investigators, showed that strains of bacteria indigenous to the human mouth could be successfully re-introduced into the oral cavity (Krasse *et al.*, 1967; Edman *et al.*, 1975; Svanberg and Loesche, 1978; and Westegren and Svanberg, 1983; Hillman *et al.*, 1985). Their studies provided information necessary for the studies that were to come involving the genetic manipulation of those indigenous strains for the purpose of replacement therapy.

The observations by Stephan of the fall and subsequent recovery of plaque pH values in the presence of sucrose (Stephan, 1944) provide one conceptual framework for strategies that might be available to us for using genetically engineered bacteria in the prevention of dental caries. Three such potential strategies are shown in the Table.

The downward slope of the Stephan curve is a result of the production of acid by plaque bacteria, specifically the oral streptococci and lactobacilli. The net result of the pH drop is the dissolution of enamel and the initiation of dental caries. Quite naturally then, the prevention of this fall in plaque pH value has been the focus of considerable attention over the last two decades. One approach to the use of micro-organisms to resist the acidification of plaque has been the exploration of mutant strains of bacteria to displace or pre-empt the colonization of teeth by native strains of cariogenic bacteria. The data of Tanzer and coworkers have suggested that non-cariogenic strains of streptococci might be capable of colonizing rats and reducing caries by preventing infection with cariogenic strains (Tanzer *et al.*, 1982; Tanzer *et al.*, 1985a).

A related approach to the use of mutant strains of *S. mutans* for the displacement of indigenous strains has been the pursuit of lactate dehydrogenase (LDH) strains. The concept has been that bacteria which do not produce lactic acid due to LDH-deficiency should be less cariogenic than wild-type strains. Thus, efforts have been made toward the isolation of stable, well-defined LDH-mutant strains that are competitive with wild-type strains of bacteria. It has been shown that implantation in rats of a spontaneously-derived LDH-defective mutant strain of *S. mutans* led to a considerable increase in the minimal infectious dose for subsequent colonization by some wild-type, cariogenic organisms (Johnson and Hillman, 1982).

In later experiments, it was shown that the implantation of such strains resulted in reduced caries scores in rats (Johnson *et al.*, 1980; Fitzgerald, *et al.*, 1989).

Thus the data on LDH-deficient strains of bacteria have indicated the potential for the use of replacement strains to control dental disease; as well as verifying the concept that lactic acid is responsible for the dissolution of enamel.

More recently, attention has turned to the use of cloned genetic material encoding LDH with which to precisely construct site-directed mutant strains for further studies. Indeed, the gene for LDH has been cloned from *S. mutans* (Hillman *et al.*, 1990) and its nucleotide sequence determined (Duncan and Hillman, 1991). A report has been presented describing the insertionally inactivation of the cloned LDH gene and its subsequent return to the *S. mutans* chromosome to create an LDH strain that is isogenic to its parental strain (Duncan and Hillman, 1991). The use of the prototroph and and the site-directed LDH strain, isogenic except at the LDH locus, should permit a clear comparison of the ability of the genetically engineered strain to compete with indigenous flora and its impact on caries.

Two other strategies for using bacteria to prevent caries are the use of streptococci to raise plaque pH values and the possibility of using the streptococci to deliver novel therapeutic agents. Both strategies, as they have evolved in our laboratories in Rochester, have involved the use of recombinant DNA technology to construct strains of the streptococci with new properties.

Before discussing those ongoing studies, however, a few questions relevant to these projects can be asked? First, why would it be desirable to manipulate the streptococcal chromosome? Secondly, can we successfully manipulate the chromosome? Finally and importantly: how effective *in vivo* and *in situ* are these recombinant strains going to be?

The answer to the first question can be found in the chapters of this volume concerning the epidemiology of caries, the summary of which is that caries is not yet eliminated. What we seek now are new instruments to be added to the armamentarium for the prevention of dental caries.

Can we manipulate the streptococcal chromosome for the prevention of dental disease? That question is being answered experimentally. With the advent of transformation protocols (Lawson and Gooder, 970; Perry and Kuramitsu, 1981; Dunny *et al.*, 1991) and shuttle vectors for cloning DNA from the streptococci into *E. coli* and moving it back into the streptococci (Macrina *et al.*, 1983; Dao and Ferretti, 1985; Murchison, *et al.*, 1986; Dunny *et al.*, 1991), the technology has progressed to the point where it is now possible to contemplate the cloning and genetic inactivation of any streptococcal gene. More importantly for this discussion, these advances have allowed us to consider adding heterologous DNA to these bacteria in order to endow them with properties not previously exhibited. Gene inactivation, via the insertion of antibiotic resistance elements, has resulted in the elucidation of the glucosyltransferase gene arrangement (see, for example, Kuramitsu, 1987). These and similar experiments with other proposed virulence factors have shown that DNA can be stably integrated into the streptococcal chromosome. Further, it has been shown that expression and secretion of the *Bacillus licheniformis* amylase can be achieved from within *S. mutans* (Lane *et al.*, 1991). In this case, the amylase gene was integrated into the chromosome as part of a transcriptional gene fusion to elements of the *S. mutans* chromosome that appear to be catabolite repressible. The stability of the gene fusions in the absence of antibiotic has not been reported; nevertheless, the data provide an important milestone in that a foreign gene product has been correctly processed and secreted in an active form from the streptococci. Other gene fusions have also been reported (Hudson and Curtiss, 1990; Sato *et al.*, 1991). The results of these experiments suggest that the introduction of foreign DNA into the streptococci with the aim of using it to produce and secrete an active enzyme is feasible. Questions remain regarding the stability of the constructions in the absence of antibiotic selective pressure. It is likely that it will become desirable to construct strains that are genetically stable in the absence of antibiotic selection and data will be shown below that indicates that progress in that area is being made.

The last of the general questions was: How effective *in vivo* and *in situ* are these recombinant strains going to be? The animal data (Johnson *et al.*, 1980; Fitzgerald, *et al.*, 1989) indicate that the answer to this question may be yes, but of necessity each strain will have to be examined carefully. For a technology that clearly is in its infancy, we believe that it is important to remember that these experiments are conducted in an environment where new knowledge concerning adherence, growth, virulence, and host-interaction is constantly accumulating and will of course contribute to the development of implantable strains.

Can we identify genes that might be useful in the prevention of dental disease? The second strategy that was eluded to above was that of using bacteria to raise plaque pH values. In this vein, Drs. Burne and Marquis have pursued the cloning and transfer of arginine deiminase from *S. sanguis* into *S. mutans*, for the purpose of exporting ammonia into the surrounding milieu of potential cariogenic plaque (Burne *et al.*, 1989). Their results are described in the chapter by Dr. Marquis.

A third possibility of using the oral streptococci to prevent dental caries might be to deliver therapeutic agents to the site where they might do the most good, namely dental plaque. One such potentially therapeutic could be an enzyme that degrades the insoluble glucan in dental plaque. This polysaccharide, a predominantly α(1- > 3)-linked glucan referred to as mutan, contributes to the ability of bacteria to adhere to the tooth surface, add to the bulk of plaque, protect the bacteria against inimical influences, may prevent diffusion of salivary materials to the tooth surface and contributes to the pathogenic potential of plaque.

Data that link dental plaque, caries, and the insoluble glucan has been obtained from experiments with bacterial mutants and by topical application of an α-(1- > 3) glucan 3-glucanohydrolase. Mutants of *S. mutans* defective in the ability to produce mutan appear to be non-cariogenic in experimental animals (Clark *et al.*, 1978; Tanzer and Freedman, 1978; Tanzer *et al.*, 1985b) , despite the observation that the *S. mutans* was still capable of persistent colonization. In seminal experiments, Guggenheim *et al.* have explored the use of a topically applied external enzyme, α-(1- > 3) glucan 3-glucanohydrolase (referred to as a mutanase) to reduce bulk plaque and dental caries in rats (Guggenheim and Haller, 1972). The enzyme, isolated from the fungus *Trichoderma harzianum* OMZ 779, could not degrade dextran, and the organism did not produce dextranase. These workers found that application of a crude preparation of mutanase led to a two-fold decrease in the number of carious lesions in rats. It also reduced the extent of dentinal fissure lesions. These data led to a study in human subjects whereby crude mutanase preparations were applied to the tooth surfaces by incorporation into chewing gum (Kelstrup *et al.*, 1978). Their double-blind study showed that less plaque had accumulated and less gingivitis developed in the experimental subjects than was found in the placebo group. Further, the bacteriologic findings indicated that the oral flora was unchanged. Importantly, as had been found in the rat study, primary skin irritations, delayed hypersensitivity, and anti-enzyme IgE were not detected in any of the subjects.

More recently, preparations of mutanase from other sources have substantiated the earlier observations in that a mutanase from the fungus *Cladosporium resinae* was highly effective in solubilizing α(1- > 3) linked mutan (Walker and Hare, 1977). Further, Inoue *et al.* observed that the mutanase prepared from a unclassified Pseudomonad species, was capable of removing insoluble glucans from glass surfaces that had been deposited by cell-free preparations of glucosyltransferase from *S. sobrinus* (Inoue *et al.*, 1988). Although these and other studies appear to suggest that mutanase may have a role in the prevention of caries, it suffers from a major drawback in that it requires frequent application to exert its therapeutic effect.

Thus, our experimental plan is to clone the gene that carries the information for the mutanase gene into *S. sanguis*. The recombinant *S. sanguis* strain will then be examined for its effect on plaque development caries in rats co-infected with *S. mutans*. To accomplish the construction of the *S. sanguis* strain, the mutanase gene will be cloned into a vector that can not replicate in the streptococci, e.g. example, the plasmid pVA891 (Macrina *et al.*, 1983). It is likely that the vector will also contain a segment of DNA that encodes a secretion signal that will permit the secretion of the mutanase or another agent, out of the cell and into the plaque milieu.

The construct will be inserted into the *S. sanguis* chromosome via homologous recombination as shown here in cartoon form where homologous DNAs (via the secretion signal) are aligned and strand exchange is catalyzed by the endogenous RecA protein, resulting in the incorporation of the plasmid into the chromosome.

In order to facilitate cloning of the gene encoding the mutanase, physical characterization of the enzymes first described by Guggenheim has been necessary. We have published preliminary results of the characterization of one of the enzymes (Quivey and Kriger, 1991). The mutanase that we have characterized has a molecular weight of approximately 80,000 and is glycosylated, though in an as yet undetermined arrangement. However, we have determined that the enzyme contains N-acetyl glucosamine and interestingly is approximately 22% serine. Polyclonal rabbit antibody directed to the protein has been developed, and it is a critical reagent for two reasons: it can be used to screen gene libraries that may be expressing the mutanase in *E. coli* as an intermediate host and secondly for demonstrating that the genetically engineered streptococci are in fact expressing and secreting the mutanase enzyme.

In addition to identifying the monomer molecular weight of the mutanase, we have determined the amino acid composition of the enzyme. The composition of the peptides provides more information that is useful to the molecular biologist. The actual composition can be used as a check against amino acid sequence that has been deduced from nucleotide sequence form the cloned mutanase gene. Further, we have found that approximately 11-12 methionines exist in the 80000 enzyme. What this means in experimental terms is that the molecule can be cleaved with cyanogen bromide at the methionines and those fragments can be fractionated by high pressure liquid chromatography (HPLC) to provide material for the direct determination of primary amino acid sequence. The actual sequence then may provide a basis for the synthesis of oligonucleotide probes which are in turn useful for screening libraries and possibly for the amplification of the gene via the polymerase chain reaction (Saiki *et al.*, 1985).

In order to facilitate the study of genetically-engineered streptococcal strains, we believe that inactivation of the *recA* gene is necessary. The *recA* gene encodes the RecA protein which is responsible for homologous DNA recombination in bacteria, including the streptococci. Elimination of *recA* gene activity will contribute significantly to the development of engineered strains that can be maintained in the absence of antibiotic pressure.

To inactivate the *recA* gene then, we have used first a technique known as the polymerase chain reaction to amplify the number of copies of that gene, *in vitro*, such that we could visualize with the naked eye a portion of the DNA encoding the RecA protein. We subsequently cloned the PCR fragment and determined its nucleotide sequence (Quivey and Faustoferri, 1992). The plasmid that resulted

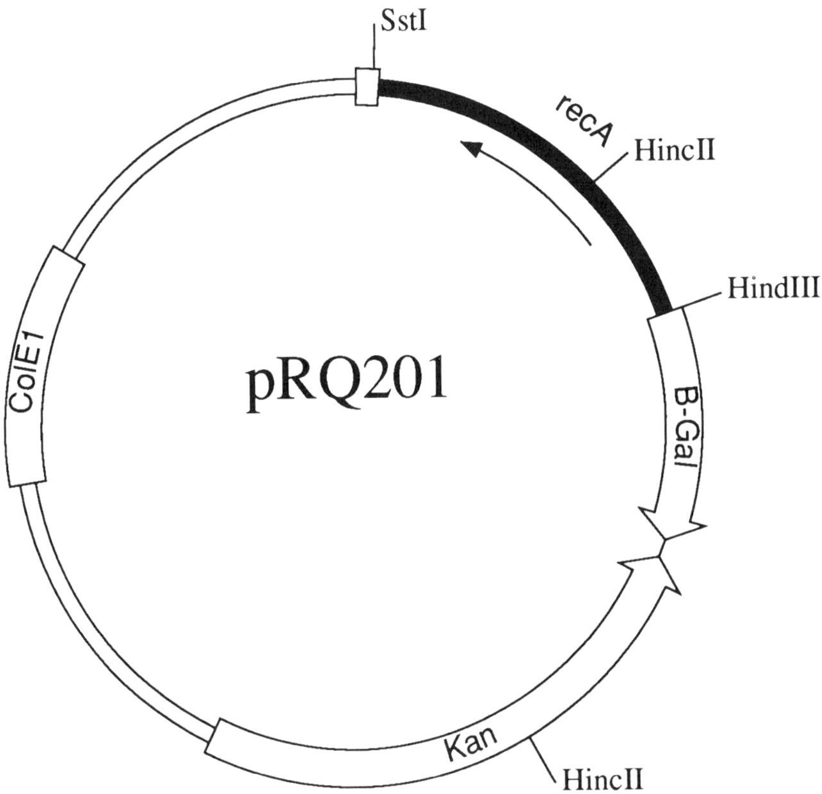

Figure 1. Map of pRQ201 containing the polymerase chain reaction amplified *recA* gene fragment from *S. mutans* (shown as the black bar). The host vector was pCR1000 (commercially available from InVitrogen, La Jolla, CA).

from those cloning experiments, pRQ201, is shown in Figure 1. Plasmid pRQ201 was found to contain a unique Hinc II restriction endonuclease site that has allowed us to insertionally inactivate the gene using an erythromycin resistance gene as shown schematically in Figure 2. The inactivated gene has been returned to the chromosome via homologous recombination, and the strains arising from erythromycin selection have been shown to be deficient in *recA* protein activity (Quivey and Faustoferri, 1991). These strains and the plasmid pRQ202, containing the inactivated *recA* gene, should now permit the construction of stable, genetically engineered strains of the streptococci. The techniques that have been discussed above may be used with any genetically-encoded element. Clearly the approaches described herein may be adapted for the development of strains containing other potentially therapeutic agents.

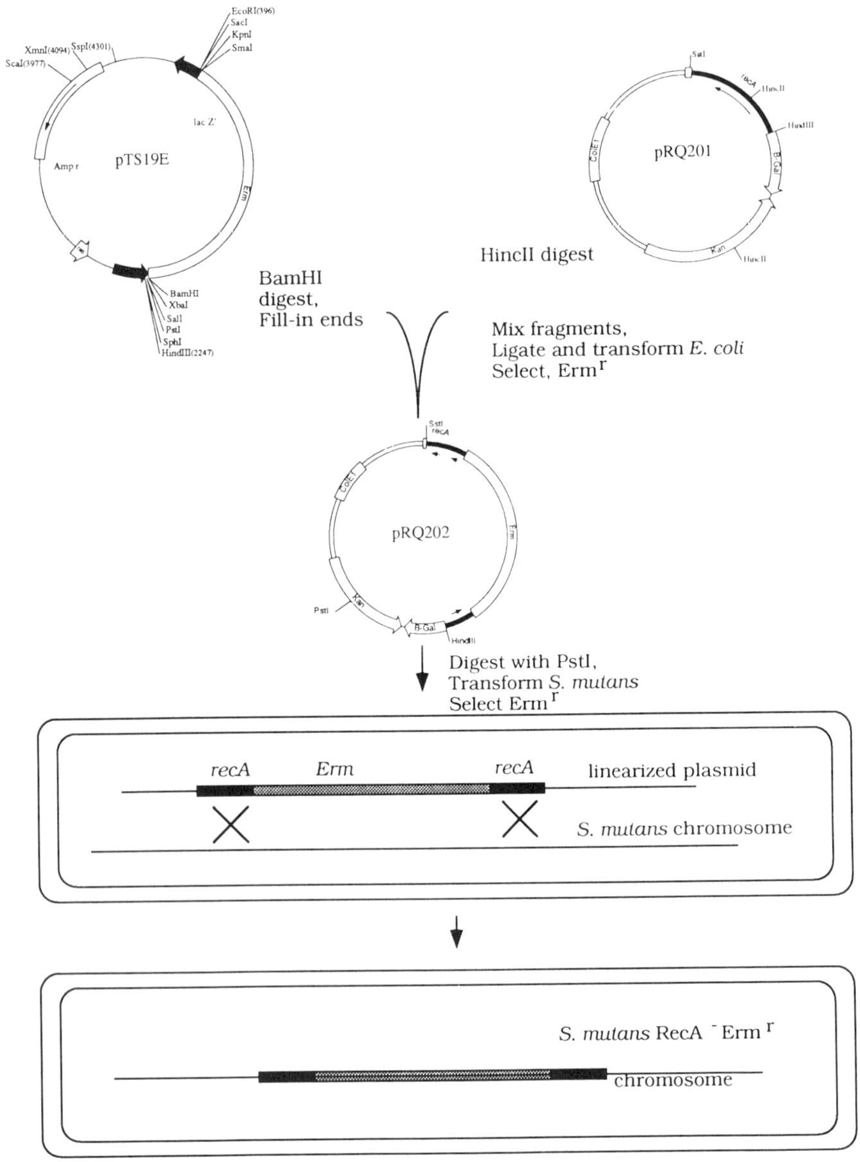

Figure 2. Schematic construction of RecA protein-deficient strains of streptococci. The *recA* gene fragment contained in plasmid pRQ201 was insertionally inactivated by digestion with HincII ligation to an erythromycin-resistance encoding element derived from plasmid pTS19E (Aoki *et al.*, 1986). The resulting plasmid, pRQ202, was digested with enzyme PstI to form linear DNA which was in turn used to transform *S. mutans*. Strains containing the Ermr marker were selected on medium containing erythromycin and were subsequently characterized for RecA-deficiency using standard techniques. Details of the construction and characterization of the strains have been described elsewhere (Quivey and Faustoferri, 1992). Figure used with the permission of Elsevier Science Publishers.

REFERENCES

AOKI, H.; SHIROZA, T.; HAYAKAWA, M.; SATO, S.; and KURAMITSU, H.K. (1986): Cloning of a *Streptococcus mutans* Glucosyltransferase Gene Coding for Insoluble Glucan Synthesis, *Infect Immun* 53:587-594.

BORIS, M.; SELLERS, T.; EICHENWALD, H.; RIBBLE, J.; and H. SHINEFELD. (1964): Bacterial Interference, *Am J Dis Child* 108:252-261.

BORIS, M.; SHINEFIELD, H.; ROMANO, P.; MCCARTHY, D.; and FLORMAN, A. (1968): Bacterial interference. Protection Against Recurrent Intrafamilial Staphylococcal Disease, *Am J Dis Child* 115:521-529.

BRUCE, A.W.; CHAN, R.C.Y.; PINKERTON, D.; MORALES, A.; and CHADWICK, P. (1983): The adherence of gram-negative uropathogens to human uroepithelial cells, *J Urol* 130:293-298.

BURNE, R.A.; PARSONS, D. T.; and MARQUIS, R.E. (1989): Cloning and Expression in *Escherichia coli* of the Genes of the Arginine Deiminase System of *Streptococcus sanguis* NCTC 10904, *Infect Immun* 57:3540-3548.

CHAN, R.C.Y.; BRUCE, A.W.; and REID, G. (1984): Adherence of cervical, vaginal and distal urethral normal microbial flora to human uroepithelial cells and the inhibition of adherence of gram-negative uropathogens by competitive exclusion, *J Urol* 131:596-601.

CHAN, R.C.Y.; REID, G.; IRVIN, R.T.; BRUCE, A.; and COSTERTON, J. W. (1985): Competitive exclusion of uropathogens from human uroepithelial cells by *Lactobacillus* whole cells and cell wall fragments, *Infect Immun* 47:84-89.

CLARK, W.B.; BAUMANN, L.L.; and GIBBONS, R.J. (1978): Ability of *Streptococcus mutans* and a glucosyltransferase defective mutant to colonize rodents and attach to hydroxyapatite surfaces, *Infect Immun* 21:681-684.

DAO, M.L. and FERRETTI, J. (1985): *Streptococcus-Escherichia coli* Shuttle Vector pSA3 and Its Use in the Cloning of Streptococcal Genes, *Appl Environ Microbiol* 49:115-119.

DUNCAN, M. J. and HILLMAN, J. D. (1991): DNA Sequence and Inactivation of the Gene Encoding the Fructose-1,6-Diphosphate-Dependent L-(+) Lactate Dehydrogenase of *Streptococcus mutans, Infect Immun* manuscript submitted.

DUNNY, G. M.; LEE, L.N.; and LEBLANC, D.J. (1991): Improved Electroporation and Cloning Vecotr System for Gram-Positive Bacteria, *Appl and Environ Microbiol* 57: 1194-1201.

EDMAN, D.C.; KEENE, H.J.; SHKLAIR, I.L.; and HOERMAN, K.C. (1975): Dental floss for implantation and sampling of *Streptococcus mutans* from approximal surfaces of human teeth, *Arch Oral Biol* 20:145-148.

FITZGERALD, R. J.; ADAMS, B. O.; SANDHAM, H. J.; and ABHYANKAR, S. (1989): Cariogenicity of a Lactate Dehydrogenase-Deficient Mutant of *Streptococcus mutans* Serotype c in Gnotobiotic Rats, *Infect Immun* 57:823-826.

GUGGENHEIM, B. and HALLER, R. (1972): Purification and Properties of an alpha-(1-3) Glucanohydrolase from *Trichoderma harzianum*, *J Dent Res* 51:394-402

HERTHELIUS, M.; GORBACH, S. L.; MÖLLBY, R.; NORD, C. E.; PETTERSSON, L.; and WINBERG, J. (1989): Elimination of Vaginal Colonization with *Escherichia coli* by Administration of Indigenous Flora, *Infect Immun* 57:2447-2451.

HILLMAN, J.D.; YAPHE, B.I.; and JOHNSON, K.P. (1985): Colonization of the human oral cavity by a strain of *Streptococcus mutans*, *J Dent Res* 64:1272-1274.

HILLMAN, J. D.; DUNCAN, M. J.; and STASHENKO, K. P. (1990): Cloning and Expression of the Gene Encoding the Fructose-1,6 Diphosphate-Dependent L-(+)-Lactate Dehydrogenase of *Streptococcus mutans*, *Infect Immun* 58:1290-1295.

HUDSON, M.C. and CURTISS, R. III. 1990. Regulation of Expression of *Streptococcus mutans* Genes Important to Virulence, *Infect Immun* 58:464-470.

INOUE, M.; YAKUSHIJI, T.; KATSUKI, M.; KUDO, N.; and KOGA, T. (1988): Reduction of the adherence of *Streptococcus sobrinus* insoluble α-D-glucan by endo-(1- > 3)-α-D-glucanase, *Carbohydr Res* 182:277-286.

JOHNSON, K. P. and HILLMAN, J. D. (1982): Competitive Properties of Lactate Dehydrogenase Mutants of the Oral Bacterium *Streptococcus mutans* in the Rat, *Arch Oral Biol* 27:513-516.

JOHNSON, C. P.; GROSS, S. M.; and HILLMAN, J. D.(1980): Cariogenic Potential *in vitro* In Man and *in vivo* In the Rat of Lactate Dehydrogenase Mutants of *Streptococcus mutans*, *Arch Oral Biol* 25:707-713.

KELSTRUP, J.; HOLM-PEDERSEN, P.; and POULSEN, S. (1978): Reduction of the formation of dental plaque and gingivitis in humans by crude mutanase, *Scand J Dent Res* 86:93-102.

KRASSE, B.; EDWARDSSON, S.; SVENSSON, I.; and TRELL, L. (1967): Implantation of caries-inducing streptococci in the human oral cavity, *Arch Oral Biol* 12:231-236.

KRIGER, P. S. and QUIVEY, R. G. (1990): Purification of Mutanase, *J Dent Res* 69(*Spec Iss*):325, *Abst* 1736.

KURAMITSU, H.K. (1987): Utilization of a mini-mu transposon to construct defined mutants in *Streptococcus mutans*, *Molec Microbiol* 1:229-231.

LANE, M.A.; BAYLES, K. W.; and YASBIN, R. E. (1991): Identification and initial characterization of glucose-repressible promoters of *Streptococcus mutans*, *Gene* 100:225-229.

LAWSON, J.W. and GOODER, H. (1970): Growth and Developement of Competence in the Group H Streptococci, *J Bacteriol* 102:820-825.

MACRINA, F.L.; EVANS, R. P.; TOBIAN, J.A.; HARTLEY, D.L.; CLEWELL, D.B.; and JONES, K.R. (1983): Novel shuttle plasmid vehicles for *Escherichia-Streptococcus* transgeneric cloning, *Gene* 25:145-150.

MURCHISON, H.H.; BARRETT, J.F.; .CARDINEAU, G.A.; and CURTISS, R. III. (1986): Transformation of *Streptococcus mutans* with Chromosomal and Shuttle Plasmid (pVA629) DNAs, *Infect Immun* 54:273-282.

PERRY, D. and KURAMITSU, H. (1981): Genetic Transformation of *Streptococcus mutans*, *Infect Immun* 32:1295-1297.

QUIVEY, R. G., Jr., and FAUSTOFERRI, R.C. (1992): *In vivo* inactivation of the *Streptococcus mutans recA* gene mediated by PCR amplification and cloning of a *recA* gene DNA fragment, *GENE* 116:35-42.

QUIVEY, R.G. JR. and FAUSTOFERRI, R. C.: Polymerase chain reaction amplification, cloning in *E. coli*, nucleotide sequence determination, and chromosomal inactivation of the *recA* gene from *S. mutans*, manuscript submitted.

REID, G.; CHAN, R.C.Y.; BRUCE, A.; and COSTERTON, J.W. (1985): Prevention of urinary tract infection in rats with an indigenous *Lactobacillus casei* strain, *Infect Immun* 99:320-324.

REID, G.; COOK, R.; and BRUCE, A. (1987): Examination of strains of Lactobacilli for properties that may influence bacterial interference in the urinary tract, *J Urol* 138: 330-335.

SAIKI, R.K.; SCHARF, S.; FALOONA, F.; MULLIS, K.B.; HORN, G.T.; ERLICH, H.A.; and ARNHEIM, N. (1985): Enzymatic amplification of b-globin genomic sequence and restriction site analysis for diagnosis of sickle cell anemia, *Science* 230:1350-1354.

SATO, Y., YAMAMOTO, Y., SUZUKI, R., KIZAKI, H. and KURAMITSU, H. K. (1991): Construction of *scrAlacZ* gene fusions to investigate regulation of the sucrose PTS of *Streptococcus mutans*, *FEMS Microbiol Letts* 79:339-346.

SHINEFIELD, H.R.; RIBBLE, J. C.; BORIS, M.; and EICHENWALD, H. F. (1963): Bacerial interference: its effect on nursery-acquired infection with *S. aureus*. I. Preliminary observations on artificial colonization of newborns, *Am J Dis Child* 105: 646-654.

SHINEFIELD, H.; WILSEN, J.; RIBBLE, J.; BORIS, M.; EICHENWALD, J.; and DITTMAR, C. (1966): Interactions of Staphylococcal Colonization, *Am J Dis Child* 111: 11-21.

SISSONS, C. H.; CUTRESS, T.W. and PEARCE, E. I. F. (1985): Kinetics and Product Stoichiometry of Ureolysis by Human Salivary Bacteria and Artificial Mouth Plaques, *Arch Oral Biol* 11/12:781-790.

STEPHAN, R. M. (1944): Intra-oral Hydrogen-ion concentration associated with dental caries activity, *J Dent Res* 23:257-264.

SVANBERG, M.L. and W.J. LOESCHE. (1978): Implantation of *Streptococcus mutans* on tooth surfaces of man, *Arch Oral Biol* 23: 551-556.

TANZER, J.M. and FREEDMAN, M.L. (1978): Genetic alterations of *Streptococcus mutans* virulence, *Adv Expt Med Biol* 107:661-672.

TANZER, J.M.; FISHER, J; and FREEDMAN, M. L. (1982): Preemption of *Streptococcus mutans* 10449S Colonization by Its Mutant 805, *Infect Immun* 35:138-142.

TANZER, J.M.; KURASZ, A.; and CLIVE, J. (1985a): Competitve Displacement of mutans streptococci and inhibition of tooth decay by *Streptococcus salivarius* TOVE-R, *Infect Immun* 48:44-50.

TANZER, J.M.; FREEDMAN, M.L.; and FITZGERALD, R.J. (1985b): Virulence of Mutants Defective in Glucosyltransferase, Dextran-Mediated Aggregation, or Dextranase Activity. In: *Molecular Basis of Oral Microbial Adhesion*, Eds., S.E. Mergenhagen and B. Rosan, ASM Press Washington, D.C. pp. 204-211.

VAN HOUTE, J.; BURGESS, R. C.; and ONOSE, H. (1976): Oral Implantation of Human Strains of *Streptococcus mutans* in Rats Fed Sucrose or Glucose Diets, *Arch Oral Biol* 21:561-564.

WALKER, G.J. and M.D. HARE. (1977): Metabolism of the polysaccharides of human dental plaque. Part II. Purification and properties of *Cladosporium resinae* (1- > 3)-α-D-glucanase, and the enzymic hydrolysis of glucans synthesized by extracellular D-glucosyltransferases of oral streptococci, *Carbohydr Res* 58:415-432.

WESTERGREN, G. and SVANBERG, M. (1983): Implantation of transformant strains of the bacterium *Streptococcus sanguis* into adult human mouths, *Arch Oral Biol* 28:729-733.

Enhancing Effects of Fluoride

J. EKSTRAND

If Little Fluoride is Good, is More Necessarily Better?

Although there has been tremendous achievement in caries research during the two last decades, fluoride is still the dominating single factor in combating dental caries. This in spite of the fact that most fluoride programs mainly are based on a questionable theory of the cariostatic mechanism of fluoride. The expression "if little fluoride is good, more is better" was for a long time an axiom among the dental profession. It was believed that maximum fluoride should be incorporated into the enamel to accomplish a cariostatic effect.

Recently, a large number of reports from the U.S. show an increasing prevalence of dental fluorosis (Leverett, 1986; Kumar *et al.*, 1989; Szpunar and Burt 1988; Pendrys and Katz 1989; Williams and Zwemer 1990). Some studies also show a close association to fluoride intake from certain dental fluoride products (Osuji *et al.*, 1988; Holm and Anderson, 1982). A too liberal prescription and usage of various fluoride preparations have thus lead to an unnecessary high fluoride exposure to many children.

It was already demonstrated in Dean's classical work in the 1940s that the "therapeutic window" for fluoride in caries prevention was very narrow. This fact has largely been disregarded and the dose/effect relationship has not been seriously discussed and monitored until recently. Hence, the classical and the fundamental pharmacological principle of a dose/effect relationship seems to have been largely ignored or forgotten when it comes to fluoride therapy.

Promotion of fluoride programs requires sound recommendations for effective and safe use of fluoridated water, fluoride supplements and other sources of fluoride in the diet of all age groups. Most of the recommendations have, so far, been empirically-based because we lack data necessary to develop scientifically based recommendations. Scientifically-based recommendations can be modified

Part of this work was supported by grants from the Swedish Medical Research Council, project no.6002 and The Swedish Patent Revenue Research Fund.

as conditions change; empirically-based recommendations generally remain in force until there is evidence that the recommended practice is either ineffective or unsafe.

Advances in fluoride research in recent years have open potentials to improve the efficacy and safety of fluoride as a cariostatic agent. Based on modern pharmacological principles and techniques the next generation of fluoride products and treatment-programs will result in a higher degree of efficacy. In addition, this seems to be accomplish with low fluoride doses.

The purpose of this presentation is to discuss ways of enhancing the effect of fluoride based on our improved knowledge of cariostatic mechanisms of fluoride and new information on the intraoral kinetics of fluoride.

The Empirical Approach to Fluoride Treatment: Is It Still an Acceptable Concept?

A relevant example of the empirical use of fluoride is the dose recommendation for fluoride supplements to infants. The current fluoride dosage schedule is solely based on the concept that children in non-fluoridated areas should ingest the same amount of fluoride as children living in an 1 PPM fluoridated area.

That the cariostatic effect of waterfluoridation mainly is a topical one has for a long time been underestimated. The effect of fluoride derived via waterfluoridation seems to be mainly related to the fluoride concentration of the oral fluids in the oral cavity and less to the fluoride dose ingested. There is no information about the amount of ingested fluoride required by the forming enamel to accomplish cariostatic protection.

The complexity of systemic fluoride administration is illustrated by results from a recent pharmacokinetic study in infants. Infants who ingest small quantities of fluoride from daily intake of fluoridated water show a different pharmacokinetic pattern of fluoride compared to when the same daily dose (0.25 mg F) is given as a single NaF dose (Ekstrand, *et al.* 1992). The fluoride retention in infants, age from 1 to 13 months, was 87 % of the ingested dose. In addition, the degree of accumulation of fluoride in the body (calcified tissues) was related to the ingested dose indicating a dose dependent mechanism for F uptake in calcified and calcifying tissues during the first year of life. Renal clearance of fluoride was also studied in all the 20 infants. Fractional renal clearance was 58 % and was related to body weight and did not change with age (Figure 1). This study demonstrates that the pharmacokinetic pattern and fluoride retention in infants reveals a complete different pattern compared to what has been found in adults. Therefore, the consequence of these findings and the relation to a proper fluoride intake needs further study. It seems however appropriate, based on these findings and the increased prevalence in dental fluorosis, to

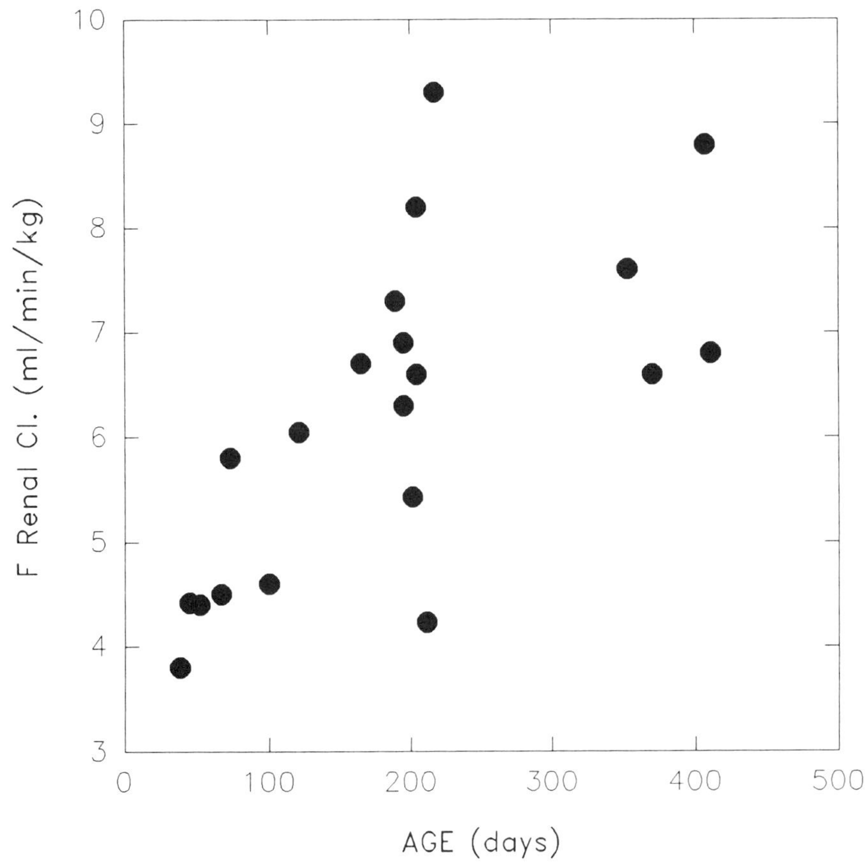

Figure 1. Fluoride renal clearance in 20 infants age 38 to 411 days of age. 0.25 mg fluoride was given as a solution 3 hours after the last meal. (Data from Ekstrand *et al.* 1992)

change the recommendation of fluoride supplementation to a more conservative dosage schedule. From a toxicological viewpoint (dose/kg bodyweight) a starting period at 3 years seems to be more pertinent. The use of a sucking tablet instead of conventional tablet certainly would be beneficial to the child in terms of the topical effect. It is apparent that more research is needed regarding the fluoride dose required to the forming enamel to accomplish cariostatic protection.

As regard topical application of fluoride, the empirical approach is somewhat more close to a dose/response concept. There seems to be both clinical as well as laboratory data to recognize that the frequency of fluoride exposure is an important factor in terms of efficacy.

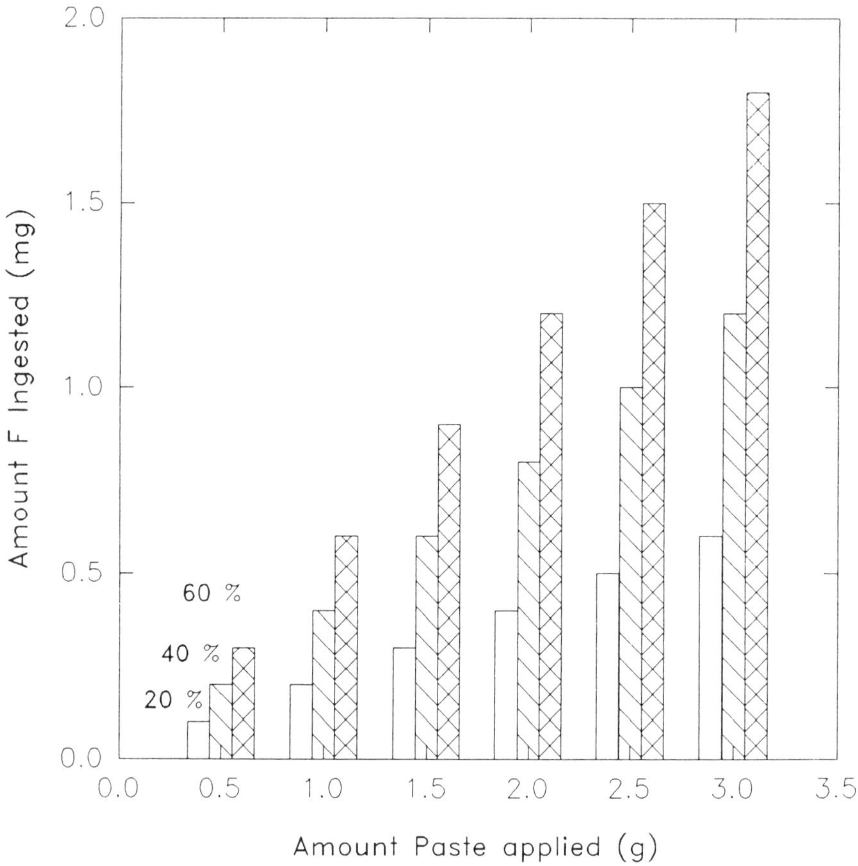

Figure 2. Amount fluoride ingested (mg) as a function of amount toothpaste applied (gram) on a toothbrush and 20, 40 or 60 % retention of applied dose. A 100 % bioavailability of the swallowed fluoride from the toothpaste is assumed.

There seems to be a general agreement among many dental researchers that the addition of fluoride to toothpaste has had a great impact of the overall decline of dental caries seen in the western world. It should be remembered that the current recommended concentration (1,000 ppm F) of fluoridated toothpaste was introduced based on toxicological considerations and not on any information of a dose/effect relationship.

The general public does not consider toothpaste as an important fluoride source. Fluoride exposure from this source is however substantial, it could be as much as 2-3 mg fluoride/day (Figure 2). It is therefore reason to believe that the reported increase in dental fluorosis among children could partly be explained by an uncontrolled intake of excessive amounts of toothpaste. The question of the appropriate fluoride concentration in toothpaste needs therefore to be looked at in great detail. It has been suggested to introduce a toothpaste for children with a lower fluoride concentration. If it would be accepted in a family to have a variety of toothpastes with different fluoride concentrations is doubtful. A better approach to this problem would be to develop a fluoridated toothpaste with low fluoride bioavailability from the gastrointestinal tract.

Cariostatic Mechanisms of Fluoride: The Theories of the Past and for the Nineties

A vast amount of research has been produced on the mechanisms of fluoride action. One of the first hypotheses to account for the cariostatic effect of fluoride was to incorporate fluoride into the enamel mineral during its formation to make the tissue more resistant to acid attack. While this holds true in an *in vitro* situation, recent research have raised doubt about its preeminence in the *in vivo* situation. Several studies indicate that a high level of fluoride in enamel does not result in any protection against caries. The most direct recent evidence is the findings that teeth consisting of shark enamel, i.e. carbonated fluorapatite, develop caries lesions during cariogenic conditions *in vivo* (Ögaard, 1990). Epidemiological studies also indicate that fluoride inhibits caries progression but has a minor effect on caries incidence (Groeneveld 1985).

A large number of both clinical and laboratory studies show that the dominating cariostatic effect of fluoride is a topical effect (for review see Fejerskov *et al.*, 1981).

The predominant factor responsible for the cariostatic effect of fluoride is the presence of fluoride in the solution at the cariogenic challenge (Larsen and Bruun 1986; ten Cate and Duijsters 1983). These findings suggest a dynamic equilibrium between fluoride in the solution and adsorbed fluoride at the crystal surface interface. The actual concentration of fluoride, calcium and phosphate and pH in the liquid in contact with the crystallite will thus determine the rate of dissolution (for review see Arends and Christoffersen 1990). This underlines the importance of fluoride in the immediate fluid environment of the teeth. Several recent studies, both in animals and in man, show that frequent exposure of the teeth to low concentration of fluoride in the oral cavity is extremely important. Not only children but also adults benefit from waterfluoridation, both as regard coronal as well as root caries. This fluoride "delivery system" leads to an exposure of relative small fluoride dose several times daily to the oral cavity, which undoubtedly results in a cariostatic effect. In rat caries experiments it has been shown (Larson and Mellberg, 1977; Whitford and Schuster, 1982) that an slight elevation of the fluoride concentration via saliva (fluoride was only given systemically and not topical) had a significant cariostatic effect. Mirth *et al.*, (1983) using a intraoral slow-release device (0.15 mg F/day) found 63 % caries reduction. Copron *et al.*, (1986) using the same type of device (0.4 mg F/day) demonstrated that acid resistance and microhardness of enamel appliances *in situ* were significantly higher when compared to controls. These and other similar *in vivo* studies confirm that an elevated fluoride level in the immediate environment of caries prone sites, "the biophase", has a cariostatic effect.

The Concentration of Fluoride at the Biophase

The concentration of fluoride in the fluid nearby the dental tissue to inhibit demineralization is difficult to define. A large number of *in vitro* studies, although they are all different in design, are all consistent in showing a decrease in the rate of demineralization with increasing fluoride concentration. (Larsen, 1973; ten Cate and Duijsters 1983). These studies indicate that a fluoride concentration of less then 1 PPM in the fluid at the cariogenic attack will slow down demineralization. ten Cate and Duijsters (1983) could demonstrate a close relationship between the fluoride concentration and calcium loss in a demineralization system *in vitro*. At a fluoride concentration of 2.4 μM (0.05 PPM) an effect of the degree of calcium loss was demonstrated. This fluoride concentration is close to the "normal" fluoride concentration in whole saliva in subjects living in a fluoridated area (Oliveby *et al.*, 1990). It should also be mentioned that demineralization of dentin is affected by fluoride in solution (Feagin and Graves, 1988).

When fluoride is applied in high concentrations it has been shown that calcium fluoride-like material is formed. (Gerould, 1945; Rölla and Ögaard, 1986; Saxegaard and Rölla, 1988; Rölla and Saxegaard, 1990; Lagerlöf *et al.* 1988). This is deposited on the enamel surfaces and in the plaque which can release fluoride during caries challenges. The calcium fluoride-like material thus acts like a biological slow-release system. Ways to improve the capacity to form calcium fluoride seem to be to lower the pH of the fluoride product. To obtain an optimum effect of the calcium-fluoride system would be to give a "booster dose" of fluoride at certain intervals resulting in high concentrations of fluoride in the oral fluids. In order to maintain the calcium fluoride "loaded" enough, frequent exposure of low concentrations seems then to be sufficient (Matsuo *et al.*, 1990).

Fluoride Kinetics at the Site of Action

The therapeutic efficacy of a pharmacological active agent is limited by its inability to gain access to the site of action at an appropriate dose and/or by its access to non-desired site of action, producing unwanted side effects (Daemen *et al.*, 1991) A cariostatic active agent like fluoride must gain access to its primary site of action and its distribution should ideally be confined to the target to produce a cariostatic effect.

At the enamel surface, fluoride is accumulated in the dental plaque and a large part is presumably in the form of calcium-like materials. This bound fluoride fraction in plaque is probably in dynamic equilibrium with the free phase of the plaque, the plaque fluid. During an acid attack a large portion of the bound fluoride seems to be released to the plaque fluid (Ophaug *et al.*, 1987) which then can interact with the demineralization process. The frequency of exposure, the fluoride dose, and the salivary flow rate will be the major factors determining the kinetics of fluoride at the site of action.

As noted above studies indicate the importance of fluoride in the fluid environment of the teeth, but very few measurements have been made of the fluoride concentration at the site of the cariogenic challenge, i.e., the extracellullar phase of the plaque (plaque fluid). In order to enhance the effect of fluoride agents such information is essential. Due to difficulty of collection and measurements such information has until recently been unknown. In a series of experiments the kinetics of fluoride in plaque fluid after fluoride exposure has been studied in detail (Vogel *et al.*, 1990; Ekstrand *et al.*, 1990).

The studies were conducted with the technique developed by Vogel (Vogel *et al.*, 1990) using the inverted-fluoride-electrode under-oil method. Following a rinse with a 0.2 % NaF solution the fluoride concentration in plaque fluid was monitored for 60 minutes at six different tooth-sites (Vogel *et al.* 1992). The results showed that the fluoride concentration was always higher than that of saliva (Figure 3). The intraoral distribution of fluoride showed that the fluoride concentration was highest in the upper incisor region which also had the slowest clearance. There was overall a large intersite and intersubject variation which could be ascribed to (1) the formation of fluorapatite or calciumfluoride on the surface of the teeth or in the plaque (Rölla and Saxegaard 1990), (2) the binding of fluoride by plaque microorganisms (Tatevossian 1978), (3) the incomplete mixing of saliva in the oral cavity (Collins and Dawes, 1987), (4) and the anatomical characteristics of the individual mouth (Weatherell *et al.*, 1988; 1986).

In a subsequent study the fluoride concentration in plaque fluid after a NaF rinse (0.2 %) was followed for 3 hours. A pharmacokinetic analysis of the plaque fluid eliminations curves revealed a bi-exponetial pattern with a T ½ of the final slope of 68 ± 21 minutes (mean ± SD, n = 7). We also found that following a rinse with a 0.2% NaF solution or a rinse with a 1,000 PPM F toothpaste slurry (NaF or MFP), the fluoride concentration in the plaque fluid was elevated (baseline = 0.4 PPM) for almost 180 minutes (Ekstrand and Vogel 1990).

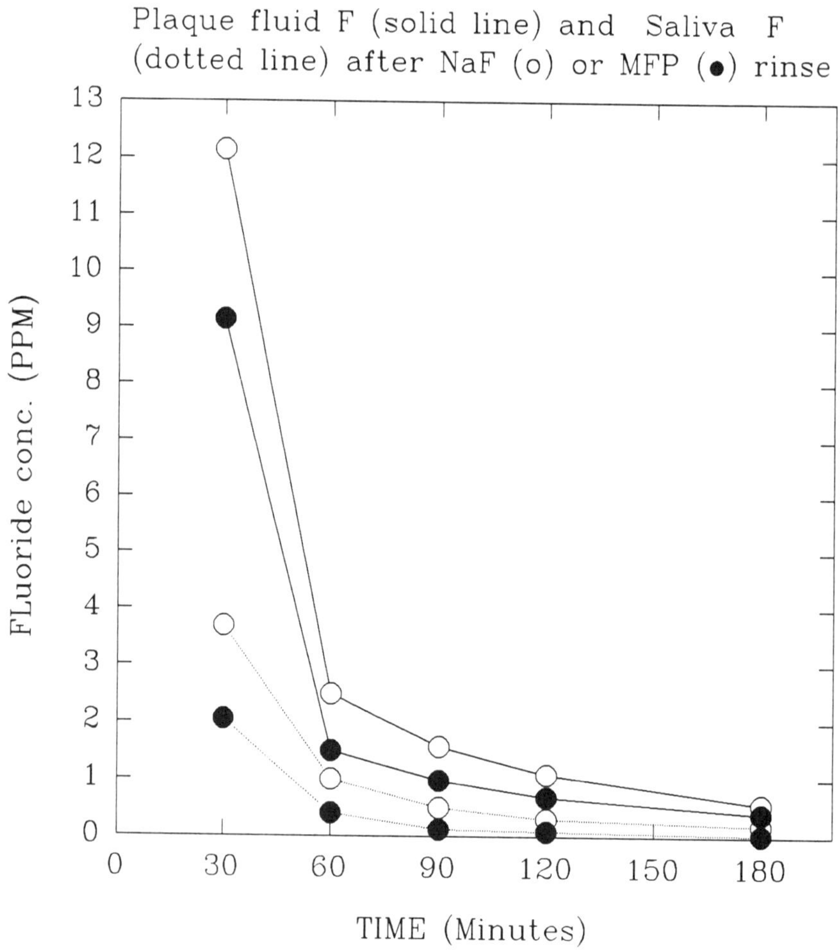

Figure 3. Fluoride concentration in plaque fluid (mean of 4 sampling sites, upper and lower left and right molars) and whole saliva after a 1 min. rinse with a 1,000 PPM F solution as NaF or MFP in one subject. (Data from Ekstrand and Vogel, 1990)

Further studies of this type should prove valuable in devising treatment modalities that deliver an appropriate fluoride concentration for a prolonged time to achieve maximum effect at the lowest fluoride dose.

Enhancing the Effect of Fluoride in Caries Treatment: Slow-Release Systems

Based on the above discussion it is evident that a prolonged elevation of the fluoride levels in the oral fluids has important cariostatic potentials. During re-

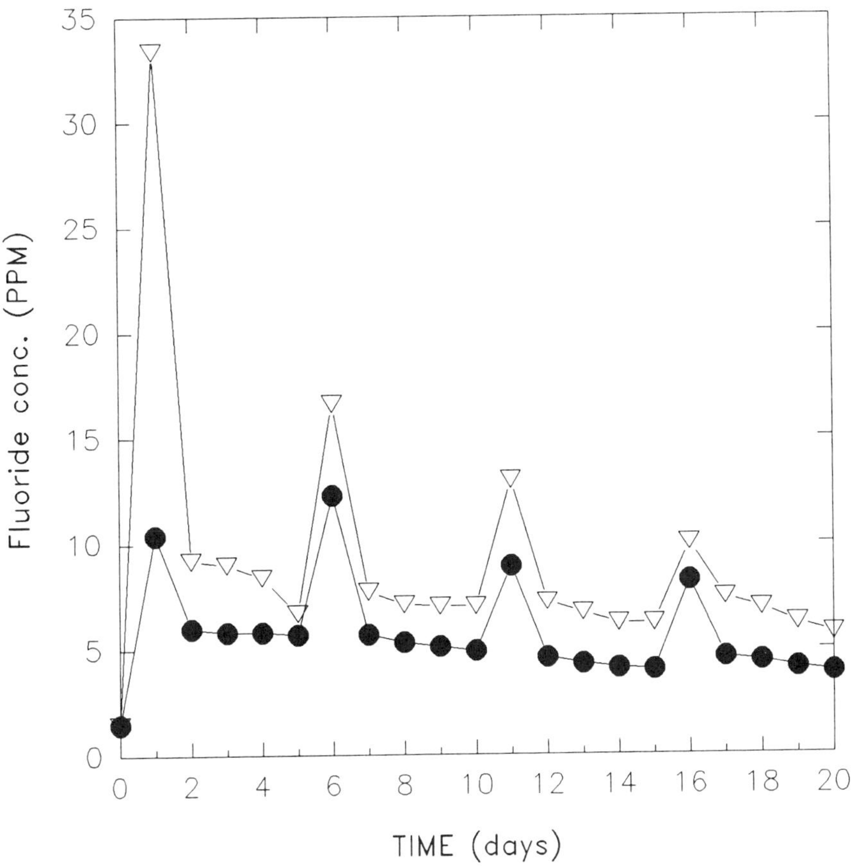

Figure 4. Fluoride release *in vitro* from a glass ionomer cement (Kerr) after repeated (on day 0, 5, 10 and 15) exposure for 10 minutes of a 0.2 (▽) or 0.02 % (●) NaF solution. (data from Hatibovic-Kofman, Koch and Ekstrand, to be published)

cent years this has also been tested by a number of investigators. In a series of experiments in rats, Mirth *et al.* (1982; 1983) tested an intraoral slow-release device on the caries incidence in a caries model. They found between 50 to 60 % caries reduction. Pharmacokinetic studies have also been done on other slow-release systems like slow-release lozenges (Ekstrand *et al.*, 1990) and bioadhesive tablets (Bottenberg, 1991).

Numerous fluoride containing dental materials have also been tested. Skartveit *et al.* (1985) tested fluoridated amalgams and reported saliva half-lives of 7 days. These authors have also reported that fluoridated amalgams have a significant effect in inhibiting secondary caries (Skartveit *et al.*, 1990).

Glass ionomer cement releases fluoride and seems to be a promising dental material in preventing secondary caries. The disadvantage of these materials is the great variation in fluoride content and the fluoride release is not constant. In an attempt to use the glass ionomer as a slow-release system we have tested the fluoride release of 5 different glass ionomer cements (Hatibovic-Kofman, Koch and Ekstrand 1992, to be published). An interesting finding was that the glass ionomers after the initial fluoride release could be re-activaited when the material was exposed to a fluoride solution at repeated intervals. The material takes up fluoride to a certain extent which is then slowly released. This is shown in Figure 4. A way to enhance the efficacy of fluoride release from this material would thus be to have the patient rinse frequently with a fluoride solution which would maintain the slow-release properties of the material.

Based on clinical experience fluoride cannot stop caries progression completely. As noted above even shark enamel which contains more than 30000 PPM fluoride will be demineralized under a thick plaque in a human oral environment (Ögaard, 1990). When the pH drop in the plaque is very low, the plaque fluid becomes undersaturated with respect to fluorapatite and dissolves and any additional fluoride will have no effect. (Rölla and Saxegaard, 1990). These authors have therefore suggested to add antibacterial substances like Sn^{2+}, Zn^{2+}, CU^{2+} or combination of these to reduce the acid production. Enhancing the cariostatic effect of, e.g. toothpastes, would therefore be to combine the effect of fluoride on demineralization with the anti-acidogenic effect of antibacterial substances.

REFERENCES

ARENDS, J. and CHRISTOFFERSEN, J. (1990): Nature and Role of Loosely Bound Fluoride in Dental caries, *J Dent Res* 69(Spec Iss): 601-605.

BOTTENBERG, P. (1991): A study of formulations for oral fluoride application. Thesis., Vrije Universität Brussel; Belgium.

COLLINS, L.M.C. and DAWES, C. (1987): The Surface Area of the Adult Human Mouth and Thickness of the Salivary Film Covering the Teeth and Oral Mucosa, *J Dent Res* 66:1300-1302.

CORPRON, R.E.; CLARK, J.W.; TSAI, A.; MORE, F.G.; MERRILL, D.F.; KOWALSKI, C.J.; TICE, T.R.; and ROWE, C.E. (1986): Intraoral Effects of a Fluoride-releasing Device on Acid-softened Enamel, *JADA* 113:383-388.

DAEMEN, M.J.A.P.; THIJSSEN, H.H.W.; and STRUYKER-BOUDIER, H.A.J. (1991): Pharmacokinetic considerations in local drug delivery, *Adv Drug Deliv Rev* 6:1-18.

EKSTRAND, J. and VOGEL, G. (1990): Kinetics of fluoride in plaque fluid and saliva after MFP and NaF rinses, *Caries Res* 24:419 (Abstract 92).

EKSTRAND, J.; ZIEGLER, E.; and FOMON, S. (1992): Pharmacokinetics of fluoride in Infants, *J Dent Res* 71 (special Issue): 522 (abstract 53).

EKSTRAND, J.; SPAK, C-J.; and VOGEL, G. (1990): Pharmacokinetics of fluoride in man and its clinical relevance, *J Dent Res* 66:550-555.

FEIGAN, F.F. and GRAVES, C.N. (1988): Evaluation of F in Acidified Gelatin Gel on Root surface Development *in vitro*, *Caries Res* 22:145-149

FEJERSKOV, O.; THYLSTRUP, A.; and LARSEN, M.J. (1981): Rational Use of Fluorides in Caries Prevention. A Concept Based on the Possible Cariostatic Mechanisms, *Acta Odontol Scand* 39:241-249.

GEROULD, C.H. (1945): Electron Microscope Study of the Mechanism of Fluorine Deposition in Teeth, *J Dent Res* 24:223-233.

GROENEVELD, A. (1985): Longitudinal Study of Prevalence of Enamel Lesions in a Fluoridated and Non-fluoridated Area, *Community Dent Oral Epidemiol* 13: 159-163.

HOLM, A.-K. and ANDERSSON, R. (1982): Enamel Mineralization Disturbances in 12 Year-Old Children with Known Early Exposure to Fluorides, *Community Dent Oral Epidemiol* 10:335-339.

KUMAR, J.V.; GREEN, E.L.; WALLACE, W.; and CARNAHAN T. (1989): Trends in dental fluorosis and dental caries prevalences in Newburgh and Kingston, NY, *Am J Public Health* 79:565-569.

LAGERLÖF, F.; EKSTRAND, J.; and RÖLLA, G. (1988): Effect of Fluoride Addition on Ionized Calcium in Salivary Sediment and Saliva, *Scand J Dent Res* 96:399-404.

LARSEN, J.J. (1973): Dissolution of Enamel, *Scand J Dent Res* 81:518-522.

LARSEN, M.J. and BRUUN, C. (1986): Enamel/Saliva-Inorganic Chemical Reactions. In: *Textbook of Cariology*, A. Thylstrup and O. Fejerskov, Eds., Copenhagen: Munksgaard, pp. 181-203.

LARSON, R.H. and MELLBERG, J.R. (1977): Experiments on Local and Systemic Action of Fluoride in Caries Inhibition in the Rat, *Arch Oral Biol* 22:437-439.

LEVERETT, D. (1986): Prevalence of dental fluorosis in fluoridated and nonfluoridated communities — a preliminary investigation, *J Public Health Dent* 46:184-187.

MARGOLIS, H.C.; MORENO, E.C.; and MURPHY, B.J. (1986) Effect of Low Levels of fluoride in Solution on Enamel Demineralization *in vitro*, *J Dent Res* 65:23-29.

MATSUO, S.; RÖLLA, G.; and LAGERLÖF, F. (1990): Effect of fluoride addition on ionized calcium in salivary sediment and in saliva containing various amounts of solid calcium fluoride, *Scand J Dent Res* 98:482-485.

MIRTH, D.B.; ADDERLEY, D.D.; AMSBAUGH, S.M.; MONELL-TORRENS, E.; LI, S.H.; and BOWEN, W.H. (1983): Inhibition of Experimental Dental Caries Using an Intraoral Fluoride-releasing Device, *JADA* 107:55-59.

MIRTH, D.B.; SHERN, R.J.; EMILSON, C.G.; ADDERLY, D.D.; LI, S-H.;GOMEZ, I.M.; and BOWEN, W.H. (1982): Clinical Evaluation of an Intraoral Device for the Controlled Release of Fluoride, *JADA* 105:791-797.

ÖGAARD, B.(1990): Effects of Fluoride on Caries Development and Progression *in vivo*, *J Dent Res* 69 (Spec Iss) :813-819.

OLIVEBY, A.; TVETMAN, S.; and EKSTRAND, J. (1990): Diurnal fluoride concentration in whole saliva in children living in a high and a low fluoride area, *Caries Res* 24:44-47.

OPHAUG, R.H.; JENKINS, S.H.; SINGER, L.; and KREBSBACH, L. (1987): Acid Diffusion Analysis of Different Forms of Fluoride in Human Dental Plaque, *Arch Oral Biol* 32:459-461.

OSUJI, O.; LEAKE, J.L.; CHIPMAN, M.L.; NIKIFORUK, G.; LOCKER, D.; and LEVINE, N.(1988): Risk factors for dental fluorosis in a fluoridated community, *J Dent Res* 67:1488-1492.

PENDRYS, D.G. and KATZ, R.V. (1989): Risk of enamel fluorosis associated with fluoride supplementation, infant formula, and fluoride dentifrice use, *Am J Epid* 130:1199-1208.

RÖLLA, G. and ÖGAARD, B. (1986): Studies on the Solubility of CaF_2 in Human Saliva. In: *Factors Relating to Demineralisation and Remineralisation of the Teeth*, S.A. Leach, Ed., Oxford: IRL Press, pp. 45-50.

RÖLLA, G. and SAXEGAARD, E. (1990): Critical Evaluation of the Composition and Use of Topical Fluorides, with Emphasis on the Role of Calcium Fluoride in Caries Inhibition, *J Dent Res* 69(Spec Iss): 780-785.

SAXEGAARD, E. and RØLLA, G. (1988): Fluoride Acquisition on and in Human Enamel during Topical Application in vitro, *Scand J Dent Res* 96:523-535.

SKARTVEIT, L.; TVEIT, A.B.; and EKSTRAND, J. (1985): Fluoride Release from a Fluoride-containing Amalgam in vivo, *Scand J Dent Res* 93:448-452.

SKARTVEIT, L.; WEFEL, J.S.; and EKSTRAND, J. (1991): Inhibition of artificial recurrent caries by F^- containing amalgam, *Scand J Dent Res* 99:287-294.

SZPUNAR, S.M. and BURT, B.A. (1988): Dental caries, fluorosis, and fluoride exposure in Michigan schoolchildren, *J Dent Res* 67:802-806.

TATEVOSSIAN, A. (1987): Distribution and Kinetics of Fluoride Ions in the Free Aqueous and Residual Phases of Human Dental Plaque, *Arch Oral Biol* 23:893-898.

TEN CATE, J.M. and DUIJSTERS, P.P.E. (1983): Influence of Fluoride in Solutions on Tooth Demineralization. I. Chemical Data, *Caries Res* 17:193-199.

VOGEL, G.L.; CAREY, C.M.; CHOW, L.C.; and EKSTRAND, J. (1990): Fluoride Analysis in Nanoliter- and Microliter-size Fluid Samples, *J Dent Res* 69(Spec Iss):522-528.

VOGEL, G.L.; CAREY, C.M.; and EKSTRAND, J. (1992):Fluoride in saliva and plaque fluid after a 0.2 % NaF rinse: Short term kinetics and distribution, *J Dent Res*. In Press.

WEATHERELL, J.A.; STRONG, M.; RALPH, J.P.; and ROBINSON, C. (1988): Availability of Fluoride at Different Sites in the Buccal Sulcus, *Caries Res* 22:129-133.

WEATHERELL, J.A.; STRONG, M.; ROBINSON, C.; and RALPH, J.P. (1986): Fluoride Distribution in the Mouth after Fluoride Rinsing, *Caries Res* 20:111-119.

WHITFORD, G.M. and SCHUSTER, G.S. (1982): Systemic versus Waterborne Fluoride and Dental Caries, IADR Prog & Abst 61:No. 324.

WILLIAMS, J.E. and ZWEMER, J.D. (1990): Community water fluoride levels, preschool dietary patterns, and the occurrence of fluoride enamel opacities. *J Puplic Health Dent* 50:276-281.

Promoting the Disposition of Acid in Dental Plaque

G. H. W. Bowden

Destruction of tooth substance by acids is basic to the pathogenisis of dental caries. Complete elimination, or even reduction in the levels of acids in dental plaque could be assumed to have a dramatic impact on the occurrence of this disease. Methods to prevent and control the progression of caries in humans are eventually directed at reducing enamel demineralization by influencing the process of demineralization and remineralization. Control of the diet and microflora; modifying the local environment and enamel solubility with fluoride or using specific rinses are all intended to shift the balance of demineralization/remineralization in favour of host tissues. It is evident that attempts to control the level of acids in plaque represent a significant aspect of caries prevention in dentistry and one which has been pursued with diligence by those interested in caries research.

This review will outline the generation of acids in plaque and their metabolism and fate. Attention will be drawn to techniques which have been used to study the biology of plaque acids and also to the methods which have been used to influence their type and level. An attempt will be made to evaluate the potential of the latter processes and hopefully to identify why methods may fail. The methods to modify acids vary in their complexity some, such as those aimed at direct neutralization of acids are very simple in their approach. However, complexity is not necessarily a virtue and elegant theory sometimes cannot easily be put into practice.

Mandel and Kleinberg (1986) have written an excellent review on methods that have been used to modify the biochemistry of dental plaque. This includes several of the topics which are considered here and it should be read in conjunction with this paper.

Deminerilization/Remineralization-A Natural Physiological Process

A high proportion of the bacteria resident in the human mouth metabolize carbohydrate. Even in the absence of dietary carbohydrate, species of bacteria will utilize salivary mucin as a substrate (Beighton *et al.* 1986; De Jong *et al.* 1987). This suggests that, even before the consumption of modern diets a certain amount of acid would be produced in dental plaque. In keeping with other physiological control systems elsewhere in the body, acid production in plaque is balanced by salivary buffer (Dawes, 1974; Lilienthal, 1955) and enamel remineralization (Wefel, 1990; Wefel *et al.* 1986; Wefel *et al.* 1987). Thus, the interaction between plaque acids and host saliva represents a natural process. A measure of the effectiveness of saliva in controlling demineralization can be gained from the increase of caries in patients with xerostomia (Brown *et al.* 1983) and also from the low incidence of caries in the lower incisors of children with nursing caries (Milnes and Bowden, 1985). In contrast to the upper incisors in these children which can develop extensive lesions in a few months, the lower incisors are protected by the tongue and bathed in saliva. It should be stated at the outset that, independent of any external agency humans possess effective physiological processes to protect against the loss of tooth mineral and control the oral flora (McNamara *et al.* 1979). One of these systems is removal and neutralization of plaque acid through the action of saliva.

The Fate of Acids in Plaque

Carbohydrate metabolism by bacteria in dental plaque results in the production of a variety of acids causing the pH to drop (Geddes, 1972). It is well recognized that lactic acid is significant among the acids and also that bacterial catabolism of acids in plaque causes a change in the acid profile with time (Cole *et al.* 1978; Geddes, 1972, 1975) Tables 1, 2. Moreover, studies in continuous culture have shown that changes in the environment of bacteria including addition of fluoride (Hamilton, 1990), and xylitol (Vadeboncoeur *et al.* 1983) can influence the amounts and types of acids produced (Hamilton, 1987). Another characteristic of the generation of acid by dental plaque is one of metabolic adaptation of bacterial populations. Bacteria may adapt to acid (Bowden and Hamilton, 1989; Hamilton and Buckley, 1991) and plaque communities can adapt to more efficiently metabolize carbohydrates which are not normal to the mouth (Kalfas *et al.* 1990).

It can be seen from the above that acids produced in plaque will be modified by the local environment and metabolized by plaque bacteria. Concomitant with these processes is loss of acid from plaque, the neutralization of acids by salivary and plaque buffer and by base produced by oral bacteria. The former two processes depend on diffusion and the latter on the availability of substrate for

TABLE 1 *Acids in Dental Plaque*

	Status of Plaque	
Resting Major Acids	*Added Carbohydrate Major Acids*	*Metabolizing Acids From Lactic*
Acetic	Acetic	
Propionic	Lactic	Acetic
N-Butyric		Propionic
		Lactic acid metabolized by *Veillonella Eubacterium Neisseria*
Minor Acids	*Minor Acids*	*Minor Acids*
Formic	+	Produced by a variety of metabolic pathways
Iso-Butyric	+	
Iso-Valeric	+	
Caproic	+	
Lactic	–	
Succinic	+	

TABLE 2 *Acids in Plaque in Relation to the Stephan Curve*
Data from Geddes, 1975
(Acids mMol × 10^{-5} mgm wet weight plaque)

State of Plaque	*Lactate*		*Volatile Acids*	
	L+	*D-*	*Acetate*	*Propionate*
Resting				
	0.19	0.31	2.05	1.18
	0.21	0.34	2.07	1.19
After Sucrose				
5 min	1.86	1.15	1.11	0.6
30 min	1.09	1.61	0.59	0.11

base production and bacteria capable of metabolizing these substrates. These processes will be considered in more detail when the approaches to the dispersal of acids from plaque are discussed.

Laboratory Methods to Study the Biology of Acids in Dental Plaque

A true measure of the outcome of any attempt to control caries by introducing changes in the generation and fate of acids in plaque can only be made from data from clinical studies. However, previous assessment of the potential of an agent or a procedure can be made in the laboratory using both *in vitro* and *in vivo* techniques. In considering the relative value of any method aimed at modification of acids in dental plaque *in vivo* it is important that one appreciate the methods which may be used to evaluate the procedure.

In Vitro Plaque Analysis and Salivary Sediment Techniques

Among the simplest of the *in vitro* techniques are those where plaque is treated *in vivo* and the effects are measured *in vitro* (Edgar, 1982; Geddes, 1972, 1975; Geddes and McNee, 1982; Lindfors and Lagerlof, 1988). A similar system is to use bacteria sedimented from saliva as representative of dental plaque Kleinberg (1970). Kleinberg and his co-workers drew attention to the significance of acid and base metabolism in the oral cavity and in plaque using these techniques (Biswas, 1982; Biswas and Kleinberg, 1971; Kleinberg *et al.* 1979a,b; Singer and Kleinberg, 1978).

Artificial Plaque/Chemostat Systems

In other systems plaque is grown as a mixed culture biofilm in an *in vitro* system and then removed and used to measure different aspects of its biology. Sissons *et al.* (1988) used an *in vitro* grown biofilm from an artificial mouth (Dibdin *et al.* 1976) to determine the kinetics of urea in plaque. Although this system uses bacteria from a biofilm, the system is little more defined than those using salivary sediment. In both systems the architecture of populations of bacteria in the biofilms is lost. While *in vitro* biofilms have been produced by inoculation of surfaces with saliva (Sissons *et al.* 1988) others have used defined inocula, either pure (Bowden *et al.* 1973) or mixed cultures (Donoghue and Perrons, 1988; Perrons and Donohue, 1990). The production and types of systems used for *in vitro* plaque models has been reviewed by Coombe *et al.* (1982). However, even with defined inocula the spatial relationships of the bacterial populations in the community are unknown and such relationships could be significant in the metabolism of bacterial biofilms (Wimpenny, 1981; Wimpenny *et al.* 1983).

A different approach has been used in study of the biology of other ecosystems. These involve stabilizing the populations of bacteria using agar gels. Macfarlane *et al.* (1984) stabilized bacteria in estuary sediments using 1.0% and 0.3% agar. Solid and semi-solid media and a sediment inoculum were layered one on another (Figure 1). After incubation, organisms from the salivary sediment had equilibrated within the 0.3% agar phase. The distribution of bacteria

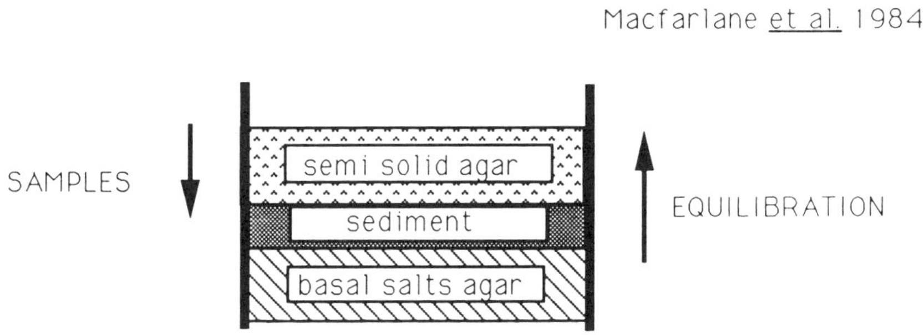

Figure 1 Ilized Model of Estuary Sediment

of different biological characteristics throughout this phase was closely similar to that in the original sediment (Table 3). Modifications of this type of system would lend themselves to the study of the bacteriology and metabolism within oral biofilms.

An approach to the study of the metabolism of urea and sucrose and acid diffusion and buffering in plaque, using gel stabilized mono-cultures has been made by Macpherson and Dawes (1991a,b) and Macpherson *et al.* (1991). These workers used an agarose stabilized gel of 0.5mm-1.5mm thickness, containing either *Streptococcus vestibularis* to examine the metabolism of urea, or *Streptococcus oralis* in studies of acid production from sucrose. It was possible to vary the concentration of organisms in the gel and also to include dead bacteria to simulate bacterial buffering (Shellis and Dibdin, 1988). Consideration of the gel-stabilized model systems suggests that they have considerable potential in analyzing the effect of spatially arranged bacterial populations on the nature and distribution of acids in biofilms (Lagerlof *et al.* 1985) such as dental plaque. Artificial biofilms can be produced where agarose stabilised populations of pure

TABLE 3 *Bacteria at Different Levels in Natural Sediments in an* in vitro *Gel Stabilized Model System*

Data from Macfarlane et al. 1984.

Depth	*Bacteria in Sediments 10^4/g*			*Bacteria in Gel 10^4ml*		
(cm)in Sediment	*Oxidising*		*Reducing*	*Oxidising*		*Reducing*
	NH_4^+	NO_2^-	*Sulphate*	NH_4^+	NO_2^-	*Sulphate*
0-1	0.7	1.6	0.38	8.2	1.0	0.11
1-2	no data	no data	4.2	0.8	0.6	4.3
2-3	0.6	0.8	61.0	nd	nd	380.0
3-4	no data	no data	43.0	nd	nd	120.0
4-5	0.3	30.0	33.0	nd	nd	18.0

nd = Not detected

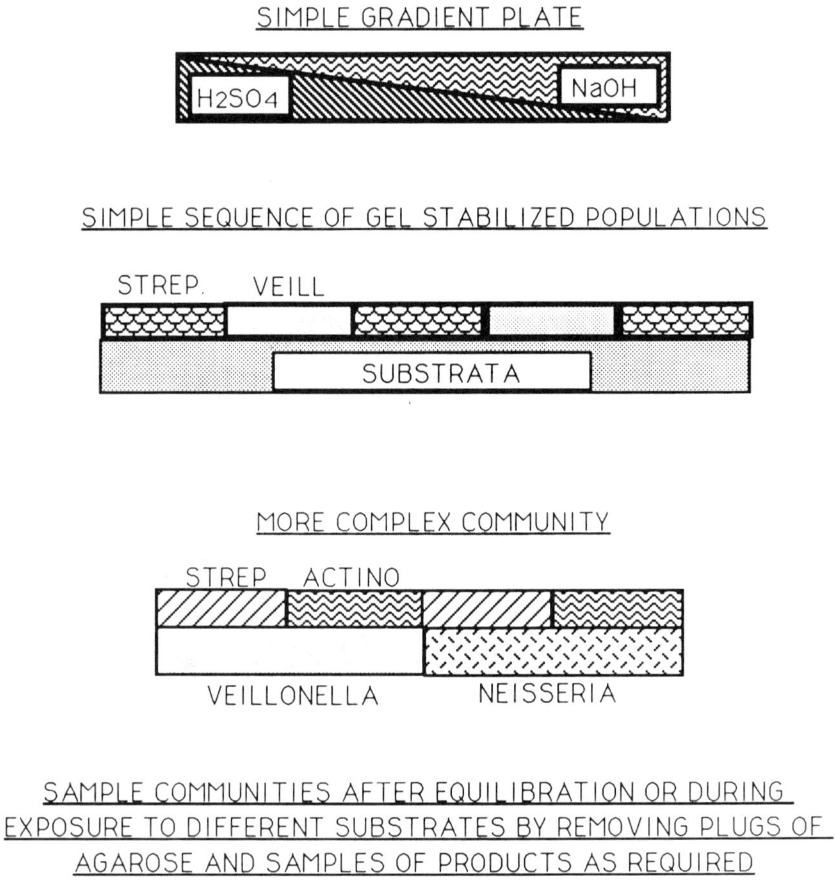

Figure 2 Gel stabilized models to study distribution of acids in biofilms

cultures of bacteria can be placed adjacent to each other in two or even three dimensional structures (Figure 2). After incubation and treatment with substrate, plugs of agarose can be removed for analysis of the bacteriology and metabolic products. Development of such systems may provide information on, for example, the distribution of acids in a simple community of *Streptococcus* and *Veillonella* and the spread of acids at the junction of two populations of bacteria in a community. In this way it would be possible to determine, *in vitro* the potential impact of agents on communities oral bacteria of known structure.

The chemostat has been used extensively in the study of the biology of oral bacteria both in pure and mixed culture, including the impact of nutrition and the environment on the production of acids (Hamilton, 1987; Marsh *et al.* 1983). Model systems using up to nine species to produce stable communities in the chemostat are well described (Bowden and Hamilton 1989; Bradshaw *et al.* 1990; Marsh *et al.* 1983; McDermid *et al.* 1986; Mikx *et al.* 1976; Mikx and Van der Hoeven, 1975; Van der Hoeven *et al.* 1985) and extensive detail need not be given here. However, it is worth noting that studies by Mikx *et al.* (1976) have compared acid metabolism in chemostat cultures to defined mixed cultures in gnotobiotic animals. Also of direct relevance to acid base metabolism in dental plaque is the study by Rogers *et al.* (1987) using mixed continuous cultures of *Streptococcus mutans* and *Streptococcus milleri* in media containing and pulsed with arginine. Arginine favored the growth of *S. milleri* as did higher pH environments (pH 7.8); low pH environments (pH 5.5) and glucose pulses favored *S. mutans*. One of the criticisms of chemostat culture is that the organisms are not in a biofilm, however, it is possible to grow organisms on surfaces in a chemostat.

In Vitro Diffusion

Studies of the diffusion of substrates and products into and from dental plaque have been of two kinds. These are *in vitro* systems, using artificial plaque (McNee *et al.* 1982a,b; Melson *et al.* 1983; Tatevossian 1985a,b) and computer models (Dawes 1983). Significant work in this area has been done by Dibdin and his co-workers (Dawes and Dibdin, 1986; Dibdin, 1981, 1984; Dibdin *et al.* 1983; Shellis and Dibdin, 1988) who have provided considered opinions and conclusions on those factors including plaque polysaccharide content, thickness, cell packing density, and permselectivity all of which can influence diffusion. Dibdin and Shellis (1988) taking data from their own work and that others, including Zero *et al.* (1986) drew attention to factors linking production of extracellular polysaccharide by plaque microorganisms and the cariogenicity of plaque. Recently Van Houte *et al.* (1989) have added support to the idea that modification of diffusion by extracellular polysaccharide could contribute to cariogenicity.

In Vivo Telemetry

The most significant of the methods which measure pH levels in plaque *in vivo* is telemetry (Imfield, 1982; Yamada *et al.* 1982). The method allows the pH to be monitored at localized sites of the dentition during normal consumption of food (Igarashi *et al.* 1988, 1989, 1990; Jensen, 1986). Telemetry probably provides the only system at this time which indicates the effectiveness of methods to modify plaque acids in areas where access is difficult. As such, it remains an important system which is available in the laboratory to stringently assess the potential of methods to control acids in dental plaque.

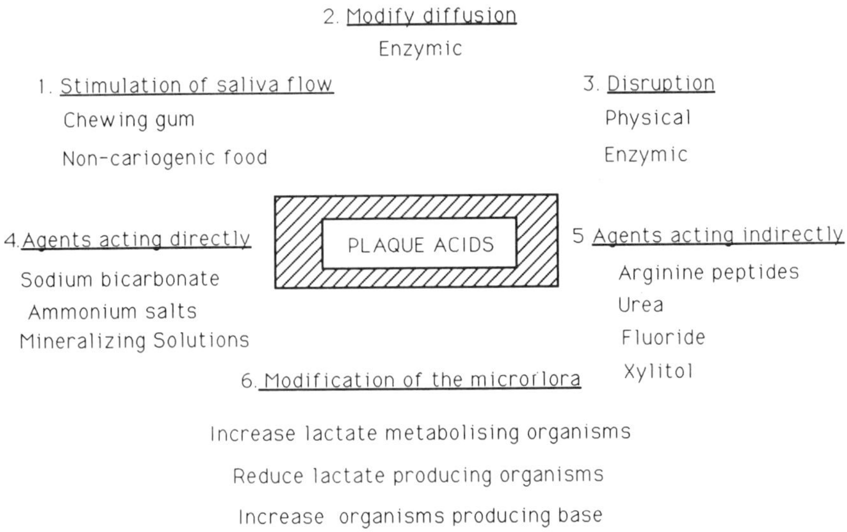

Figure 3 Approaches to the modification of acid metabolism in dental plaque

Animal Studies

Gnotobiotic animals have been used to study the ecology of dental plaque including the production of acid. Early studies by Mikx *et al.* (1976) and Mikx and Van der Hoeven (1975) demonstrated the potential of animal experiments in studies of the production and fate of acids in plaque. Mono or di-associated gnotobiotic animals provide a valuable model for analyzing the impact of different agents on plaque acid production (Van der Hoeven and Franken 1984) as well as analysis of acids from plaque of defined microbial composition.

Approaches to Promoting the Disposition (Dispersal) of Acids in Dental Plaque

Several methods have been proposed to influence the levels and/or metabolism of acids in plaque and affect the balance of demineralization and remineralization in favour of the host. Examples of these methods are shown in Figure 3. Generally the techniques can be subdivided as shown below.

1) Stimulation of salivary flow.
2) External application of methods to disrupt plaque.
3) External application of agents to act directly on plaque
4) External aplication of agents acting indirectly through the metabolic activities of plaque

5) Modification of the microflora of plaque to reduce its ability to produce acid or increase its capacity to produce base.
6) Modification of diffusion in plaque.

Stimulation of Salivary Flow

Salivary flow is increased during eating and consumption of non-cariogenic food (Jenkins,1979) could influence plaque pH. However, perhaps one of the more interesting agents for stimulating salivary flow is chewing gum. Chewing gum has been used extensively for this purpose and as a vehicle for a wide range of agents intended to influence plaque including mutanase (Kelstrup *et al.* 1978). A recent review by Edgar and Geddes (1990) provides details on the relationship between chewing gum and dental health. Various aspects of the relationship between saliva and caries are covered in the publication ''Saliva and Dental Caries'' edited by Kleinberg *et al.* (1979a) and Dawes (1979) has discussed the possibility of enhancing the anticaries effect of saliva.

External Agents to Disrupt Plaque

Physical disruption of plaque obviously results in the dispersion of plaque acid. Holmen *et al.* (1987, 1988) have shown that mechanical disturbance of plaque prevents demineralization. Another method proposed to disrupt plaque by lysing its matrix was to use enzymes like dextranase. The literature on dextranase and other enzymes has been reviewed by Mandel and Kleinberg (1986). While enzymes may not cause disintegration of plaque they may modify its characteristics with regard to diffusion. It must also be remembered that members of the plaque community produce extracellular enzymes including those which will hydrolyse glucose polymers (Staat *et al.* 1973).

External Agents Acting Directly on Plaque Acid

Several alkaline chemicals have been proposed as agents to increase plaque pH. These include a variety of agents which have been included into tooth powders and pastes (Regolati, 1971). Sodium carbonate included into chewing gum has been used in pH telemetry of human interproximal plaque (Igarashi *et al.* 1988), where it produced an increase in pH relative to a control. Recently Pearce and Nelson (1988) have used a mouthrinse to increase the level of plaque mineral, it is likely that such mouthrinses would also impact on the acids in plaque. Given adequate access these types of agents should increase plaque pH although the duration of their effects may vary.

External Agents Acting Indirectly on Plaque Acids

It is apparent that the bacteria in dental plaque exhibit a wide range of metabolic potential. It has been suggested that components of this potential be used to cause increases in plaque pH. The metabolic capabilities of bacterial populations in plaque may be constituitive or inducible. Perhaps the best known of these agents are urea (Regolati, 1971; Mandel and Kleinberg, 1986) and peptides containing arginine (Kleinberg *et al.* 1979b; Kanapka and Kleinberg 1983; Mandel and Kleinberg, 1986). There have been different opinions on the metabolic pathways involved in ureolysis in dental plaque (Biswas and Kleinberg, 1971), although it now seems most likely that bacterial urease is mainly responsible (Sissons and Nelson 1985). Little is known of the intrinsic ability of plaque to degrade proteins to liberate base or which organisms are involved.

Among the non-fermentable carbohydrates proposed as sweeteners xylitol has been shown to have an impact on carbohydrate metabolism, reducing acid production (Vadeboncoeur *et al.* 1983) Similarly, fluoride is known to impact on bacterial metabolism and plaque ecology. These topics recently have been reviewed in detail (Bowden 1990: Hamilton 1990).

Modifying the Microflora of Dental Plaque

Caries results from changes in the microbiology of local areas of dental plaque which promote demineralization of enamel (Bowden 1991; Loesche 1986). These changes reflect in part the characteristics of the local environment, which provide an ecological advantage to organisms such as the 'mutans streptococci' (Loesche 1986). This group of organisms includes the most significant of those bacteria which are cariogenic in humans (Bowden 1991). The selective pressure for 'mutans streptococci' is most likely to be a low pH (acid) (Svanberg, 1980).

Changing the Environment of the Local Ecosystem

It seems reasonable to propose that if pathogenic organisms develop in bacterial communities (dental plaque) in response to the environment, modification of the environment could reverse the process. Similarly, organisms beneficial to health could be encouraged by introducing the necessary factors into the environment.

Geddes (1975) showed that lactate was mainly responsible for the drop in pH early in the Stephan curve. She proposed that this phenomenon could be controlled either by reducing lactate production or enhancing lactate catabolism. In his studies of diffusion Tatevossian (1985a) noted that live plaque deposits metabolized ^{14}C lactate and organisms such as *Veillonella* and *Eubacterium alactolyticum* are know to metabolize lactate. However, relatively little is know of the numbers or diversity of lactate utilizing bacteria in dental plaque. Further support for an effect of lactate catabolism came from Mikx *et al.* (1976) who demonstrated that *Veillonella* modified the cariogenicity of *Streptococcus mutans* in experimental animals. However, it should be noted that very often *Veillonella* are found in high numbers associated with caries lesions in humans (Boyar and Bowden, 1985; Milnes and Bowden 1985) possibly as a result of the presence of lactate. Although it cannot be said that these bacteria are not reducing the rate of caries, they have not prevented the development of a lesion.

If it was intended to increase the level of lactate utilizing organisms in plaque it could be suggested that a mouth rinse containing lactate would be effective. A pilot study where young adults rinsed their mouths daily with a buffered solution of sodium lactate for 14 days did not show any significant increases in *Veillonella* in their plaque (Bowden and Brownstone, unpublished).

However, Kalfas *et al.* (1990) have shown that plaque can adapt to new carbon sources and that specific bacteria increase in numbers. Ingestion of sorbitol by humans resulted in adaptation of plaque, such that metabolism of sorbitol by the community became more efficient and *S. mutans* (which metabolizes sorbitol) increased in numbers. The acids produced by the plaque were modified by sorbitol, giving a higher ratio of weak to strong acids than that from glucose, although this tendency was reduced the longer sorbitol was ingested. This study is an excellent example of adaptation of the community of plaque bacteria to a nutritional change in their environment.

Urea is a normal component of saliva, and its levels may be increased in patients with renal defects (Mandel and Kleinberg,1986). Some species of oral bacteria produce urease which will convert urea to ammonia (Macpherson and Dawes, 1991a). This process is the basis for proposals that ureolysis in plaque will neutralize acids causing an increase in pH. Apparently there is little information on the ability of plaque to adapt to more efficiently metabolize urea or the bacteria which are involved (Gallagher *et al.* 1984). Resolution of these questions is well within the technologies available today and should provide valuable data on the potential for ecological approaches to modify plaque acid as a means of caries control. Controlling of the amounts and patterns of acids in plaque, through modification of the environment of the microflora, remains an interesting concept that deserves further study.

Genetic Modification of Plaque Bacteria

This topic is discussed in detail elsewhere in this meeting and details of methods and the types of genetic modifications envisaged need not be given here. However, if it were possible to introduce organisms into the mouth which possessed enhanced capacities to produce base or other characteristics intended to modify the metabolism of plaque they would have a major advantage over other methods mentioned above. These organisms would be included into plaque during its formation and would not suffer from the problem of access to sites at risk.

Modifying Plaque Matrix to Enhance Diffusion of Acids

It might seem reasonable to propose, that if the rate of diffusion of acids from plaque could be increased demineralization would be reduced. This might be achieved by treatment of plaque with enzymes to modify the plaque matrix. However, the evidence suggests that plaque, unless it is thick, with packed cells, or in a protected area does not limit diffusion to a great extent (Dawes and Dibdin, 1986; Dibdin 1984; Dibdin and Shellis, 1988; Igarashi *et al.* 1989, 1990). In addition, any change in diffusion will apply to substrate entering plaque, and other factors, including the possibility of metabolism of diffusing species (Bowden *et al.* 1973; Tatevossian 1985a,b) will influence the final outcome of acid diffusion. Tatevossian (1985a) observed the metabolism of lactate in artificial plaque and Bowden *et al.* (1973) demonstrated the uptake and binding of phosphorus by biofilms of *Streptococcus sanguis* growing on bovine enamel. Modification of plaque to enhance diffusion may also produce an effect similar to increasing the proportion of extracellular polysaccharide with the risk of promoting its cariogenicity (Dibdin and Shellis 1988; Van Houte *et al.* 1989).

Consideration of the Problems in Modifying the Levels of Acids in Dental Plaque

The concentration of acids in plaque and the duration of the associated lowering of the pH is dependent on the interaction between a variety of factors (Figure 4). The composition of the microflora (Loesche, 1986; Bowden 1991) dictates acid and base production and catabolism. Coupled to these variables is the rate of diffusion,which is in itself modified by plaque thickness, matrix and tortuosity. Including the activity of salivary and plaque buffers, further complicates the process of deciding on the fine details of the outcome of the metabolism of carbohydrate by plaque. Computer models have been very valuable in this respect, particularly when it has been possible to test them *in vivo* and *in vitro* (Dawes, 1983; Dawes and Dibdin, 1986; Lagerlof *et al.* 1985; Lindfors and Lagerlof, 1988).

Given the complexity of the factors involved is it possible to influence the levels and metabolism and acids in dental plaque? Certainly, fluoride has the capacity to influence caries in part by its impact on plaque ecology and acid metabolism (Bowden 1990; Hamilton, 1990). Moreover, the effect of urea and

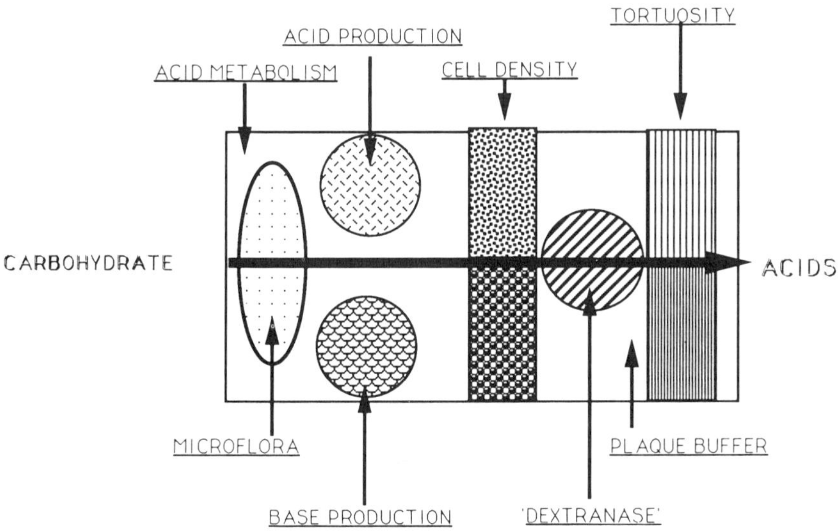

Figure 4 Some factors influencing the level of acids and pH in dental plaque

arginine peptides on plaque pH has been demonstrated in several *in vitro* systems and *in vivo*. Thus, given an effective agent, plaque pH and acid production can be modified, particularly when tested in *in vitro* models. Modification of the microflora of plaque occurs naturally, albeit to our detriment, in caries. It should also be possible to introduce beneficial modifications which cause reductions in plaque acids. Perhaps a clue to a significant problem in modifying the acids in dental plaque lies in the location of caries in humans. Caries most often occurs at protected sites where there is little physical disturbance, ie. sites with reduced access (McNamara *et al.* 1979) by externally applied agents. Given adequate access it seems likely that many of the agents proposed to modify acids directly, or influence the microflora could be as effective *in vivo* as they are shown to be *in vitro*. The patterns of pH response revealed by telemetry at interproximal and fissure sites illustrate the problem of access and its impact on the duration of effect of a protective agent. The environmental pressures which enhance acid production in plaque (carbohydrate) are applied over long periods of time. In addition, the factors which allow cariogenic bacteria to develop, include nutritional (carbohydrate) and environmental (pH) which form a powerful selective pressure, beneficial to organisms such as *Streptococcus mutans*. Regular application of urea might enhance the ureolytic bacteria in plaque but urea does not influence the pH of the environment to the extent that carbohydrate does and may not give ureolytic bacteria a strong selective advantage. *Streptococcus vestibularis* which actively metabolizes urea, obtains its energy from carbohydrate and produces acid. However, chemostat studies by Rogers *et al.* (1987) where

S. mutans and *Streptococcus milleri* were grown together in a medium with arginine have shown that high pH may place *S. mutans* at a disadvantage relative to *S. milleri*.

It seems therefore, that if one wishes to influence acids in plaque either directly or indirectly gaining access to sites at risk is of prime importance. This suggests that many of the procedures discussed here should be used in conjunction with physical agents which enhance access (flossing) or vehicles for delivery which can be used easily and repetitively (chewing gum). The fissures of teeth present a special case in prevention as physical methods may not enhance access, however, their susceptibility to caries can be reduced by fissure sealants. Any procedure proposed to enhance the disposition of acids in dental plaque, used as a preventive measure, can best be seen as an adjunct to physical methods enhancing access to sites at risk.

REFERENCES

BEIGHTON, D.; SMITH, K.; and HAYDAY, H. (1986): The growth of Bacteria and the Production of Exoglycosidic Enzymes in the Dental Plaque of Macaque Monkeys, *Arch Oral Biol* 31:829-835.

BISWAS, S. D. (1982): Effect of Urea on pH, Ammonia, Amino Acids and Lactic Acid in the Human Salivary Sediment System Incubated with Varying Levels of Glucose, *Arch Oral Biol* 27:683-691.

BISWAS, S. D. and KLEINBERG, I. (1971): Effect of Urea Concentration on its Utilization, on the pH and The formation of Ammonia and Carbon Dioxide in a Human Salivary Sediment System, *Arch Oral Biol* 16:759-780.

BOWDEN G. H. W. (1990): Effects of Fluoride on the Microbial Ecology of Dental Plaque, *J Dent Res* 69(Spec Iss):653-659.

BOWDEN, G. H. W. (1991): Which Bacteria are Cariogenic in Humans? In: *Risk Markers for Oral Diseases*, Vol 1 Dental Caries, N. W. Johnson Ed, pp. 266-286, Cambridge, England: Cambridge University Press.

BOWDEN G. H. W. and HAMILTON, I. R. (1989): Competition between *Streptococcus mutans* and *Lactobacillus casei* in Mixed Continuous Culture, *Oral Microbiol Immunol* 6:65-71.

BOWDEN, G. H.; NASH, R. L.; and SPIERS, R. L. (1973): The Localization and Retention of ^{32}P and ^{45}Ca within Surface Deposits of *Streptococcus sanguis* and the Influence of such Deposits on the Release of these Isotopes from enamel, *Caries Res* 7:185-200.

BOYAR, R. M. and BOWDEN, G. H. W. (1985): The Microflora Associated with the Progression of Incipient Lesions in Teeth of Children Living in a Water Fluoridated Area, *Caries Res* 12:298-306.

BRADSHAW, D. J.; MCKEE, A. S.; and MARSH, P. D. (1990): Prevention of Population Shifts in Oral Microbial Communities *in vitro* by Low Fluoride Concentrations, *J Dent Res* 69:436-441.

BROWN, L. R.; WHITE, J. O.; HORTON, I. M.; DRIEZEN, S.; and STREKFUSS, J. L. (1983): Effect of Continuous Fluoride Gel Use on Plaque Fluoride Retention and Microbial Activity, *J Dent Res* 62:746-751.

COLE, M. F.; BOWDEN, G. H.; KORTS, D. C.; and BOWEN, W. H. (1978): The Effect of Pyridoxine, Phytate and Invert Sugar on Production of Plaque Acids *in situ* in the Monkey (*M. fascicularis*), *Caries Res* 12:190-201.

COOMBE, R. A.; TATEVOSSIAN,; and WIMPENNY, J. W. T. (1982): Bacterial Thin Films as *in vitro* Models for Dental Plaque. *Surface and Colloid Phenomena in the Oral Cavity: Methodological Aspects*, R. M. Frank and S. A. Leach Eds. London: IRL Press, pp. 239-249.

DAWES, C. (1974): The Effects of Flow Rate and Duration of Stimulation on the Concentrations of Protein and the Main Electrolytes in Human Submandibular Saliva, *Arch Oral Biol* 19:887-895.

DAWES, C. (1979): Augmentation and Supplementation of Natural Salivary Constituents- in Caries Control. In *Saliva and Dental Caries*, I. Kleinberg, S. A. Ellison, and I. D. Mandel Eds. pp. 505-513 New York: Information Retrieval.

DAWES, C. (1983): A Mathematical Model of Salivary Clearance of Sugars from the Oral Cavity, *Caries Res* 17:321-334.

DAWES, C. and DIBDIN, G. H. (1986): A Theoretical Analysis of the Effects of Plaque Thickness and Initial Salivary Sucrose Concentration on Diffusion of Sucrose into Dental Plaque and its Conversion to Acid During Salivary Clearance, *J Dent Res* 65:89-94.

DEJONG, M. H. and VAN DER HOEVEN, J. S. (1987): The Growth of Oral Bacteria on Saliva, *J Dent Res* 66:498-505.

DIBDIN, G. H. (1981): Diffusion of Sugars and Carboxylic Acids through Human Dental Plaque *in vitro*, *Arch Oral Biol* 26:515-523.

DIBDIN, G. H. (1984): A Brief Survey of Recent *in vitro* Work on Diffusion of Small Ions and Molecules in Dental Plaque, In *Cariology Today*, B. Guggenheim Ed, pp. 191-198 Basel: Karger.

DIBDIN, G. H. and SHELLIS, R. P. (1988): Physical and Biochemical Studies of *Streptococcus mutans* Sediment Suggest New Factors Linking the Cariogenicity of Plaque with its Extracellular Polysaccharide Content, *J Dent Res* 67:890-895.

DIBDIN, G. H.; SHELLIS, R. P.; and WILSON, C. M. (1976): An Apparatus for the Continuous Culture of Micro-organisms with Special Reference to Dental Plaque, *J Appl Bact* 40:261-268.

DIBDIN, G. H.; WILSON, C. M.; and SHELLIS, R. P. (1983): Effect of Packing Density and Polysaccharide to Protein Ratio of Plaque Samples Cultured in vitro upon their Permeability, *Caries Res* 17:52-58.

DONOGHUE, H. D. and PERRONS, C. J. (1988): Establishment of Defined Mixed Bacterial Plaques on Teeth in a Laboratory Microcosm (Model Mouth), *Microb Ecol Health Dis* 1:193-200.

EDGAR, W. M. (1982): Methodological Considerations Affecting the determination of pH in Tooth Surface Plaque. In *Surface and Colloid Phenomena in the Oral Cavity: Methodological Aspects* R. M. Frank and S. A. Leach, Eds. London: IRL Press, pp. 131-142

EDGAR, W. M. and GEDDES, G. A. M. (1990): Chewing Gum and Dental Health, *Br Dent J* 168:173-177.

GALLAGHER, I. H. C.; PEARCE, E. I. F.; and HANCOCK, E. M. (1984): The Ureolytic Microflora of Imature Dental Plaque before and after Rinsing with a Urea-based Mineralizing Solution, *J Dent Res* 63:1037-1039.

GEDDES, D. A. M. (1972): The Production of L(+) and L(-) Lactic Acids and Volatile acids by Human Dental Plaque and the Effect of Plaque Buffering and Acidic Strength on pH, *Arch Oral Biol* 17:537-545.

GEDDES, D. A. M. (1975): Acids produced by Human Dental Plaque Metabolism *in situ*, *Caries Res* 9:98-109.

GEDDES, D. A. M. and McNEE, S. G. (1982): The Effect of 0.2 percent (48mM) NaF Rinses Daily on Human Plaque Acidogenicity in situ (Stephan Curve) and Fluoride Content, *Arch Oral Biol* 27:765-769.

HAMILTON, I. R. (1987): Effect of Changing Environment on Sugar Transport and Metabolism by Oral Bacteria. In *Sugar Transport and Metabolism by Oral Bacteria*, J. Reizer and A. Peterkofsky, Eds Chichester, England: Ellis Horwood, pp. 94-133.

HAMILTON, I. R. (1990): Biochemical Effects of Fluoride on Oral Bacteria, *J Dent Res* (Spec Iss) 69:660-667.

HAMILTON, I. R. and BUCKLEY, N. D. (1991): Adaptation by *Streptococcus mutans* to Acid Tolerance, *Oral Microbiol Immunol* 6:65-71.

HOLMEN, L.; MEJARE, J.; MALMGREN, B.; and THYLSTRUP, A. (1988): The Effect of Regular Professional Plaque Removal on Dental Caries in vivo. A Polarized Light and Scanning Electron Microscope Study, *Caries Res* 22:250-256.

HOLMEN, L.; THYLSTRUP, A.; and ARTUN, J. (1987): Surface Changes During the Arrest of Active Enamel Carious Lesions in vivo, A Scanning Electron Microscope Study, *Acta Odont Scand* 45:383-390.

IGARASHI, K.; LEE, I. K.; and SCHACHTELE, C. F. (1988): Effect of Chewing Gum Containing Sodium Bicarbonate on Human Interproximal Plaque pH, *J Dent Res* 67:531-535.

IGARASHI, K.; LEE, I. K.; and SCHACHTELE, C. F. (1989): Comparison of *in vivo* Human Dental Plaque pH Changes within Artificial Fissures and at Interproximal Sites, *Caries Res* 23:417-422.

IGARASHI, K.; LEE, I. K.; and SCHACHTELE, C. F. (1990): Effect of Dental Plaque Age and Bacterial Composition on the pH of Artificial Fissures in Human Volunteers, *Caries Res* 24:52-58.

IMFELD, T. (1982): Interdental Plaque -pH-Telemetry. In: *Surface and Colloid Phenomena in the Oral Cavity: Methodological Aspects* R. M. Frank and S. A. Leach, Eds. London: IRL Press, pp. 143-156.

JENKINS, G. N. (1979): Salivary effects on plaque pH. In: *Saliva and Dental Caries*, I. Kleinberg, S. A. Ellison, and I. D. Mandel Eds., New York: Information Retrieval, pp. 307-322

JENSEN, M. E. (1986): Effects of Chewing Sorbitol Gum and Paraffin on Human Interproximal Plaque pH, *Caries Res* 20:503-509.

KALFAS, S.; SVENSATER, G.; BIRKHEAD, D.; and EDWARDSSON, S. (1990): Sorbitol Adaptation of Dental Plaque in People with Low and Normal Salivary-secretion rates, *J Dent Res* 69:442-446.

KANAPKA, J. A. and KLEINBERG, I. (1983): Catabolism of Arginine by the Mixed Bacteria in Human Salivary Sediment under Conditions of Low and High Glucose Concentration, *Arch Oral Biol* 28:1007-1015.

KELSTRUP, J.; HOLM-PEDERSON, P.; and POULSEN, S. (1978): Reduction of the Formation of Dental Plaque and Gingivitis in Humans by Crude Mutanase, *Scand J Dent Res* 86:93-102

KLEINBERG, I. (1970): Biochemistry of Dental Plaque. In: *Advances in Oral Biology* Vol 4, P. H. Staple, Ed. New York: Academic Press, pp. 43-70.

KLEINBERG, I.; KANAPKA, J. A.; CHATTERJEE, R.; CRAW, D.; D'ANGELO, N.; and SANDHAM, H. J.(1979a): Metabolism of Nitrogen by the Oral Mixed Bacteria. In *Saliva and Dental Caries*, I. Kleinberg, S. A. Ellison, and I. D. Mandel, Eds., New York: Information Retrieval, pp. 357-377.

KLEINBERG, I.; ELLISON, S. A.; and MANDELL, I. D. (1979b) Eds. *Saliva and Dental Caries*. New York: Information Retrieval.

LAGERLOF, F.; DAWES, R.; and DAWES, C. (1985): The Effect of Different Concentrations of Sucrose, Fructose, and Glucose on pH changes by *Streptococcus mitior* in an Artificial mouth, *J Dent Res* 64:405-410.

LILIENTHAL, B. (1955): An Analysis of the Buffer Systems in Saliva, *J Dent Res* 34:516-530.

LINDFORS, B. and LAGERLOF, F. (1988): Effect of Sucrose Concentration in Saliva after a Sucrose Rinse on the Hydroxonium Ion Concentration in Dental Plaque, *Caries Res* 22:7-10.

LOESCHE, W. J. (1986): Role of *Streptococcus mutans* in Dental Decay, *Microbiol Rev* 50:353-380.

MACFARLANE, G. T.; RUSS, M. A.; KEITH, S. M.; and HERBERT, R. A. (1984): Simulation of Microbial Processes in Estuarine Sediments using Gel Stabilised systems, *J Gen Microbiol* 130:2927-2933.

MACPHERSON, L. M. D. and DAWES C. (1991a): Urea Concentration in Minor Mucous Gland Secretion and the Effect of Salivary Film Velocity on Urea Metabolism by *Streptococcus vestibularis* in an Artificial Plaque, *J Periodont Res* 26: 395-401.

MACPHERSON, L. M. D. and DAWES C. (1991b): Effects of Salivary Film Velocity on pH Changes in an Artificial Plaque Containing *Streptococcus oralis* After Exposure to Sucrose, *J Dent Res* 70:1235-1238.

MACPHERSON, L. M. D.; CHEN, W. Y.; and DAWES, C. (1991): Effects of Salivary Bicarbonate Content and Film Velocity on pH changes in an Artificial Plaque Containing *Streptococcus oralis*, After Exposure to Sucrose, *J Dent Res* 70:1230-1234.

MANDEL, I. D. and KLEINBERG, I (1986): Methods for Plaque Biochemistry Alteration, In *Dental Plaque Control and Oral Hygiene Practices*, H. Loe and D. Kleinman Eds, Oxford, England: IRL Press.

MARSH, P. D.; HUNTER, J. R.; BOWDEN, G. H.; HAMILTON, I. R.; MCKEE, A. S.; HARDIE, J. M.; and ELLWOOD, D. C. (1983): The Influence of Growth Rate and Nutrition Limitation on the Microbial Composition and Biochemical Properties of a Mixed Culture of Oral Bacteria Grown in a Chemostat, *J Gen Microbiol* 129:755-770.

MCNAMARA, T. F.; FRIEDMAN, B. K.; AND ROTH, P. (1979): Salivary Access as an Ecological Determinant. In *Saliva and Dental Caries*, I. Kleinberg, S. A. Ellison, and I. D. Mandel Eds. New York: Information Retrieval, pp. 211-225.

MCDERMID, A. S.; MCKEE, A. S.; ELLWOOD, D. C.; and MARSH, P. D. (1986): The Effect of Lowering the pH on the Composition and Metabolism of a Community of Nine Oral Bacteria Grown in a Chemostat, *J Gen Microbiol* 132:1205-1214.

MCNEE, S. G.; GEDDES, D. A. M.; and WEETMAN, D. A. (1982a): Diffusion of Sugars and Acids in Human Dental Plaque *in vitro*, *Arch Oral Biol* 27:975-979.

MCNEE, S. G.; GEDDES, D. A. M.; WEETMAN, D. A.; SWEENEY, D.; and BEELEY, J. A. (1982b): Effect of Extracellular Polysaccharide on Diffusion of NaF and (^{14}C) Sucrose in Human Dental Plaque and Sediments of the Bacterium *Streptococcus sanguis* 804 (NCTC 10904), *Arch Oral Biol* 27:981-986.

MELSON, B.; KAAE, O.; AND ROLLA, G. (1983): Penetration of Fluoride and Chlorhexidine into Human Dental Plaque *in vitro*, *Caries Res* 17:113-117.

MIKX, F. H. M. and VAN DER HOEVEN, J. S. (1975): Symbiosis of *Streptococcus mutans* and *Veillonella alcalescens* in Mixed Continuous Culture, *Arch Oral Biol* 20:407-410.

MIKX, F. H. M.; VAN DER HOEVEN; J. S.; and WALKER, G. J. (1976): Microbial Symbiosis in dental Plaque Studied in Gnotobiotic Rats and in the Chemostat. In *Microbial Aspects of Dental Caries* Vol 3, H. M. Stiles, W. J. Loesche and T. C. OBrien, Eds, Washington: Information Retrieval.

MILNES, A. R. and BOWDEN, G. H. W. (1985) : The MIcroflora Associated with Developing Lesions of Nursing Caries, *Caries Res* 19:289-297.

PEARCE, E. I. F. and NELSON, D. G. A. (1988): *In vivo* Comparison of Caries Inhibition by a Plaque Mineral Enriching mouthrinse and a Fluoride Dentifrice, *Caries Res* 22:362-370.

PERRONS, C. J. and DONOGHUE, H. D. (1990): Colonization Resistance of Defined Bacterial Plaques to *Streptococcus mutans* Implantation on Teeth in a Model Mouth, *J Dent Res* 69:483-488.

REGOLATI, B. (1971): Ammonia and Urea in oral Pathophysiology- a Literature Review, *Helv Odont Acta* 15:139-146.

ROGERS, H.; ZILM, P.S.; and GULLY, N.J. (1987): Influence of Arginine on the Coexistence of *Streptococcusmutans* and *S. milleri* in Glucose-Limited Mixed Continuous Culture, *Microb Ecol* 14:193-202.

SHELLIS, R. P. and DIBDIN, G. H. (1988): Analysis of the Buffering System in Dental Plaque, *J Dent Res* 67:438-446.

SINGER, D. L. and KLEINBERG, I. (1978): Ammonia and Urea Content of Human Incisor Tooth Plaque, *Arch Oral Biol* 23:1083-1087.

SISSONS, C. H.; CUTRESS, T. W.; and PEARCE, E. I. F. (1985): Kinetics and Product Stoichiometry of Ureolysis by Human Salivary Bacteria and Artificial Mouth Plaque, *Arch Oral Biol* 30:781-790.

STAAT, R. H.; GAWRONSKI, T. H.; and SCHACHTELE, C. F. (1973): Detection and Preliminary Studies on Dextranase Producing Microorganisms from Human Dental Plaque, *Infect Immun* 45:1009-1016.

SVANBERG, M. (1980): *Streptococcus mutans* in plaque after rinsing with buffers of varying pH, *Scand J Dent Res* 88:76-78.

TATEVOSSIAN, A. (1985a): Some Factors Affecting the Diffusion of (^{14}C) Lactate in Human Dental Plaque, *Arch Oral Biol* 30:141-146.

TATEVOSSIAN, A. (1985b): The Effects of Heat Inactivation, Tortuosity, Extracellular Polyglucan and Ion Exchange Sites on the Diffusion of (^{14}C) Sucrose in Human Dental Plaque Residue *in vitro*, *Arch Oral Biol* 30:365-371.

VADEBONCOEUR, C.; TRAHAN, L.; MOUTON, C.; and MAYRAND, D. (1983): Effect of Xylitol on the Growth and Glycolysis of Acidogenic Oral Bacteria, *J Dent Res* 62:882-884.

VAN DER HOEVEN, J. S. and FRANKEN, H. C. M. (1984): Effect of Fluoride on Growth and Acid Production by *Streptococcus mutans* in Dental Plaque, *Infect Immun* 45:356-359.

VAN DER HOEVEN, J. S.; DE JONG, M. H.; CAMP, P. J. M.; and VAN DER KIEBOOM, C. W. A. (1985): Competition between Oral *Streptococcus* Species in the Chemostat under Alternating Conditions of Glucose Limitation and Excess, *FEMS Microbiol Ecol* 31:373-379.

VAN HOUTE, J.; RUSSO, J.; and PROSTAK, K. S. (1989): Increased pH lowering Ability of *Streptococcus mutans* Cell Masses Associated with Extracellular Glucan-rich Matrix Material and the Mechanisms Involved, *J Dent Res* 68:451-459.

WEFEL, J. S. (1990): Effects of Fluoride on Caries Development and Progression Using Intra-Oral Models, *J Dent Res* (Spec Iss) 69:626-633.

WEFEL, J. S.; MAHARY,M. E.; HAYES, P.; and CLARKSON, B. H. (1986): In vivo Demineralization and Remineralization of Enamel and Root Surfaces. In: *Factors Relating to Demineralization and Remineralization of The Teeth*, S. A. Leach, Ed., Oxford: IRL Press Ltd, pp. 181-190.

WEFEL, J. S.; MAHARRY, G.; JENSEN, M. E.; and HARLESS, J. D. (1987) : Development of an Intra-oral Single Section Remineralization Model, *J Dent Res* 66:1485-1489.

WIMPENNY, J. W. T. (1981): Spatial Order in Microbial Ecosystems. *Biological Reviews* 56:295-342.

WIMPENNY, J. W. T.; LOVITT, R. W.; and COOMBS, J. P. (1983): Laboratory Model Systems for the Investigation of Spatially and Temporally organized microbial ecosystems, *Symposia of the Society of General Microbiology* 34:67-117.

YAMADA, T.; IGARASHI, K.; and KAMIYAMA, K. (1982): Advantages and Disadvantages of using an Ion-sensitive Transistor Electrode for Measuring pH in Human Dental Plaque *in vivo*. In *Surface and Colloid Phenomena in the Oral Cavity: Methodological Aspects* R. M. Frank and S. A. Leach, Eds., London: IRL Press, pp. 157-166.

ZERO, D. T.; VAN HOUTE, J.; and RUSSO, J. (1986): The Intra-oral Effect on Enamel Demineralization of Extracellular Matrix Material Synthesized from Sucrose by *Streptococcus mutans*, *J Dent Res* 65:918-923.

Vaccination: A Cariostatic Option?

Martin A. Taubman and Daniel J. Smith

The concept of vaccination in the oral cavity appeared incongruous since no easy immunization method existed to interfere with pathogens that were essentially outside the body. The concept was strengthened by 3 major findings: 1. The transmissible and infectious nature of dental caries, 2. The discovery and understanding of the secretory immune system, and 3. The vaccine studies performed in the late 1960's and early 1970's indicating that dental caries, as an infectious disease, was amenable to immunological intervention. Since those initial demonstrations, many strategies have been developed and are being employed in clinical trials. The application of the vaccine approach is primarily as a preventive measure. However, active, or passive induction of oral immunity may also have promise as a cariostatic option. These options will be discussed.

Preventive Aspects of Vaccines in Dental Caries

Immunologic Protection and Dental Caries

The discovery of a separate and unique mucosal immune system in 1965 (Tomasi *et al.*), suggested that one might be able to interfere with caries by stimulating salivary antibodies to appropriate antigens (Bowen, 1969; Taubman & Smith, 1974; McGhee *et al.*, 1975). Initial studies of the potentially protective effects of the immune system utilized whole cells of mutans streptococci as antigens. A variety of routes (intravenous, intraductal, subcutaneous, submucosal, or per os immunization) have resulted in protection in animal systems. Most significant were the initial studies designed to stimulate directly the gut-associated lymphoreticular tissues (GALT) by ingestion of killed mutans streptococci,

The research reported in this manuscript was supported by grants DE 04733, DE 07009 and DE 06153 from the National Institute of Dental Research. We thank Donna Freedman for expert secretarial assistance.

(Michalek *et al.*, 1976; Smith *et al.*, 1980). These studies demonstrated that consistent induction of secretory IgA antibody to a dental pathogen resulted in reductions in both disease and cariogenic infection. Importantly, the previous notion that salivary IgA antibody was a protective principle was reinforced by these investigations since virtually no serum (IgG) antibody could be detected.

Immunization with intact streptococcal cells would elicit immune responses to an array of cell-bound components likely to be involved in several of the phases of colonization, accumulation, or acid production. Antibody to the serotype carbohydrate is uniformly distributed on the mutans cell surface (Iacono *et al.*, 1976). Conceivably, antibody to this or any antigen at or near the cell surface could interfere with important bacterial pathogenic features or result in clearance by virtue of steric hindrance. Furthermore, injection of whole cells may induce unwanted cross-reactive responses (Russell and Wu, 1990).

Vaccine Approach Related to Mutans Streptococci

Several steps in the colonization, accumulation, or acid production of the mutans streptococci may be vulnerable to immunological attack (See Taubman and Smith, 1989). The initial interaction in colonization takes place with the pellicle-coated tooth surface. The components on the mutans streptococci that participate in pellicle binding appear to be protein (Staat *et al.*, 1980). Following the initial attachment phase, mutans streptococci accumulate. These streptococci produce glucosyltransferases (GTFs), which then synthesize water-soluble and water-insoluble glucans from sucrose. Mutans streptoccoci and certain other oral streptococci express cell surface proteins which serve as binding sites for these extracellular glucans. The interactions between GTF, glucans and cell-bound glucan-binding proteins appear to be fundamental to the accumulation process. This mechanism results in an increase in numbers of potentially cariogenic bacteria in plaque and can be inhibited in vitro by specific antibody to GTF (Taubman *et al.*, 1983; Taubman and Smith, 1989).

There has been a focus on identifying safe and effective antigens from the mutans streptococci for use in experimental immunization. Examples of such antigens are the cell wall antigen I/II (Russell and Lehner, 1978) also known as SpaA, SpaP, B or P1, which may be involved in the initial attachment phase, and components of the GTF enzyme system that participate in the accumulation phase (See Krasse *et al.*, 1987; Taubman and Smith, 1989; Michalek and Childers, 1990).

Development of New Types of Vaccines

The best way to influence pathogens in the oral cavity may be by means of vaccination. Vaccination is a simple, generally safe, and most effective form of preventing infectious disease, and has achieved remarkable success in eliminating pathogens such as small pox virus from the human flora. Vaccination has not been a top priority of researchers for use as a preventive method for dental caries. Past generations of non oral vaccines have had adverse side effects. Some of the side-effects of these older vaccines can be serious enough to constitute a risk not worth taking for non-life-threatening diseases such as dental caries. This reluctance has changed since present strategies promise to provide safe, and effective vaccines. Most of the strategies involve active immunization.

Active Immunization

Oral Immunization

Most oral immunization studies in humans have utilized intact *S. mutans* or *S. sobrinus* cells as antigen (Table 1). The first investigations (Mestecky *et al.*, 1978) demonstrated a pronounced secretory immune response both after primary and secondary oral immunization regimes using mutans streptococci administered in capsules. Detection of salivary IgA antibody was facilitated by using subjects without detectable antibody prior to immunization. These studies demonstrated induction of a salivary IgA response by stimulation of GALT in humans, and reinforced observations from animals suggesting the presence of an IgA anamnestic response. Although, subsequent studies (Table 1) using a variety of modest changes in the protocols, have not shown such pronounced elevated salivary IgA antibody levels, alterations in levels of implanted or indigenous mutans streptococci have been quite consistent (see Table 1, Krasse *et al.*, 1978; Gahnberg and Krasse, 1983; Cole *et al.*, 1984).

Studies of oral immunization with indigenous mutans streptococci (Gregory & Filler, 1987) resulted in elevated saliva IgA antibody and decreased indigenous *S. mutans*. The presence of specific IgA antibody-producing mononuclear cells in peripheral blood after oral administration of mutans streptococci in enterically coated gelatin capsules has been demonstrated (Czerkinsky *et al.*, 1987). These predominantly IgA antigen-specific precursor cells peaked in blood 10-12 days after oral immunization and specific IgA antibodies were found in saliva by 2 to 3 weeks. These experiments provided strong support for the generation of IgA precursor cells after oral immunization followed by emigration of these precursors to selected secretory sites. Oral passive immunization was also effective (Ma *et al.*, 1987) and is described below.

Initial uptake of antigen may take place in the small intestine in gut-associated lymphoreticular tissues. Particulate antigen administered by gastric intubation to rodents elicited a higher salivary IgA response than an equivalent dose of the soluble form of the same antigen (Cox and Taubman, 1984). These findings may be partially attributed to the enhanced uptake of particulate material by antigen sampling M cells in Peyer's patches (Wolf *et al.*, 1982). Particulate forms of GTF also promote enhanced salivary responses after

TABLE 1 *Oral Immunization Studies in Humans*

Study	*Number of Subjects*	*Vaccine (Serotype)*	*Frequency*	*Route*	*Results*
Mestecky *et al*, 1978	4	Cells (d)	14d	Oral	Increased antibody, anamnestic response.
Krasse *et al*, 1978	3	Cells (c)	8d	Topical	No detectable change in antibody.
Gahnberg Krasse, 1983	11	Cells (d)	14d	Oral	No change in antibody, fewer bacteria.
Cole *et al*, 1984	8	Cells (d)	3(7)d	Oral	No change in antibody, fewer bacteria reductions in levels and duration.
Gregory Filler, 1987	5	Indigenous cells	10d	Oral	Specific salivary IgA antibody and decreased indigenous *S. mutans*.
Czerkinsky *et al*, 1987	6	Cells (c)	7d	Oral	Specific IgA antibody producing cells peripheral blood, antibody increase in saliva, tears, fewer bacteria.
Ma *et al*, 1987	8	Anti-SA I/II MAb	3X	Passive Oral	Decreased colonization with implanted *S. mutans*.
Smith Taubman 1987	25	GTF (g) with aluminum phosphate	13X 17d	Oral	Specific IgA antibody in parotid saliva and retardation of indigenous streptococcal accumulation.
Smith Taubman 1990	23	GTF (g) aluminum phosphate	5X 5d	Topical	Delays in reaccumulation associated with parotid IgA antibody.

intragastric immunization of rodents (Ebersole *et al.*, 1983, 1986). We (Smith and Taubman, 1987) orally administered a vaccine containing GTF prepared from *S. sobrinus*, suspended in aluminum phosphate, in capsules to 25 adult males aged 18-36 years. The subjects were assigned to a vaccine or placebo group. Saliva samples were taken during an initial screening and antibody levels were compared with those in the parotid saliva of these same individuals taken prior to the immunization procedure. Parotid saliva SIgA antibody rose after oral antigen ingestion. A unique feature of this study was the use of a defined soluble antigen combined with a suspension of aluminum phosphate. We also found that GTF administration resulted in retardation of reaccumulation of indigenous mutans streptococci after a dental prophylaxis (Smith and Taubman, 1987). Presumably these effects were related to the salivary IgA antibody to *S. sobrinus* GTF which inhibits GTF of other serotypes. Antibody to water-insoluble glucan synthesizing GTF can markedly inhibit glucan synthesis and subsequent accumulation of mutans streptococci *in vitro* (Taubman *et al.*, 1983) and *in vivo*. This effect may result from direct inhibition of GTF-mediated glucan synthesis giving rise to alteration in the nature of dental plaque and restrictions in availability of glucan to binding sites for accumulation of mutans streptococci.

Local application of GTF (combined with aluminum phosphate) onto lower labial surfaces was investigated in 23 subjects (Smith and Taubman, 1990). GTF (or placebo) was administered to the lower lip daily for five days (Table 1). The delay in reaccumulation of indigenous mutans streptococci was significantly associated ($p < 0.025$) with elevations in parotid IgA antibody levels of all subjects. These results indicate that labial application of GTF-AP can modify the salivary immune environment to retard the reaccumulation of indigenous mutans streptococci after a dental prophylaxis. Salivary tissues contain the principal cellular components required for immune response to antigen (Pappo *et al.*, 1988). Deposited antigen could be captured by resident mononuclear phagocytes after endocytosis by ductal epithelium or other specialized cells. Antigen could be presented directly to immunologically competent cells in the labial gland, or be transported into local lymphatics. In either case, the recirculating IgA precursor cell population could be expanded and migrate to the parotid gland.

New Vaccine Strategies

Recent advances have resulted in new types of vaccines (Table 2). These include: internal image anti-idiotype vaccines, recombinant regulatory molecules, synthetic peptide vaccines, subunit vaccines, recombinant vaccines and recombinant infection vectors. Three exceptionally novel strategies which may be utilized for dental caries vaccines in the future are also listed in Table 2. These speculative strategies include transgenic approach, directed colonization, host cell replacement and are discussed in more detail in Taubman *et al.*, (1989).

TABLE 2 *Novel Vaccine Strategies.*

Strategy	*Used in Caries Vaccine*	*Potential use in Caries Vaccine*
Internal image anti-idiotypes	+	+
Recombinant regulatory molecules	–	?
Synthetic peptides	+	+
Subunit vaccines	–	+
Recombinant vaccines	+	+
Recombinant infectious vectors	+	+
Transgenic approach	–	?
Directed colonization	–	?
Host cell replacement therapies	–	?

Anti-idiotype Vaccines

The antibody combining site consists of diverse amino acid sequences on hypervariable regions unique for each antibody. This antibody-combining site itself is an antigen, or idiotype, and an immunogen potentially capable of inducing anti-idiotypic antibodies. The activity of the immune network is also postulated to generate a variety of internal image anti-idiotypes (some may recognize idiotypes, while others will mimic the epitope against which the idiotype was directed). Anti-idiotypes behave like the original epitope, since they can share the identical amino acid sequence with the immunogenic epitope (Gaulton and Greene, 1986). The epitope can also be recognized by the anti-idiotype antibody at the stereochemical level. This is particularly significant for poor immunogens such as carbohydrates. Thus, certain anti-idiotypes can be used as substitute antigens for inducing specific immunity to replace antigens that are unsafe or toxic, or for inducing anti-carbohydrate immunity. Idiotype vaccines that are proteins could be used to induce a protective immune response. Such vaccines could be of significance in affecting the developing flora of the oral cavity, where many important molecules in adherence and colonization are carbohydrates. Recently rabbit anti-rat idiotypic antibody has been used to immunize rats with a resulting 53% reduction in *S. mutans* and a 20% reduction in caries (Michalek *et al.*, 1990a).

Regulatory Molecules

Cytokines are products of various cells of the immune system that appear to be involved in regulating a variety of host cellular immune functions (Balkwill and Burke, 1989). Several of these human factors have been produced by recombinant technology or by protein synthetic means and are available for use. However, the use of any of these individual cytokines in isolated fashion has usually not resulted solely in beneficial effects, because some of the cytokine's multiple biologic activities may be deleterious to the host. A more complete understanding of the structure-function relationship of portions of the cytokine molecules will facilitate selective synthesis of those portions with beneficial effects for use in amplifying desired host responses of specific isotype.

Synthetic Peptides

The concept of synthetic vaccines for infectious bacterial or viral diseases emanates from the demonstration that chemically synthesized peptides can elicit antibodies which react with the original protein (Steward and Howard, 1987). Two characteristics of critical importance in investigations of synthetic peptide vaccines are immunogenicity and T cell recognition. Immunogenicity is dependent on the quality of Th cell function, immunization protocol, nature of T-cell, B-cell interactions and the genetics of the immunized animal. Dual recognition of antigen by T cells and MHC molecules is determined by an individual's phenotype. High percentages of human T lymphocytes proliferate to single peptides (Berzofsky *et al.*, 1988).

Several factors can be managed in synthetic vaccine design which increase its desirability as a vaccine over the parent protein. For example, one can theoretically include epitopes which trigger protective aspects of the immune response and omit those epitopes which trigger suppressive responses. Synthetic vaccines can also be designed to avoid host tissue cross-reactive epitopes which may exist on the parent molecule. The in vivo effectiveness of the synthetic vaccine approach has been realized for several infectious diseases such as influenza, cholera and group A streptococcal infections. Multicomponent vaccines can incorporate epitopes from separate regions of the same molecule or epitopes from different bacterial species. Most importantly, peptides have been actually used as experimental oral vaccines (Lehner *et al.*, 1989) to elicit secretory antibody and to confer immunity to humans (Schmidt *et al.*, 1988).

Studies have deduced the B and T cell regions of the amino terminal epitope of a 3,000 dalton streptococcal peptide. The minimal peptide containing 17 amino acids as a dimer will elicit both B-cell and T-cell immunity. Most individuals appear to be capable of responding to this material with serum and salivary antibody and also with CD4+ T cell proliferative responses (Childerstone *et al.*, 1990). The 17 amino acid peptide, (as a dimer) in dimethyl sulphoxide, was applied directly to the gingivae of monkeys and appeared to initiate both gingival IgG and salivary IgA antibodies (Lehner *et al.*, 1989a). Other studies (Takahashi *et al.*, 1991) employed peptides from the US. mutans PAc antigen coupled to cholera toxin B subunit for intranasal immunization. The immunization suppressed colonization of mouse teeth after a challenge of mutans streptococci (Table 2). Synthetic peptide technology and various passive immunization strategies are mechanisms that could also avert any potential heart reactive antibody formation. We (Smith *et al.*, 1991) have recently synthesized a 22 residue peptide whose sequence surrounds a GTF catalytic region, DSIRVDAVD, described by Mooser and coworkers (1990). This peptide contains nearly complete homology between GTFs from *S. sobrinus* and *S. mutans*. Furthermore, extensive sequence homology exists between GTFs which synthesize insoluble and soluble glucan in this region. Thus, epitopes contained on this peptide are likely to elicit cross-reactive immune responses among GTFs from the most common mutans streptococci that infect man. We have shown this peptide (CAT) to be antigenic in humans and immunogenic in rodents and have synthesized another peptide (GLUa), derived from a putative glucan-binding region of GTF. Twenty nine human sera and salivas were screened for IgG or IgA antibody activity, to this peptide. Five sera and four salivas contained significant reactivity. The GTF-inhibitory activity of four of the five sera could be significantly diminished by preincubation with the GLUa. Furthermore, antibody to intact GTFs from both *S. sobrinus* and *S. mutans* react with both the GLUa and CAT peptides, indicating shared epitopes between the synthetic peptides and native GTF and that antibody to epitopes on these peptides may significantly affect GTF-mediated activities in vivo which lead to plaque formation.

The immunogenicity of the CAT and GLUa synthetic peptides was measured after injection of Sprague-Dawley rats. These peptides elicited vigorous serum IgG antibody responses (ELISA titer > 1:10:000). Sera from rats immunized with CAT or GLUa reacted with intact GTF from both *S. mutans* and *S. sobrinus* in ELISA and Western blot. Also, incubation of splenocytes from peptide-injected rats with GTF induced significant proliferative responses after 5 days. These combined observations support the presence of T cell epitopes and the existence of shared epitopes between CAT and GLUa peptides and intact mutans streptococcal GTF.

Recombinant Bacterial Vectors

A novel modification to this approach (Table 2) has been described in which a recombinant vector involved expression of *S. mutans* antigens on an avirulent *Salmonella typhimurium* (Curtiss *et al.*, 1988). This *Salmonella* attaches to, and invades, Peyer's patches (Carter and Collins, 1974) presumably through M cells and therefore should generate a prominent mucosal immune response to the expressed antigen. Other studies (Iwaki *et al.*, 1990) have transformed the PAc protein from *S. mutans* into *Streptococcus lactis* by joining the gene to shuttle vector pSa3. Oral administration of formalin killed cells of *S. lactis* recombinant induced salivary IgA and serum IgG antibody to PAc in mice.

Antigen Placement

Another major approach has involved more direct antigen placement on or in oral mucosa or salivary glands to stimulate local or distant (GALT) elements to provide a salivary IgA response. Direct instillation of mutans streptococci antigen into parotid ducts resulted in elevated antibody production and interference with bacterial colonization (Emmings *et al.*, 1975). Further efforts involved intramucosal injection of monkeys with *S. mutans* antigen and resulted in serum but no detectable salivary antibody. More successful were studies employing topical application of a small *S. mutans* antigen (3.8Kd) and DMSO to monkey gingival tissues (Lehner *et al.*, 1989a). Immunization of monkeys in this fashion resulted in crevicular IgG, no serum IgG antibody, and whole saliva IgA antibody, and in reduced caries and proportions of plaque *S. mutans* (Lehner *et al.*, 1986). The mechanism of this IgA induction remains unclear although the antibody could have been derived from crevicular fluid. Other studies of topical mucosal application in rodents with whole *S. mutans* did not result in detectable antibody but did appear to reduce colonization (Krasse and Jordan, 1977). Questions of duration remain.

Passive Immunization

Murine Monoclonal Antibody

Recently, passive immunization using the oral route has received attention as a means of interfering with dental caries. Usually this interference is assumed to occur during the microbial colonization or accumulation steps. One approach has utilized murine monoclonal IgG antibody to streptococcal antigen I/II applied to monkey gingiva (Ma *et al.*, 1987). This approach resulted in decreased colonization of implanted *S. mutans*, reduced caries and did not require active immunization with this antigen, which may have tissue-reactive properties.

Immune Bovine Milk

Other creative passive immunization approaches in rodents have involved ingestion of food supplemented with immune bovine milk to four mutans streptococcal serotypes, and suckling on locally immunized rat dams (Michalek and McGhee, 1977; Michalek *et al.*, 1987). These procedures resulted in diminished *S. mutans*, less plaque and reduced caries activity. Thus, while infection with mutans streptococci can lead to dental caries, the immune system can regulate the extent of this infection.

Egg Yolk Antibody

Recently a cell associated GTF has also been used as an antigen in passive immunization studies (Otake *et al.*, 1991). This novel approach involved immunization of hens, with the GTF, purification of the antibody-enriched IgG from egg yolks, and experimental use of this enriched antibody as a dietary additive in studies of rodent dental caries after infection with the homologous strain of mutans streptococcus. Dental caries was decreased by more than 50%.

Target Populations for Development of a Caries Vaccine

Animal studies have shown that several different types of mutans streptococcal antigens can stimulate protective antibody responses. Both human serotype prevalence and salivary antibody data suggest that salivary antibody may interfere with colonization of mutans streptococci. The indication that IgA antibody can be protective has underscored the importance of the scientific basis for developing a mucosal-based human dental caries vaccine but most studies that have been performed have not demonstrated prevention. Is it possible to demonstrate complete prevention of dental caries by using immunologic means? It is conceivable that previous investigations of host immune capability and dental caries have focused on the wrong population to demonstrate complete prevention.

The target population for the caries vaccine might very well be a young age group. The most appropriate age for immunization remains a major question that must take into account the ontogeny of the secretory immune system and the host age of initial colonization with mutans streptococci. The secretory immune system is not fully developed at birth (Cooper *et al.*, 1974). At this time, salivary IgA concentrations are very low but increase dramatically during the first year of life. Secretory IgA levels are somewhat lower in chidren less than 2 years of age than adult levels. However, these children demonstrate secretory antibody responses to viral antigens that are quite similar to those of older children and also show immunologic memory (Wright *et al.*, 1983). Furthermore, most infants less than three months old have measurable levels of salivary IgA antibody to antigens of bacteria that colonize the oral cavity after birth (Smith *et al.*, 1990). Therefore infants can demonstrate secretory immune responses to antigens that are actually encountered. The colonization of the oral cavity with many oral streptococci, including those that are cariogenic, requires the presence of teeth. *Streptococcus sanguis*, a prominent component of dental plaque, can be found in nearly all children by the end of the first year of life (Carlsson *et al.*, 1975). Salivary antibody to *S. sanguis* GTF is present in many 3 to 5 year old children (Gahnberg *et al.*, 1985). Mutans streptococci are not consistently found in the oral cavity until the third year of life or later (Carlsson *et al.*, 1975; Gahnberg *et al.*, 1985). Salivary antibody to *S. mutans* GTF is not detectable in the great majority of children 4 years of age, although most adults demonstrate detectable IgA antibody to this antigen. Therefore, antibody to *S. mutans* GTF is not present when children are colonized with mutans streptococci.

Theoretically, immunization with GTF at approximately 12 months of age would encounter a competent immune system. Salivary IgA antibody to GTF formed at this time would be present to interfere with subsequent colonization and accumulation of mutans streptococci in children. Clinical control of the level of mutans streptococcal infection in mothers (Kohler *et al.*, 1983) has been shown to limit or virtually eliminate the infectious challenge. Children with no detectable mutans streptococci do not have dental caries (Kohler *et al.*, 1988). Reduction of infection coupled with the presence of appropriate salivary antibody before permanent colonization by mutans streptococci should ultimately result in caries prevention. This strategy promises to provide a more effective mucosal approach for prevention of certain dental infections. Development and testing of further strategies utilizing information derived from the molecular pathogenesis of dental infections and the ontogeny and capabilities of the host immune response promise to result ultimately in the complete prevention of dental infections.

Cariostatic Options of Vaccine Approach

Recent experiments have shown that congenitally athymic rats develop more dental caries and are more extensively colonized with mutans streptococci than control euthymic rats (Stack *et al.*, 1990). These data, along with the human experiments in which immunization was accompanied by a reduction in indigenous cariogenic bacteria (Smith and Taubman, 1987; Smith and Taubman, 1990) were interpreted to indicate that antibody could be viewed as regulating the colonization or accumulation of the mutans streptococci. This notion can be extended to suggest that antibody can maintain a static condition of oral infection. Such a concept for a vaccine strategy might be best applied to situations where filling cavities is not practical, or to keep an existent infection in check. While this concept has not directly been tested, there are several compelling experiments and data which suggest, indirectly, that such may be the case. The data have accumulated both for root and coronal surfaces, and for IgA and IgG antibodies.

Evidence that Antibody Can be a Means of Cariostatic Maintenance

Serum IgG Antibody

Most cross sectional studies have concluded that high levels of serum IgG antibody to mutans streptococci in young subjects are associated with low caries experience (Challacombe *et al.*, 1980, 1984; Gregory *et al.*, 1986). The assumption is that this antibody, via the gingival crevice is keeping mutans levels reduced or static. However, the relationship between antibody and mutans streptococci may have been changed when older subjects are studied. In an investigation of IgG antibody to ten supra- and subgingival microorganisms in an older population at risk for root surface caries (recessed gingivae), we (Kent *et al.*, 1991) found that only serum IgG antibody to *S. mutans* showed a significant positive correlation with subject DMF scores.No strong associations were found with serum antibody to other supragingival bacteria. Elevated crevicular fluid IgG antibody levels to *S. mutans* could be associated with presently active or previously restored root caries on the respective tooth. The results support the involvement of mutans streptococci in the root caries processes and suggest that substantial antibody has been formed in response to infection. For purposes of this discussion we will consider that the presence of such antibody can still exert a regulatory effect on the cariogenic bacteria and will present additional evidence to support this contention.

Salivary IgA Antibody

Studies (Gregory *et al.*, 1985) have suggested that the presence of preexisting indigenous antibody to a particular serotype can result in rapid elimination of that serotype, but not of serotypes to which little or no salivary IgA antibody is present. An increased clearance of labelled *S. mutans* challenge has been observed in subjects with high salivary IgA antibody to *S. mutans* antigens (Krasse and Gahnberg, 1983). Also, IgA antibody to *S. mutans* was significantly higher in children with no caries experience (n = 22) when compared to children (n = 17) with more than 2 df surfaces (Camling and Kohler, 1987). Conceivably salivary IgA can interfere with colonization or accumulation of mutans streptococci on more coronal surface aspects, whereas serum or gingival crevice IgG may influence the areas most approximating the gingivae.

Gingival Crevice Fluid IgG Antibody

Camling *et al.* (1991) have demonstrated a tendency to higher recovery of *S.mutans* in GCF from surfaces with low IgG antibody than in GCF from surfaces with high antibody activity. We have investigated (Smith *et al.*, 1991) the effect of preexistent levels of gingival crevicular fluid (GCF) antibody to mutans streptococci on recolonization and accumulation of indigenous microbiota after cleaning of exposed root surfaces. The increase in indigenous mutans streptococci was monitored 24 hours after the cleaning. Sites were ranked with respect to the increase in the respective organism. Gingival crevice fluids containing antibody were significantly associated with root surfaces having low increases in mutans streptococcal colony forming units (CFU). In a total of 46 sites examined, 74% of the sites with antibody to mutans streptococci showed an increase of 10-fold or less, while 64% of the sites with no GCF antibody showed increases greater than 10-fold (Table 3). Also, 50% of the sites with antibody showed an increase of mutans streptococci equal to, or less than 2-fold whereas only 29% of sites with no detectable antibody showed such a low increase. These findings provide preliminary evidence that early recolonization of exposed root surfaces can be regulated to some extent, by the level of GCF IgG antibody to mutans streptococci on a site-specific basis. Some indication as to the mechanism(s) of this regulatory effect of antibody is suggested by the demonstration (Gregory *et al.*, 1990) that levels of salivary IgA and serum IgG antibodies to *S. mutans* antigens were significantly higher in caries resistant (CR) subjects than in caries susceptible (CS) subjects. Salivas and sera from CR significantly inhibited *S. mutans* growth, adherence, acid production and GTF and

TABLE 3 *Mutans Streptococcal Reaccumulation and Recolonization after Cleaning Root Surfaces.*

	Mutans Increase $\leq$ *10 fold*	*after 24 hours ** > *10 fold*
Sites with Antibody to mutans streptococci	74%	26%
Sites with No Antibody to mutans streptococci	36%	64%

*$p < 0.05$, Chi Square analysis.

glucose-phosphotransferase activities more than salivas or sera from CS. Inhibition of one or more of these pathogenic processes in vivo could result in stasis of *S. mutans* infection and/or cariogenesis.

REFERENCES

BALKWILL, F.R. and BURKE, F. (1989): The Cytokine Network. *Immunol Today* 10:299-304.

BERZOFSKY, J.A.; BENUSASSAN, A.; CEASE, B.; BOURGE, J.F.; CHEYNIER, R.; LURHUMA, Z.; SALAUND, J.J.; GALLO, R.E.; and ZAGURY, D. (1988): Antigenic Peptides Recognized by T Lymphocytes From AIDS Viral Envelope-Immune Humans. *Nature* 334:706-708.

BOWEN, W.H.; COHEN, B.; and COLMAN, G. (1975): Immunization Against Dental Caries. *Br Dent J* 139:45-58.

BOWEN, W.H. (1969): A Vaccine Against Dental Caries. A Pilot Experiment in Monkeys (*Macaca irus*). *Br Dent J* 126:159-160.

CAMLING, E. and KOHLER, G. (1987): Infection With the Bacterium *Streptococcus mutans* and Salivary IgA Antibodies in Mothers and Their Children. *Infect Immun* 32:817-823.

CARLSSON, J.; GRAHNEN, H.; JONSSON, G. (1975): Lactobacilli and Streptococci in the Mouths of Children. *Caries Res* 9:333-339.

CARTER, P.B. and COLLINS, F.M. (1974): The Route of Enteric Infection in Normal Mice. *J Exp Med* 139:1189-?.

CHALLACOMBE, S.J. (1980): Serum and Salivary Antibodies to *Streptococcus mutans* in Relation to the Development and Treatment of Human Dental Caries. *Arch Oral Biol* 25:495-502.

CHALLACOMBE, S.J.; BERGMEIER, L.A.; CZERKINSKY, C. and REES, A.S. (1984): Natural Antibodies in Man to *Streptococcus mutans*: Specificity and Quantitation. *Immunology* 52:143-150.

CHILDERSTONE, A.; HARON, J.; and LEHNER, T. (1990): The Reactivity of Naturally Sensitized Human CD4 Cells and IgG Antibodies to Synthetic Peptides Derived From the Amino Terminal Sequences of a 3899 MW *S. mutans* Antigen. *Immunology* 69:177-183.

COLE, M.F.; EMILSON, C.G.; HSU, S.D.; LI S-H.; and BOWEN, W.H. (1984): Effect of Peroral Immunization of Humans with *Streptococcus mutans* on Induction of Salivary and Serum Antibodies and Inhibition of Experimental Infection. *Infect Immun* 46:703-709.

COOPER, M.D.; KINCADE, P.W.; BOCKMAN, D.E.; and LAWTON, A.R. (1974): Origin, Distribution and Differentiation of IgA-producing Cells. *Adv Exp Med Biol* 45:13-22.

COX, D.S. and TAUBMAN, M.A. (1984): Oral Induction of the Secretory Antibody Response by Soluble and Particulate Antigens. *Int Arch Allergy Appl Immunol* 75:126-131.

CURTISS, R., III; GOLDSCHMIDT, R.; KELLY, S.; LYONS, M.; MICHALEK, S.; PASTIEN; and STEIN, S. (1988): Recombinant a Virulent *Salmonella* for Oral Immunization to Mucosal Immunity to Bacterial Pathogens, In: *Vaccines: New Concepts and Developments*, Kohler, A. and Lovede, P.T., Eds. Longman Scientific and Technical, Harlow Essex, UK, pp. 261-271.

CZERKINSKY. C.; PRINCE, S.J.; MICHALEK, S.M.; JACKSON, S.; RUSSELL, M.W.; MOLDOVEANU, Z.; MCGHEE, J.R.; and MESTECKY, J. (1987): IgA Antibody-producing Cells in Peripheral Blood After Antigen Ingestion: Evidence for a Common Mucosal Immune System in Humans. *Proc Natl Acad Sci* USA 84:2449-2453.

EBERSOLE, J.L.; TAUMBAN, M.A.; and SMITH, D.J. (1983): Adjuvants, Glucosyltransferases and Caries Vaccine. In: *Glucosyltransferase, Glucans, Sucrose and Dental Caries*. Special Supplement, Chemical Sense, Doyle R.J., Ciardi, J.E., Eds. Washington, DC, pp. 241-248.

EBERSOLE, J.L.; TAUBMAN, M.A.; SMITH, D.J.; and FREY, D.E. (1986): Regulation of Salivary SIgA Antibody. In: *Molecular Microbiology and Immunology of Streptococcus mutans*, Hamada, S., Michalek, S.M., Kiyono, H., Menaker, L., McGhee, J.R. Elsevier, Amsterdam, pp 329-336.

EMMINGS, F.G.; EVANS, R.T.; and GENCO, R.J. (1975): Antibody Response in the Parotid Fluid and Serum of Irus Monkeys (*Macaca fascicularis*) After Local Immunization with *Streptococcus mutans*. *Infect Immun* 12:281-292.

GAHNBERG, L. and KRASSE, B. (1983): Salivary Immunoglobulin A Antibodies and Recovery from Challenge of *Streptococcus mtuans* After Oral Administration of *Streptococcus mutans* Vaccine in Humans. *Infect Immun* 39:514-519.

GAHNBERG, L.; SMITH, D.J.; TAUBMAN, M.A.; and EBERSOLE, J.L. (1985): Salivary IgA Antibody to Glucosyltransferase of Oral Microbial Origin in Children. *Arch Oral Biol* 30:551-556.

GAULTON, G.N. and GREENE, M.I. (1986): Anti-idiotypic Antibodies of Reoviruses as Biochemical and Immunological Mimics. *Int Rev Immunol* 1:79-90.

GREGORY, R.L.; KINDLE, J.C.; HOBBS, L.C.; FILLER, S.J.; and MALMSTROM, H.S. (1990): Function of Anti-*Streptococcus mutans* Antibodics: Inhibition of Virulence Factors and Enzyme Neutralization. *Oral Microbiol Immunol* 5:181-188.

GREGORY, R.L. and FILLER, S.J. (1987): Protective Secretory Immunoglobulin A Antibodies in Humans Following Oral Immunization with *Streptococcus mutans*. *Infect Immun* 55:2409-2415.

GREGORY, R.L.; FILLER, S.J.; MICHALEK, S.M. and MCGHEE, J.R. (1986): Salivary Immunoglobulins A and Serum Antibodies to *Streptococcus mutans* Ribosomal and Preparations in Dental Caries-Free and Caries-Susceptible Human Subjects. *Infect Immun* 51:348-351.

GREGORY, R.L.; MICHALEK, S.M.; FILLER, S.J.; MESTECKY, J.; and MCGHEE, J.R. (1985): Prevention of *Streptococcus mutans* Colonization by Salivary IgA Antibodies. *J Clin Immunol* 5:55-61.

IACONO, V.J.; TAUBMAN, M.A.; SMITH, D.J.; GARRANT, P.R.; and POLLACK, J.J. (1976): Structure and Function of the Type Specific Polysaccharide of *Streptococcus mutans* 6715. *Immunol Abst* Spec Suppl: 75-90.

IWAKI, M.; OKAHASHI, N.; TAKAHASHI, I.; KANAMOTO, T.; SUGITA-KONISHI, Y.; AIBARA, K.; and KOGA, T. (1990): Oral Immunization with Recombinant *Streptococcus lactis* Carrying the *Streptococcus mutans* Surface Protein Antigen Gene. *Infect Immun* 58:2929-2934.

KENT, R.; SMITH, D.J.; JOSHIPURA, K.; and TAUBMAN, M.A. (1991): Associations Among Serum IgG Antibody Specificities and Clinical Variables in a Population at Risk for Root Surface Caries. *J Dent Res* 70:317.

KOHLER, B.; BRATTHALL, D.; and KRASSE, B. (1983): Preventive Measures in Mothers Influence the Establishment of the Bacterium *Streptococcus mutans* in Their Infants. *Arch Oral Biol* 28:225-231.

KOHLER, B.; ANDREEN, I.; and JONSSON, B. (1988): The Earlier the Colonization by Mutans Streptococci, the Higher the Caries Prevalence at 4 Years of Age. *Oral Microbiol Immunol* 3:14-17.

KRASSE, B.; GAHNBERG, L. and EMILSON, C.G. (1987): An Anticaries Vaccine: Report on the Status of Research. *Caries Research* 21:255-276.

KRASSE, B.; GAHNBERG, L.; and BRATTHALL, D. (1978): Antibodies Reacting With *Streptococcus mutans* in Secretions from Minor Salivary Glands in Humans. *Adv Exp Med Biol* 107:349-354.

KRASSE, B. and JORDAN, H.V. (1977): Effect of Orally Applied Vaccines on Oral Colonization by *Streptococcus mutans* in Rodents. *Arch Oral Biol* 22:479-484.

LEHNER, T.; CALDWELL, J.; and SMITH, R. (1985): Local Passive Immunization by Monoclonal Antibodies Against Streptococcal Antigen I/II in the Prevention of Dental Caries. *Infect Immun* 50:796-799.

LEHNER, T.; MEHLERT, A.; and CALDWELL, J. (1986): Local Active Gingival Immunization by a 3,800 Molecular-Weight Streptococcal Antigen in Protection Against Dental Caries. *Infect Immun* 52:682-687.

LEHNER, T.; WALKER, P.; BERGMEIER, L.A.; and HARON, J.A. (1989a): Immunogenicity of Synthetic Peptides Derived from the Sequences of an *S. mutans* Cell Surface Antigen in Nonhuman Primates. *J Immunology* 143:2699-2705.

LEHNER T.; HARON, J.; BERGMEIER, L.A.; MEHLERT, A.; BEARD, R.; DODD, M.; MIELNIK, B.; and MOORE, S. (1989): Local Oral Immunization with Synthetic Peptides Induces a Dual Mucosal IgG and Salivary IgA Antibody Responses and Prevents Colonization of *S. mutans*. *Immunology* 67:419-424.

LUO, Z.; SMITH, D.J.; TAUBMAN, M.A.; and KING, W.F. (1988): Cross Sectional Analyses of Serum Antibody to Oral Streptococcal Antigens in Children. *J Dent Res* 67:554-560.

MA, JK-C; SMITH, R.; and LEHNER, T. (1987): Use of Monoclonal Antibodies in Local Passive Immunization to Prevent Colonization of Human Teeth by *Streptococcus mutans*. *Infect Immun* 55:1274-1278.

MCGHEE, J.R.; MICHALEK, S.M.; WEBB, J.; NAVIA, J.M.; RAHMAN, A.F.R.; and LEGLER, D.W. (1975): Effective Immunity to Dental Caries: Protection of Gnotobiotic Rats by Local Immunization with *Streptococcus mutans*. *J Immunol* 16:300-305.

MESTECKY, J.; MCGHEE, J.R.; ARNOLD, R.R.; MICHALEK, S.M.; PRINCE, S.J.; and BABB, J.L. (1978): Selective Induction of an Immune Response in Human External Secretions by Ingestion of Bacterial Antigen. *J Clin Invest* 61:731-737.

MICHALEK, S.M. and CHILDERS, N.K. (1990): Development and Outlook for a Caries Vaccine. *Crit Rev Oral Biol Med* 1:37-54.

MICHALEK, S.M.; CHILDERS, N.K.; JACKSON, S.; KATZ, J.; and MESTECKY, J. (1990): Oral *Streptococcus mutans* Vaccines: Diversity of Approaches for the Induction of Mucosal Responses. In: *Advances in Mucosal Immunology*, MacDonald, TT, Challacombe, S.J., Bland, P.W., Stokes, C.R., Heatly, R.V. and Mowat, A.M., Eds. Kluwer, London, pp. 340-344.

MICHALEK, S.M.; GREGORY, R.L.; HARMON, C.C.; KATZ, J.; RICHARDSON, G.J.; HILTON, T.; FILLER, S.T. and MCGHEE, J.R. (1987): Protection of Gnotobiotic Rats Against Dental Caries by Passive Immunization With Bovine Milk Antibodies to *S. mutans*. *Infect Immun* 55:2341-2345.

MICHALEK, S.M. and MCGHEE, J.R. (1977): Effective Immunity to Dental Caries: Passive Transfer to Rats of Antibodies to *Streptococcus mutans* Elicits Protection. *Infect Immun* 17:644-650.

MICHALEK, S.M.; MCGHEE, J.R.; ARNOLD, R.R.; and BOZZO, L. (1976): Ingestion of *Streptococcus mutans* Induces Secretory IgA and Caries Immunity. *Science* 192:1238-1240.

MOOSER, G.; PAXTON, R.J.; HEFTA, S.A.; SHIVELY, J.E.; and LEE, T. (1990): Sequence of a Catalytically Significant Active Site Peptide from Two *S. sobrinus* Glucosyltransferases. *J Dent Res* 69:325.

OTAKE, S.; NISHIHARA, Y.; MAKIMURA, M.; HATTA, H.; KIM, M.; YAMAMOTO, T.; and HIRASAWA, M. (1991): Protection of Rats Against Dental Caries by Passive Immunization with Hen Egg Yolk Antibody (IgY). *J Dental Res* 70:162-166.

RUSSELL, M.W. and WU, H. (1990): *Streptococcus mutans* and the Problem of Heart Cross-Reactivity. *Crit Rev Oral Biol Med* 1:191-205.

RUSSELL, M.W. and LEHNER, T. (1978): Characterization of Antigens Extracted from Cells and Culture Fluids of *Streptococcus mutans* Serotype C. *Arch Oral Biol* 23:7-15.

SCHMIDT, M.A.; O'HANLEY, P.; LARK, D.; and SCHOOLNIK, G.K. (1988): Synthetic Peptides Corresponding to Protective Epitopes of *E. coli* in a Murine Pyelonephritis Model. *Proc Nat Acad Sci* 85:1247-1251.

SMITH, D.J.; VAN HOUTE, J.; ALI-SALAAM, P.; KING, W.F. and TAUBMAN, M.A. (1991): Effect of Crevicular Fluid Antibody on Colonization of Exposed Root Surfaces by Mutans Streptococci and *A. viscosus*. *J Dent Res* 70:317.

SMITH, D.J.; KING, W.F.; and TAUBMAN, M.A. (1990): Salivary IgA Antibody to Oral Streptococcal Antigens in Predentate Infants. *Oral Microbiol Immunol* 5:57-62.

SMITH, D.J. and TAUBMAN, M.A. (1990): Effect of Deposition of Antigen on Salivary Immune Responses and Reaccumulation of Mutans Streptococci. *J Clin Immunol* 10:273-281.

SMITH D.J. and TAUBMAN, M.A. (1987): Oral Immunization of Humans With *Streptococcus sobrinus* Glucosyltransferase. *Infect Immun* 55:2562-2569.

SMITH, D.J.; TAUBMAN, M.A.; and EBERSOLE, J.L. (1980): Local and Systemic Antibody Response to Oral Administration of Glucosyltransferase Antigen Complex. *Infect Immun* 28:441-450.

STAAT, R.H.; LANGLEY, S.D.; and DOYLE, R.J. (1980): *Streptococcus mutans* Adherence: Presumptive Evidence for Protein-mediated Attachment Followed by Glucan-dependent Cellular Accumulation. *Infect Immun* 27:675-681.

STACK, W.E.; TAUBMAN, M.A.; TSUKUDA, T.; SMITH, D.J.; EBERSOLE, J.L.; and KENT, R. (1990): Dental Caries in Congenitally Athymic Rats. *Oral Microbiol Immunol* 5:309-314.

STEWARD, M.W. and HOWARD, C.R. (1987): Synthetic Peptides: A Next Generation of Vaccines. *Immunol Today* 8:51-58.

TAKAHASHI, I.; OKAHASHI, N.; MATSUSHITA, K.; TOKUDA, M.; KANAMOTO, T.; MUNEKATA, E.; RUSSELL, M.W.; and KOGA, T. (1991): Immunogenicity and Protective Effect Against Oral Colonization by *Streptococcus mutans* of Synthetic Peptides of a Streptococcal Surface Protein Antigen. *J Immunol* 146:332-336.

TAUBMAN, M.A.; GENCO, R.J.; and HILLMAN, J.D. (1989): The Specific Pathogen-Free Human: A New Frontier in Oral Infectious Disease Research. *Adv Dent Res* 3:58-68.

TAUBMAN, M.A. and SMITH, D.J. (1989): Oral Immunization for the Prevention of Dental Diseases. In: *Current Topics In Microbiology and Immunology*, Vol 146, J. Mestecky and J.R. McGhee Eds., Berlin, Springer Verlag, pp. 187-195.

TAUBMAN, M.A.; SMITH, D.J., EBERSOLE, J.L.; and HILLMAN, J.D. (1983): Protective Aspects of Immune Response to Glucosyltransferase in Relation to Dental Caries. In: *Glucosyltransferase, Glucans, Sucrose and Dental Caries*, Special Supplement, Chem Senses, Doyle R.J. and Ciardi, J.E. Eds., Washington, DC, p. 249.

TAUBMAN, M.A. and SMITH, D.J. (1974): Effects of Local Immunization with *Streptococcus mutans* on Induction of Salivary Immunoglobulin A Antibody and Experimental Dental Caries in Rats. *Infect Immun* 9:1079-1091.

TOMASI, T.B. JR.; TAN, E.M.; SOLOMON, A.; and PRENDERGAST, R.A. (1965): Characteristics of an Immune System Common to External Secretions. *J Exp Med* 121:10-24.

WOLF, J.L.; RUBIN, D.H., FINBERG, R.; KAUFFMAN, R.S.; SHARPE, A.H.; TRIER, J.S.; and FIELDS, B.N. (1982): Intestinal M cells: A Pathway of Entry for Reovirus into the Host. *Science* 212:471-472.

WRIGHT, P.F.; MURPHY, B.R.; KERVINA, M.; LAWRENCE, E.M.; PHELAN, M.A.; and KARZON, D.T. (1983): Secretory Immunological Response After Intranasal Inactivated Influenza A Virus Vaccination: Evidence for Immunoglobulin A Memory. *Infect Immun* 40:1092-1095.

Index